Pathology for the
Health Professions

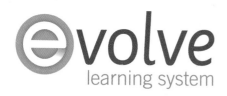 **evolve**
learning system

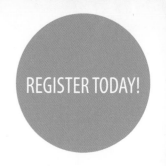

To access your Student Resources, visit:

http://evolve.elsevier.com/Damjanov/pathologyHP/

Register today and gain access to:

Evolve Student Learning Resources for Pathology for the Health Professions offer the following features:

- ## Prepare for Class, Clinical, or Lab
  Body Spectrum Electronic Anatomy Coloring Book
  Archie Animations
  PowerPoint Lecture Notes

- ## Content Updates
  The latest content updates from the author to keep you current with recent developments in this area.

- ## WebLinks
  Links to places of interest on the web, specific to your classroom needs.

 ELSEVIER
SAUNDERS

Pathology for the Health Professions

Fourth Edition

Ivan Damjanov, MD, PhD

Professor
Department of Pathology and Laboratory Medicine
The University of Kansas
School of Medicine
Kansas City, Kansas

ELSEVIER
SAUNDERS

3251 Riverport Lane
St. Louis, Missouri 63043

PATHOLOGY FOR THE HEALTH PROFESSIONS, FOURTH EDITION   ISBN: 978-1-4377-1676-4
Copyright © 2012, 2006, 2000, 1996 by Saunders, an imprint of Elsevier Inc.

Notice

Knowledge and best practice in this field are constantly changing. As new research and experience broaden our understanding, changes in research methods, professional practices, or medical treatment may become necessary.

Practitioners and researchers must always rely on their own experience and knowledge in evaluating and using any information, methods, compounds, or experiments described herein. In using such information or methods they should be mindful of their own safety and the safety of others, including parties for whom they have a professional responsibility.

With respect to any drug or pharmaceutical products identified, readers are advised to check the most current information provided (i) on procedures featured or (ii) by the manufacturer of each product to be administered, to verify the recommended dose or formula, the method and duration of administration, and contraindications. It is the responsibility of practitioners, relying on their own experience and knowledge of their patients, to make diagnoses, to determine dosages and the best treatment for each individual patient, and to take all appropriate safety precautions.

To the fullest extent of the law, neither the Publisher nor the authors, contributors, or editors, assume any liability for any injury and/or damage to persons or property as a matter of products liability, negligence or otherwise, or from any use or operation of any methods, products, instructions, or ideas contained in the material herein.

Library of Congress Cataloging-in-Publication Data

Damjanov, Ivan.
  Pathology for the health professions / Ivan Damjanov. — 4th ed.
    p. ; cm.
  Includes index.
  ISBN 978-1-4377-1676-4 (pbk. : alk. paper)
  1. Pathology. I. Title.
  [DNLM: 1. Pathologic Processes. QZ 140]
  RB25.D26 2012
  616.07—dc22

                                                        2010042972

Managing Editor: Billie Sharp
Developmental Editor: Kathleen Sartori
Publishing Services Manager: Julie Eddy
Project Manager: Jan Waters
Designer: Kim Denando
Illustrations: Eighteen new illustrations provided by Jim Perkins

Printed in China

Last digit is the print number: 9 8 7 6 5 4 3 2 1

To my agathodemons, Ivana and Milena,
with a quote from Gandhi:
*"Almost anything you do will be insignificant,
but it is very important that you do it."*
Of course, because the circle is never entirely round.

TATA

Reviewers

Debra Adams, MEd, CHI, CCMA, CET, CPT, CPCT, CPCT, CPhT, CMAA, CPC, CBCS
Denar Enterprises, LLC
Manchester, New Hampshire

Allen W. Barbaro, MS, RRT
Department Chair, Respiratory Care Education
St. Luke's College
Sioux City, Iowa

Ron Gerrits, PhD
Associate Professor
Milwaukee School of Engineering
Milwaukee, Wisconsin

Cheri Goretti, MA, MT(ASCP), CMA(AAMA)
Professor and Coordinator, Medical Assisting & Allied
    Health Department
Quinebaug Valley Community College
Danielson, Connecticut

Nathanial Gray, MS, PA(ASCP)
Instructor
Mount Sinai Hospital
North Chicago, Illinois

Suezette R. Hicks, ThB, RRT, CPFT
Program Director for Respiratory Care
Black River Technical College
Pocahontas, Arkansas

Leslie J. Lovett, MS, MT(ASCP)
Professor
Pierpont Community and Technical College
Fairmont, West Virginia

Douglas E. Masini, EdD, RPFT, RRT-NPS, AE-C, FAARC
Associate Professor and Director, Respiratory Therapy
Armstrong Atlantic State University
Clinical Assistant Professor of Internal Medicine
Mercer University College of Medicine
Savannah, Georgia

Peter A. McCue, MD
Professor of Pathology
Thomas Jefferson University
Philadelphia, Pennsylvania

Debra Morrison, RN, BScN, MN
Academic Coordinator
Faculty, Practical Nursing
Faculty, Critical Care
Durham College
Oshawa, Ontario, Canada

Paula Denise Silver, BS Biology, PharmD
Medical Instructor
Medical Careers Institute—Newport News Campus
Newport News, Virginia

Brandi NiCole Woodard, MS, PA(ASCP)^{CM}
Instructor and Director of Clinical Education
Rosalind Franklin University of Medicine and Science
North Chicago, Illinois

Nancy H. Wright, RN, BS, CNOR
Adjunct Instructor
Jefferson State Community College
Birmingham, Alabama

Preface

Almost 15 years have passed since the first edition of this book appeared in print. The book sales and the comments made by my colleagues and by students across the country indicate that it was well received. I was most gratified by this response, and I readily accepted the invitation from the publisher to prepare a fourth edition.

The first edition that appeared in 1996 was prepared for students in allied health professions. As the popularity of the book grew, I discovered that the book was used not only by students of laboratory medicine, future nurses, and radiology technicians but also by students preparing themselves to become pathology assistants, physician assistants, pharmacists, veterinarians, and other health care professionals. Their comments and suggestions helped me prepare the new edition and I hope that it will meet with their approval and expectations.

Like the previous three editions, this book covers both general and systemic pathology. The material is presented in a standard manner to enable students to study efficiently and gain knowledge systematically. The book is divided into 23 chapters, grouped into two major sections: general pathology and organ system pathology. More pages and emphasis are given to systemic pathology to meet the requirements of most curricula.

Each chapter is a self-contained teaching unit. Each begins with an outline and a list of key terms and concepts. Learning objectives are provided to guide students and help them focus on the core material. Students should return to these opening pages for review after reading each chapter. Students who can discuss comprehensively, in their own words, all the learning objectives should be assured that they know the material.

OVERVIEW OF MAJOR DISEASES

The most important diseases of the cardiovascular system can be classified into the following categories:
- Congenital heart disease
- Ischemic vascular disease
- Hypertension-related disease
- Inflammatory disease (infectious and autoimmune disorders)
- Metabolic disease

At the beginning of each chapter, students are reminded that pathologic processes occur in organs and tissues that were normal before the disease began. A brief review of the normal structure and function of each organ is included to emphasize the most important aspects of normal anatomy, histology, and physiology that are essential to an understanding of pathology. Diagrams of the normal organs are also included, and these will help students refresh their knowledge of material that was covered in anatomy and physiology courses.

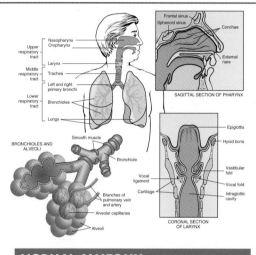

NORMAL ANATOMY AND PHYSIOLOGY

The upper respiratory tract comprises the *nose,* including the nasal cavity and the nares; the paranasal sinuses; the pharynx; and the larynx (Figure 8-1). The primary function of these structures is to provide entry for inhaled air, thus enabling respiration. The mucus covering the nasal mucosa serves as a trap for bacteria and foreign particles. Air passing through the upper respiratory tract is warmed and moistened and partially

This book contains so many new facts and concepts that students might easily get lost in details. To enable students to keep their perspective, the beginning of each chapter on systemic pathology is devoted to an overview of major diseases and how they relate to the normal organ. The core information in each chapter is presented in these sections. Students are advised to keep these brief statements in mind as they study the material in greater detail later in the chapter. Students should spend as much time as possible thinking about these concepts because they are essential to an understanding of the details. These statements are the actual take-home messages that should remain with the student a long time after most of the minutiae are forgotten. Students should avoid at any cost memorizing details taken out of context. An understanding of general principles and concepts is encouraged.

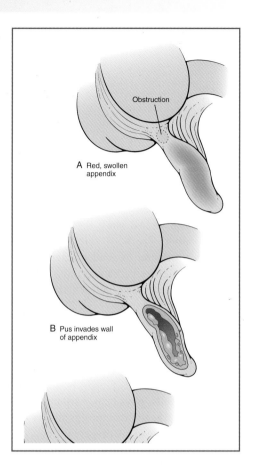

A Red, swollen appendix

B Pus invades wall of appendix

Pathology is too vast a subject to be covered in one semester. To produce a book that could be read in a time frame mandated by most current curricula, I had to eliminate many diseases and concentrate on a few salient pathologic processes and entities that could serve as prototypes or instructional paradigms. These diseases, which are discussed in detail, were chosen either because they are common and thus frequently encountered in practice or because they illustrate important principles and thus provide significant insight into the reaction pattern of an injured organ. Understanding the principles of these paradigmatic diseases will facilitate the understanding of other similar or related disorders.

Each major disease is presented in a standardized format that includes a comprehensive **D**efinition or description of basic features of a disease; discussions on **E**tiology, **P**athogenesis, **P**athology, and **C**linical features; as well as a brief comment about **T**herapy or prognosis. I advise students to use this approach (which I call **DEPPiCT**) in their studies of pathology, as well as in their studies of clinical medicine in general. It is a didactic approach that has repeatedly proved its validity and usefulness in practice.

Because the students reading this text will practice clinical medicine rather than pathology, all the data presented here have a clinical slant and were included with the ultimate goal of preparing students for their work with living patients and enabling them to understand various clinical aspects of specific diseases. To this end, we have included a plethora of illustrations. Colorful diagrams and photographs of pathologic lesions contain important information, and students should spend time studying them. Illustrations can reinforce the written message, and often a concept can be made more vivid with figures than with words. To reinforce the message, at the end of each chapter, students will find review questions pertaining to the main topics covered in that chapter.

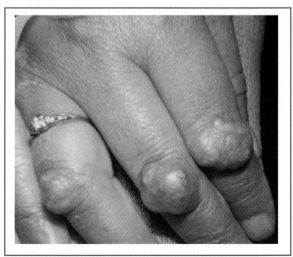

PERITONITIS

Acute **peritonitis,** an inflammation of the peritoneal lining of the abdominal cavity, can be localized or diffuse. Chronic *tuberculous peritonitis* was common previously but is rare today.

Etiology and Pathogenesis

Peritonitis is classified as *infectious* or *sterile.* Infectious peritonitis is usually caused by bacterial invasion of the abdominal cavity, which is secondary to one of the following events:

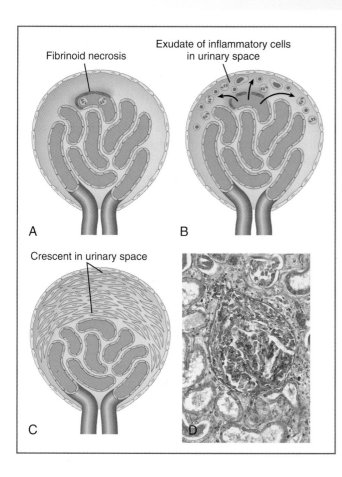

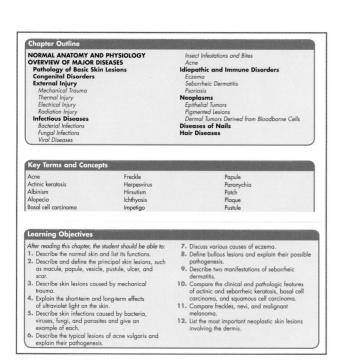

Students of pathology are asked to master a new vocabulary and memorize hundreds of new words. Most of these new pathologic terms are explained when they are first mentioned in the text. Additional definitions and explanations can be found in the glossary at the end of the book.

REVIEW QUESTIONS

1. List the main components of the central and peripheral nervous systems.
2. Describe the functions of the four major lobes of the brain.
3. Compare the functions of the midbrain, pons, and medulla oblongata with that of the cerebellum.

The contemporary layout and multicolor print were designed to facilitate reading and comprehension and to keep students' attention focused on important concepts during long hours of study. To enliven the text, material of human interest was inserted in boxes titled "Did You Know?" The brief stories and curious facts presented here should serve as a reminder that, although pathology is a clinical discipline, the knowledge acquired from this book can be used not only in a medical setting but in everyday life as well.

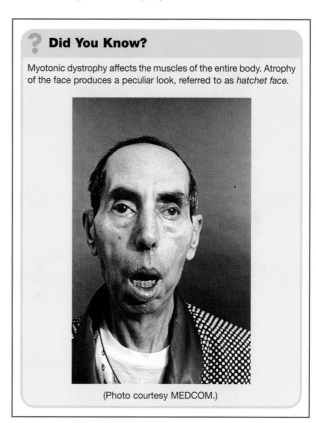

? Did You Know?

Myotonic dystrophy affects the muscles of the entire body. Atrophy of the face produces a peculiar look, referred to as *hatchet face*.

(Photo courtesy MEDCOM.)

My task in revising the original work was facilitated by the input of "users"—that is, teachers and students who have sent me suggestions and have pointed out typos, misspellings, and inaccuracies. Under ideal circumstances I would list them all, but that is almost impossible; thus, I hope that they will accept this brief note as my heartfelt thank you note.

In addition to making the necessary corrections, I have updated the text to include new concepts and discoveries. At the suggestion of several teachers, I have inserted at the end of each chapter a set of review questions. To stimulate students to actively use these questions, I have not included the answers in the textbook. However, the professors may find them in the *Instructor's Manual* (IM) on the Evolve site that accompanies this text. The IM also contains clinicopathologic reviews. Some professors use these clinicopathologic case studies to enrich small group discussions or as material for students' homework assignments. The IM includes matching and multiple-choice questions, as well.

For the student, we've included an anatomy review coloring book and PowerPoint lecture notes for valuable review.

With the generous support of the publisher, I was able to add new illustrations and update some of the artwork from previous editions. To help my fellow teachers prepare their lecture presentations, the image collection for this text can be found in the instructor resources on the text's Evolve site. These lectures contain the material in the form in which it is presented in the textbook. We've also embedded images into the PowerPoint slides, along with wonderful video animations.

The PowerPoint slides reflect my own approach to pathology, and they can be readily altered or custom-adapted to reflect each professor's personal style of lecturing. This edition features Audience Response System questions embedded within the PowerPoints as appropriate. I hope that the professors and the students will appreciate this novelty. This student assessment tool is in the form of questions to be used for quick feedback or the review of the material.

All of these materials can be found on the text's accompanying Evolve website: http://evolve.elsevier.com/Damjanov/pathologyHP/. I was reminded by a friend that good textbooks share some common features with the best Hollywood movies but differ from them in one important aspect: Textbook sequels are almost always better than the original. I hope that I have maintained this tradition. I also invite the users of this book to help me continue to improve it even more. I can be reached by e-mail at IDAMJANO@KUMC.EDU, and I eagerly await your input.

Ivan Damjanov

Acknowledgments

It is my pleasure to acknowledge the contributions of my St. Louis–based Elsevier technical support team who made this edition possible. Above all, my thanks go to the Managing Editor Billie Sharp and Developmental Editor Kathleen Sartori, who were there from the beginning to the very end with their guidance, cheers, and most valuable suggestions. They also coordinated and organized anonymous external reviews from experts who advised me on how to revise and improve the text. They provided valuable insight on how to make the text more useful didactically; some factual and textual inconsistencies and inaccuracies were also corrected. Jim Perkins, the artist who illustrated the first three editions and is by now one of the leading medical illustrators in the entire world, contributed additional new art to this edition. I would also like to thank my Croatian Editor Ms. Andja Raič for allowing me to reproduce the following figures from the book: Damjanov I, Jukić S, Nola M: Patologija, Medicinska naklada, Zagreb, Croatia, 2007: Fig. 1-18, Fig. 2-11, Fig. 2-17, Fig. 2-24, Fig. 5-14, Fig. 10-2, Fig. 14-15. Finally, I must thank my professional colleagues at the University of Kansas, and my wife, Andrea, for allowing me to arrange my schedule and take time off to write and edit this book.

Ivan Damjanov

Contents

1. CELL PATHOLOGY — 1

STRUCTURE AND FUNCTION OF NORMAL CELLS — 2
- Nucleus — 2
- Cytoplasm — 3
  - Mitochondria — 4
  - Ribosomes — 4
  - Endoplasmic Reticulum — 4
  - Golgi Apparatus — 4
  - Lysosomes — 4
- Plasma Membrane — 6
- Integration and Coordination of Cell Functions and Response to Injury — 6
  - Integration of Function of Normal Cells — 6
  - Reversible Cell Injury — 8
  - Irreversible Cell Injury — 9
  - Causes of Cell Injury — 10
CELL ADAPTATIONS — 12
- Atrophy — 12
- Hypertrophy and Hyperplasia — 13
- Metaplasia — 14
- Intracellular Accumulations — 14
  - Anthracosis — 15
  - Hemosiderosis — 15
  - Lipid Accumulation — 15
- Aging — 15
DEATH — 16
- Cell Death — 17
  - Necrosis — 17
  - Apoptosis — 18

2. INFLAMMATION — 21

- Signs of Inflammation — 22
  - Pathogenesis of Inflammation — 23
- Cellular Events in Inflammation — 27
  - Emigration of Leukocytes — 27
  - Phagocytosis — 27
  - Cells of Inflammation — 28
- Classification of Inflammation — 30
  - Duration — 30
  - Etiology — 30
  - Location — 30
- Pathology of Inflammation — 30
  - Serous Inflammation — 30
  - Fibrinous Inflammation — 31
  - Purulent Inflammation — 31
  - Ulcerative Inflammation — 32
  - Pseudomembranous Inflammation — 32
  - Chronic Inflammation — 33
  - Granulomatous Inflammation — 33
- Clinicopathologic Correlations — 34
- Healing and Repair — 34
  - Wound Healing — 35

3. IMMUNOPATHOLOGY — 40

- Immune Response — 41
  - Innate Immunity — 41
  - Acquired Immunity — 42
- Cells of the Immune System — 43
  - Lymphocytes — 43
  - Plasma Cells — 44
- Antibodies — 45
  - Antibody Production — 46
  - Major Histocompatibility Complex — 46
  - Antigen-Antibody Reaction — 46
- Hypersensitivity Reactions — 47
  - Type I Hypersensitivity — 47
  - Type II Hypersensitivity — 50
  - Type III Hypersensitivity — 51
  - Type IV Hypersensitivity — 52
- Transplantation — 53
  - Transplant Rejection — 54
  - Clinical Use of Transplantation — 55
  - Graft-Versus-Host Reaction — 55
- Blood Transfusion — 55
  - Rh Factor Incompatibility — 56
- Autoimmune Diseases — 58
  - Systemic Lupus Erythematosus — 58
- Immunodeficiency Diseases — 59
  - Primary Immunodeficiency Diseases — 60

CONTENTS

Acquired Immunodeficiency Syndrome 61
Amyloidosis 64

4. NEOPLASIA 67

Terminology 68
Classification of Tumors 69
Benign and Malignant Tumors 69
Metastasis 71
Histologic Classification of Tumors 72
Tumor Staging and Grading 75
Biology of Tumor Cells 75
Biochemistry of Cancer Cells 75
Growth Properties in Cell Culture 76
Causes of Cancer 77
Identification of Human Carcinogens 78
Chemical Carcinogens 79
Physical Carcinogens 80
Natural Biologic Carcinogens 81
Viral Carcinogens 81
Human Oncogenes 83
Tumor Suppressor Genes 84
Hereditary Cancer 84
Immune Response to Tumors 86
Clinical Manifestations of Neoplasia 86
Local Symptoms 87
Systemic Symptoms 88
Cancer Epidemiology 88
Incidence 89
Prevalence 89
Mortality 90

5. GENETIC AND DEVELOPMENTAL DISEASES 91

NORMAL EMBRYONIC DEVELOPMENT 92
DEVELOPMENTAL MALFORMATIONS 94
Genetic Factors 94
Exogenous Teratogens 95
Physical Teratogens 95
Chemical Teratogens 95
Microbial Teratogens 95
Chromosomal Abnormalities 96
Structural Chromosomal Abnormalities 96
Numerical Chromosomal Abnormalities 96
Abnormalities of Sex Chromosomes 98
Single-gene Disorders 99
Autosomal Dominant Disorders 100
Autosomal Recessive Disorders 102
X-linked Recessive Disorders 105
Multifactorial Inheritance 107
Anencephaly 108
Diabetes Mellitus 108
Prenatal Diagnosis 109

Prematurity 109
Neonatal Respiratory Distress Syndrome 110
Birth Injury 111
Sudden Infant Death Syndrome 112

6. FLUID AND HEMODYNAMIC DISORDERS 113

Edema 115
Forms of Edema 115
Hyperemia 117
Active Hyperemia 117
Passive Hyperemia 117
Hemorrhage 117
Cardiac Hemorrhage 117
Aortic Hemorrhage 117
Arterial Hemorrhage 118
Capillary Hemorrhage 118
Venous Hemorrhage 118
Thrombosis 119
Embolism 122
Infarction 124
White or Pale Infarcts 124
Red Infarcts 124
Shock 125
Cardiogenic Shock 125
Hypovolemic Shock 125
Hypotonic Shock 125

7. THE CARDIOVASCULAR SYSTEM 129

NORMAL ANATOMY AND PHYSIOLOGY 130
Heart 130
Blood Vessels 131
Lymphatics 133
OVERVIEW OF MAJOR DISEASES 133
Congenital Heart Disease 134
Septal Defects 135
Tetralogy of Fallot 136
Atherosclerosis 137
Atherosclerosis of the Aorta 140
Peripheral Vascular Disease 141
Coronary Heart Disease 142
Hypertension and Hypertensive Heart Disease 147
Rheumatic Heart Disease 150
Infectious Diseases of the Heart 151
Endocarditis 152
Myocarditis 154
Pericarditis 154
Cardiomyopathy 154
Cardiac Tumors 155
Iatrogenic Heart Lesions 155
Arterial Diseases 156
Polyarteritis Nodosa 156

Giant Cell Arteritis 156
Raynaud's Disease 156
Diseases of the Veins 157
Lymphatic Diseases 158

8. THE RESPIRATORY SYSTEM 160

NORMAL ANATOMY AND PHYSIOLOGY 161
OVERVIEW OF MAJOR DISEASES 164
Infectious Diseases 165
Upper Respiratory Infections 165
Middle Respiratory Syndromes 166
Pneumonia 167
Pulmonary Tuberculosis 171
Fungal Diseases 173
Lung Abscess 173
Chronic Obstructive Pulmonary Disease 173
Chronic Bronchitis 173
Bronchiectasis 174
Emphysema 174
Immune Diseases 175
Allergic Rhinitis 175
Asthma 176
Sarcoidosis 178
Hypersensitivity Pneumonitis 179
Pneumoconioses 180
Coal-Workers' Lung Disease 181
Silicosis 181
Asbestosis 182
Ventilatory Disturbances, Acute Respiratory
Distress Syndrome, and Atelectasis 183
Disturbances of Ventilation 183
Acute Respiratory Distress Syndrome 184
Atelectasis 186
Neoplasms of the Respiratory Tract 187
Carcinoma of the Larynx 187
Lung Carcinoma 188
Metastatic Cancer 191
Pleural Diseases 191
Pneumothorax 191
Pleural Effusions 191
Pleural Tumors 192

9. THE HEMATOPOIETIC AND LYMPHOID SYSTEMS 194

NORMAL ANATOMY AND PHYSIOLOGY 195
Peripheral Blood 197
OVERVIEW OF MAJOR DISEASES 198
Anemia 200
Aplastic Anemia 203
Iron Deficiency Anemia 203
Megaloblastic Anemia 204
Hemolytic Anemias 206
Immune Hemolytic Anemia 210

Polycythemia 211
Leukocytic Disorders 212
Leukopenia 212
Leukocytosis 212
Malignant Diseases of White Blood Cells 212
Leukemias 213
Lymphoma 216
Multiple Myeloma 219
Bleeding Disorders 221
Normal Hemostasis 221
Major Bleeding Disorders 222

10. THE GASTROINTESTINAL SYSTEM 227

NORMAL ANATOMY AND PHYSIOLOGY 228
OVERVIEW OF MAJOR DISEASES 230
Diseases of the Oral Cavity 232
Developmental Abnormalities 232
Inflammation 232
Oral Cancer 234
Salivary Gland Diseases 234
Sialadenitis 234
Neoplasms 234
Diseases of the Esophagus 235
Developmental Abnormalities 235
Hiatal Hernia 235
Motility Disorders of the Esophagus 235
Esophagitis 235
Circulatory Disturbances 236
Carcinoma of the Esophagus 236
Diseases of the Stomach and Duodenum 237
Developmental Abnormalities 237
Gastritis 238
Peptic Ulcer 238
Gastric Neoplasms 240
Diseases of the Small and Large Intestine 241
Developmental Abnormalities 241
Diverticulosis 241
Intestinal Vascular Diseases 242
Inflammatory Bowel Disease 243
Gastrointestinal Infections 246
Intestinal Obstruction 249
Malabsorption Syndromes 250
Intestinal Neoplasms 253

11. THE LIVER AND BILIARY SYSTEM 260

NORMAL ANATOMY AND PHYSIOLOGY 261
OVERVIEW OF MAJOR DISEASES 263
Jaundice 265
Acute Viral Hepatitis 267
Forms of Hepatitis 267
Cirrhosis 271

Drug- and Toxin-induced Liver Diseases 276
Alcoholic Liver Disease 276
Hereditary Diseases of the Liver 277
    Gilbert's Disease 277
    Hemochromatosis 277
    Wilson's Disease 277
    Alpha$_1$-Antitrypsin Deficiency 278
Immune Disorders 278
    Autoimmune Hepatitis 278
    Primary Biliary Cirrhosis 278
    Primary Sclerosing Cholangitis 279
Bacterial, Protozoal, and Parasitic Infections 280
Gallstones 280
Hepatobiliary Neoplasms 282
    Hepatocellular Carcinoma 283
    Bile Duct Cancer 283
    Carcinoma of the Gallbladder 283
    Metastases to the Liver 285
Liver Transplantation 285

12. THE PANCREAS — 287

NORMAL ANATOMY AND PHYSIOLOGY 288
OVERVIEW OF MAJOR DISEASES 289
Pancreatitis 290
    Acute Edematous Pancreatitis 290
    Acute Pancreatitis 290
    Chronic Pancreatitis 293
Pancreatic Neoplasms 295
    Adenocarcinoma of the Pancreas 295
    Tumors of the Endocrine Pancreas 296
Diabetes Mellitus 297

13. THE URINARY TRACT — 302

NORMAL ANATOMY AND PHYSIOLOGY 303
OVERVIEW OF MAJOR DISEASES 304
    Localized Symptoms 305
    Systemic Symptoms 306
Developmental Disorders 306
    Polycystic Kidney Disease 306
Glomerular Diseases 307
    Classification 307
    Multiple Mechanisms 308
    Acute Glomerulonephritis 308
    Crescentic Glomerulonephritis 309
    Membranous Nephropathy 310
    Lipoid Nephrosis 310
    Focal Segmental Glomerulosclerosis 311
    Chronic Proliferative Glomerulonephritis 311
    End-stage Glomerulopathy 312
Metabolic Diseases 313
    Diabetes Mellitus 313
    Urinary Tract Infections 314

Circulatory Disturbances 315
    Acute Tubular Necrosis 315
    Nephroangiosclerosis 316
    Hypertension 316
Neoplasms 316
    Renal Cell Carcinoma 317
    Urothelial Carcinoma of the Renal Pelvis 318
    Wilms' Tumor 318
    Carcinoma of the Urinary Bladder 318

14. THE MALE REPRODUCTIVE SYSTEM — 321

NORMAL ANATOMY AND PHYSIOLOGY 322
OVERVIEW OF MAJOR DISEASES 324
    Infertility 324
    Infections 324
    Tumors 324
Congenital Abnormalities 325
    Cryptorchidism 325
Infections 325
    Sexually Transmitted Diseases 326
Neoplasms 328
    Tumors of the Testis 328
    Prostatic Hyperplasia and Neoplasms 332
    Carcinoma of the Prostate 335
    Carcinoma of the Penis 337

15. THE FEMALE REPRODUCTIVE SYSTEM — 338

NORMAL ANATOMY AND PHYSIOLOGY 339
OVERVIEW OF MAJOR DISEASES 340
Developmental Abnormalities 343
Inflammatory Diseases 343
    Clinically Important Infections 345
Hormonally Induced Lesions 346
    Endometrial Hyperplasia 346
Neoplasia and Related Disorders 347
    Carcinoma of the Vulva 347
    Carcinoma of the Vagina 348
    Carcinoma of the Cervix 348
    Tumors of the Uterus 351
    Tumors and Tumor-like Conditions of the Ovary 355
PATHOLOGY OF PREGNANCY 359
Pathology of Fertilization 359
Pathology of Implantation 360
    Ectopic Pregnancy 360
Pathology of Placentation 360
    Placental Anomalies 360

16. THE BREAST 364

NORMAL ANATOMY AND PHYSIOLOGY 365
OVERVIEW OF MAJOR DISEASES 366
Developmental Anomalies 366
Inflammation of the Breast 366
Hormonally Induced Changes 367
Pubertal Changes 367
Gynecomastia 367
Fibrocystic Change 368
Proliferative Breast Disease with Atypia 369
Benign Tumors 369
Malignant Tumors 370
Lesions of the Male Breast 376

17. THE ENDOCRINE SYSTEM 377

NORMAL ANATOMY AND PHYSIOLOGY 378
OVERVIEW OF MAJOR DISEASES 380
Pituitary Diseases 381
Syndromes of Pituitary Hyperfunction 381
Pituitary Hypofunction 382
Nonfunctioning Pituitary Tumors 382
Thyroid Diseases 383
Hyperthyroidism 383
Hypothyroidism 384
Nodular Goiter 385
Thyroid Neoplasms 385
Diseases of the Parathyroid Glands 386
Hyperparathyroidism 386
Hypoparathyroidism 388
Diseases of the Adrenal Cortex 388
Adrenocortical Hyperfunction 388
Adrenocortical Hypofunction 391
Diseases of the Adrenal Medulla 391
Neuroblastoma 391
Pheochromocytoma 392

18. THE SKIN 394

NORMAL ANATOMY AND PHYSIOLOGY 395
OVERVIEW OF MAJOR DISEASES 396
Pathology of Basic Skin Lesions 397
Congenital Disorders 397
External Injury 398
Mechanical Trauma 398
Thermal Injury 398
Electrical Injury 399
Radiation Injury 399
Infectious Diseases 400
Bacterial Infections 400
Fungal Infections 401
Viral Diseases 402
Insect Infestations and Bites 402
Acne 402

Idiopathic and Immune Disorders 403
Eczema 403
Seborrheic Dermatitis 404
Psoriasis 404
Neoplasms 404
Epithelial Tumors 404
Pigmented Lesions 406
Malignant Melanoma 407
Dermal Connective Tissue Tumors 408
Dermal Tumors Derived from
Bloodborne Cells 408
Diseases of the Nails 409
Hair Diseases 409

19. BONES AND JOINTS 411

NORMAL ANATOMY AND PHYSIOLOGY 412
OVERVIEW OF MAJOR DISEASES 414
Developmental and Genetic Disorders 415
Achondroplasia 415
Osteogenesis Imperfecta 415
Infectious Diseases 416
Osteomyelitis 416
Circulatory Disturbances 417
Metabolic Disorders 417
Osteoporosis 417
Osteomalacia 419
Renal Osteodystrophy 420
Paget's Disease 421
Traumatic Injuries 421
Bone Fractures 422
Joint Dislocations 422
Bone Tumors 423
Benign Bone Tumors 423
Malignant Bone Tumors 423
Joint Diseases 425
Osteoarthritis 426
Rheumatoid Arthritis 428
Infectious Arthritis 430
Gout 430

20. MUSCLES AND PERIPHERAL NERVES 433

NORMAL ANATOMY AND PHYSIOLOGY 434
OVERVIEW OF MAJOR DISEASES 436
Neurogenic Atrophy 437
Myasthenia Gravis 439
Muscular Dystrophies 441
Duchenne's Muscular Dystrophy 441
Other Dystrophies 442
Congenital Myopathies 443
Acquired Myopathies 444
Diabetic Myopathy 444
Cancer Myopathy 444

CONTENTS

Mechanical Injury of Muscles 444
Myositis 444
   Infectious Myositis 445
   Immune Myositis 445
Soft Tissue Tumors 446

21. THE NERVOUS SYSTEM 449

NORMAL ANATOMY AND PHYSIOLOGY 450
  Histology of the Brain 452
OVERVIEW OF MAJOR DISEASES 453
  Developmental Disorders 455
    Anencephaly and Dysraphic Disorders 455
  Intracranial Hemorrhages 455
    Epidural Hemorrhages 455
    Subdural Hematomas 456
    Subarachnoid Hemorrhages 457
    Intracerebral Hemorrhage 457
  Cerebrovascular Diseases 458
    Global Ischemia 458
    Cerebral Infarct 459
    Intracerebral Hemorrhage 459
  Trauma 460
    Brain Injury 460
    Neck and Spinal Cord Injuries 460
  Infections 461
  Autoimmune Diseases 463
    Multiple Sclerosis 463
  Metabolic and Nutritional Diseases 464
    Inborn Errors of Metabolism 464
    Nutritional Diseases 464
    Alcoholism 465
  Neurodegenerative Diseases 465
    Alzheimer's Disease 466
    Parkinson's Disease 467
    Huntington's Disease 468
    Amyotrophic Lateral Sclerosis 468
  Epilepsy 469
  Neoplasms 469
    Gliomas 471
    Tumors of Neural Cell Precursors
    and Undifferentiated Cells 472

Meningioma 472
Tumors of the Cranial and Spinal Nerves 472
Metastases to the Brain 473

22. THE EYE 474

NORMAL ANATOMY AND PHYSIOLOGY 475
OVERVIEW OF MAJOR DISEASES 476
  Developmental Disorders 477
  Trauma 478
  Infections 478
  Immunologic Disease 479
  Circulatory Disorders 479
    Hypertensive Retinopathy 479
    Diabetic Retinopathy 479
  Glaucoma 480
  Cataract 481
  Neoplasms 482
    Retinoblastoma 482
    Malignant Myeloma 482

23. THE EAR 484

NORMAL ANATOMY AND PHYSIOLOGY 485
OVERVIEW OF MAJOR DISEASES 485
  Diseases of the External Ear 486
  Diseases of the Middle Ear 486
    Otitis Media 486
    Otosclerosis 488
  Diseases of the Inner Ear 488
    Ménière's Disease 488
  Deafness 488
    Classification 488

GLOSSARY 490

INDEX 507

Introduction

WELCOME TO THE WONDERFUL WORLD OF PATHOLOGY!

In this book you will read about pathology—the basic medical science concerned with diseases. The term *pathology* is derived from two Greek words: *pathos,* meaning disease, and *logos,* meaning science. Thus, *pathology* is the science that studies diseases. It is also a medical specialty traditionally divided into anatomic and clinical pathology. Anatomic pathology—or, as the British like to call it, *morbid anatomy*—deals with the dissection and microscopic examination of human tissues removed from cadavers at postmortem autopsies or from biopsies taken from living patients to diagnose tumors and other diseases. Clinical pathology, on the other hand, is a vast field that includes medical chemistry, microbiology, immunopathology, hematopathology, and blood banking. It is therefore also called *laboratory medicine.* All of you will interact with and come to know pathologists, and some of you will work in pathology laboratories. To assist you in becoming knowledgeable of and conversant in pathology, this book is presented to you in the hope that it provides you with the medical knowledge essential for the understanding of diseases.

The primary goal of this book is to teach you the basic concepts underlying various pathologic processes. You will study the *pathogenesis* of diseases, learn their mechanisms, and understand how they develop. You will learn the *etiology* of pathologic changes and understand the causes of many diseases. However, it is important for you to know that, although many diseases are well delineated, such as cancer and AIDS, others are still shrouded in mystery and only poorly understood.

You will be shown gross and microscopic specimens of human organs and tissues affected by various diseases in order to visualize the *morphology* of various lesions. These pathoanatomic facts that you learn will be correlated with biochemical and immunologic findings, as well as with the clinical symptoms with which a specific disease presents in the living patient. Through *clinicopathologic* correlations, you will see how important the understanding of pathology is for your future medical practice.

Some of you will be caring for living patients and will encounter pathology every day in different guises. Others of you will be working in laboratories examining pathologic specimens on a daily basis. Nonetheless, all of you will be involved with people, and to understand and fully appreciate their problems, you will have to know pathology. Why? Because pathology is the basis of all medical practice. Dr. William Osler, the famous clinician who worked in the great hospitals of Baltimore, Philadelphia, and Boston at the turn of the twentieth century, noted that our clinical practice is only as good as our understanding of pathology. This adage is the motto of our textbook. Remember that you are laying the scientific foundations of your future medical career. Be sure that they are solid.

In the end, you will recall that the greatest pleasure from having done a job well stems from having done it at all. Nothing worthwhile ever comes easily. Persevere and your efforts will be rewarded.

Good Luck and Enjoy Your Studies!

Cell Pathology

Chapter Outline

STRUCTURE AND FUNCTION OF NORMAL
  CELLS
  Nucleus
  Cytoplasm
    Mitochondria
    Ribosomes
    Endoplasmic Reticulum
    Golgi Apparatus
    Lysosomes
  Plasma Membrane
  Integration and Coordination of Cell
    Functions and Response to Injury
    Integration of Function of Normal Cells
    Reversible Cell Injury
    Irreversible Cell Injury
    Causes of Cell Injury

CELL ADAPTATIONS
  Atrophy
  Hypertrophy and Hyperplasia
  Metaplasia
  Intracellular Accumulations
    Anthracosis
    Hemosiderosis
    Lipid Accumulation
  Aging
DEATH
  Cell Death
    Necrosis
    Apoptosis

Key Terms and Concepts

Adaptations
Aging
Anoxia
Anthracosis
Alanine aminotransferase (ALT)
Apoptosis
Aspartate aminotransferase
  (AST)
Atresia
Atrophy
Autophagosomes
Calcification
Chromatin
Cytoplasmic organelles
Cytoskeleton

Death
Gangrene
Golgi apparatus
Hemosiderin
Heterophagosomes
Homeostasis
Hyaloplasm
Hydropic change
Hyperplasia
Hypertrophy
Hypoxia
Intermediate filaments
Intracellular accumulations
Lactate dehydrogenase (LDH)
Lipofuscin

Lysosomes
Metaplasia
Microfilaments
Microtubules
Mitochondria
Necrosis
Nucleus
Oxygen radicals
Plasma membrane
Rough endoplasmic reticulum
  (RER)
Smooth endoplasmic reticulum
  (SER)
Syndactyly
Ubiquitin

Learning Objectives

After reading this chapter, the student should be able to:

1. Describe the essential components of a typical cell and their functions.
2. Explain homeostasis and the integrated response of cell to external stimuli.
3. Define reversible cell injury.
4. Explain the cytoplasmic changes in reversible cell injury and the concept of hydropic change.
5. Compare and contrast reversible and irreversible cell injury.
6. List the most important causes of cell injury.
7. Describe three types of cell adaptations.
8. Give three examples of atrophy.
9. Define and explain hypertrophy and hyperplasia and give appropriate examples of each.
10. Compare and contrast metaplasia and dysplasia and give appropriate examples of each.
11. Define various forms of intracellular accumulation.
12. Explain the pathogenesis of fatty liver.
13. Explain the significance of cellular aging.
14. Compare two forms of cell death: necrosis and apoptosis.
15. List examples of coagulative, liquefactive, caseous, and enzymatic necrosis.
16. Understand the difference between dystrophic and metastatic calcification.

The foundation of modern pathology can be traced to the nineteenth century, when German scientists realized that the cell represented the basic functional unit of the body and that all diseases could be related to disturbances in cell function. Rudolf Virchow (1821-1902), the scientist who introduced the concept of cellular pathology, is thus the father of modern pathology.

The concepts of cellular pathology have been expanded and modified since Virchow's times, but most remain unchallenged. Today, we know that the cells consist of smaller functional units, cellular organelles, which can be seen with an electron microscope. Organelles consist or molecules that can be further dissected and studied by using the techniques of molecular biology. These research endeavors are laying the groundwork for *molecular pathology,* a science that will encompass all living phenomena and provide explanations for pathologic processes at the level of the basic units of living nature: molecules, atoms, and their elementary particles. However, until this longtime goal of pathologists becomes a reality, we limit our discussions to cells *(cell pathology),* tissues *(histopathology),* and organs *(organ pathology).*

STRUCTURE AND FUNCTION OF NORMAL CELLS

Almost all normal cells of the human body have some common features and consist of the same basic components. These include the nucleus, the cytoplasm, and the cell (plasma) membrane (Figure 1-1).

NUCLEUS

All human cells, except the red blood cells and platelets, need a nucleus for survival. The **nucleus** is the essential part of most living cells. It consists of nucleic acids, such as deoxyribonucleic acid (DNA) and ribonucleic acid (RNA), and

nuclear proteins. In resting cells, these components are arranged into aggregates known as **chromatin** and a specialized organelle composed primarily of RNA known as the *nucleolus.* In the dividing of cells—that is, during *mitosis*—the chromatin is restructured and the strands of DNA condense into *chromosomes.* The resting cells have a nuclear membrane, which delimits the nucleus from the cytoplasm. This membrane disappears in mitosis and reappears after cell division is completed.

The DNA of the nucleus contains essential genetic material that is identical for all somatic cells that form various

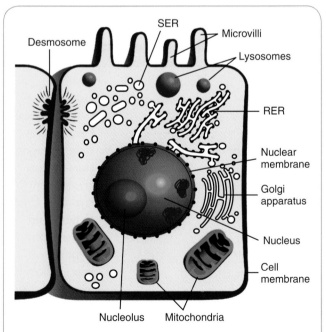

Figure 1-1 Normal cells have a nucleus and a cytoplasm. On the outside, the cell is delimited by a plasma membrane. In the cytoplasm, there are organelles, such as mitochondria, smooth and rough endoplasmic reticulum (SER and RER, respectively), Golgi apparatus, and lysosomes.

tissues and organs of the body. This genetic material consists of genes that are differentially expressed in various tissues and organs. Differential expression of genes allows the cells to assume unique features in various tissues and organs and to perform specialized functions. Such cells are called *differentiated,* in contrast to embryonic cells, which have not undergone specialization and which are therefore termed *undifferentiated.*

The genetic information encoded in the DNA is transcribed into the nuclear RNA. From the nuclear RNA, the message is transmitted by transfer RNA (tRNA) and messenger RNA (mRNA) into the cytoplasm (Figure 1-2). The ribosomal RNA (rRNA) serves as a template for translating the genetic messages into amino acids, which are assembled into polypeptides and proteins. Protein synthesis is essential for the maintenance of life. Proteins are needed for cellular growth, replication, metabolism, respiration, and other essential functions. Proteins also act as structural elements, maintaining the cell's shape and the internal organization of the cytoplasm. None of these

elementary functions (and many others that we mention later) would be possible without the nucleus, which acts as the main overseer of all critical cytoplasmic events.

CYTOPLASM

All cells have cytoplasm. However, the amount of cytoplasm and its structure vary from one cell to another. In embryonic cells, the cytoplasm is scant and contains few organelles. In specialized, highly differentiated cells, such as liver or kidney cells, the cytoplasm is more abundant and is replete with organelles. The ratio of the nucleus to the cytoplasm, the so-called *nucleocytoplasmic (N:C) ratio,* is high in undifferentiated embryonic cells and much lower in differentiated cells of adult tissues. As we shall see later, many tumor cells are also undifferentiated and have a high N:C ratio.

The principal **cytoplasmic organelles** are the *mitochondria, ribosomes, endoplasmic reticulum, Golgi apparatus,*

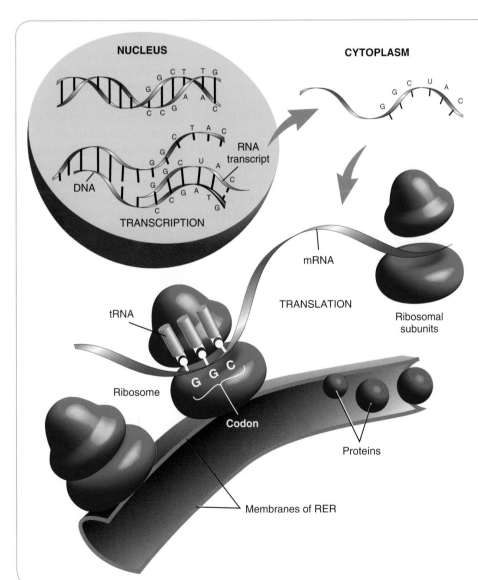

Figure 1-2 Transcription and translation by RNA of the genetic code stored in the DNA leads to protein synthesis on ribosomes. mRNA, messenger RNA; RER, rough endoplasmic reticulum; tRNA, transfer RNA.

and *lysosomes*. In addition to these, some cells have organelles for specialized functions. For example, muscle cells have myofilaments composed of actin and myosin, which are essential for contraction; glandular cells have secretory granules, which contain enzymes or mucus destined for excretion. Furthermore, it is important to note that the cytoplasmic ground substance of all cells consists of an amorphous matrix called *hyaloplasm* and a fibrillar meshwork called *cytoskeleton*. Each cell is also enclosed by an outer *plasma membrane,* which forms the border between the cytoplasm and the extracellular space.

MITOCHONDRIA

Mitochondria are cytoplasmic organelles involved primarily in the generation of energy (see Figure 1-1). Hence, mitochondria contain oxidative enzymes (e.g., cytochrome oxidase) that participate in cellular respiration and the formation of energy-rich compounds like adenosine triphosphate (ATP). Because the process uses oxygen, it is called oxidative phosphorylation. ATP generated by the mitochondria is essential for all other cellular functions. Cells with complex functions, such as liver cells and nerve cells, require a considerable amount of energy and therefore contain numerous mitochondria. By comparison, undifferentiated cells, including many malignant tumor cells, have few mitochondria.

RIBOSOMES

Ribosomes are small granules composed of RNA. They may be arranged into aggregates that float freely in the cytoplasm, called *polysomes* or *free ribosomes,* or they may be attached to the membranes of the **rough endoplasmic reticulum (RER).** The ribosomes are involved in protein synthesis. Structural proteins and enzymes needed for the maintenance of basic cell functions ("proteins for internal purposes") are synthesized on the free ribosomes. Those intended for excretion ("export or luxury proteins") are synthesized on the RER and discharged from the cells through the cisternae lined by the membranes of the RER.

ENDOPLASMIC RETICULUM

The endoplasmic reticulum is a meshwork of membranes that is in continuity with the outer plasma membranes on one side and the nuclear membrane on the other. With use of electron microscopy, one can distinguish two forms of endoplasmic reticulum: the RER and the **smooth endoplasmic reticulum (SER).** As stated earlier, the RER is the site of protein synthesis for export and secretion. Cells producing large amounts of proteins for export have a well-developed RER. For example, liver cells, which synthesize blood proteins such as albumin and the clotting factors, and plasma cells, which synthesize immunoglobulins, contain prominent stacks of RER.

SER has complex metabolic functions, the most important of which are the catabolism (i.e., metabolic degradation) of drugs, hormones, and various nutrients and the synthesis of steroid hormones. To perform these functions, liver cells have a well-developed SER, which takes part in the metabolic degradation and transformation of many chemicals, including drugs and hormones. Likewise hormone-secreting gonadal cells of the testis and ovary and the adrenocortical cells that synthesize steroid hormones (e.g., estrogens, androgens, and corticosteroids) also have prominent SERs.

GOLGI APPARATUS

The **Golgi apparatus** is a synthetic organelle adjacent to the nucleus (see Figure 1-1). Its tubules and flattened cisternae give rise to secretory granules and lysosomes. Many proteins synthesized in the endoplasmic reticulum pass through the Golgi apparatus, where they are biochemically modified before being packaged into secretory granules or lysosomes. Proteins to be incorporated into the internal cell membranes (e.g., endoplasmic reticulum) or the outer plasma membrane are also glycosylated in the Golgi apparatus.

LYSOSOMES

Lysosomes are membrane-bound digestive cytoplasmic organelles that are rich in lytic enzymes. The lysosomes originate as small vesicles budding from enzymes on the lateral sides of the Golgi apparatus (Figure 1-3). These primary lysosomes contain acid hydrolases, which are digestive enzymes that are maximally active in an acidic milieu (i.e., at low pH levels). Under normal circumstances, the lytic enzymes are tightly enclosed by a lysosomal outer membrane and do not harm the cell. Even if some lysosomal content is spilled into the cytoplasm, the acid hydrolases would cause little damage in normal cytoplasm, which has a neutral pH. However, if the cell is injured and the pH of the cytoplasm becomes acidic, enzymes released from the lysosomes could cause damage, as we will see in the section on cell injury.

The primary lysosomes fuse with other cytoplasmic vesicles to form secondary lysosomes. Typically they fuse with the absorptive vesicles originating from the invaginated plasma membrane to form secondary lysosomes, which are also called **heterophagosomes.** Secondary lysosomes that are involved in the digestion of a cell's own organelles are called **autophagosomes.** The digestive enzymes in secondary lysosomes degrade the material enclosed within its membrane. The metabolites obtained through this intracellular digestion are reutilized within the cell's cytoplasm. The undigested residues are extruded from the cytoplasm into the extracellular spaces by reverse endocytosis or exocytosis. Some of the undigested material, mostly complex lipids derived from cell membranes, may remain within the cytoplasm as "residual bodies." These residual bodies typically contain lipid-rich brown pigment known as **lipofuscin,** a term derived from the Greek word *lipos* (meaning "fat") and the Latin word *fuscus* (meaning "brown"). Lipofuscin is also known as the *brown pigment of aging* because it is commonly found in aging cells. With aging, all cellular processes become less efficient.

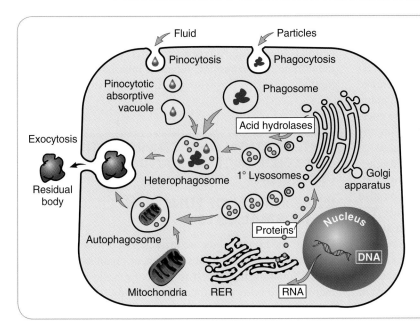

Figure 1-3 Lysosomes. Primary (1°) lysosomes, which originate from the Golgi apparatus, give rise to heterophagosomes and autophagosomes. Undigested material in phagosomes is extruded from the cell or remains in the cytoplasm as lipofuscin-rich residual bodies. RER, rough endoplasmic reticulum.

Energy-dependent processes, such as lysosomal digestion and exocytosis, are especially affected. Therefore, cells in an old organism contain more lipofuscin than those in a metabolically active, more vigorous young body.

The function of lysosomes and the formation of phagocytic vacuoles are well controlled in healthy cells. Most importantly, the cells must control the inadvertent leakage of lysosomal enzymes into the hyaloplasm, because these enzymes could damage other organelles. Formation of autophagosomes and the incorporation of cytoplasmic organelles into these digestive vacuoles are also fully regulated by intracellular signaling. If not adequately controlled, autophagy may cause cell death.

Hyaloplasm and Cytoskeleton

The **hyaloplasm,** which is the ground substance of the cytoplasm, has no distinct structure and appears as an "empty" space on electron microscopic studies. Biochemically hyaloplasm consists predominantly of water, but it also contains minerals, proteins, carbohydrates, and lipids that keep its osmolarity constant. The hyaloplasm is the fluid phase of the cell that contains the organelles. In between the organelles, the hyaloplasm is traversed by a network of filaments that form the **cytoskeleton.** Three types of filaments are recognized: **microfilaments,** composed of actin and myosin and measuring 5 nm in diameter; **microtubules,** which are 22-nm thick and composed of tubulin; and **intermediate filaments,** named so because their diameter (10 nm) is intermediate between that of microfilaments and microtubules.

In contrast to microfilaments and microtubules, which have the same biochemical composition in all cells, the intermediate filament proteins are cell-type–specific proteins (Table 1-1). The *intermediate filaments* of epithelial cells contain *keratins,* mesenchymal cells contain *vimentin,* muscle cells contain *desmin,* glial cells contain *glial acidic fibrillary*

protein (GAFP), and neural cells contain *neurofilament* proteins. Intermediate filament proteins are useful markers for those cell types. Pathologists use antibodies to intermediate filaments for typing of tumors because tumor cells retain the same intermediate filament proteins as the normal cells from which they arise. For example, carcinomas, which are tumors of epithelial cells, express keratin, whereas sarcomas, which are tumors of mesenchymal cells, express vimentin. In diagnostic pathology laboratories antibodies to these intermediate filament proteins are widely used to establish whether a tumor is a carcinoma or sarcoma.

The function of the cytoskeleton is to maintain cell shape and to enable the cell to adapt to external mechanical pressure. Cytoskeletal filaments are also important for cell movement and the traffic of organelles in the cytoplasm. Microtubules also form the mitotic spindle during cell division.

TABLE 1-1 Proteins of Cytoskeletal Filaments

Type of Filament	Diameter (nm)	Protein
Microfilaments	5	Actin, myosin
Intermediate filaments	10	Epithelial—keratins Mesenchymal—vimentin Muscle—desmin Glia—GFAP Nerve—neurofilaments
Microtubules	22	Tubulin

GFAP, glial fibrillary acidic protein.

PLASMA MEMBRANE

The **plasma membrane** forms the outer surface of the cell (Figure 1-4). The plasma membrane is composed of proteins, lipids, and carbohydrates arranged in a polarized complex bilayer that has an internal and external surface. On the internal side, the plasma membrane is in continuity with the membrane of the endoplasmic reticulum. Invaginations of the plasma membrane give rise to endocytotic vesicles, which fuse with primary lysosomes to form heterophagosomes. The cytoplasmic surface of the cell membrane also serves as an anchorage site for cytoskeletal filaments. For example, intermediate filaments composed of keratin aggregate at the site of desmosomes, the typical intercellular bridges that interconnect epithelial cells of the oral or vaginal mucosa. Microtubules are integral parts of cilia, which are specialized parts of the cell surface that have the ability to move and propel the cell (e.g., sperm) or to move the external secretions of the cell. For example, mucus is moved by the cilia of the bronchial ciliated cells; dysfunction of these cilia may predispose an individual to bronchial infection (bronchitis).

The external surface of the plasma membrane serves as the site of contact between the cell and the environment. This interaction between the cell and the environment is maintained through the action of specialized portions of the cell membrane that serve as receptors, adhesion molecules, transducers of signals, or metabolic channels. The complexity of the plasma membrane varies from one cell type to another.

The plasma membrane of cells is a living structure that is maintained by active expenditure of energy and a constant supply of ATP. The structural integrity of the plasma membrane is a prerequisite for the maintenance of all essential cellular functions. Rupture or major damage of the cell membrane that cannot be repaired invariably leads to *cell death*.

INTEGRATION AND COORDINATION OF CELL FUNCTIONS AND RESPONSE TO INJURY

INTEGRATION OF FUNCTION OF NORMAL CELLS

Cells of the human body are arranged into tissue, and these tissues form organs. Organs are part of organ systems, all of which function in concert to meet the basic vital requirements of the body and to enable the body to perform many complex functions. The integration of cells, tissues, and organs into functional units is achieved through several mechanisms, best illustrated by the response of cells to growth-stimulating factors (Figure 1-5).

The simplest form of integration occurs at the level of single cells. For example, T lymphocytes secrete *cytokines,* which stimulate the growth of other cells, such as fibroblasts, but at the same time act on the cells that have produced them—that is, act as their own growth factors. This self-stimulation, known as an *autocrine stimulation,* is feasible because T lymphocytes have surface receptors for their own secretory product. Interleukins that are released from the cell bind to the surface of the same cell and stimulate its receptors to transmit signals for cell growth.

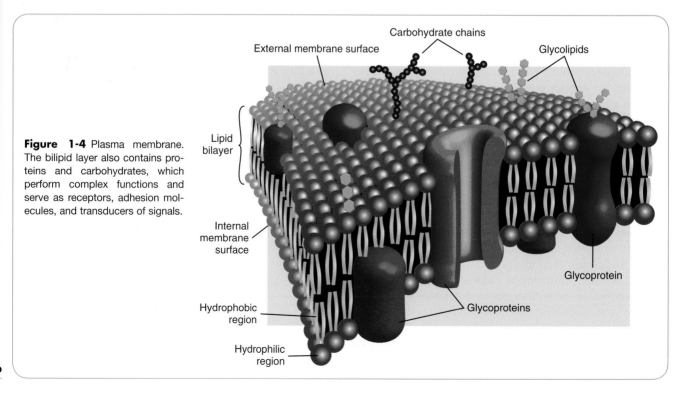

Figure 1-4 Plasma membrane. The bilipid layer also contains proteins and carbohydrates, which perform complex functions and serve as receptors, adhesion molecules, and transducers of signals.

Carbohydrate chains

External membrane surface

Glycolipids

Lipid bilayer

Internal membrane surface

Glycoprotein

Hydrophobic region

Glycoproteins

Hydrophilic region

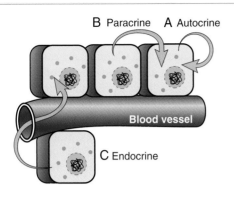

Figure 1-5 Integration of cell functions occurs through interaction with other cells in the body. *A,* Autocrine stimulation. Secretions from the cell may attach to the cell's own surface receptors, providing autocrine stimulation. *B,* Paracrine stimulation. Closely adjacent cells act on each other. *C,* Endocrine stimulation. Hormones secreted by endocrine cells reach target cells via the blood.

More complex integration of cells requires transmission of hormonal signals from one cell to another. This is done through the release of mediators from one cell and their uptake by another, a process called *paracrine stimulation.* Paracrine stimulation is typically mediated by biogenic amines (e.g., epinephrine) and neuropeptide hormones (e.g., glucagon and gastrin). The best example is the release of hydrochloric acid from gastric chief cells under the influence of gastrin. Gastrin is a hormone released from neuroendocrine G cells, which are located in the gastric mucosa, adjacent to the hydrochloric acid–secreting chief cells. Gastrin extruded from neuroendocrine cells attaches to receptors on the chief cells, triggering hydrochloric acid release.

Endocrine stimulation is achieved by hormones released into the blood circulation. This is clearly a higher form of integration of cell functions, because it may involve cells in several anatomically distinct organs. For example, insulin secreted by the islet cells of the pancreas affects the liver, muscle, fat cells, and many others. A similarly high level of integration of cell functions can be achieved through *neural stimulation.* The central and autonomic nervous systems are the ultimate coordinators of body functions.

From the point of view of cell pathology, each cell is best considered as a distinct functional unit in a defined *internal milieu* formed by the intercellular fluids. To maintain its life and normal functions, the cell must be in homeostasis with its environment. **Homeostasis** (derived from the Greek words *homoios,* "steady," and *stasis,* "state") is defined as the state of balance between opposing pressures operating in and around a cell or tissue. From the environment, the cell receives nutrients, oxygen, water, and essential minerals. The cell generates energy by burning some of the calories derived from the nutrients. This energy is used for the upkeep of the nucleus and the integrity and function of the cytoplasm, cell organelles, and plasma membranes. By maintaining its own

integrity, the cell contributes to the stability of the internal milieu. A normal internal milieu is essential for the normal function of the cell; likewise, the milieu remains normal only if all the cells are functioning properly.

The supply of essential minerals and the water in which these minerals are dissolved are also of paramount importance for the maintenance of homeostasis. The essential minerals include sodium, chloride, potassium, calcium, and iron. Magnesium, zinc, copper, and selenium—known as *oligominerals* because they are needed in minute amounts—are also required. The oligominerals are essential for the function of several important enzymes.

The cell is also critically dependent on a constant supply of oxygen and nutrients, provided to cells by the circulation of the fluids that surround cells. At the same time, the circulating fluids carry away the degradation products of cellular metabolism.

When an equilibrium between the cells and their environment is achieved and maintained, the cells are said to be in a *steady state* (Figure 1-6). External stimuli may alter this equilibrium. If the demands are increased, the cell may shift its metabolism to a higher level, achieving a new steady state. Similarly, the cell may shift to a lower steady state if the demands are decreased. In both instances, the adaptation is temporary, and the cell may revert to the original steady state after the external demands cease. However, if the demands exceed the capacity of the cell to adapt, a permanent disequilibrium may ensue. Similar to a pulled muscle that has exceeded its ability to stretch and has ruptured and cannot contract any more, the cell that has passed beyond the *point of no return* has been irreparably

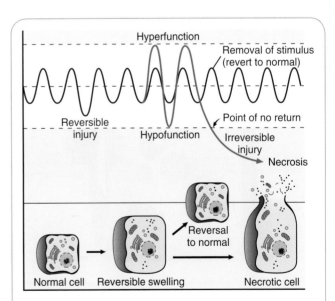

Figure 1-6 Steady state. The range of the steady state is determined by the reactivity of each cell and the ability of the cells to respond to increased demands or stimuli. The increased or decreased functional adaptations are reversible. However, once response passes beyond the point of no return, the cell injury becomes irreversible.

damaged and cannot return to the original steady state. Such a cell cannot maintain homeostasis and will die.

REVERSIBLE CELL INJURY

If the adverse environmental influences evoke a cellular response that remains within the range of homeostasis, the changes produced are called *reversible cell injury.* Cessation of injury results in the return of the cell to the original steady state.

Reversible cell injury is typically mild or short lived. It can be induced by exposure to toxins in low concentration. Brief *hypoxia* or *anoxia* (i.e., decreased oxygen supply or complete deprivation of oxygen) can induce the same changes, which are best described as swelling of the cytoplasm and cytoplasmic organelles (Figure 1-7).

Cellular swelling, known as **hydropic change,** reflects an increased influx of water into the cytoplasm. The water crosses the plasma membrane, enters the hyaloplasm, and accumulates within the mitochondria ("mitochondrial swelling") and membrane-bound vacuoles formed from the invaginations of the plasma membrane and endoplasmic reticulum. This vacuolization of the cytoplasm is best appreciated by electron microscopy. After the insult is over, the cell recovers by pumping out the water, reverting to the original steady state.

The pathogenesis of cellular swelling is relatively easy to explain in terms of altered permeability of the plasma membrane. The plasma membrane is a selectively permeable membrane that maintains gradient in the concentration of minerals—primarily, sodium (Na^+), potassium (K^+), and chloride (Cl^-)—inside and outside the cell. This is achieved through the function of the Na^+/K^+–adenosine triphosphatase

(ATPase) pump, which acts as a sodium pump, constantly pumping Na^+ ions from the cytoplasm into the extracellular space (Figure 1-8). The pump keeps the intracellular concentration of potassium high. Chloride generally follows Na^+ ions and accordingly, the concentration of Na^+ and Cl^- is higher in the extracellular space than in the cytoplasm, whereas the concentration of K^+ is higher inside than outside the cell. Because the ATPase is fueled by high-energy compounds such as ATP, anoxia or any other form of energy deprivation causes dysfunction of this enzyme. Without functioning ATPase, the cell membrane loses its capacity to maintain the gradient of intracellular and extracellular minerals. A high concentration of sodium in the extracellular space results in an influx of sodium and chloride into the cell. This is followed by an influx of water and concomitant cellular swelling. Once ATPase function is restored, the sodium and the water are pumped out of the cell and the swelling disappears.

Reversible cell injury is associated with many functional changes (Figure 1-9), the most important of which are as follows:

- *Reduced energy production.* Swollen mitochondria generate less energy. Instead of oxidative ATP production, the cell reverts to less efficient anaerobic glycolysis, which also results in excessive production of lactic acid.
- *Decreased protein synthesis.* The pH of the cell becomes acidic, which further slows down the entire cell metabolism. The consequent dilation and fragmentation of RER and the loss of membrane-attached ribosomes ("degranulation of the RER") result in decreased protein synthesis.
- *Increased autophagy.* Damaged proteins and potentially toxic intermediary products formed during cell injury are sequestered in autophagosomes. The hydrolytic lysosomal enzymes that take part in the degradation of sequestered material may leak from overdistended phagosomes into the

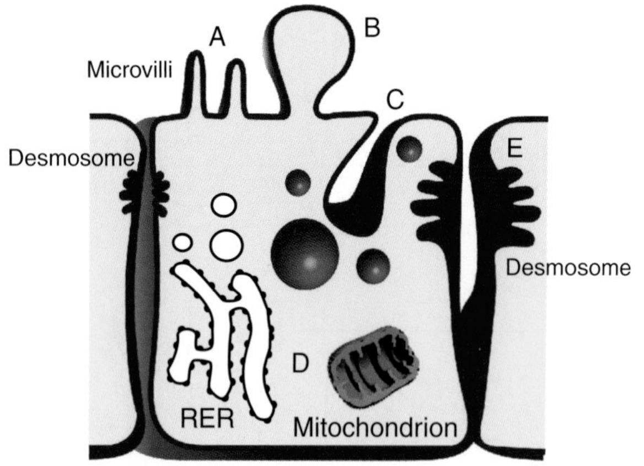

Figure 1-7 Cellular swelling. *A,* Normal microvilli. *B,* Swollen microvilli are the consequence of an influx of water in the cytoplasm. *C,* Invagination of the cell membrane gives rise to fluid-filled cytoplasmic vacuoles that account, in part, for the changes known as *vacuolar degeneration. D,* Swollen mitochondria and dilated rough endoplasmic reticulum (RER) are also part of vacuolar degeneration. *E,* Swollen cells lose contact with adjacent cells at the site of cell-to-cell junctions, such as desmosomes.

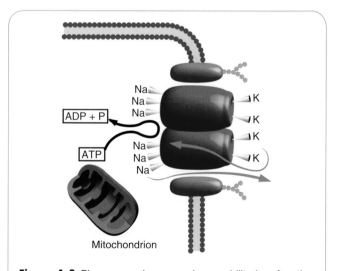

Figure 1-8 Plasma membrane semipermeability is a function of the Na^+/K^+–ATPase pump. ADP, adenosine diphosphate; ATP, adenosine triphosphate; P, phosphorus.

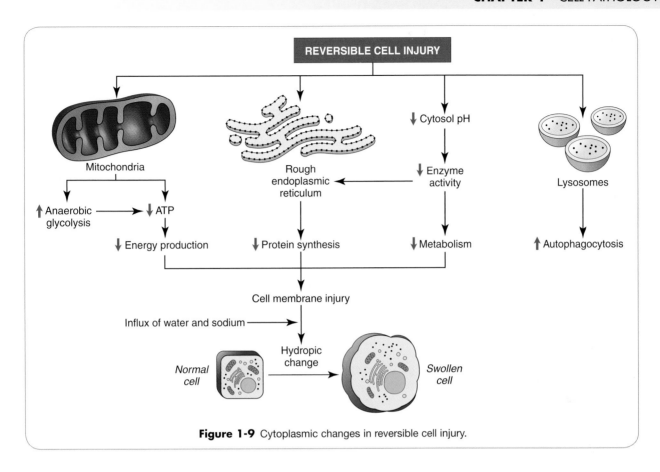

Figure 1-9 Cytoplasmic changes in reversible cell injury.

acidified cytoplasm, contributing to the damage of other cellular components.

Hydropic change is reversible, and if the energy source is restored or toxic injury is neutralized, the cell will revert to its normal state.

IRREVERSIBLE CELL INJURY

Cells exposed to heavy doses of toxins, anoxia or severe or prolonged hypoxia, or other overwhelming insults cannot recover from the injury, hence the term *irreversible cell injury.* Morphologically, irreversible cell injury may be recognized by typical changes in the nucleus or by a loss of cell integrity and rupture of the cell membrane. Functional tests will show that the nuclear functions have been disrupted, the energy production within mitochondria has fallen below the essential minimum needed for cell function and cannot be restored to normal levels, and the plasma membrane functions are irrevocably lost.

Irreversible cell injury is characterized by typical ultrastructural changes, many of which can be recognized by light microscopy as well. The most characteristic are *nuclear changes;* clearly, without a viable nucleus, the cell cannot survive. Damage to the nucleus can present in three forms:

- *Pyknosis,* marked by condensation of the chromatin (*pyknos* means "dense" in Greek).
- *Karyorrhexis,* characterized by fragmentation into smaller particles, colloquially called *nuclear dust. (Karyorrhexis* is

a term derived from the Greek words *karyon,* meaning "nucleus," and *rrhexis,* meaning "disruption.")
- *Karyolysis,* which involves dissolution of nuclear structure and lysis of chromatin by enzymes, such as DNAase and RNAase (Figure 1-10).

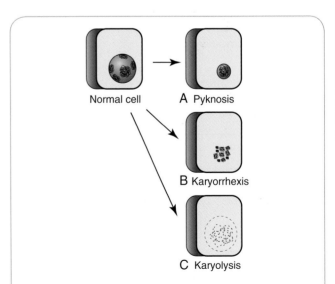

Figure 1-10 Nuclear changes in irreversible cell injury. *A,* Pyknosis (condensation of chromatin). *B,* Karyorrhexis (fragmentation of nucleus). *C,* Karyolysis (lysis of chromatin).

Dead cells release their contents into the extracellular fluid, whereby they reach the circulation. Cytoplasmic enzymes, such as **aspartate aminotransferase (AST), alanine aminotransferase (ALT)**, or **lactate dehydrogenase (LDH),** which are released from damaged cells, can be measured in blood and are clinically useful signs of cell injury. Levels of AST, ALT, and LDH are typically elevated in the serum of patients with myocardial infarct or viral hepatitis. These enzymes are widely used as clinical laboratory evidence of cell injury and cell death.

CAUSES OF CELL INJURY

Cell injury may be induced by numerous pathogenetic mechanisms, the most important of which are hypoxia, toxins, microbial pathogens, endogenous mediators of inflammation and immune reactions, and genetic and metabolic disturbances. Depending on the severity of the insult, the cell injury may be reversible or irreversible. The causes of cell injury as they relate to pathogenesis are listed, together with clinical examples, in Table 1-2.

HYPOXIA AND ANOXIA

Hypoxia, a reduced availability of oxygen, and **anoxia,** the complete lack of oxygen, are among the most important and most common causes of cell injury. Oxygen is essential for cellular respiration, and a lack of oxygen results in cessation of energy production. Without energy, the cell cannot survive. Short-term anoxia induces reversible cell injury. However, if the oxygen supply is interrupted for long periods, the injury becomes irreversible. Of course, not all cells respond the same way to injury, and the final outcome of anoxia will depend on many factors. For example, brain cells cannot survive without oxygen for more than a few minutes, heart cells can survive 1 to 2 hours, and kidney cells can survive for several hours. Connective tissue cells are most resistant to anoxia; indeed, viable fibroblasts can be obtained from a cadaver even 1 day after death.

In clinical practice, hypoxia or anoxia may occur under many circumstances (Figure 1-11), including (1) obstruction of the airways (e.g., suffocation secondary to drowning), (2) inadequate transport of oxygen across the respiratory surfaces of the lung (e.g., pneumonia), (3) inadequate transport of oxygen in the blood (e.g., anemia), or (4) an inability of the cell to use oxygen for cellular respiration (e.g., cyanide poisoning). Cyanide inhibits oxidative enzymes in the cell and prevents oxidative phosphorylation.

Short-lived reversible cell injury secondary to hypoxia may be repaired completely on reoxygenation. For example, a patient who suffers a heart block and loses consciousness as a result of brain anoxia can resume a normal life if resuscitation is timely and adequate. Ischemic myocardial injury caused by coronary artery thrombosis can be minimized, and sometimes even completely prevented, by the angioplastic removal of the thrombus with thrombolytic enzymes. However, reoxygenation of the tissue carries an additional risk because the oversupply of oxygen may have a deleterious effect on the reversibly damaged cells (Figure 1-12). Oxygen toxicity results in such cases from activated **oxygen radicals.** These toxic compounds are formed in tissues in several ways from oxygen activated by ionized iron or in chemical reactions that produce hydrogen peroxide (H_2O_2) and superoxide (O_2^-). Under normal circumstances, these activated oxygen radicals are formed in small amounts and are inactivated by the cellular enzymatic scavenger mechanisms. However, if oxygen consumption in the tissues is decreased and scavenger enzyme systems (e.g., *catalase* or *superoxide dismutase*) are inoperative, excessive formation of oxygen radicals may result in additional tissue loss. In patients with myocardial infarction, this is called *postperfusion myocardial injury.*

TOXIC INJURY

Toxic injury may be induced by substances known for their *direct* toxic effects on cells and by those that are not directly toxic but that must be metabolically activated to become

TABLE 1-2 Major Causes of Cell Injury

Cause	Pathogenesis	Clinical Examples
Hypoxia and anoxia	Circulatory disturbances Inadequate oxygen intake	Myocardial infarct Strangulation
Toxin	Direct toxicity Indirect toxicity	Mercury poisoning Carbon tetrachloride poisoning
Microbes	Bacterial exotoxins Direct (viral) cytopathic effect Indirect (immune-mediated cytotoxicity)	Food poisoning Viral infection
Inflammation and immune reactions	Action of cytokines and complements	Autoimmune diseases
Genetic and metabolic disorders	Disruption of metabolic pathways	Lysosomal storage disease (e.g., Tay-Sachs disease)
	Abnormal metabolism	Diabetes

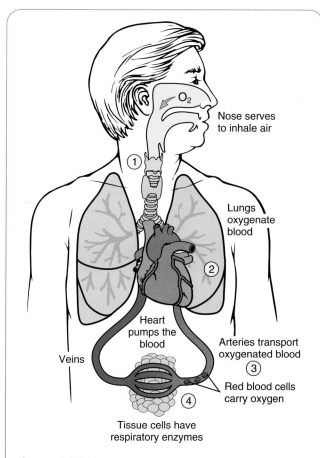

Figure 1-11 The major causes of hypoxia-anoxia include (1) interruption of the oxygen supply, (2) inhibition of blood oxygenation in the lungs, (3) inadequate transport of oxygen in circulation, and (4) inhibition of cellular respiration.

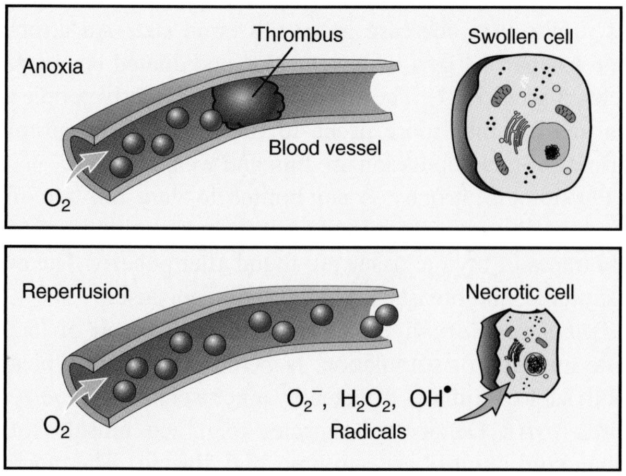

toxins *(indirect toxicity)*. Heavy metals, such as mercury, are *directly* toxic because they inactivate cytoplasmic enzymes by disrupting the sulfhydryl (S-S) groups that hold the polypeptide chains of an enzyme together in an active state. Carbon tetrachloride (CCl_4), a component of commercial metal-cleaning solutions (metal polish), is the best-studied *indirect* toxin. On ingestion, CCl_4 is metabolized to CCl_3, which acts as a toxic free radical, damaging cell membranes.

Many drugs and their metabolites cause cell injury, especially if given in large amounts. Although the mechanism of cell injury varies from one drug to another, the end results are usually comparable. However, because various drugs affect various organs, the clinical presentations vary considerably. The effect of drugs is also dose dependent. In large amounts, most drugs may be toxic and many are even lethal. Suicide by drug overdose is probably the best example of drug-induced toxicity.

> **? Did You Know?**
>
> Potassium cyanide is a potent toxin and has been used as a poison. In Germany, during World War II, many high-ranking Nazi officials carried a capsule of cyanide placed into a hole in their teeth that they could use for suicide in case they were captured by Allied soldiers. As you know from history, however, for whatever reasons, the Nazi suicide plan was never implemented and most German officials were captured alive.
>
> Cyanide is found naturally in fruit pits. Apricot seeds were used by quack doctors for production of an alleged anticancer drug called *laetrile*. Laetrile did not cure any cancers, and it is not known how many patients developed cyanide toxicity from this so-called treatment.

MICROBIAL PATHOGENS

Microbial pathogens cause cell injury in several ways. Bacteria most often produce *toxins,* which may inhibit various cell functions, such as respiration or protein synthesis. For example, food poisoning from spoiled, unrefrigerated leftover food is caused by *exotoxins,* which are released by bacteria growing on contaminated food. Ingestion of these exotoxins in spoiled food produces nausea, vomiting, and diarrhea. All these symptoms are a consequence of "cell poisoning"—that is, the adverse effects of bacterial exotoxins on the gastrointestinal cells.

Viruses that are directly cytopathic invade cells and "kill from within" by disturbing various cellular processes or by disrupting the integrity of the nucleus or plasma membrane (Figure 1-13). Other viruses that are not directly cytopathic integrate themselves into the cellular genome. The genetic material of these viruses encodes the production of foreign proteins, which are mixed with the cell's own proteins and incorporated into the cell's membrane. The body's immune system will recognize the foreign viral proteins in the cell membrane and attack it. By attacking the foreign protein, the immune system will at the same time damage and ultimately kill the virus-infected cell.

Figure 1-12 Postperfusion injury by oxygen radicals.

Anoxia

Thrombus

Swollen cell

Blood vessel

O_2

Reperfusion

Necrotic cell

O_2

O_2^-, H_2O_2, $OH^\bullet$
Radicals

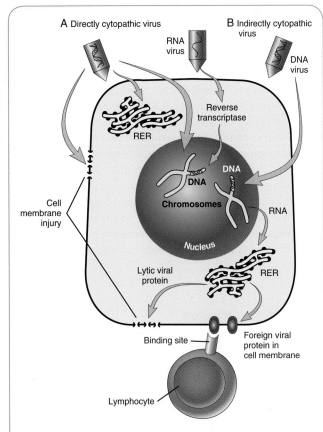

Figure 1-13 Viral cell injury. *A,* Direct cytopathic effect. *B,* Indirect cytopathic effect mediated by immune mechanisms. *RER,* rough endoplasmic reticulum.

MEDIATORS OF INFLAMMATORY AND IMMUNE REACTIONS

Mediators of inflammation and immune reactions, such as cytokines, interferons, or complement proteins, may injure cells in several ways. These biologically active substances are produced by the body in response to infection or in various immune reactions. Although such substances are valuable for eliminating the infectious agents, often they kill not only the microbes but also the body's own cells as well. These substances are discussed in greater detail in Chapters 2 and 3.

GENETIC AND METABOLIC DISTURBANCES

Genetic and metabolic disturbances are important causes of cell injury. Many genetic inborn errors of metabolism cause disturbances of intermediate metabolism and subsequent accumulation of toxic metabolites in the cells. For example, in *Tay-Sachs disease* (a genetic deficiency of hexosaminidase A), gangliosides accumulate in the lysosomes of nerve cells and eyes. Severe mental deficiency and blindness develop, and those with Tay-Sachs usually die in early childhood.

Metabolic disturbances of adulthood also may cause various forms of cell injury. In some instances, the injury affects the cells directly, whereas in others the injury is indirect. For example, *diabetes mellitus,* a disease caused by insulin deficiency, is characterized by hyperglycemia (excess of glucose in blood), which alters the metabolism of liver or kidney cells. At the same time, diabetes produces pathologic changes in the small blood vessels, which in turn cause additional pathologic changes in tissues receiving blood through the altered vessels. In most instances such changes are a consequence of ischemia, the most prominent complication of diabetic small-vessel disease *(diabetic microangiopathy).*

CELL ADAPTATIONS

Prolonged exposure of cells to adverse or exaggerated normal stimuli evokes various **adaptations** at the level of individual cells, tissues, or organs. Once the cause is removed, most cells that have adapted to chronic stimulation revert to normalcy again. However, some forms of adaptation, especially those associated with cell loss (e.g., bone loss in osteoporosis), are irreversible.

ATROPHY

Atrophy denotes a decrease in the size of a cell, tissue, or organ or the entire body. *Atrophy* can refer to the reduced size of individual cells, reduced number of cells in a tissue or organ (also known as *involution*), or a combination of these two processes. Like all adaptations, atrophy can be classified as physiologic or pathologic.

Physiologic atrophy occurs with age and involves essentially the entire body. For example, in the brain, a certain number of cells is lost every day from birth on; over the years, this results in a decrease in overall brain size. An atrophic brain has narrow gyri, widened sulci, and dilated lateral ventricles (Figure 1-14). The atrophic bones of elderly people are thin and are thus more prone to fracture, and the atrophic muscles of this population are thin and weak.

Physiologic atrophy is not limited to very old age. The thymus undergoes physiologic atrophy during childhood, and only traces of thymic tissue are found after puberty. The ovaries, uterus, and breasts atrophy after menopause.

Pathologic atrophy typically occurs as a result of inadequate nutrition or stimulation. Ischemic organs are typically small, such as kidneys affected by atherosclerosis *(nephroangiosclerosis).* Denervated muscles (e.g., leg muscles after spinal cord injury) are atrophic and flaccid. The general cachexia caused by cancer or malnutrition is marked by muscle wastage and atrophy of muscle fibers.

Atrophy of individual cells is associated with obvious reduction of cell size and reduced metabolism. The cytoplasm of atrophic cells contains fewer mitochondria and endoplasmic

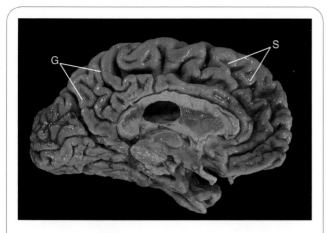

Figure 1-14 Atrophic brain. The gyri (G) are narrow and the sulci (S) are wide.

reticulum. Effete, aging, and damaged organelles are taken up by autophagosomes. Inside the autophagosomes these organelles are digested and lyzed. Undigested residues remain in the cytoplasm in the form of lipid-rich brown pigment residues (*lipofuscin*), which impart a brown color to atrophic organs (e.g., brown atrophy of the heart or brown atrophy of the testis).

Proteins released from damaged organelles, as well as those that are no longer needed in the cytoplasm of atrophic cells, are bound to a scavenger protein called **ubiquitin.** Ubiquitin marks them for destruction in *proteasomes,* large protease complexes specializing in degradation of effete proteins.

HYPERTROPHY AND HYPERPLASIA

Hypertrophy is an increase in the size of tissues or organs caused by an enlargement of individual cells. Etymologically the term is related to the Greek word *trophe,* meaning "food," and thus actually means enlargement of "overfed" cells. By contrast, **hyperplasia** is an increase in the size of tissues and organs caused by an increased number of cells (Figure 1-15). Etymologically it means "increased proliferation or formation

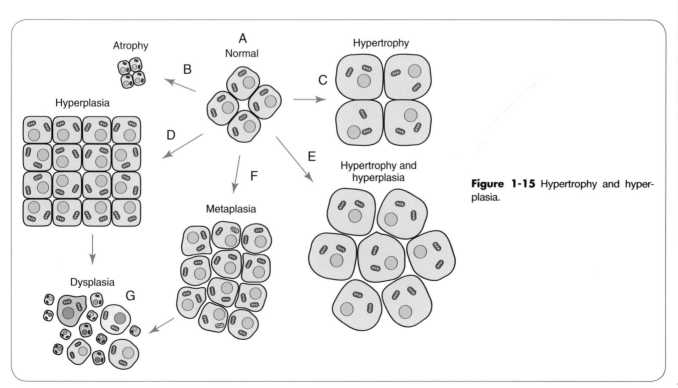

Figure 1-15 Hypertrophy and hyperplasia.

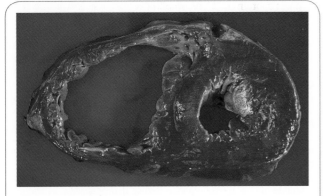

Figure 1-16 Hypertrophy of the left ventricle of the heart caused by hypertension.

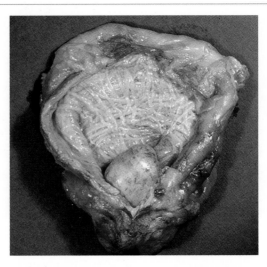

Figure 1-17 Hyperplasia of the prostate with secondary thickening of the obstructed urinary bladder. The enlarged prostate (P) is seen protruding into the lumen of the bladder, which appears trabeculated (T). These "trabeculae" result from hypertrophy and hyperplasia of smooth muscle cells that occurs in response to increased intravesical pressure caused by urinary obstruction.

of cells." Hypertrophy and hyperplasia are often combined. Pure hypertrophy occurs only in the heart and striated muscles, because these organs consist of cells that cannot divide.

Hypertrophy of the heart is a common pathologic finding that occurs as an adaptation of heart muscle to increased workload (Figure 1-16). Hypertrophy of the left ventricle of the heart is a typical complication of hypertension. The increased pressure in the outflow side of the left ventricle requires more force to be overcome, and this is achieved by hypertrophy of muscle fibers. Hypertrophic heart cells increase in size. Such cells contain more myofilaments, which allow them to contract more efficiently. *Hypertrophy of skeletal muscles* is commonly induced by exercise and is typically found in bodybuilders.

Hypertrophy with hyperplasia occurs under a variety of conditions. For example, smooth muscle cells in the wall of the urinary bladder, when obstructed by a hyperplastic prostate, increase in size and number. This contributes to thickening of the wall of the urinary bladder (Figure 1-17). Physiologic hypertrophy of uterine smooth muscle cells during pregnancy is also accompanied by hyperplasia.

Pure hyperplasia typically occurs as a result of hormonal stimulation. For example, when continuously stimulated by estrogen, the endometrium may become very thick *(endometrial hyperplasia)*. Histologic examination reveals an increased number of glandular and stromal cells. In benign prostatic hyperplasia (a common cause of prostatic enlargement in elderly individuals, which is also hormonally induced), hyperplasia of epithelial and stromal cells leads to the formation of grossly visible nodules.

Hyperplasia may also occur in response to chronic injury. In some cases, the cause is obvious. For example, tight shoes may cause chronic irritation of the skin. In such cases, the epidermal cells undergo hyperplasia and form a callus or corn. However, some hyperplastic lesions have no obvious cause and probably represent early neoplasia. Examples of such lesions are *hyperplastic polyps* of the large intestine and foci of *nodular hyperplasia* in the liver. Some forms of

endometrial hyperplasia may undergo additional genetic changes and if left untreated may progress to neoplasia.

METAPLASIA

Metaplasia is a form of adaptation characterized by the change of one cell type into another. For example, columnar cells of the bronchial mucosa, when irritated by cigarette smoke, change into stratified squamous epithelium.

Metaplasia represents a reversible change. If the smoker stops smoking, the squamous epithelium will revert back to ciliated columnar cells. If the stimulus that has induced squamous metaplasia persists (i.e., if the smoker does not stop smoking), the squamous metaplasia may progress to *dysplasia*. In contrast to the regular layering of normal squamous cells that is typical of metaplasia, dysplasia is characterized by a disorderly arrangement of cells and nuclear atypia. Dysplasia may still be reversible if the stimulus is discontinued, but more often than not it progresses to *neoplasia* (discussed in Chapter 4; also see Chapter 8 for content on lung carcinoma in smokers).

INTRACELLULAR ACCUMULATIONS

Intracellular accumulations may occur as a result of an overload of various metabolites or exogenous material, or they may be attributable to metabolic disturbances that prevent excretion of metabolic byproducts or normal secretions from cells. In most instances, the underlying mechanisms are complex and involve both an overload and underutilization or reduced excretion.

ANTHRACOSIS

Anthracosis (accumulation of coal particles) is the best example of exogenous material accumulation. The term is derived from the Greek word *anthrax,* meaning "carbon." Severe anthracosis is seen in the lungs of people who work in coal mines. Coal particles are released into the air from chimneys; in essence, any air pollution could cause anthracosis. Pulmonary anthracosis is also caused by cigarette smoke.

HEMOSIDEROSIS

Hemosiderosis is an accumulation of blood-derived brown pigment called **hemosiderin** (derived from the Greek words *haima,* "blood," and *sideros,* "iron"). Hemosiderin is usually derived from hemolyzed blood. Remember that red blood cells contain iron-rich hemoglobin, which disintegrates into globin and heme. Heme gives rise to micelles of ferritin, which aggregate into hemosiderin. Iron in hemosiderin can be demonstrated in tissues with the so-called Prussian blue reaction. Hemosiderosis of the liver is a constant feature of a genetic disorder of iron absorption from food called *hereditary hemochromatosis* (Figure 1-18).

LIPID ACCUMULATION

Lipid accumulation in the liver is an example of intracellular accumulation of intermediate metabolites. Fat is normally stored in liver cells in the form of triglycerides. Obese people have fatty livers because of an overload of fat. Fat accumulation in the liver, also known as *steatosis,* is a typical finding in persons suffering from chronic alcohol abuse or from diabetes mellitus.

As shown in Figure 1-19, alcohol stimulates accumulation of fat in the liver through several mechanisms. The fat is derived, in part, from free fatty acids mobilized from peripheral stores at an accelerated rate. Alcohol has a high caloric content and serves as a substrate for new fat formation in liver cells *(neolipogenesis).* It also inhibits several hepatic lypolitic enzymes and thus impedes utilization of intrahepatic fat. Finally, alcohol inhibits apoprotein synthesis and the export of fat from the liver in the form of lipoproteins.

The clinical consequences of cytoplasmic storage are variable. For example, fatty change of liver cells has almost no functional consequences, and the accumulation of carbon particles in the lung and lymph node cells in anthracosis is also innocuous. On the other hand, congenital lysosomal storage diseases usually have serious and even lethal consequences. Accumulation of iron pigment in hereditary hemochromatosis causes liver damage and may lead to cirrhosis (end-stage liver disease).

AGING

The **aging** of cells includes many complex adaptations and, unfortunately, many cellular events that are irreversible. Aging cannot be avoided or prevented; the best we can do is to retard it or minimize its adverse effects on the body.

The process of aging is poorly understood. There are many theories of aging, none of which explains in full the essence of this complex biologic phenomenon. Everybody is aware of the remarkable differences between an old and a young person, but our understanding of these differences is still very shallow.

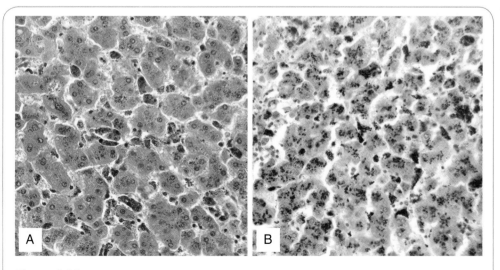

Figure 1-18 Hereditary hemochromatosis. *A,* The disease is characterized by an accumulation of hemosiderin, an iron-rich brown pigment, in liver and Kupffer cells. B, The so-called Prussian blue reaction gives hemosiderin a blue hue.

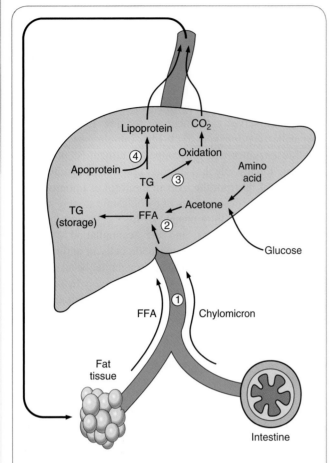

Figure 1-19 Pathogenesis of alcoholic fatty liver. Triglycerides (TG) in the liver cell are formed through several mechanisms, all of which contribute to the accumulation of fat: (1) increased influx of free fatty acids (FFA) from peripheral stores; (2) increased neolipogenesis from glucose, amino acids, and alcohol; (3) decreased utilization of triglycerides because of the inhibition of enzymes. (4) Decreased synthesis of apoprotein, which is essential for the formation of lipoproteins, reduces export of lipids from the liver.

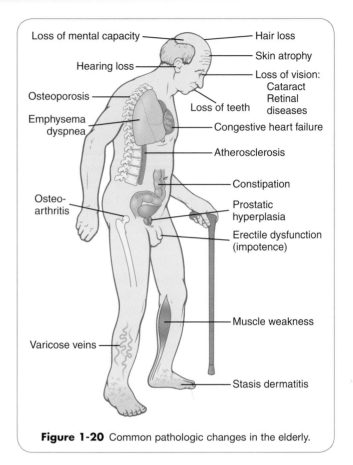

Figure 1-20 Common pathologic changes in the elderly.

Pathologic changes associated with aging vary from one individual to another. Overall, most organs undergo atrophy and have a reduced functional reserve. Resistance to infection declines with advancing age. On the other hand, the incidence of cardiovascular diseases and cancer is increased. Typical pathologic changes encountered in the elderly are illustrated in Figure 1-20.

Scientists studying old age (gerontologists) favor two major hypotheses as an explanation for aging: the *wear-and-tear hypothesis* and the *genetic hypothesis.* Because cells represent the basic living units of all tissues and organs, it is thought that cellular aging represents the critical event in the aging of the organism and that the decline of complex integrative and specialized functions of the body results from dysfunctions at the cellular level. In organs composed of cells that cannot regenerate, such as the brain and heart, the wear-and-tear hypothesis accounts, to a great extent, for the decline in function of these organs. However, because all people do not lose brain cells at the same speed, the genetic theory of aging also has merit. This hypothesis asserts that aging is a genetically predetermined process. Hormonal, immune, and neural theories blame all the calamities of aging on the dysfunction of these integrative processes.

DEATH

Death, even more so than aging, is an inevitable feature of life. All the cells in the human body have a finite life span, and when the life span comes to an end, cells die. Some of the cells may be replaced from stem cells in that tissue, whereas others are irreplaceable. Heart cells belong to the latter category. However, even if all heart cells die, the life of a person can be extended today with heart transplantation. If the neural cells of the vital centers of the brain die, death is inevitable. Thus we use the term *brain death,* which for legal purposes means cessation of vital brain functions and an absence of electrical activity in the brain as detected by electroencephalography. In practical terms the noncerebral body functions in a "brain dead" person cannot be maintained on their own and typically require medical support, including mechanical ventilation, assisted feeding, and special long-term care.

CELL DEATH

Cell death occurs in several forms. We have already mentioned that the irreversible cell injury caused by anoxia or toxins leads to cell death with typical nuclear changes (pyknosis, karyorrhexis, karyolysis), rupture of the cell membrane, and cessation of cellular respiration. This form of exogenously induced cell death is called *necrosis* (from the Greek term *necros,* meaning "dead"). By contrast, *apoptosis* (Greek for "dropping out") refers to endogenously programmed cell death. Necrosis and apoptosis represent the death of single cells or groups of cells within a living organism. Death of cells and tissues in a dead organism that occurs as a result of cessation of respiration and heartbeat is called *autolysis* (from the Greek terms *autos,* meaning "self," and *lysis,* meaning "dissolution").

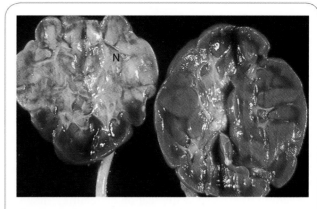

Figure 1-21 Coagulative necrosis of the kidney of an infant caused by ischemia. The necrotic area (N) is pale yellow, in contrast to the normally perfused parenchyma of the kidney on the right, which is reddish brown.

 Did You Know?

The Greek word *necros,* meaning "dead corpse," is also used to construct many other medical words. For example, the postmortem examination of human or animal bodies performed by pathologists is called a *necropsy.* However, the same linguistic root can be found in other words as well. According to Greek mythology, *nectar,* sweet juice consumed by Greek gods, could bestow immortality. Nectarines, although good for our health, are unfortunately not a remedy for our mortality.

NECROSIS

In contrast to autolysis, which is a postmortem event and is therefore of little significance for clinicians, **necrosis** is clinically important. It occurs in several forms: coagulative, liquefactive, caseous, and enzymatic fat necrosis.

Coagulative Necrosis

Coagulative necrosis is the most common form of necrosis. Coagulative necrosis is marked by rapid inactivation of cytoplasmic hydrolytic enzymes. This prevents lysis of tissues, which retain their original form and firm consistency. Coagulative necrosis typically involves solid internal organs such as the heart, liver, or kidneys (Figure 1-21). Most often it is caused by anoxia (e.g., myocardial infarct).

Liquefactive Necrosis

Liquefactive necrosis is characterized by the dissolution of tissues, which become soft and diffluent. It occurs most often in the brain. The brain cells lose their contours and are "liquefied" (i.e., transformed into semifluid mush). Liquefactive necrosis is typical of a brain infarct, which is usually soft and ultimately becomes transformed into a fluid-filled cavity (Figure 1-22).

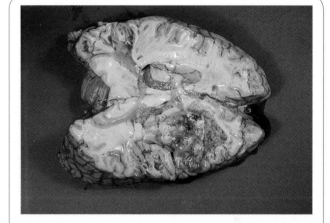

Figure 1-22 Cerebral infarct. The area of infarction is softened as a result of liquefaction necrosis (LN).

Coagulative necrosis may liquefy, usually through the action of leukocytes that invade the necrotic tissue to remove the dead cells. Leukocytes release lytic enzymes, which in turn transform the solid tissue into liquid pus. Pus is a viscous yellow fluid composed of leukocytes and cell debris. Myocardial infarcts that initially show coagulative necrosis are invaded by leukocytes and undergo *secondary liquefaction,* usually 4 to 6 days after the blood vessel occlusion.

Caseous Necrosis

Caseous necrosis, which is typically found in patients with tuberculosis, is a special form of coagulative necrosis with limited liquefaction. The center of a tuberculous granuloma becomes necrotic and the cells fall apart. The tissue is yellow-white and "cheesy," hence the name caseous necrosis (in Latin, *caseum* means "cheese"). Caseous necrosis is not unique to tuberculosis; it may also be found in fungal infections such as histoplasmosis.

Enzymatic Fat Necrosis

Enzymatic fat necrosis is a special form of liquefactive necrosis caused by the action of lipolytic enzymes. It is limited to fat tissue, usually around the pancreas. Pancreatic enzymes released into the adjacent fat tissue (e.g., after rupture of the pancreas caused by seat belt trauma following a traffic accident) degrade the fat into glycerol and free fatty acids. The free fatty acids rapidly bind with calcium, forming calcium soaps. Therefore the area of fat necrosis appears like liquefied fat with whitish specks of calcium soap scattered throughout.

Necrotic tissue, especially that on extremities, may undergo secondary changes that produce specific morphologic features. Bacterial infection of coagulated tissue leads to inflammation and a secondary liquefaction that is clinically known as *wet gangrene.* If the necrotic tissue dries out, it becomes dark black and mummified, just as the ancient Egyptian mummies dried in the hot air of the sand desert. Such lesions are called *dry gangrene* (Figure 1-23). Both forms of **gangrene** are most often seen on the toes and lower extremities and are usually caused by peripheral vascular disease (atherosclerosis). Gangrene of the toes or the entire foot is especially common in diabetic patients.

Necrotic tissue attracts calcium salts and often undergoes **calcification.** Calcification of necrotic tissue is called *dystrophic calcification,* in contradistinction to *metastatic calcification,* which is typically a consequence of hypercalcemia. Dystrophic calcification is seen in atherosclerotic arteries, damaged heart valves (Figure 1-24), or necrotic tumors. Metastatic calcification is a feature of metabolic hypercalcemia secondary to hyperparathyroidism or vitamin D toxicity. It most often involves the kidneys, presumably because the fluctuating pH levels in the renal parenchyma and the high concentration of calcium predispose the individual to deposition of calcium salts in the tissue.

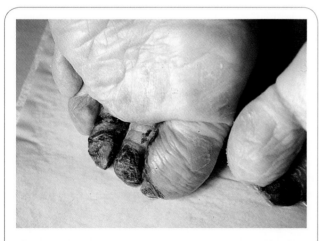

Figure 1-23 Dry gangrene involving several toes, which appear black.

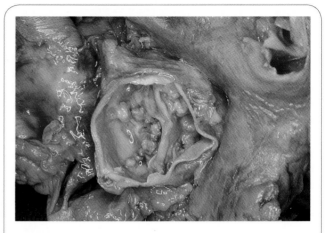

Figure 1-24 Calcified aortic valve. Nodules on the valves are examples of dystrophic calcification.

APOPTOSIS

Apoptosis is an "active" form of *cell death.* Because it is energy dependent and requires activation of a specific set of genes and enzymes, it is also known as *programmed cell death.* The genes activated in apoptosis are popularly known as *suicide genes,* and accordingly, apoptosis is best compared with a suicide. The initial event could be *endogenous* or *exogenous.* In cellular terms, this could mean a long-lasting viral infection (exogenous; e.g., chronic viral hepatitis C) or a lack of necessary growth factors in a brain cell (endogenous). Like a person who has decided to die rather than to live, the cell entering the apoptosis pathway will use its "brain" (i.e., its nucleus) and "decide" how to activate a certain set of killer genes and how to inactivate other life-sustaining genes. In analogy with the suicide, the cell also chooses the tools for suicide; that is, it synthesizes specific killer enzymes that attack the cell's vital structures, such as the nucleus and the mitochondria.

Apoptosis is a form of cell death that typically affects single cells (Figures 1-25 and 1-26). During apoptosis, an energy-requiring process, there is active transcription and translation of genetic material, and the enzyme activity of the cytoplasm remains high. The cell subdivides into smaller apoptotic bodies, which contain fragments of the nucleus and metabolically active mitochondria and other organelles. Ultimately, these fragments are taken up by macrophages or adjacent living cells in the tissue, which act as "nonprofessional phagocytes." In contrast to apoptosis, necrosis affects groups of cells or an entire organ. Toxic stimuli or ischemia causing necrosis lead to the inhibition of vital processes such as gene activity and cellular respiration. The nucleus disintegrates or undergoes lysis, the cytoplasm swells, and the cell membrane ruptures. The fragments are typically taken up by polymorphonuclear neutrophils. The main differences between apoptosis and necrosis are listed in Table 1-3.

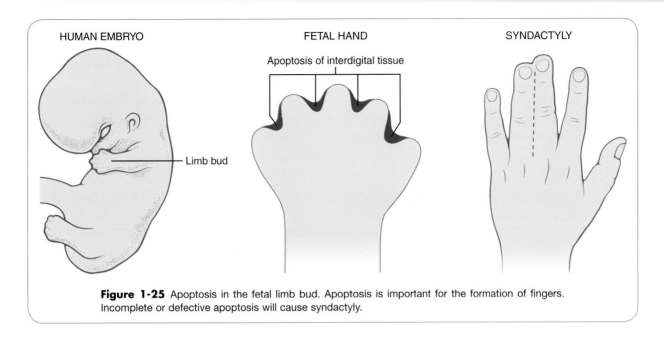

Figure 1-25 Apoptosis in the fetal limb bud. Apoptosis is important for the formation of fingers. Incomplete or defective apoptosis will cause syndactyly.

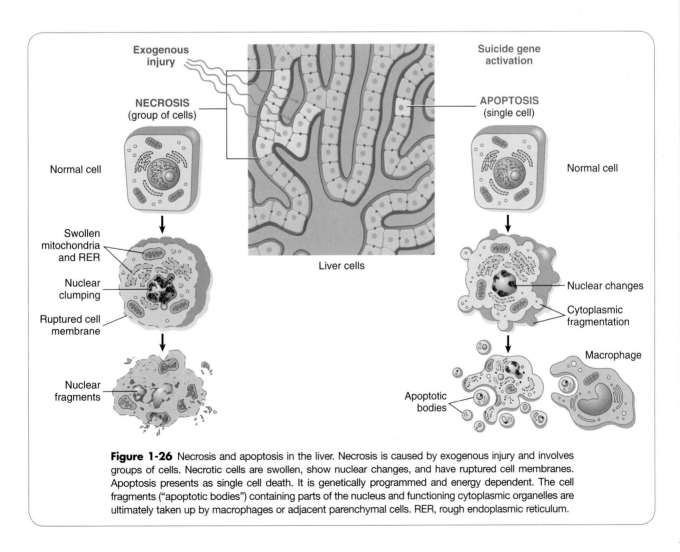

Figure 1-26 Necrosis and apoptosis in the liver. Necrosis is caused by exogenous injury and involves groups of cells. Necrotic cells are swollen, show nuclear changes, and have ruptured cell membranes. Apoptosis presents as single cell death. It is genetically programmed and energy dependent. The cell fragments ("apoptotic bodies") containing parts of the nucleus and functioning cytoplasmic organelles are ultimately taken up by macrophages or adjacent parenchymal cells. RER, rough endoplasmic reticulum.

TABLE 1-3 Comparison of Necrosis and Apoptosis

Feature	Necrosis	Apoptosis
Cause	Exogenous injury	May be exogenous or endogenous
Mechanisms	Vital processes inhibited	Energy dependent, vital processes active
Cells affected	Multiple	Single
Cell morphology	Swollen, ruptured	Rounded up, fragmented (apoptotic bodies)
Cell membrane	Ruptured	Functionally intact
Outcome	Phagocytosis by neutrophils	Phagocytosis by macrophages and "nonprofessional macrophages"

Like all other cellular functions, apoptosis is a highly regulated process. Life and death are intricately interconnected; certain cells must die so that others can live. Accordingly, apoptosis occurs during the entire human life span, from early embryonic stages to old age. Apoptosis can also be induced by adverse exogenous events, and accordingly, it is customary to classify apoptosis as physiologic or pathologic.

Physiologic apoptosis plays an important role in the formation of many, if not all, body parts. For example, in the fetal limb buds, apoptosis of the soft tissues between the primordia of the digits ensures that the fingers and toes are normally formed (Figure 1-25). Without apoptosis, such limbs will be abnormally shaped—for example, the digits may be fused together (**syndactyly**). If apoptosis does not occur during the formation of the esophagus or the intestines, there will be no lumen and these organs will show **atresia** (obliteration of the lumen).

Pathologic apoptosis may be a consequence of endogenous intracellular events, or it may be caused by adverse exogenous stimuli. For example, in muscular dystrophy, a group of genetic diseases characterized by a deficiency of specific cell components, the skeletal muscle cells that lack those proteins undergo apoptosis. Organs transplanted from one person to another show signs of apoptosis because the transplanted cells are attacked by the host's immune cells. Liver cells infected with hepatitis viruses also undergo apoptosis (Figure 1-26).

Lack of apoptosis also can cause pathologic changes. As mentioned previously, congenital intestinal atresia and syndactyly are salient examples of how lack of apoptosis can cause pathologic changes. Chronic lymphocytic leukemia or lymphoma is related to a lack of apoptosis. In this disease, a mutation of the proapoptotic gene (known as *BCL2*) adversely affects the lymphocytes, making them "forget to die." Because lymphocytes do not die at their normal rate, they remain in the lymph nodes (thus enlarging the lymph nodes) and also spill into the blood, causing leukemia.

REVIEW QUESTIONS

1. What are the main components of the nucleus and the cytoplasm?
2. Which components of the cell contain RNA?
3. Compare mitochondria with endoplasmic reticulum and Golgi apparatus.
4. What is the difference between primary and secondary lysosomes, autophagosomes, and heterophagosomes?
5. Compare intermediate filaments with microfilaments and microtubules.
6. Explain autocrine, paracrine, and endocrine cell stimulation.
7. What is homeostasis?
8. How is cellular steady state maintained, and what does it mean when a cell reaches the point of no return?
9. Explain the pathogenesis of hydropic change and the role of Na^+/K^+–ATPase in cellular swelling.
10. What are the microscopic signs of irreversible cell injury?
11. Explain the pathogenesis of hypoxia or anoxia and give clinical examples of these conditions.
12. What are oxygen radicals, and how do they damage cells?
13. How do toxins, microbes, and chemical mediators of inflammation kill cells?
14. Compare acute cell injury with cellular adaptations.
15. Compare atrophy with hypertrophy and hyperplasia and give clinical examples of each condition.
16. Explain the significance of smoking-induced metaplasia of the bronchial epithelium in the pathogenesis of bronchial neoplasia.
17. Compare anthracosis and hemosiderosis.
18. Explain the pathogenesis of fatty liver induced by alcohol.
19. Discuss the merits of the wear-and-tear and genetic hypotheses of aging.
20. What is meant by the term *brain death*?
21. Compare the gross appearances of various forms of necrosis.
22. What is the difference between dry and wet gangrene?
23. Compare metastatic calcification and dystrophic calcification.
24. What is apoptosis?
25. Provide two examples of physiologic apoptosis and two examples of pathologic apoptosis.
26. Compare apoptosis with necrosis.

Inflammation

2

Chapter Outline

Signs of Inflammation
Pathogenesis of Inflammation
Cellular Events in Inflammation
Emigration of Leukocytes
Phagocytosis
Cells of Inflammation
Classification of Inflammation
Duration
Etiology
Location
Pathology of Inflammation
Serous Inflammation

Fibrinous Inflammation
Purulent Inflammation
Ulcerative Inflammation
Pseudomembranous Inflammation
Chronic Inflammation
Granulomatous Inflammation
Clinicopathologic Correlations
Healing and Repair
Wound Healing

Key Terms and Concepts

Abscess
Adhesion molecules
Anaphylatoxins
Angioblasts
Arachidonic acid
Bacteremia
Basophils
Bradykinin
Chemotaxis
Collagens
Complement
Contractures
Cyclooxygenase
Cytokines
Empyema
Fever
Fibrinous inflammation
Fibroblasts
Fibronectin

Fibrosis
Fistula
Furuncle
Granulation tissue
Granuloma
Hageman factor
Histamine
Hyperemia
Keloids
Leukocytes
Leukotrienes
Lymphocytes
Macrophages
Mast cells
Membrane attack complex (MAC)
Mitosis
Multinucleated giant cells
Myofibroblasts
Opsonin

Phagocytosis
Plasma cells
Platelets
Polymorphonuclear leukocytes
Prostacyclin
Prostaglandins
Pseudomembranous inflammation
Pus
Scar
Sepsis
Serous inflammation
Sinus
Ulceration
Wound dehiscence
Wound healing
Wounds

Learning Objectives

After reading this chapter, the student should be able to:

1. Define inflammation.
2. List the main components of acute inflammation.
3. Describe the vascular changes in acute inflammation.
4. Describe the cellular events in acute inflammation.
5. Define the following terms pertaining to leukocytes involved in an inflammatory response: *margination, diapedesis, emigration, exudation, chemotaxis, phagocytosis,* and *microbicidal substances.*
6. List two cell-derived and three plasma-derived mediators of inflammation.
7. Explain the function of proteins of the complement system and the clotting system in inflammation.
8. Explain the role of arachidonic acid metabolites in inflammation.
9. Explain the main functions of cytokines released in inflammation.
10. Describe possible outcomes of acute inflammation.
11. Describe three pathogenetic pathways leading to chronic inflammation.
12. List the principal cells of acute and chronic inflammation.
13. Describe the formation of granuloma.
14. Describe the typical complications of granulomatous inflammation.
15. Define the following pathologic terms: *serous inflammation, fibrinous inflammation, purulent inflammation, abscess, ulcer, wound, scar,* and *keloid.*
16. Describe the typical local and systemic symptoms of inflammation.
17. Explain the pathogenesis of fever.
18. Describe wound healing and repair.
19. List three factors that may delay healing and repair.
20. List two complications of wound healing.

Inflammation is a nonspecific but predictable response of living tissues, or the entire body, to injury. The injury may be caused by chemical agents, physical forces, living microbes, or many other physiologic or pathologic (exogenous or endogenous) stimuli that disturb the normal steady state. It is important to note the following with regard to inflammation:

- Inflammation includes a series of interconnected events. Thus inflammation is a dynamic process, evolving through several phases that last from a few minutes to days or even months and years. Inflammation of sudden onset and short duration is characterized as acute inflammation, in contrast to chronic inflammation, which lasts a long time.

- Inflammation occurs only in multicellular organisms that are capable of mounting a neurovascular and cellular response to injury. Thus in contrast to cell injury, which occurs at the level of single cells, inflammation is a coordinated reaction of the animal and human body, and it involves nerves, vessels, blood cells, and soluble mediators of inflammation.

- Inflammation has a protective role and is generally beneficial to the body. However, the side effects of inflammation may be noxious. For example, fever, which initially has a beneficial effect, may be so high that it causes death. Sometimes the process may become uncontrollable, producing more harm than good. For example, pulmonary tuberculosis elicits a protective tissue reaction. This inflammatory response may erode pulmonary vessels and cause massive bleeding.

- Inflammation occurs only in living tissues. Necrotic or dead tissue cannot mount an inflammatory response. For example, a gangrenous foot cannot become inflamed. Because the body cannot combat infection in necrotic tissue, a foot that is affected by gangrene must be amputated. From a forensic point of view, inflammation is considered a *vital reaction.* If histologic signs of inflammation are found in tissues recovered at autopsy, this indicates that injury occurred before death, because inflammation cannot develop postmortem.

SIGNS OF INFLAMMATION

The Roman physician Celsus (circa 30 BCE–38 CE) described the *four cardinal signs of inflammation*: *calor* (heat), *rubor* (redness), *tumor* (swelling), and *dolor* (pain) (Figure 2-1).

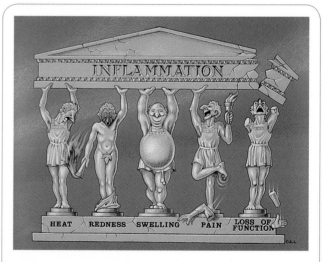

Figure 2-1 The cardinal signs of inflammation were described in Roman times. (Reprinted by permission of Professor Peter Cull, London University.)

Rudolf Virchow (1821–1902), the father of modern pathology, is credited with adding *functio laesa,* or *disturbed function,* as the fifth classical symptom of inflammation. However, the pathology of inflammation remained poorly understood until the scientific advances of the nineteenth century made possible microscopic studies of inflamed tissues.

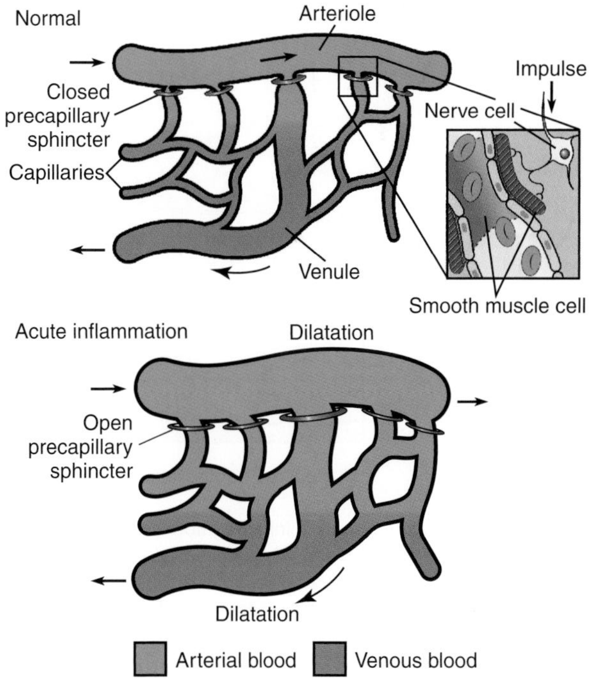

> **? Did You Know?**
>
> A forensic pathologist examined the decomposing body of a child who froze to death in an unheated apartment. The skin showed numerous small holes. The forensic pathologist thought that these holes might have been caused by rats who tried to eat the dead body. Histologic examination showed signs of inflammation around every skin wound. The pathologist concluded that the animal bites must have occurred before death because inflammation is a "vital reaction," occurring only in living organisms.

Microscopic studies of the nineteenth century have been supplemented and expanded by biochemical and molecular biology investigations of the past and this century. Today we know that inflammation is a complex process that involves (1) changes in circulation of blood, (2) changes in vessel wall permeability, (3) a white blood cell response, and (4) the release of soluble mediators.

PATHOGENESIS OF INFLAMMATION

Circulatory Changes

Hemodynamic (vascular) changes—that is, changes in blood flow—represent the body's first response to injury. The redness and swelling of the skin following a gentle slap on the arm or the face are typical of such a vascular response. The mechanical stimulus stimulates nerves that transmit signals to smooth muscle cells on precapillary arterioles. The smooth muscle cells act as sphincters, regulating the inflow of blood into the capillaries (Figure 2-2).

The relaxation of smooth muscle cells allows the blood to rush into the capillaries, and this accounts for the redness, swelling, and warmth of the tissue. The first response of arterioles to an injurious stimulus is vasoconstriction, which lasts only a few seconds. This is followed by vasodilation (i.e., relaxation of the precapillary sphincter), which results in flooding of the capillary network with arterial blood, manifested by redness and mild swelling of the tissue engorged by blood. The arterial blood is warm, and because it is pumped into the area in large quantities, the inflamed tissue also becomes warm. This is called **hyperemia** (from the Greek, meaning "too much blood"). The influx of blood dilates the capillaries, which consist only of endothelial cells and a basement membrane and thus cannot actively regulate blood flow. From the capillaries, the pressure is transmitted to venules, which also do not have a capacity to contract. Increased pressure in the capillaries

Figure 2-2 Circulatory changes in inflammation. Relaxation of the precapillary sphincter in the arterioles results in flooding of the capillary network and dilation of capillaries and postcapillary venules.

and venules forces plasma filtration through the vessel wall, leading to edema.

The blood flow in dilated capillaries and venules is slow, which leads to *congestion* (the Latin root of which means "heaping together") and other hemodynamic changes. The distribution of the cellular elements of the blood (i.e., the white blood cells, red blood cells, and platelets) changes in the bloodstream. In the central part of the stream, the erythrocytes form stacks, called *rouleaux,* which impede the circulation even more, contributing to the turbulent flow of the blood. The white blood cells (**leukocytes**) are marginalized and become attached to the endothelium, a phenomenon called *pavementing* (Figure 2-3). These leukocytes develop elongated protrusions of their surface cytoplasm and become sticky, adhering to the endothelial cells lining the capillaries and particularly those of the postcapillary venules. This adhesion is accomplished by surface **adhesion molecules,** such as selectins and integrins. These molecules are normally present on leukocytes and endothelial cells in an inactive form and become activated during inflammation. Adhesion molecules are activated through the action of **cytokines,** soluble mediators of inflammation, such as interleukins (ILs) or tumor necrosis factor (TNF). Small amounts of IL and TNF are normally present in the blood. However, their concentration is increased at the site of inflammation, as they are released from endothelial cells, leukocytes, platelets, and macrophages in the adjacent connective tissue. These cytokines play

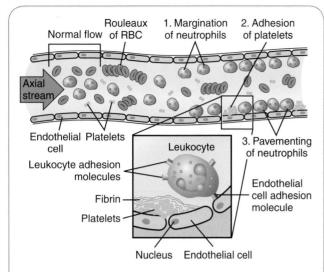

Figure 2-3 Cellular changes in inflammation. (1) Margination of neutrophils brings these inflammatory cells in close contact with the endothelium. (2) Adhesion of platelets results in the release of mediators of inflammation and coagulation. Fibrin strands are the first signs of clot formation. (3) Pavementing of leukocytes is mediated by adhesion molecules activated by the mediators of inflammation released from platelets and leukocytes. RBC, red blood cell.

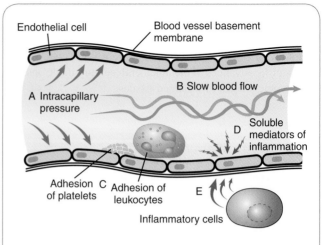

Figure 2-4 Increased permeability of blood vessels, the most important causes of which are increased intracapillary pressure *(A)*, relative hypoxia secondary to slow blood flow *(B)*, adhesion of leukocytes and platelets to endothelial cells *(C)*, the action of soluble mediators of inflammation in the plasma *(D)*, and mediators of inflammation released from inflammatory cells in the tissue surrounding the blood vessel *(E)*.

a major role in maintaining and amplifying inflammation and, as we will see later, also have a major role in immune reactions.

The complexity of processes that occur during inflammation has been a subject of numerous studies. Numerous new anti-inflammatory drugs have been developed, but the search for new inhibitors of inflammation still goes on. Scientists are also looking for stimulators of inflammation and ways of controlling the adverse consequences of inflammatory processes.

Vessel Wall Changes

The permeability of the vessel wall of capillaries and postcapillary venules changes in response to inflammation because of (1) increased pressure inside the congested blood vessels; (2) slowing of the circulation, which reduces the supply of oxygen and nutrients to endothelial cells; (3) adhesion of leukocytes and platelets to endothelial cells; and (4) release of soluble mediators of inflammation from inflammatory cells, platelets, endothelial cells, and plasma (Figure 2-4).

Mediators of Inflammation

The following brief summary contains three primary messages about the chemical mediators of inflammation:

- The mediators of inflammation belong to two classes: *plasma-derived* and *cell-derived* substances. Plasma-derived mediators circulate in an inactive form and must be transformed into an active form by an activator. There are numerous specific and nonspecific activators. All activators have natural inactivators keeping them in balance. The cell-derived mediators may be preformed and stored in granules of platelets and leukocytes, or they may be synthesized *de novo* on demand. Preformed

mediators (e.g., **histamine**) are released quickly, whereas the others (e.g., **bradykinin, leukotrienes,** cytokines) require time to be produced. This lag period from onset of inflammation until the mediators are released may last several hours or even a day or two. The action of these newly synthesized mediators usually lasts longer than the action of preformed mediators.

- Mediators of inflammation are biochemically heterogeneous. The most important are biogenic amines (e.g., histamine), proteins (e.g., **complement**), and **arachidonic acid** derivatives (e.g., prostaglandins).
- Mediators of inflammation are multifunctional and thus have numerous effects on blood vessels, inflammatory cells, and other cells in the body. The most important effects relevant to an understanding of inflammation are vasodilation or vasoconstriction, altered vascular permeability, activation of inflammatory cells, chemotaxis, cytotoxicity, degradation of tissue, pain, and fever.

HISTAMINE

Early in inflammation, the vessels become leaky because of the action of biogenic amines, such as histamine, and inflammatory proteins, such as bradykinin. Histamine that is released from platelets and mast cells provokes a contraction of the endothelial cells of venules. This leads to formation of gaps, which increase blood vessel permeability and allow fluids and blood cells to exit into the interstitial spaces. This effect occurs quickly but lasts less than half an hour because histamine is rapidly inactivated by *histaminase*. It is therefore called an *immediate transient reaction.*

BRADYKININ

Bradykinin, a plasma protein formed through the action of the enzyme kallikrein on its precursor kininogen, has effects similar to those of histamine, but these become evident at a slower pace (in Greek, *bradys* means "slow" and *kinein* means "acting"). Bradykinin is formed in the plasma through the activation of **Hageman factor,** also known as *coagulation factor XII.* Hageman factor serves at the same time as an activator of intravascular coagulation and *plasminogen.* The latter acts as a thrombolytic factor and also activates the complement system (Figure 2-5). Apparently, this important initiator of inflammation leads to activation of several biologic systems in the circulating blood, all of which may act on the wall of blood vessels and on the inflammatory cells to amplify and sustain the response to injury. Finally, bradykinin is capable of inciting pain

and is one of the mediators of inflammation that account for *dolor,* the fourth cardinal sign of inflammation.

COMPLEMENT SYSTEM

Another important source of mediators of inflammation is the complement system, consisting of several proteins that are activated in a cascade, acting one on another. These complement proteins are numbered from 1 to 9 (e.g., C1, C5, C9). Activation of the complement cascade can occur through three pathways:

- The *classical* pathway is typically activated by antigen-antibody complexes formed in immune reactions. It is called classical because it was first discovered during the study of classical immune reactions. However, today we know that other stimuli can also initiate it. For example, proteolytic enzymes released from leukocytes or uric acid deposited in the tissue during an attack of gout also can activate complement through this pathway.
- The *alternative pathway,* called "som" because it has nothing to do with the immune reactions, is activated by bacterial endotoxins, fungi, snake venom, and some other substances.
- The *lectin pathway* is activated by the binding of plasma mannose–binding lectin to carbohydrates on bacteria.

All three pathways converge toward a common terminal pathway (Figure 2-6), which finally leads to the formation of

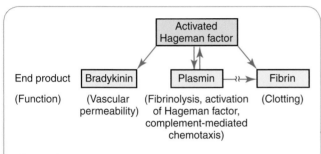

Figure 2-5 Activation of Hageman factor leads to synthesis of bradykinin, plasmin, and fibrin, resulting in increased vascular permeability, thrombolysis, complement activation, and clotting, respectively.

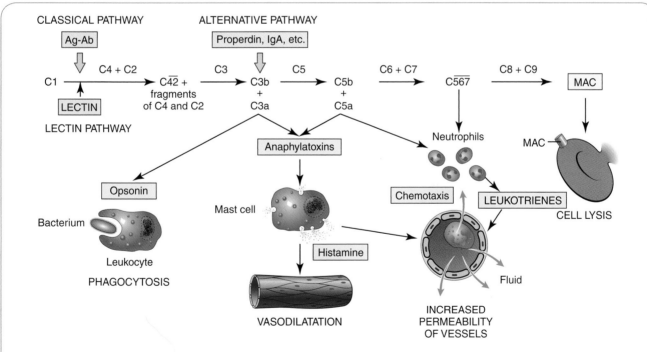

Figure 2-6 Complement activation. Activation of the classical (antigen [Ag] and antibody [Ab] mediated), alternative, or lectin pathways leads to a common terminal pathway from C5 to C9. These complement components form the final membrane attack complex (MAC). Other intermediate complexes and fragments are also biologically active: opsonins facilitate phagocytosis; anaphylatoxins act on mast cells and mediate a release of histamine, which acts on blood vessels; and chemotactic fragments and intermediate complexes attract leukocytes to the site of inflammation. Activated neutrophils secrete other mediators, such as leukotrienes, which amplify the inflammatory response.

the **membrane attack complex (MAC).** The MAC is enzymatically active and is able to destroy cells by literally boring holes in membranes. For example, in hemolytic anemia, the MAC perforates the cell membrane of red blood cells and causes their lysis. Other biologically active complexes are formed along the common terminal pathway of the complement cascade. Furthermore, the activated complement components are cleaved into fragments (e.g., labeled C3a or C5b), which are also biologically active. Intermediate complement complexes and fragments act on leukocytes and endothelial cells directly or by activating other mediators of inflammation (e.g., C3b binds to the surface of bacteria, whereupon it acts as **opsonin,** facilitating phagocytosis). Some complement fragments are considered **anaphylatoxins** because they mediate the release of histamine from mast cells, thus causing vasodilation and increased vascular permeability. Complement fragments promote *chemotaxis* of neutrophils and also activate these cells. Activating neutrophils produces leukotrienes from arachidonic acid, thus contributing to the propagation of inflammation. These main aspects of complement activation are illustrated in Figure 2-6.

ARACHIDONIC ACID DERIVATIVES

Arachidonic acid metabolites represent an important group of mediators of inflammation. Arachidonic acid is derived from the phospholipids of cell membranes through the action of phospholipase. Once formed, it is further metabolized through one of two possible metabolic pathways (Figure 2-7).

The lipoxygenase *pathway* leads to the formation of leukotrienes and lipoxins. *Leukotrienes* promote chemotaxis and increase vascular permeability, as typically found in *anaphylactic shock.* They also cause bronchospasm in asthma by contracting the smooth muscles in the bronchi. Lipoxins inhibit chemotaxis of leukocytes and apparently serve as negative regulators of leukotriene-mediated reactions.

The **cyclooxygenase** pathway leads to formation of the prostaglandins (including *prostacyclin*), which causes vasodilation and formation of thromboxane. **Prostaglandins** stimulate vasodilation and increased vascular permeability and also mediate pain and fever. Thromboxane promotes platelet aggregation, thrombosis, and vasoconstriction, whereas **prostacyclin** counteracts these effects.

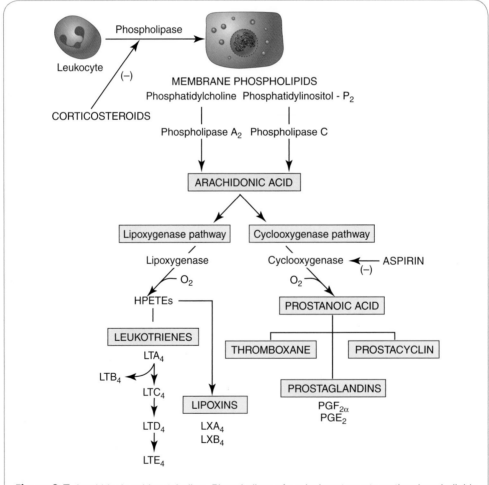

Figure 2-7 Arachidonic acid metabolism. Phospholipase from leukocytes acts on the phospholipids in cell membranes, forming the arachidonic acid pool. The cyclooxygenase and lipoxygenase pathway metabolites actively mediate all aspects of inflammation. HPETEs, hydroperoxyeicosatetraenoic acid compounds.

The synthesis of arachidonic acid and its derivatives can be inhibited by several drugs. For example, corticosteroid hormones have an inhibitory effect on *phospholipase,* which is involved in generating arachidonic acid from cell membrane phospholipids. Cyclooxygenase can be inhibited by aspirin, a drug known to have anti-inflammatory and antipyretic effects. Newer selective inhibitors of cyclooxygenase and lipoxygenase have been synthesized and are used for the treatment of chronic inflammatory diseases such as rheumatoid arthritis and asthma.

CELLULAR EVENTS IN INFLAMMATION

EMIGRATION OF LEUKOCYTES

The increased permeability of the vessel walls of postcapillary venules and capillaries lasts from several hours to several days. It is usually accompanied by leakage of fluid from the vessels into the interstitial spaces. This process is called *transudation* and typically accounts for the formation of *edema,* which is rich in protein but contains few cells. Emigration of cells across the vascular wall leads to the formation of exudate. Exudate contains much more protein than transudate and, in addition, contains inflammatory cells. In acute inflammation, most of these cells are **polymorphonuclear leukocytes,** also called *polymorphonuclear neutrophils* (PMNs).

As the inflammation evolves, PMNs are joined by other cells, such as *monocytes* and *eosinophils,* which become apparent in the exudate within the first 48 hours. As the inflammation proceeds into chronic stages, the PMNs, which have a life span of only 2 to 4 days, become less prominent and are replaced by macrophages, lymphocytes, and **plasma cells.**

The emigration of PMNs through the vessel wall is an active process that occurs in several phases. These phases include (1) adhesion of PMNs to the endothelial cells, (2) insertion of cytoplasmic pseudopods between the junctions of endothelial cells, (3) passage through the basement membrane, and (4) ameboid movement away from the vessel toward the cause of inflammation (e.g., bacteria) (Figure 2-8).

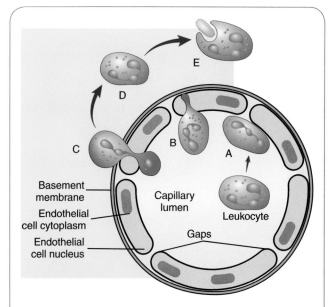

Figure 2-8 The emigration of leukocytes from blood vessels comprises several steps: adhesion *(A),* insertion of pseudopods between the endothelial cells *(B),* passage through the basement membrane *(C),* ameboid movement toward the source of chemotactic stimuli *(D),* and phagocytosis of bacteria that were the source of chemotactic stimuli *(E).*

> **? Did You Know?**
>
> Did the ancient Greeks use aspirin? Aspirin is a drug that was introduced in the nineteenth century. It contains acetylsalicylic acid, which is an inhibitor of cyclooxygenase that has anti-inflammatory properties.
>
> Today, aspirin is used to treat headaches and fever. The ancient Greeks did not have the necessary knowledge to produce acetylsalicylic acid. However, they used the bark of the willow tree, which contains the same chemical, for medicinal purposes. Aspirin could therefore be considered one of the oldest medicinal substances still in use.

Active movement of PMNs along a concentration gradient is called **chemotaxis** (in Greek, *taxis* means "order"). The *chemoattractant* is derived from bacteria or tissues destroyed by inflammation or from activated complement. Chemotactic substances stimulate PMNs to move along a chemical concentration gradient until they reach its source or the site that has the highest concentration. In this respect, the movement of PMNs resembles the attraction that bees have for flowers or that male insects have toward a sexually receptive female that is releasing pheromones.

Red blood cells do not migrate actively like the neutrophils. Nevertheless, if the vascular wall defect is large enough, the red blood cells will be carried through it into the interstitial spaces. This is called *diapedesis* (in Greek, *dia* means "through" and *pedesis* means "passage").

PHAGOCYTOSIS

PMNs that reach the bacteria or other sources of chemotactic substances lose their mobility and begin acting as scavengers. This is accomplished through **phagocytosis** (in Greek, *phagein* means "to eat"), or active uptake of bacteria and other cellular debris.

To illustrate phagocytosis, assume that a PMN encounters a bacterium (Figure 2-9). The bacterium is recognized as a foreign particulate material by the pseudopods extending from the surface of the PMN. This recognition is followed by attachment of the cell membrane of the PMN to the bacterial wall. The attachment can be facilitated by immunoglobulin or complement, which may act like *opsonins* (derived from the Greek word for "catering"). Many leukocytes have receptors for C3 complement and the Fc portion of the immunoglobulin. These receptors mediate the contact of bacteria and leukocytes.

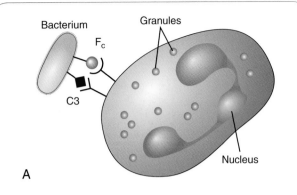

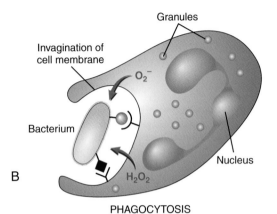

PHAGOCYTOSIS

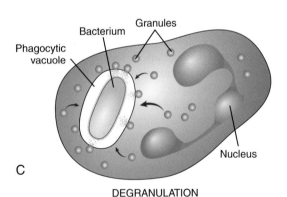

DEGRANULATION

Figure 2-9 Phagocytosis of bacteria. *A,* The bacterium that was opsonized (i.e., coated with IgG and complement [C3]) binds to the F$_c$ and complement receptors on the surface of the leukocytes. *B,* Engulfment of the bacterium into an invagination of surface membrane is associated with an oxygen burst and formation of oxygen radicals that are bactericidal and thus kill the bacterium. *C,* Inclusion of the bacterium into a phagocytic vacuole is associated with the fusion of the vacuole with lysosomes and specific granules of the leukocyte. The contents of the lysosomes and specific granules are bactericidal and contribute to final inactivation and degradation of the bacterium in the heterophagosome. The cytoplasm of the leukocyte is therefore devoid of granules ("degranulation of leukocytes").

Engulfment of the bacterium is a process by which the cytoplasm of the PMN surrounds the foreign particle and encloses it into an invagination of the cell membrane. Inside the nascent vacuole, the bacterium is killed by bactericidal substances released from the cytoplasm of the PMN. The bacterium is internalized into a phagocytic vacuole, which fuses with lysosomes. The content of specific leukocytic granules and lysosomes is discharged into the lumen of this phagocytic vacuole. This degranulation of the PMN is the final step in the fight against bacteria. Lysosomal enzymes also kill bacteria that have survived earlier stages of phagocytosis. These lytic enzymes digest bacteria and dissolve them into harmless elementary components.

Many PMNs die in their fight with bacteria. Dead and dying leukocytes, admixed with tissue debris and lytic enzymes released from their granules, form a viscous yellow fluid known as **pus.** Inflammations dominated by pus formation are called *purulent* or *suppurative.*

CELLS OF INFLAMMATION

PMNs are the primary cells that respond to bacterial infection. Platelets are also present from the earliest stages of inflammation. Other cells are recruited shortly thereafter. These latecomers include eosinophils, **basophils**, macrophages, lymphocytes, and plasma cells (Figure 2-10).

Polymorphonuclear Neutrophils

PMNs are the most numerous white blood cells in the circulating blood, accounting for 60% to 70% of all white blood cells. They are the first cells to appear in acute inflammation. PMNs have a segmented nucleus and a well-developed cytoplasm filled with granules. The term *PMN* is used because the nucleus may have one to five segments—that is, it is polymorphous (variably shaped). Because the granules of PMNs stain with both hematoxylin and eosin, the PMNs are considered neutral. These cells are also known as *neutrophilic granulocytes* or simply *neutrophils.*

The most important features of PMNs include the following:

- *Mobility.* PMNs are highly mobile and are therefore the first cells to reach the site of inflammation in response to chemotactic substances.
- *Phagocytosis.* PMNs are scavenger cells capable of ingesting bacteria and other cellular debris.
- *Bactericidal activity.* Granules in the cytoplasm of PMNs contain substances that kill bacteria. Toxic oxygen radicals generated during the activation of PMNs are also bactericidal.
- *Cytokine production.* PMNs secrete and release various mediators of inflammation. These biologically active substances promote inflammation, recruit new leukocytes, and also cause systemic symptoms. For example, the release of interleukin-1 (IL-1) from PMNs serves as an endogenous *pyrogen,* which acts on the hypothalamic thermoregulatory centers and causes fever.

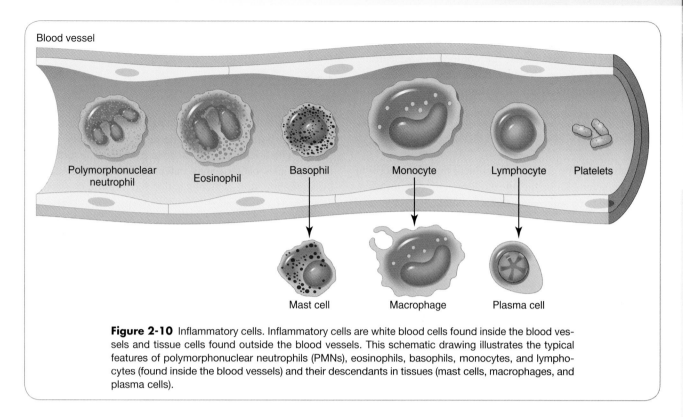

Figure 2-10 Inflammatory cells. Inflammatory cells are white blood cells found inside the blood vessels and tissue cells found outside the blood vessels. This schematic drawing illustrates the typical features of polymorphonuclear neutrophils (PMNs), eosinophils, basophils, monocytes, and lymphocytes (found inside the blood vessels) and their descendants in tissues (mast cells, macrophages, and plasma cells).

Eosinophils

Eosinophils, or eosinophilic leukocytes, account for 2% to 3% of circulating white blood cells. In the zone of inflammation, eosinophils appear 2 to 3 days after the PMNs. This is in part because of their slower mobility and their comparatively slower reaction to chemotactic stimuli.

The term *eosinophils* is derived from their cytoplasmic granules, which stain pink with eosin. Like PMNs, they are mobile, phagocytic, and bactericidal. In contrast to a PMN, however, an eosinophil has a single nucleus, which is usually divided into two lobes located at opposite sides of the cytoplasm.

Eosinophils interact with basophils and are prominent in allergic reactions, such as hay fever and asthma. They also participate in the inflammatory response to parasitic infections. Eosinophils live longer than PMNs and therefore may be seen in chronic inflammations.

Basophils

Basophils account for less than 1% of circulating white blood cells. Nevertheless, these cells are important participants in inflammatory reactions and are most prominent in allergic reactions mediated by immunoglobulin E (IgE). Basophils have a bean-shaped single nucleus and are somewhat larger than PMNs. Their cytoplasm contains granules rich in vasoactive substances, such as histamine. Basophils are precursors of **mast cells,** which have similar functions and are best considered as tissue basophils.

Macrophages

Macrophages are tissue mononuclear cells (histiocytes) derived from blood monocytes. They have a bean-shaped nucleus and are larger than PMNs. Macrophages appear at the site of inflammation 3 to 4 days after the onset of infection or tissue destruction. Macrophages are long-lived cells and therefore are typically present in chronic inflammation.

Macrophages, as their name implies, are capable of phagocytosis and are active in bacterial killing, albeit not as efficiently as the PMNs are. Macrophages also secrete mediators of inflammation (cytokines) that act locally on other cells and the body as a whole.

Platelets

Platelets are fragments of cytoplasm released from megakaryocytes in the bone marrow. They do not have a nucleus, and their cytoplasm contains vacuoles and membrane-bound granules. These granules contain various biologically active substances such as histamine; coagulation proteins; cytokines; and growth factors, such as *platelet-derived growth factor* (PDGF).

Platelets release their granules on contact with extracellular matrix, endothelial cells, or thrombin formed in early thrombi. The release of histamine increases vascular permeability in the early stages of inflammation. Other substances released on degranulation promote blood clotting. PDGF promotes the proliferation of connective tissue cells.

Other Cells

Lymphocytes and plasma cells are components of chronic inflammation. However, because these cells have immune functions, they are described in greater detail in Chapter 3.

CLASSIFICATION OF INFLAMMATION

Inflammations can be classified in clinical practice according to four parameters. These include duration, etiology, location, and morphology or pathologic characteristics.

DURATION

Inflammations can be classified according to their duration as acute or chronic. *Acute inflammation* has usually a sudden onset and lasts from a few hours to a few days, like an acute inflammation of the nasal mucosa *(acute rhinitis)* in common cold. Chronic inflammation lasts longer, usually weeks or months to years.

Overall, chronic inflammation may represent (1) extension of an acute inflammation, (2) prolonged healing of an acute inflammation, or (3) persistence of causative agents. Some chronic inflammations evolve without a typical acute phase and represent slow-smoldering processes from their onset. For example, tuberculosis has a gradual onset and lasts a long time. Typically, patients complain of fatigue and have a low-grade fever. Often they cannot pinpoint the exact onset of their symptoms and do not remember any acute phase of their disease.

Chronic inflammations also develop in response to foreign substances. For instance, a foreign body granuloma will develop around thorns in subcutaneous tissue. Likewise, persons exposed to dust containing silica particles develop chronic lung silicosis, which does not have a recognizable acute phase. Autoimmune diseases, such as rheumatoid arthritis, also are characterized by a chronic course, although these diseases tend to have periodic flare-ups (exacerbations).

Middle ear inflammations *(otitis media)* in small children tend to recur and are a common health problem. Usually it is impossible to decide whether such a *recurrent* otitis media is a flare-up of a persistent infection or a new infection *(reinfection).*

ETIOLOGY

Inflammations are caused by infectious pathogens or by chemical, physical, and immune factors. Infections are classified as bacterial, viral, protozoal, fungal, or helminthic. *Chemical causes* can be classified as organic or inorganic, industrial or medicinal, and exogenous or endogenous. *Physical causes* of inflammation, which act on the tissue by transmitting upon them measurable energy, include heat, irradiation, and trauma. Foreign bodies also may cause inflammation, which is typically seen around a thorn wedged into the skin or in the subcutaneous tissue around surgical sutures. The *immune causes* of inflammation are discussed in Chapter 3.

LOCATION

Inflammation may be *localized* or *widespread (systemic).* For example, a boil or **furuncle** is a localized skin infection. Disseminated boils, a condition termed *furunculosis,* occur in people with a reduced resistance to bacterial infections. From the furuncles bacteria may enter the bloodstream and cause systemic infection, which is called **bacteremia** or **sepsis.**

> **? Did You Know?**
>
> The Bible mentions Job as a pious man whose body was covered with boils by Satan. In reference to this Biblical story, physicians have named a hereditary susceptibility to bacterial infections "Job's syndrome." Children affected by this disease typically have numerous skin furuncles, which are often complicated by pneumonia and infections of other internal organs. Scientists have isolated the gene that accounts for the defective defense against bacterial infections in this syndrome.

PATHOLOGY OF INFLAMMATION

Several forms of inflammation can be recognized on gross examination of the affected tissues. These changes are readily seen in clinical practice. Physical examination of the patient may reveal typical signs of inflammation on the skin, eyes, oral mucosa, or genital organs. During surgery, it is possible to see the inflamed internal organs. These organs can also be visualized without surgery by using a fiberoptic instrument, such as a laparoscope, which is used to inspect the abdominal cavity.

The terms for the various forms of inflammation are usually descriptive. Most terms are formed by adding a suffix *-itis* to the Latin or Greek names for various organs. For example, *hepatitis* denotes inflammation of the liver, and *appendicitis* signifies inflammation of the appendix. Additional terms are used for greater precision. For example, *post-transfusion viral hepatitis B* indicates that the disease was acquired by transfusion and that it is caused by hepatitis B virus.

SEROUS INFLAMMATION

Serous inflammation, considered the mildest form of inflammation, is characterized by the *exudation of serum* (i.e., the acellular clear fluid portion of the blood [in Latin, *serum* means "whey"]). Serous inflammation occurs in the early stages of most inflammations. In pneumonia, it can be recognized as a proteinaceous material inside the alveolar space that contains only a few inflammatory cells. As the inflammation progresses, these inflammatory cells proliferate in the fluid. However, if the disease is diagnosed early and the

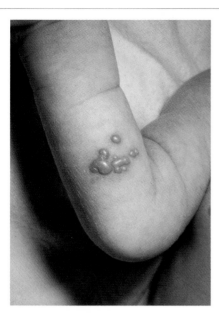

Figure 2-11 Serous inflammation. Herpes infections present with vesicles filled with serous fluid.

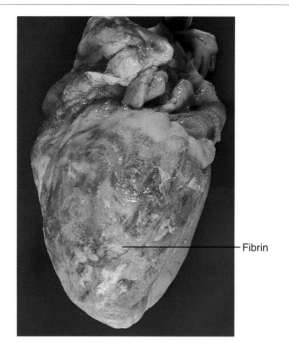

— Fibrin

Figure 2-12 Fibrinous pericarditis. The epicardium is covered with a shaggy layer of fibrin.

causative bacterium is eliminated, serous fluid is restored and the inflammation resolves.

Serous inflammation is typical of many viral infections. The skin vesicles caused by herpes virus are perhaps the best examples of a serous inflammation (Figure 2-11). These vesicles are filled with proteinaceous fluid. Autoimmune diseases affecting serosal surfaces are also serous. Serous pericarditis, pleuritis, or peritonitis is characterized by an accumulation of clear, yellowish fluid in these cavities. Joint swelling secondary to fluid accumulation is typical of rheumatoid arthritis, the most common autoimmune disorder. Blisters of the skin caused by second-degree burns are yet another example of serous inflammation. The serous fluid is readily reabsorbed, and if the cause of the inflammation is eliminated, the lesions heal without any obvious consequences.

FIBRINOUS INFLAMMATION

Fibrinous inflammation is characterized by an exudate that is rich in fibrin. Fibrin is formed from long strands of polymerized fibrinogen, which is one of the largest plasma proteins. In contrast to serous exudate, which contains predominantly albumin and immunoglobulins that have leaked from intact but permeable blood vessels or through small vascular defects, extravasation of fibrin occurs only through larger defects. Fibrinous exudate is therefore indicative of relatively severe inflammation.

Fibrinous inflammation is seen in many bacterial infections, such as "strep throat" or bacterial pneumonia. In bacterial pericarditis, the surface of the heart is covered with shaggy, yellowish layers of fibrin (Figure 2-12).

Fibrinous exudate does not resolve as easily as does serous exudate. Macrophages that invade the exudate have

the capacity to lyse fibrin and thrombi. Blood vessels grow into the exudate, probably to provide a route for scavenger cells and the removal of the debris. These blood vessels fill the space occupied by fibrin and further obliterate it, a process termed *organization* of the exudate. Macrophages in the exudate also stimulate the ingrowth of fibroblasts, contributing further to formation of fibrous tissue obliterating the tissue spaces (e.g., organizing pneumonia).

PURULENT INFLAMMATION

Purulent inflammation is typically caused by pus-forming bacteria, such as streptococci and staphylococci. Pus is viscous yellow fluid composed of dead and dying PMNs and necrotic tissue debris. It is rich in lytic enzymes released from leukocytes, destroyed cells, and bacteria. Purulent exudate that is also rich in fibrin is said to be fibrinopurulent.

Pus may accumulate on the mucosa or skin or in internal organs (Figure 2-13). A localized collection of pus within an organ or tissue is called an **abscess** (Figure 2-14). The central portion of an abscess is liquid or is composed of pus. In chronic abscesses, the wall of the cavity is composed of a capsule, which consists of fibrotic granulation tissue. Abscesses do not heal spontaneously and must be evacuated surgically.

Large abscesses tend to rupture, forming a *sinus* or *fistula* (Figure 2-15). A **sinus** is a cavity, usually occupied previously by an abscess, that drains through a tract to the surface of the body. A **fistula** (Latin, meaning "tube") is a similar channel formed between two preexisting cavities or hollow organs or between a hollow organ or preexisting cavity and the surface

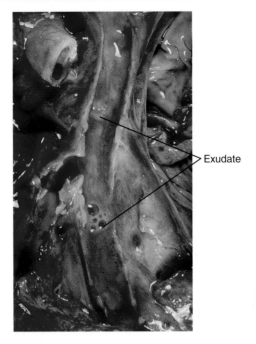

Figure 2-13 Purulent tracheobronchitis. The trachea is filled with pus, which appears as a turbid yellow exudate.

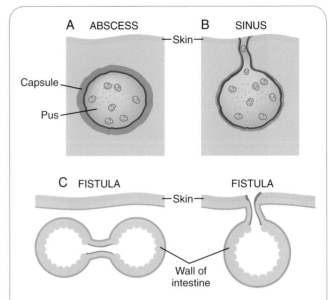

Figure 2-15 Diagram of an abscess, sinus, and fistula. *A,* An abscess is a localized, purulent inflammation. Older abscesses are surrounded by a capsule that consists of granulation tissue. *B,* A sinus forms a tract connecting the abscess with the skin. This allows the drainage of pus outside the body. *C,* A fistula is an inflammatory tract that connects either two hollow organs or a hollow organ with the skin.

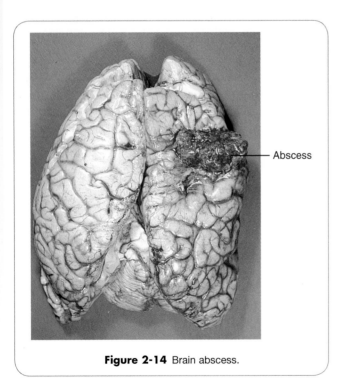

Figure 2-14 Brain abscess.

of the body. A fistula may be formed, for example, between two loops of intestine that have been fused together by inflammation, as we will see in the discussion of Crohn's disease in Chapter 10. Inflammatory cells create a hole in the intestinal wall, allowing the passage of pus and intestinal contents from one loop to another.

Accumulation of pus in a preformed cavity is called **empyema.** For example, empyema of the gallbladder occurs when drainage of pus from the gallbladder is obstructed by an impacted gallstone. Thoracic empyema denotes an accumulation of pus in the pleural cavity.

ULCERATIVE INFLAMMATION

Inflammation of body surfaces or the mucosa of hollow organs, such as the stomach or intestines, may result in **ulceration,** or a loss of epithelial lining. An *ulcer* is defined as a defect involving the epithelium, but it may extend into the deeper connective tissues as well. A peptic ulcer typically occurs in the stomach or duodenum (Figure 2-16).

PSEUDOMEMBRANOUS INFLAMMATION

Pseudomembranous inflammation is a particular form of ulcerative inflammation that is combined with fibrinopurulent exudation. The exudate of fibrin, pus, cellular debris, and mucus forms a pseudomembrane on the surface of the ulcers (Figure 2-17). For example, *Clostridium difficile* causes pseudomembranous colitis. This bacterial overgrowth, which is secondary to intake of broad-spectrum antibiotics, may affect the entire large intestine. These pseudomembranes can be scraped away to expose ulcerated defects that bleed profusely. Pseudomembranes can also form in the throat in diphtheria, a previously lethal childhood infection that has been almost completely eradicated in the Western world by specific immunization.

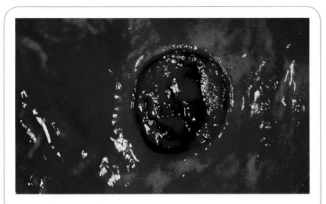

Figure 2-16 Peptic ulcer. An ulcer represents a defect of the epithelial lining.

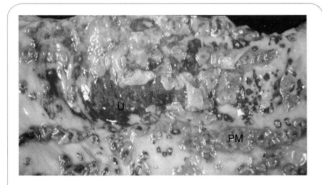

Figure 2-17 Pseudomembranous inflammation. The mucosa of the large intestine is partially ulcerated and red (U), but in other parts it is covered with greenish-yellow material corresponding to the pseudomembranes (PM).

CHRONIC INFLAMMATION

Chronic inflammation is best defined by its duration—it lasts a long time. Because of its prolonged duration, such an inflammation produces more extensive tissue destruction, heals less readily, and is associated with more serious functional deficiencies than an acute inflammation.

Chronic infections are marked by an exudate that on histologic examination is found to contain lymphocytes, macrophages, and plasma cells. The secretory products of chronic inflammatory cells stimulate proliferation of fibroblasts and also perpetuate the inflammation by constantly recruiting new inflammatory cells. Thus loss of parenchymal cells is accompanied by scarring (i.e., the replacement of normal cells with fibroblasts and collagen), which may distort the organs involved. For example, fallopian tubes affected by chronic pelvic inflammatory disease (PID) are twisted and obliterated. Kidneys affected by chronic disease are small and shrunken and do not function properly, accounting for the clinical symptoms of uremia, also known as end-stage kidney disease.

The functional consequences of chronic inflammation cause many clinical symptoms. For example, the **fibrosis** (hardening of tissue) associated with chronic lung disease causes thickening of the alveolar walls, which impairs the passage of oxygen from the air into the blood and causes *dyspnea* (shortness of breath). Constrictive pericarditis prevents dilation of the heart during diastole and adversely affects the pumping function of the heart. Chronic myocarditis with scarring may prevent the normal transmission of electrical signals from the atrioventricular node to the myocardium and may cause cardiac block. Loss of pancreatic parenchyma causes severe digestive problems because of the resultant deficiency of pancreatic enzymes.

> **? Did You Know?**
>
> Pelvic inflammatory disease (PID) is the most common cause of infertility in women. Inflammation of the fallopian tubes interferes with fertilization, which normally takes place there. The passage of ova from the ovary into the uterus is also impeded. However, because the function of the ovary is preserved, gynecologists can harvest ova directly from the ovary, fertilize them *in vitro,* and implant them into the uterus.

GRANULOMATOUS INFLAMMATION

A **granuloma** is a special form of chronic inflammation that typically is not preceded by an acute, PMN-mediated inflammation. It may be caused by antigens that evoke a cell-mediated hypersensitivity reaction or by antigens that persist at the site of inflammation. Granulomas are typically formed in tuberculosis but are also found in tissues infected with fungi, such as *Histoplasma capsulatum, Blastomyces dermatitidis,* and others. Granulomas found in advanced stages of syphilis are known as *gummas.*

Granulomatous reactions are formed of macrophages and T lymphocytes. These cells accumulate at the site of injury, aggregating into nodules. Under the influence of cytokines secreted by lymphocytes, the macrophages transform into so-called epithelioid cells. Epithelioid cells may fuse and thus form **multinucleated giant cells** (Figure 2-18).

The granulomas of tuberculosis and other infectious granulomas are often associated with central caseous necrosis. In contrast, the immunologically mediated granulomas of *sarcoidosis,* a disease of unknown origin, do not show central caseating necrosis (and are thus termed *noncaseating granulomas*).

Granulomas destroy tissue and tend to persist for a long time. In the lungs, confluent necrotizing granulomas may cause cavities, erode blood vessels, and ultimately destroy the entire lung. Bleeding from eroded blood vessels into the cavities is a well-known complication of pulmonary tuberculosis. Fibrosis induced by chronic inflammation may destroy the organ and completely incapacitate the patient.

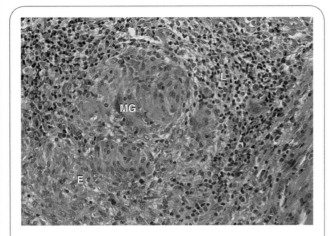

Figure 2-18 Granulomatous reaction. The lesion is composed of epithelioid cells (E), lymphocytes (L), and multinucleated giant cells (MG).

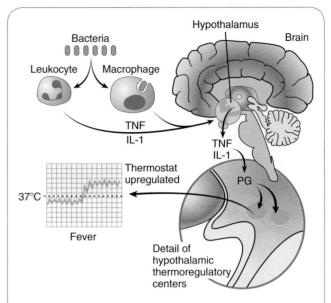

Figure 2-19 Pathogenesis of fever. Interleukin-1 (IL-1) and tumor necrosis factor (TNF) are endogenous pyrogens released from leukocytes or macrophages during inflammation. The action of IL-1 and TNF on the thermoregulatory centers in the hypothalamus is mediated by prostaglandins (PGs). This can be inhibited by aspirin, which blocks prostaglandin synthesis by inhibiting cyclooxygenase.

CLINICOPATHOLOGIC CORRELATIONS

The classical symptoms of inflammation are still the most important local findings and most useful indicators in the diagnosis of inflammation. For example, acute inflammation of the nail fold *(paronychia)* presents with redness *(rubor)*, swelling *(tumor)*, warmth *(calor)*, and pain *(dolor)*. Movement may also be limited by pain *(functio laesa)*.

Similar symptoms could characterize an acute attack of appendicitis, but this organ is hidden from sight, so all the symptoms cannot immediately be recognized. The swollen hyperemic appendix may produce pain, or the pain may be elicited by the physician palpating the abdominal wall in the right lower quadrant. Clearly, one cannot see the appendix through the skin; thus the other signs of inflammation do not become evident until the surgeon intervenes and removes the affected organ. At the time of the operation, the appendix is typically swollen, red, and warm.

Localized inflammations like appendicitis typically produce two important clinical findings: fever and leukocytosis. **Fever**—an elevation in body temperature that exceeds 37°C—is a typical response to acute inflammation caused by *endogenous pyrogens*. These substances—primarily IL-1 and TNF—act on the thermoregulator centers in the hypothalamus, which serves as a thermostat (Figure 2-19). If the threshold of the thermostat (like the heating sensor in a house) is raised, the temperature of the body rises.

Fever is mediated by prostaglandins that are released by pyrogens in the hypothalamic center. Prostaglandin synthesis can be inhibited by antipyretic drugs, such as aspirin. However, in most cases the fever will abate on its own as soon as the inflammation is eradicated.

Leukocytosis, an increase in the number of leukocytes in the blood, is another important sign of inflammation. Normal blood has 4,500 to 11,000 white blood cells per μL. Mediators of inflammation act on the bone marrow and stimulate a rapid release of leukocytes, resulting in leukocytosis (i.e., leukocytes in the blood exceed 11,000 per μL). Leukocytosis is usually transient except in certain forms of chronic inflammation, when it may be prolonged. Such chronic leukocytosis is associated with overstimulation of the bone marrow by leukocytic growth factors.

Other symptoms of inflammation are mostly nonspecific and are called *constitutional.* These include fatigue, weakness, depression, lack of appetite, generalized pain, and exhaustion. The pathogenesis of these symptoms is not understood but could be related to the action of mediators of inflammation, such as IL-1 or TNF. These cytokines and others, known as *acute phase reactants,* act adversely on various cells and also stimulate the metabolism in general. This hypermetabolism may then cause fatigue and exhaustion.

HEALING AND REPAIR

Acute inflammation may heal without any consequences, or it may progress to chronic inflammation. Mild inflammation usually resolves spontaneously after the inciting stimuli have disappeared and the mediators of inflammation are no longer being secreted. However, if the inflammation was accompanied by considerable destruction of tissue, complete healing may be postponed or never accomplished.

Tissue loss has different consequences in different organs, depending primarily on the nature of the cells forming those tissues. In general, cells can be classified into three groups according to their capacity to proliferate (Figure 2-20):

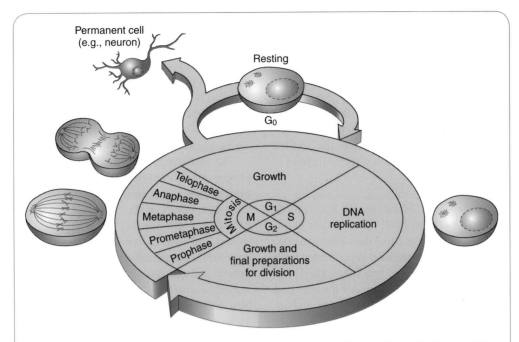

Figure 2-20 Three cell types in relation to the mitotic cell cycle. Mitotic cells may be in any of the four phases of the normal mitotic cycle. Facultative mitotic cells are arrested in the G_0 phase but can enter the cycle if necessary. Postmitotic cells have left the mitotic cycle and cannot reenter it. Mitosis, marked in red, is a relatively short phase of the mitotic cycle. Following mitosis, the mitotic cells enter the G_1 (gap) phase, which is of variable duration. The facultative mitotic cells enter a G_0 phase, during which they perform various specialized functions. The G_1 phase is followed by the DNA synthetic phase (S) and a second gap (G_2).

1. *Continuously dividing* or *mitotic cells* (also known as *labile cells*) are cells that divide throughout the entire life span. Such cells are typically known as *stem cells* and are found in the basal layer of the skin or in the mucosa of internal organs. These cells divide at a regular rate and give rise to more differentiated cells. Their descendants replace the superficial epithelial cells that have been shed after having reached the end of their predetermined life span.
2. *Quiescent, facultative mitotic cells* (also known as *stable cells*) do not divide regularly but can be stimulated to divide if necessary. Such cells form the parenchymal organs (e.g., the liver or kidney). Loss of liver parenchyma following partial hepatectomy stimulates the remaining liver cells to enter **mitosis** and, by dividing, to replace the loss. Once the liver has regenerated, the cells become quiescent again and do not proliferate.
3. *Nondividing, postmitotic cells,* also known as *permanent cells,* do not have the capacity to proliferate under any circumstances. This category includes neurons and myocardial cells. Loss of postmitotic myocardial cells cannot be compensated; instead, the defect is repaired by fibrous scarring. Loss of brain cells is also irreversible.

Thus it is clear that continuously dividing cells can easily repair a defect in the epithelial covering. Likewise, skin **wounds** or *mucosal ulcers* heal readily under appropriate conditions as the superficial layers are replenished from the descendants of cycling stem cells in the basal layer or the

intestinal crypts. Loss of liver or kidney tubular cells may be replenished by regeneration to complete the healing. However, necrosis of heart muscle or brain cells leads to permanent defects that cannot be remedied by the proliferation of equivalent, highly specialized cells.

WOUND HEALING

Wound healing is an important event that takes place at many anatomic sites. It is perhaps best illustrated by the sequence of events following skin incision. Similar changes occur during the healing of internal wounds, at the site of internal surgical incisions, or following surgical removal of organs or tumors. Even a small tissue defect caused by an endoscopic biopsy will be repaired by passing through the typical stages of wound healing.

CELLS PARTICIPATING IN HEALING

The most important cells that are involved in wound healing are leukocytes, macrophages, various connective tissue cells, and epithelial cells. PMNs play a brief role in scavenging the initial site of injury. *Macrophages* are much more important. These cells stay long at the site of healing and produce many cytokines, growth factors, and mediators that act on other connective tissue cells, most notably myofibroblasts, angioblasts, and fibroblasts.

Myofibroblasts

Myofibroblasts, as their name implies, have hybrid properties of smooth muscle cells and fibroblasts. This enables them to contract like muscle cells and secrete matrix substances like fibroblasts. The contraction of myofibroblasts that occurs within the first few days of healing reduces the defect and holds the margins of tissue in close approximation. This enables the proliferating epithelial cells to cover the surface defect and to restore the integrity of the surface epithelium.

Angioblasts

Angioblasts are the precursors of blood vessels. They proliferate like sprouts from the several small blood vessels at the margins of the wound. These appear 2 to 3 days after incision, and by the fifth or sixth day the entire field is permeated with newly formed blood vessels that serve two functions: (1) to provide a route for the scavenger cells to remove the scab and tissue debris and (2) to allow the influx of blood and its accompanying oxygen and nutrients.

Fibroblasts

Fibroblasts are the cells that produce most of the extracellular matrix. Of the numerous matrix components, the most important are fibronectin and collagen. **Fibronectin** has numerous functions in wound healing, the most important of which are the formation of scaffold, the provision of tensile strength, and the ability to "glue" other substances and cells together. **Collagens** form fibrils in the interstitial spaces. More than 20 different collagens have been isolated and characterized thus far, and it is likely that several others will be identified in the near future. Initially, fibroblasts synthesize predominantly type III collagen, which is typical of "young" or "immature" connective tissue temporarily formed in the wound. Later, type III collagen is replaced by type I collagen, which is the most common form of collagen in the body, providing tensile strength for all tissues.

The secretion of collagen is rather complex and requires several essential elements, such as zinc and copper, and vitamin C (ascorbic acid). Furthermore, collagen does not acquire its full strength until it is laid down in the extracellular spaces. This occurs several weeks after injury, when the collagen fibers are cross-linked with each other to form a dense meshwork.

> ### ❓ Did You Know?
>
> Vitamin C is called ascorbic acid, which in Latin means that it prevents scurvy. Today we all know that scurvy is a consequence of vitamin C deficiency. However, it took many years until this fact became so well known. It all began some 250 years ago when the Scottish captain James Lind forced his sailors to take a spoonful of citrus juice during long sea voyages. Thereafter he wrote a book on how lemon can prevent scurvy. Before Lind's discovery, scurvy was a deadly disease that claimed the lives of millions of sailors on transoceanic trips. Today vitamin C is added routinely to many commercial foods; it not only prevents scurvy but also helps wound healing.

CLINICAL WOUND HEALING

Healing of sterile surgical wounds occurs by *first intention* (Figure 2-21). The incision site initially contains coagulated blood that forms a scab. The scab is invaded by PMNs, whose function is to scavenge debris. These are replaced 2 to 4 days later by macrophages. The cytokines and growth factors secreted by macrophages promote the ingrowth of myofibroblasts, angioblasts, and fibroblasts.

The vascularized connective tissue that is rich in macrophages, myofibroblasts, angioblasts, and fibroblasts is called **granulation tissue** (Figure 2-22). Granulation tissue represents a temporary, makeshift structure that changes over time. Initially it contains many myofibroblasts, which contract the wound and then disappear. Macrophages also become less prominent, and the blood vessels that are initially prominent slowly collapse. As a result, if everything goes well, the wound becomes less inflamed and, by the second week, starts blanching. The interstitial spaces that were initially filled with extravasated blood become edematous and finally are filled with matrix. With time, the composition of this matrix changes from fibronectin and fibrin to type III collagen and, finally, to predominantly type I collagen. This final collagenous structure is called a **scar.**

Changes in the dermis are accompanied by a proliferation of epithelial cells from the margins of the wound. These cells cover the defect within 3 to 7 days. Under ideal

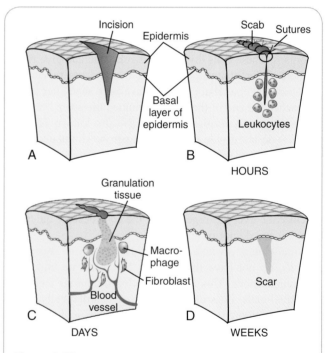

Figure 2-21 Wound healing by first intention. The sequence of events includes formation of a scab *(A)* and scavenger action of polymorphonuclear leukocytes *(B)*, formation of the granulation tissue *(C)*, and scarring *(D)*.

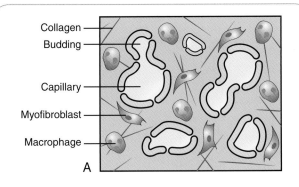

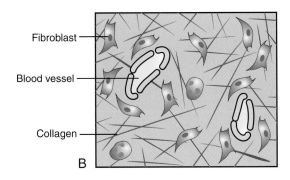

Figure 2-22 Diagram of the histologic appearance of granulation tissue. *A,* In the early stages it contains numerous macrophages, myofibroblasts, and blood vessels. *B,* In the late stages the granulation tissue is less vascular. Moreover, it contains more matrix and fibroblasts and only scattered macrophages.

2. *Mechanical factors.* Wounds heal faster if the margins can be juxtaposed neatly by a surgeon and the field can be kept immobile. Tension at the wound margins, if the skin had to be stretched to cover the gap, will impede healing. Movement may slow healing, which is why patients often remain confined to bed for some time after an operation. Foreign particles in the wound also retard healing.

3. *Size of the wound.* Small wounds heal faster than large ones.

4. *Presence or absence of infection.* Sterile wounds heal faster than those that are infected. Unfortunately, infections are sometimes inevitable. Indeed, wound infections develop in approximately 5% of hospitalized patients postoperatively. Antibiotic treatment is therefore important for all patients with wounds, especially when the surgeon operates in an infected field.

5. *Circulatory status.* Wounds involving ischemic tissues heal poorly. Diabetes mellitus, a disease marked by chronic ischemia secondary to small blood vessel disease *(diabetic microangiopathy),* is typically associated with poor wound healing.

6. *Nutritional and metabolic factors.* General well-being promotes wound healing. Proteins are essential for wound healing; thus malnutrition delays wound healing, as does vitamin C deficiency. Metabolic disturbances, such as those caused by diabetes mellitus, also cause delayed wound healing. An excess of endogenous corticosteroids, caused by endocrine oversecretion or exogenous intake for medicinal purposes, adversely affects scar formation.

7. *Age.* Wounds heal faster in children than in elderly patients.

COMPLICATIONS OF WOUND HEALING

Wound healing may be less than optimal as a result of the factors just discussed. In general, these complications may lead to the following:

- *Deficient scar formation.* Sluggish formation of granulation tissue occurs in diabetic patients, partly as a result of the ischemia caused by diabetic microangiopathy and partly as a consequence of the metabolic disturbances of diabetes. Inadequate collagen production has been reported in patients treated with corticosteroid hormones. Scars in such patients may not have sufficient tensile strength, and **wound dehiscence** (separation of tissue margins) may occur.

- *Excess scar formation.* Excessive scarring leads to the formation of **keloids,** hypertrophic scars, which may cause disfigurement of extremities or parts of the body (Figure 2-24). Large scars, especially those caused by skin burns, tend to be irregularly shaped, which can give rise to **contractures** (an exaggeration of wound contraction). Contractures over the joints may impede movement and in some cases may even completely immobilize an extremity.

circumstances, the granulation tissue filling the skin defect in the wound is transformed into a scar within 3 to 6 weeks. The scar is then remodeled, and most of the disorderly formed collagen is replaced with collagen that is indistinguishable from that in the normal skin.

In contrast to the orderly sequence of events that characterizes the healing of sharp, sterile, surgical wounds by first intention (primary union), large defects and essentially all infected wounds heal by *secondary intention* (Figure 2-23). Large defects cannot readily be bridged, and the surgeon cannot juxtapose the gaping tissue margins. Wound contraction cannot be accomplished by myofibroblasts in such cases, and the granulation tissue remains exposed to the external world. Wound healing by secondary intention is usually prolonged, and some wounds never heal completely.

DELAYED WOUND HEALING

Wound healing may be complicated by local or systemic influences. Overall, the most important determinants of wound healing are as follows:

1. *Site of the wound.* Skin wounds heal well, whereas brain wounds do not heal at all.

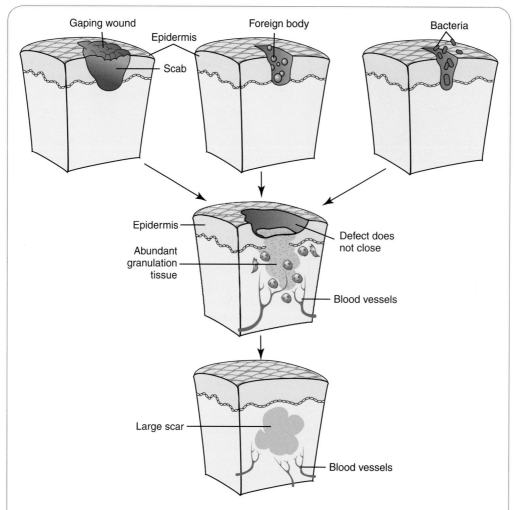

Figure 2-23 Wound healing by secondary intention occurs in wounds that are marked by a large defect of tissue, that contain foreign material, or that are infected. The healing is slower because the epithelial cells proliferating from the wound margin take longer to cover the defect. Granulation tissue is more abundant; consequently, scarring is more prominent.

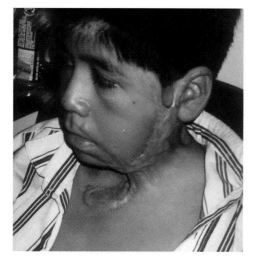

Figure 2-24 Keloid. Healing of a deep burn is characterized by formation of an irregular and hypertrophic scar.

REVIEW QUESTIONS

1. Explain why inflammation cannot occur in an ameba or in a dead body.

2. Does inflammation have beneficial or noxious effects on the human body?

3. What are the cardinal signs of inflammation?

4. Explain the sequence of events that leads to active hyperemia in inflamed tissues.

5. What happens to the leukocytes inside the blood vessels in inflamed tissue?

6. Why does the permeability of blood vessels increase during acute inflammation?

7. Describe the consequences of activation of Hageman factor in acute inflammation.

8. Why are some complement fragments called opsonins, anaphylatoxins, or chemotactic factors?

9. How is membrane attack complex (MAC) formed, and how does it damage red blood cells?

10. Explain the formation of leukotrienes and prostaglandins in acute inflammation.

11. How does a transudate differ from an exudate?

12. How do polymorphonuclear neutrophils emigrate from blood vessels toward bacteria in the tissue?

13. What are the most important chemotactic substances, and how do they promote inflammation?

14. How do polymorphonuclear neutrophils engulf and kill bacteria?

15. What is pus, and how is it formed?

16. Why are polymorphonuclear neutrophils best suited to combat acute bacterial infection?

17. How do eosinophils differ from polymorphonuclear neutrophils?

18. Which inflammatory reactions are mediated by eosinophils and basophils?

19. What are the main functions of macrophages?

20. How do platelets differ from other white blood cells?

21. Compare acute with chronic inflammation.

22. Compare cellular inflammatory response to a typical viral infection with that occurring in bacterial infection.

23. What are the main causes of inflammation?

24. Give an example of both a localized and a systemic inflammation.

25. Give an example of a serous inflammation and describe the pathologic findings.

26. Give an example of fibrinous inflammation and describe the pathologic findings.

27. Give an example of a purulent inflammation and describe the pathologic findings.

28. Give clinical examples of an abscess, sinus, fistula, and empyema.

29. What is the difference between an ulcerative and pseudomembranous inflammation?

30. Describe tissue changes in chronic inflammation, such as pelvic inflammatory disease.

31. Describe possible chemical symptoms of chronic inflammation involving the lungs, heart, and pancreas.

32. What are the main features of a granulomatous inflammation?

33. Compare caseating and noncaseating granulomas with gummas.

34. Correlate the typical clinical features of acute appendicitis with the pathologic changes found at surgery.

35. What are endogenous pyrogens, and how do they act on the hypothalamus?

36. Explain the differences between continuously dividing, quiescent, and nondividing cells and give examples of each.

37. Which cells participate in wound healing?

38. What is granulation tissue, and how does it evolve during wound healing?

39. Compare wound healing by primary and secondary intention.

40. Explain why various adverse factors delay wound healing.

41. Compare wound dehiscence with keloid formation.

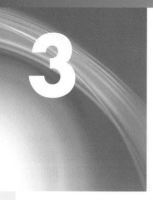

3

Immunopathology

Chapter Outline

Immune Response
Innate Immunity
Acquired Immunity
Cells of the Immune System
Lymphocytes
Plasma Cells
Antibodies
Antibody Production
Major Histocompatibility Complex
Antigen-Antibody Reaction
Hypersensitivity Reactions
Type I Hypersensitivity
Type II Hypersensitivity
Type III Hypersensitivity
Type IV Hypersensitivity

Transplantation
Transplant Rejection
Clinical Use of Transplantation
Graft-versus-Host Reaction
Blood Transfusion
Rh Factor Incompatibility
Autoimmune Diseases
Systemic Lupus Erythematosus
Immunodeficiency Diseases
Primary Immunodeficiency Diseases
Acquired Immunodeficiency Syndrome
Amyloidosis

Key Terms and Concepts

Acquired immunodeficiency
  syndrome (AIDS)
Allografts
Amyloidosis
Anaphylactic shock
Antibodies
Antigen-presenting cells (APCs)
Antigen
Arthus phenomenon
Asthma
Autograft
Autoimmune diseases
B cells
Bone marrow
Contact dermatitis
Cytokines

DiGeorge syndrome
Goodpasture's syndrome
Graft-versus-host (GVH) reaction
Graves' disease
Haptens
Hay fever
Hemolytic anemia
Homografts
Human immunodeficiency viruses
  (HIVs)
Hydrops fetalis
Hypersensitivity reactions
IgA deficiency
Immunity
Immunodeficiency, congenital
Immunoglobulins

Kaposi's sarcoma
Lymph nodes
Lymphocytes
Myasthenia gravis
Natural killer (NK) cells
Opportunistic infections (in AIDS)
Polyarteritis nodosa
Poststreptococcal glomerulonephritis
Rh incompatibility, maternofetal
Serum sickness
Severe combined immunodeficiency
Systemic lupus erythematosus (SLE)
T cells
Thymus
Transplant rejection
Xenografts

Learning Objectives

After reading this chapter, the student should be able to:

1. Define and distinguish between natural immunity and acquired immunity.
2. List the main organs and cells that participate in the immune response.
3. Describe the main differences between subsets of lymphocytes: B cells, T cells, and natural killer (NK) cells.
4. Describe the antigen-presenting cells and discuss their functions.
5. Describe the functions of lymphokines.
6. Describe the basic features of immunoglobulins and their reaction with antigen.
7. Describe the role of major histocompatability complex (MHC) in antigen presentation.
8. List four mechanisms of hypersensitivity reactions.
9. Describe type I hypersensitivity reaction and how it induces hay fever and asthma.
10. Describe type II hypersensitivity reaction and how it induces hemolytic anemia, myasthenia gravis, and Graves' disease.
11. Describe type III hypersensitivity reaction and how it induces glomerulonephritis.
12. Describe the cell-mediated hypersensitivity reaction and how it induces granuloma formation.
13. Describe the main forms of transplants: homograft, isograft, autograft, and xenograft.
14. Discuss the medical uses of transplantation and give three examples.
15. Discuss the principles of blood transfusion.
16. Describe Rh incompatibility between the mother and the fetus.
17. Discuss the pathogenesis of autoimmune diseases.
18. List three congenital immunodeficiency diseases and three acquired immunodeficiency states.
19. Explain the pathogenesis of acquired immunodeficiency syndrome (AIDS) and list its most important complications.
20. List the three forms of amyloid and relate them to clinical presentations of amyloidosis.

Immunity, derived from the Latin term denoting exemption from duty (*munus,* meaning "duty" or "service") was originally defined as resistance to infections. Immune persons would be "exempt from suffering" inflicted by the infectious diseases. Subsequently, it became apparent that immune reactions are not elicited only by bacteria but also by many other substances, as long as they are perceived as foreign by the immune system. Furthermore, we have learned that these reactions occur in many forms and that immunity not only provides protection but also can cause diseases. To appreciate the beneficial and not-so-beneficial consequences of immunity, a review of the basic mechanisms of immunity is provided and then discussed in relation to immunopathology. The secondary immune reactions that accompany most infectious diseases, many systemic diseases, and tumors are not presented here. However, there are few human diseases that do not affect the immune system.

Immunologic techniques are useful in research but are also used daily in clinical laboratories. This applied immunology forms the basis for immunodiagnostics. Finally, immunotherapy should be mentioned because it provides new modalities for the treatment of diseases. Immunopreventive techniques, such as vaccination and active and passive immunization, have contributed enormously to the fight against diseases in humans and animals. It is fair to say that immunization has probably saved more human lives than all other drugs together.

IMMUNE RESPONSE

The immune response has two different forms: a relatively primitive, nonspecific set of innate protective mechanisms and a complex system of cellular and humoral reactions that evolve in response to repeated exposures to foreign substances, known as *acquired immunity.* In this chapter we will mostly deal with the pathology of acquired immunity.

INNATE IMMUNITY

Innate protective mechanisms are inherited and operational at the time of birth. They are relatively nonspecific, and in contrast to acquired immunity these mechanisms rely on antigenic stimulation—that is, they do not depend on previous exposure to foreign substances (Figure 3-1). These innate defense mechanisms include the following:

- Various mechanical barriers (e.g., the epidermis or the ciliated cells in the mucosa of the nose or bronchus)
- Phagocytic cells, such as neutrophils and macrophages
- Natural killer (NK) cells
- Protective proteins found in tissues and plasma, such as complement, properdin, and lysozyme. (*Complement* was discussed in the previous chapter. *Properdin* is a plasma protein that activates the alternative complement pathway, thus generating a set of protective substances. *Lysozyme* is a basic protein of low molecular weight found in tears and in nasal and intestinal secretions. It is

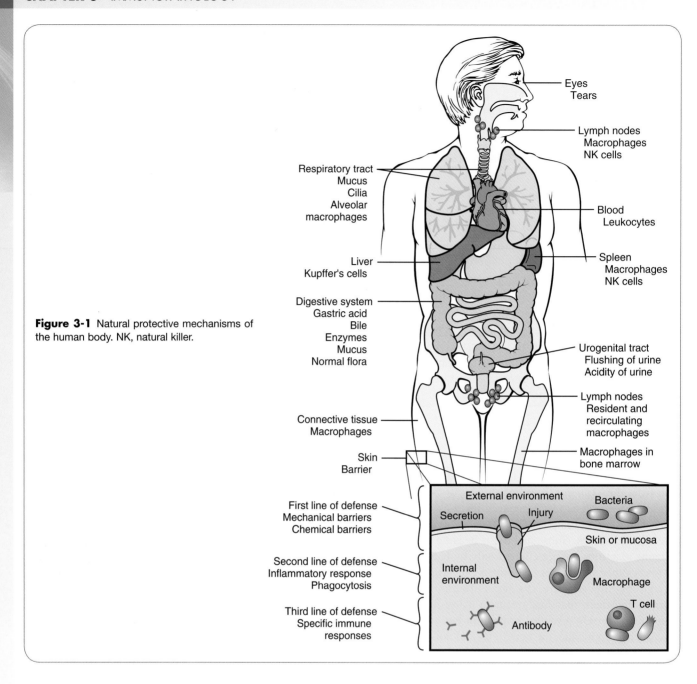

Figure 3-1 Natural protective mechanisms of the human body. NK, natural killer.

Eyes
Tears

Lymph nodes
Macrophages
NK cells

Respiratory tract
Mucus
Cilia
Alveolar
macrophages

Blood
Leukocytes

Liver
Kupffer's cells

Spleen
Macrophages
NK cells

Digestive system
Gastric acid
Bile
Enzymes
Mucus
Normal flora

Urogenital tract
Flushing of urine
Acidity of urine

Lymph nodes
Resident and
recirculating
macrophages

Connective tissue
Macrophages

Macrophages in
bone marrow

Skin
Barrier

First line of defense
Mechanical barriers
Chemical barriers

External environment

Bacteria

Secretion

Injury

Skin or mucosa

Second line of defense
Inflammatory response
Phagocytosis

Internal
environment

Macrophage

Third line of defense
Specific immune
responses

Antibody

T cell

a potent bactericidal agent that nonspecifically kills many bacteria.)

ACQUIRED IMMUNITY

Acquired immunity is based on specific responses elicited by substances that act as antigens. An **antigen** is any chemical substance that can induce a specific immune response—that is, a reaction to production of specific antibodies or specifically sensitized immune cells. Acquired immunity is based on the ability of the body's immune system to distinguish *self* from *non-self,* to generate an immunologic memory, and to mount

an integrated reaction of various cells. As will be shown later, acquired immunity is based on the reaction of the immune system but also involves other cells (auxiliary [helper] cells), such as *macrophages, basophils,* and *eosinophils.*

The body's ability to mount an appropriate immune response is termed *immunocompetence.* Immunocompetence depends on adequate structural and functional development of the immune system and on the coordinated action of its components. A brief description of the organs and cells that constitute the immune system is presented, along with a review of their function. Then various pathologic changes mediated by immune mechanisms are discussed.

CELLS OF THE IMMUNE SYSTEM

All cells of the immune system are descendants of primitive hematopoietic stem cells originally found in the bone marrow (Figure 3-2). The **bone marrow** stem cells give rise to two major cell lineages: lymphoid cells and all other hematopoietic cells. In this context, note that macrophages are descendants of the nonlymphoid premyeloid stem cells in the bone marrow that give rise to other leukocytes. Lymphoid cells are the primary cells of the immune system, whereas the other cells may or may not contribute to

immune reactions and are in this context considered as helper cells.

LYMPHOCYTES

Lymphocytes are small cells, only slightly larger than erythrocytes. They have a round nucleus and very little cytoplasm. All lymphocytes are derived from bone marrow prelymphoid stem cells, which give rise to two distinct cell lineages. Descendants of one lineage migrate to the thymus and mature into T lymphocytes. B lymphocytes, descendants of the other lineage, remain in the bone marrow, from which they colonize

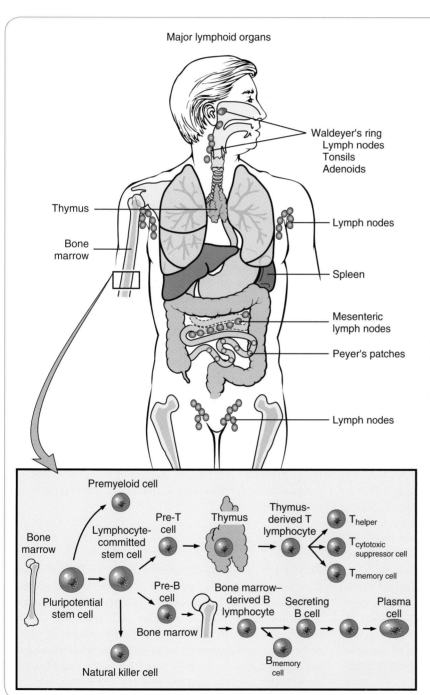

Figure 3-2 Immune system. Lymphocytes, like all other hematopoietic cells, are derived from a common pluripotential bone marrow stem cell. These stem cells give rise to myeloid cell precursor and the stem cell committed to lymphocytic lineages. Three lymphoid cell lineages lead to mature T and B cells (plasma cells) or natural killer cell formation.

the peripheral lymphoid tissues. The *bone marrow* and **thymus** are called *primary lymphoid organs,* and the differentiation of **T cells** and **B cells** in them is developmentally programmed and unrelated to antigenic stimulation. From the primary lymphoid organs, the T and B lymphocytes enter the blood circulation and colonize various *secondary lymphoid organs.* Among these, the most prominent are the **lymph nodes** and spleen, in which lymphocytes constitute a significant percentage of the total cell population. Lymphocytes are also present in other organs and are most prominent in the gastrointestinal and bronchial mucosa, where they form the so-called mucosa-associated lymphoid tissue (MALT). In contrast to encapsulated lymph nodes and spleen, MALT has no capsule, and its cells are an integral part of the mucosa.

T and B lymphocytes have distinct functions, although morphologically they cannot be distinguished by light or electron microscopy. Subtle differences between T and B lymphocytes can be recognized by immunochemical techniques designed to identify unique marker molecules on the surface of these cells. In practice, this can be done by immunocytochemical staining of tissue sections or cell smears with specific, color-coded antibodies. Antibodies to so-called cluster differentiation (CD) antigens have been most useful in this regard. CD antigens are selectively expressed during specific stages of lymphocyte development. Some CD antigens are selectively expressed on T cells, whereas others are selectively expressed on B cells. Several subsets of T and B lymphocytes and their immature precursors can be recognized by using this approach. With use of cell sorters, such as the fluorescence-activated cell sorter (FACS), it is possible to distinguish T from B lymphocytes or to determine their ratio in circulation or in various lymphoid organs. FACS also can be used for separation of subsets of T lymphocytes, which is important for the diagnosis of immunodeficiency diseases, such as **acquired immunodeficiency syndrome (AIDS).**

T Lymphocytes

T lymphocytes are lymphocytes that have matured in the thymus. They account for two-thirds of all lymphocytes in the blood and also are found in the paracortical zone of the lymph nodes and the periarteriolar sheath of the spleen. There are several subsets of T cells, the most important of which are the *T helper* and *T suppressor/cytotoxic* cells. T helper cells actively participate in the immune responses to antigens, helping B cells produce antibodies, which is discussed in the next section. T suppressor/cytotoxic cells suppress unwanted antibody production and mediate killing of virus-infected cells or tumor cells that are recognized by the body as foreign.

Common to all T cells is the surface T-cell receptor (TCR), which is linked to a membrane protein known as *CD3.* T cells use TCR for recognition of antigens. TCR-CD3 complex is thus essential for the activity of T cells. Like all other genes inherited from our parents, the gene for TCR is in all the cells of the body. However, the gene is activated only in T cells. TCR gene activation occurs through rearrangement of parts of the gene. Because TCR rearrangement occurs only in T cells,

it is a unique genetic marker for T lymphocytes. This is important to note because 10% to 15% of peripheral lymphocytes have the same surface markers as T lymphocytes but do not have TCR gene rearrangement. These cells are known as **natural killer (NK) cells.** NK cells mediate innate immune reactions and are not involved in T- and B-cell–mediated immune reactions. Their function is to react against virus-infected cells and to kill tumor and foreign cells without previous sensitization.

T helper cells express CD4 on their surface, whereas the T suppressor/cytotoxic cells express the CD8 antigen on their surface. CD4 and CD8 are used as markers for these lymphocytes and for the counting of T helper and T suppressor/cytotoxic cells in blood. In normal blood, CD4-positive cells predominate, and the cell ratio of CD4 to CD8 is approximately 2:1. In individuals with AIDS, CD4 cells are selectively lost and the cell ratio of CD4:CD8 is less than 1.

CD4-positive helper cells can be activated to secrete **cytokines** (group of proteins). T helper cells can be subdivided into two major groups on the basis of which cytokines they produce: T helper-1 (T_H1) cells that synthesize interleukin-2 (IL-2) and interferon-gamma (IFN-g) and T helper-2 (T_H2) cells that synthesize IL-4, IL-5, and IL-13. T_H1 cells stimulate macrophages to become phagocytic and mediate the formation of granulomas, whereas the cytokines secreted by T_H2 cells are important for secretion of IgE and other immunoglobulins and activation of eosinophils.

B Lymphocytes

B cells are lymphocytes that are primed to differentiate into immunoglobulin-producing plasma cells. This differentiation occurs in a stepwise manner. Each of these intermediate stages is characterized by distinct cell surface and cytoplasmic changes that can be recognized by immunohistochemical methods. However, some features are shared by all B cells and their mature descendants, the plasma cells. The most important shared feature is the activation of the immunoglobulin gene, which occurs only in the B-cell lineage. The immunoglobulin gene is similar to TCR, and its activation also occurs through a rearrangement of parts of the gene. The immunoglobulin gene rearrangement enables B cells to produce immunoglobulins that are incorporated into the B-cell antigen receptor complex on the plasma membrane. Antigen-stimulated B lymphocytes differentiate subsequently into plasma cells.

PLASMA CELLS

Plasma cells are fully differentiated descendants of B lymphocytes. These cells have an oval shape and an eccentrically located round nucleus. The cytoplasm of plasma cells is basophilic because it contains an abundance of ribosomes. On electron microscopy, the cytoplasm of plasma cells contains numerous stacks of rough endoplasmic reticulum (RER) (Figure 3-3). The RER is the site of synthesis of **immunoglobulins,** the primary secretory products of plasma cells.

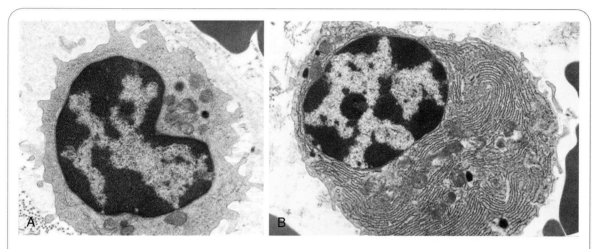

Figure 3-3 Electron microscopic photograph of a lymphocyte and a plasma cell. *A,* The cytoplasm of the lymphocyte is scant and contains few organelles. *B,* The cytoplasm of the plasma cell is well developed and contains prominent rough endoplasmic reticulum (RER). The RER serves as the site for production of immunoglobulins.

ANTIBODIES

Antibodies are proteins of the immunoglobulin class that are secreted by plasma cells. They can be defined operationally as proteins reacting with antigens. Chemically they can be classified into five classes: IgG, IgM, IgA, IgE, and IgD.

These immunoglobulins share some common features:

- All immunoglobulins are composed of light and heavy chains (Figure 3-4). All immunoglobulins have the same light chains, which are either kappa or lambda. A single molecule contains either two kappa or two lambda chains. Heavy chains are immunoglobulin class specific. These are called *gamma, mu, alpha, epsilon,* and *delta* and correspond to IgG, IgM, IgA, IgE, and IgD, respectively. Heavy chains are the primary determinants of the class of each immunoglobulin, their properties, and their function.

- Each chain has a constant and a variable part. The *constant* part extends from the C terminal (so called because it ends with a COO$^-$ [carboxy] group) across the *hinge* region to the *variable* part, which occupies the N terminal (so called because it ends in an NH$_3^+$ [amino] group).

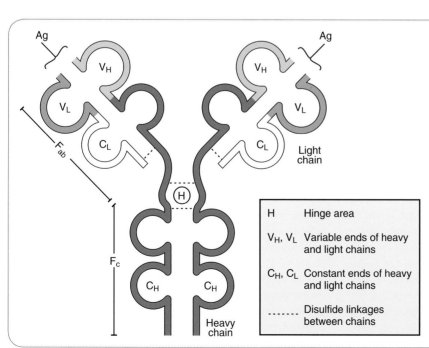

H	Hinge area
V$_H$, V$_L$	Variable ends of heavy and light chains
C$_H$, C$_L$	Constant ends of heavy and light chains
------	Disulfide linkages between chains

Figure 3-4 Diagram of an immunoglobulin. The F$_{ab}$ and F$_c$ portions are also indicated. Ag, antigen.

Thus distinct domains include variable portions of the heavy and light chain (V_H, V_L) and constant parts of the heavy and light chain (C_H, C_L).

- Each antibody is made up of domains of about 110 amino acids that form loops held together by disulfide bonds on cysteine residues.
- Each antibody can be cleaved enzymatically into two fragments: the F_c portion, which contains the constant region, and the F_{ab} fragment, which contains the variable region. F_c binds to specific F_c receptors that are expressed on macrophages, polymorphonuclear neutrophils (PMNs), and other cells. F_{ab} serves as the antigen-binding site.

IgM is composed of five basic units and is thus the largest immunoglobulin (macroglobulin) held together with a linker–J chain. Its function is to neutralize microorganisms. It is an avid complement activator because it has five complement-binding sites. IgM is the first immunoglobulin to appear after immunization, and it is a natural antibody against blood group antigens ABO.

IgG has the smallest molecular weight of the immunoglobulins but is nevertheless the most copious immunoglobulin. It is produced in small amounts on initial immunization, but its production is boosted by reexposure to the antigen. F_c receptors for IgG exist on macrophages, PMNs, lymphocytes, eosinophils, and platelets and in the placenta. This allows the passage of IgG across the placenta into the fetus. IgG acts as an opsonin; that is, it coats bacteria and thus facilitates their phagocytosis.

IgA is predominantly found in mucosal secretions (e.g., tears and nasal mucus), breast milk, and intestinal contents, where it functions as a primary protective immunoglobulin. It is usually joined into a dimer with a J chain. The dimers usually carry a secretory piece that protects the immunoglobulin that is discharged into the intestine from the action of digestive enzymes.

IgE is present in trace amounts in serum. This immunoglobulin is secreted by sensitized plasma cells in tissues and is locally attached to mast cells. IgE mediates allergic *type I hypersensitivity reactions,* also known as atopic or anaphylactic reactions. *IgD* is a cell membrane–bound immunoglobulin found exclusively on B cells. It participates in the antigenic activation of B cells and is not released into serum or body fluids.

ANTIBODY PRODUCTION

Antibody production begins with contact between an antigen and the cells of the immune system. All substances identified by the body as foreign may serve as antigens and incite an immune response. This activation of B cells culminates in the production of specific antibodies that can react with the antigen. Antigens that can elicit an immune response are called *complete antigens,* in contrast to incomplete antigens, or haptens. **Haptens** are low-molecular-weight substances that are not immunogenic by themselves. However, if attached to a larger carrier molecule, haptens become immunogenic. Once the antibodies have been induced against a hapten, they will react with this hapten, even if the hapten is not linked to the carrier.

To elicit antibody production, the antigen must bind to the B-lymphocyte antigen receptor complex. This complex includes IgM or IgD, which binds the antigen, and several membrane molecules that do not participate in antigen binding but are essential for signal transduction and initiation of antibody production. Antibody production requires the support of T helper cells. It is worth noting that B cells can internalize the antigens and thereafter function as **antigen-presenting cells (APCs)** by presenting the internalized antigens to T cells.

MAJOR HISTOCOMPATIBILITY COMPLEX

All processed antigens are presented to T cells in the context of the major histocompatibility complex (MHC) proteins expressed on the surface of APCs. These MHC proteins, first identified on leukocytes, are also known as *human leukocyte antigens* (HLAs), although they are expressed on other nucleated cells in the body. A unique set of MHC antigens determines the individuality of each person. Only identical twins have the same MHC antigens. In immune reactions, the MHC antigens regulate the cell-to-cell contact during antigen presentation.

Human MHC antigens belong to two groups. Type I MHC proteins, found on all nucleated cells of the body, serve as the receptors for CD8, thus linking macrophages to suppressor and/or cytotoxic T lymphocytes. Type II MHC molecules react with CD4, mediating the attachment of macrophages to helper T lymphocytes. Type II molecules serve for presentation of exogenous antigens (e.g., bacteria and soluble antigens) that are first internalized and processed before presentation to T cells.

The main function of the MHC is presentation of antigens to T cells. It is worth remembering that T cells can react only to membrane-bound antigens; thus without the APC there is no T-cell reaction to antigens. The MHC is also important for organ transplantation, and most transplant rejection reactions result from the HLA incompatibility of the host and the donor.

ANTIGEN-ANTIBODY REACTION

Most antigens carry more than one antigenic site, or *epitope,* and are thus able to bind more than one antibody to their surface. Antigens are thus multivalent. Antigens and antibodies are bound to each other by complex physical and chemical bonds, forming *antigen-antibody complexes.* If the antigen is soluble and circulating in the blood, the complexes will also be soluble and will circulate in the plasma, the fluid portion of blood. However, these complexes tend to enlarge as more and more antibodies and antigen molecules are included in the meshwork. Finally, the complexes reach the size of small particles, which are phagocytized in the spleen and the liver by fixed macrophages. The smaller complexes may remain in the circulation, depending on their overall solubility, size, and electrical charge. Depending on these three properties, the immune complexes may remain suspended in circulation for a long time; alternatively, they may be attached to red blood cells (RBCs) or endothelial cells or filtered through the capillary walls with other proteins.

Antibodies to insoluble antigens, such as cell surface antigens, become fixed to the cell membrane (Figure 3-5). This is best illustrated by the antibodies to RBCs that typically coat the cell surface. Antibodies bind RBCs to one another, which is recognized as *agglutination*—that is, clumping of RBCs and their separation from serum. If the antigen-antibody complex activates the complement cascade, cell lysis will occur *(hemolysis)*. This occurs almost invariably with all IgM- and IgG-containing complexes because these immunoglobulins fix complement.

Complement activation results from circulating, soluble, or cell-surface–fixed immune complexes inside the blood vessels. Antigen-antibody complexes formed outside the vessels, or those that are pathologically deposited in tissues, also activate complement. As previously stated, antigen binds to the F_{ab} region of the antibody. The F_c region that protrudes on the opposite side serves as a binding site for complement. At the same time, F_c can attach to all cells that have F_c receptors. The most important among these are the macrophages and PMNs, which act as scavengers of immunoglobulin-coated (opsonized) bacteria. RBC membrane fragments that are coated with antibodies and the large soluble immune complexes are taken in the same way by macrophages and removed from circulation.

In summary, the antibody response has many biologically important features. These can be recognized in the living organism and reproduced experimentally in animals or *in vitro* in the test tube. Immune reactions primarily have a protective role, which can be fully realized only in the context of the coordinated participation of APCs and T and B lymphocytes, which interact one with another. The critical role of MHC in antigen presentation and the complex regulatory role of cytokines produced by T lymphocytes and macrophages should not be forgotten. Finally, the process of antibody production and the nature of antibodies must be fully appreciated to understand the protective and the potentially pathologic consequences of antigen-antibody reactions.

HYPERSENSITIVITY REACTIONS

An abnormal immune response to exogenous antigens or a reaction to endogenous autoantigens is called a **hypersensitivity reaction.** Hypersensitivity reactions are the basis of hypersensitivity diseases, which are also known as *allergic disorders.*

Hypersensitivity diseases are pathogenetically classified into four major groups, each of which is mediated by distinct mechanisms:

Type I—anaphylactic or atopic reaction
Type II—cytotoxic antibody–mediated reaction
Type III—immune complex–mediated reaction
Type IV—cell-mediated, delayed-type reaction

TYPE I HYPERSENSITIVITY

Type I hypersensitivity, also known as anaphylactic or atopic reaction, is primarily mediated by IgE and mast cells or basophils. IgE is produced by plasma cells derived from B lymphocytes that are sensitized to foreign antigens, such as pollen. The antibody, which is produced in tissues exposed to antigens, diffuses locally toward mast cells and

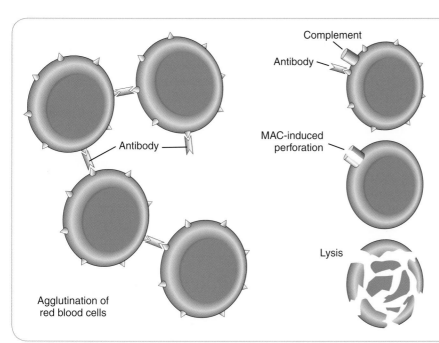

Figure 3-5 Reaction of antibody with antigen on the surface of red blood cells (RBCs). This could lead to agglutination of RBCs or hemolysis mediated by activated complement. MAC, membrane attack complex.

Complement

Antibody

MAC-induced perforation

Antibody

Lysis

Agglutination of red blood cells

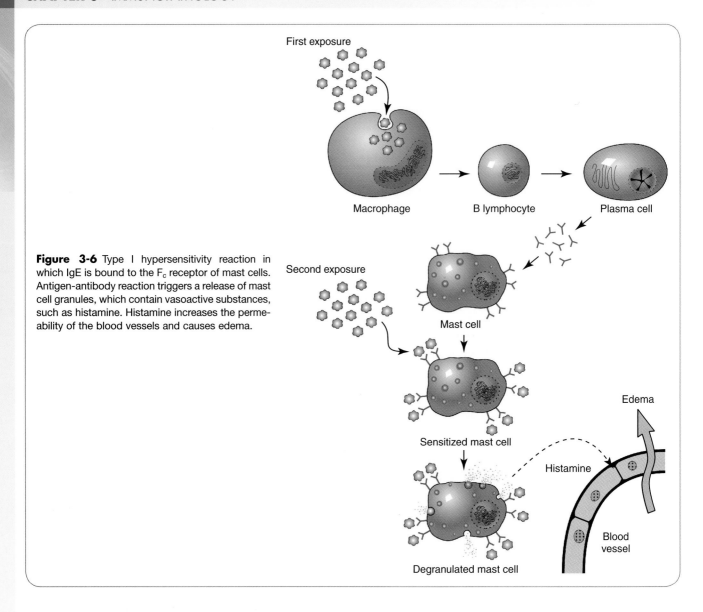

First exposure

Macrophage   B lymphocyte   Plasma cell

Second exposure

Mast cell

Sensitized mast cell

Edema

Histamine

Blood vessel

Degranulated mast cell

Figure 3-6 Type I hypersensitivity reaction in which IgE is bound to the F_c receptor of mast cells. Antigen-antibody reaction triggers a release of mast cell granules, which contain vasoactive substances, such as histamine. Histamine increases the permeability of the blood vessels and causes edema.

is fixed to the F_c receptors on their surface (Figure 3-6). Reexposure to the antigen leads to the formation of antigen-antibody complexes on the surface of mast cells. This triggers the release of vasoactive substances stored in mast cell granules. The most important among these is histamine, the well-known vasoactive biogenic amine. The release is instantaneous, as any sufferer of hay fever can testify. It is accompanied by increased vascular permeability, edema, and accumulation of inflammatory cells, most notably eosinophils. *Eosinophilia*—an increased number of eosinophils in the blood—is a common systemic feature of type I hypersensitivity reactions.

Type I hypersensitivity reactions also produce a late-phase response that usually occurs 4 to 6 hours after exposure to allergens. Basophils and mast cells play an important role in this reaction, but other inflammatory cells also partake and are important for prolonging the tissue reaction to antigens. The late-phase response is mediated by *slow-reacting substances of anaphylaxis*

(SRS-As). SRS-As are arachidonic acid derivatives classified as leukotrienes. Late-phase response is typical of bronchial asthma, a chronic respiratory disease prone to frequent exacerbations in the form of asthmatic attacks, characterized by coughing and shortness of breath as a result of bronchospasm and excessive mucus production in the bronchi.

The most important clinical examples of type I hypersensitivity are as follows:

- Hay fever
- Atopic dermatitis
- Bronchial asthma
- Anaphylactic shock

Hay Fever

Hay fever, or allergic rhinitis, occurs typically as a seasonal allergy to pollens (Figure 3-7). It may also be caused by other foreign substances, such as cat dander, and it is not always seasonal.

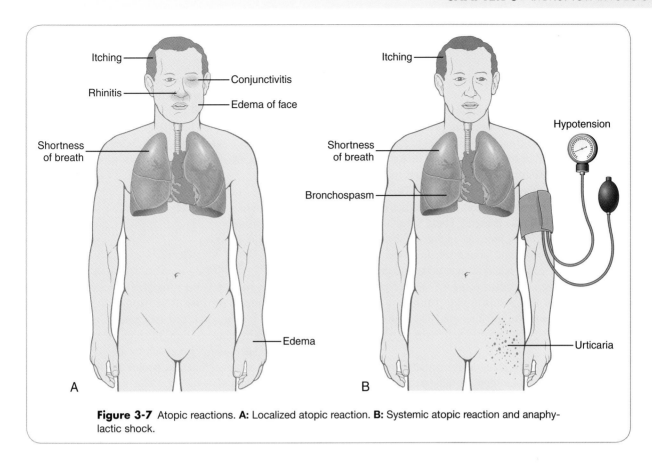

Figure 3-7 Atopic reactions. **A:** Localized atopic reaction. **B:** Systemic atopic reaction and anaphylactic shock.

Exposure to inhaled allergen causes nasal itching and sneezing. Swelling and inflammation of the nasal mucosa (rhinitis) is often associated with similar irritation and inflammation of the conjunctiva *(conjunctivitis)*. All symptoms can be attributed to the effects of histamine and can be neutralized with antihistamines. Drugs that stabilize mast cells and prevent the discharge of their granules are also effective. Long-term relief can be achieved through desensitization to specific allergens. This treatment is based on repeated prophylactic injections of antigen, which induce a neutralizing IgG response. When a desensitized patient encounters the allergen again, the IgG that is bound to the antigen prevents its contact with the IgE in the sensitized tissue. The adverse response of mast cells is thus prevented.

Atopic Dermatitis

Atopic dermatitis is typically a disease of childhood, presenting as a chronic skin irritation known as *eczema* (derived from the Greek term for "boiling over" or erupting). Eczema affects approximately 10% of all children, 50% of whom have a family history of similar problems. This genetic predisposition is associated with hyperproduction of IgE in response to potential environmental allergens. However, a nonfamilial form of atopic dermatitis can occur as well.

Exposure to allergen usually occurs through direct skin contact. Other allergens may be inhaled or ingested in food. Atopic dermatitis improves with age, although affected

children have a tendency to develop other type I hypersensitivity diseases in adulthood, such as asthma or hay fever.

Asthma

Asthma is considered a type I hypersensitivity reaction affecting the bronchi. However, as presented in Chapter 8, there are several forms of asthma, not all of which are immunologically mediated. Asthma caused by hypersensitivity to inhaled antigens is mediated by SRS-As and usually affects children. Attacks of asthma are marked by coughing and wheezing related to the constriction of bronchi and overproduction of mucus by bronchial glands.

Anaphylactic Shock

Anaphylactic shock is a life-threatening, severe, systemic response to an allergen to which the body was previously sensitized. Anaphylactic shock following a bee sting in a person sensitized to bee venom is a typical example. In hospitals it is most often encountered after intravenous injection of anesthetics, opioids or antiseizure drugs, or radiographic contrast media. Shock develops as a result of a massive release of histamine and other vasoactive substances into the circulation. Typical symptoms include *stridor* (high-pitched sound during breathing) caused by vocal cord spasm; choking secondary to laryngeal edema and narrowing; wheezing and shortness of breath resulting from bronchial spasm; and pulmonary edema and systemic circulatory collapse with fainting, caused by hypotension secondary to vasodilation and increased leakage of fluid from the hyperpermeable blood vessels.

TYPE II HYPERSENSITIVITY

Type II hypersensitivity is mediated by cytotoxic antibodies that react with antigens in cells or tissue components, such as basement membranes. The antigen may be extrinsic or intrinsic, as is often the case in some autoimmune diseases. Intrinsic antigens include macromolecules, such as proteins, RNA, or DNA. The reasons these body components become antigenic are not known. Foreign antigens include drugs or simple chemicals that usually act as haptens. These substances bind to soluble plasma proteins or proteins on the surface of RBCs or other cells in the body and immunize the body. Foreign substances released from bacteria and cells infected with viruses may provoke a similar response. Hypersensitivity reaction occurs upon reexposure to the pathogenic antigen. Persistent antigens, as in chronic infection, and a slow release of endogenous autoantigens provoke deleterious hypersensitivity reactions.

Type II hypersensitivity reaction is mediated by IgG or IgM, which forms antigen-antibody complexes on cell membranes or extracellular matrix, such as basement membranes (Figure 3-8). These complexes activate complement, which is the major effector mechanism accounting for the cell lysis that occurs, for instance, in the acute hemolytic reaction caused by transfusion of mismatched blood. Immunoglobulins attached to the antigen also may evoke an *antibody-dependent, cellular, cytotoxic* (ADCC) *reaction.* The antibody typically binds to the antigen with the F_{ab} end, whereas the F_c portion is free and serves as the attachment site for various effector cells, such as NK cells, macrophages, and other leukocytes. Finally, some type II hypersensitivity reactions do not require either complement or an ADCC reaction. Such reactions are based on the binding of antibodies to the receptors on cell surfaces. The binding of antibodies to receptors may stimulate or inhibit the function of such cells.

Following are the best examples of type II hypersensitivity reaction:
- Hemolytic anemia
- Goodpasture's syndrome
- Graves' disease
- Myasthenia gravis

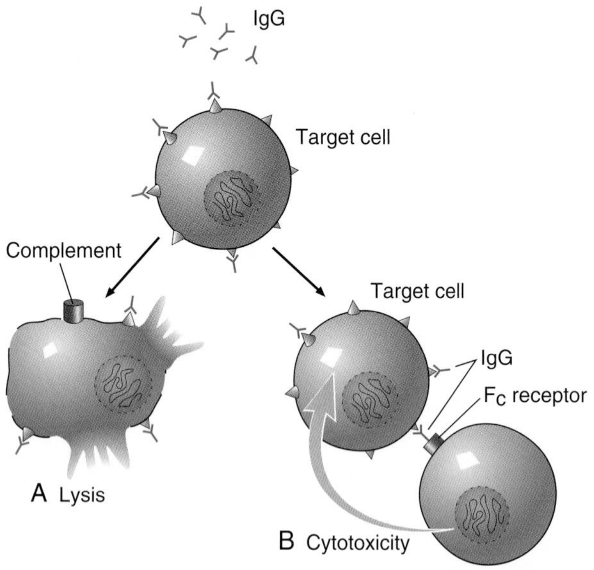

Hemolytic Anemia

Hemolytic anemia is the prototype of a cytotoxic antibody–mediated reaction. The RBC antigens of these patients become antigenic and are recognized as foreign by the body's own immune system. In some circumstances, foreign chemicals, such as drugs, attach to the surface of the RBCs and act as haptens. The antibodies against haptens on the RBCs cause hemolysis.

Goodpasture's Syndrome

Goodpasture's syndrome is marked by renal and pulmonary pathologic changes. These develop because of autoimmunity to a component of collagen type IV in the basement membranes of the glomeruli and alveoli. An epitope, which is normally hidden, becomes inappropriately exposed, allowing the circulating antibodies to attack the kidneys and lungs (Figure 3-9). "Membranotoxic" antibodies cause destruction of glomeruli and consequent renal failure, as well as massive pulmonary hemorrhage that may be lethal.

Figure 3-8 Pathogenesis of type II hypersensitivity. *A,* Binding of the antibody to the antigen on the surface of the cell activates complement, resulting in cell destruction. *B,* An antibody-dependent, cellular, cytotoxic (ADCC) reaction involves effector killer cells, which destroy the target cell coated with the antibody.

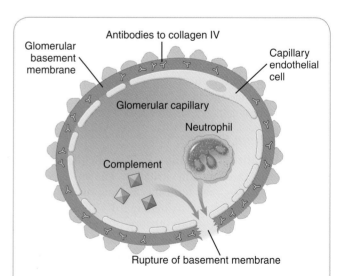

Figure 3-9 Goodpasture's syndrome. Antibodies to collagen type IV activate complement and attract polymorphonuclear neutrophils (PMNs) that contribute to the damage and rupture the glomerular basement membrane.

Graves' Disease

Graves' disease is a form of hyperthyroidism that typically develops in women who have autoantibodies to the thyroid-stimulating hormone (TSH) receptor on the surface of their own follicular cells of the thyroid. The binding of the antibody to the receptor leads to the stimulation of the cells, which is similar to the action of TSH. This results in hyperthyroidism, or overproduction of thyroid hormones.

Myasthenia Gravis

Myasthenia gravis is a muscle disease marked by severe muscle weakness. This autoimmune disease is mediated by antibodies to the receptor for acetylcholine on the surface of striated muscle cells. Acetylcholine is the neurotransmitter released from the nerves at the neuromuscular junction, and it mediates the transmission of signals for muscle contraction. Blockade of acetylcholine receptors prevents the binding of the neurotransmitter, causing progressive muscle weakness and even paralysis.

TYPE III HYPERSENSITIVITY

Type III hypersensitivity is mediated by immune complexes that are formed between antigens and appropriate antibodies. In systemic reactions to soluble antigens, the immune complexes are in the circulation, whereas in localized reactions the immune complexes are formed in tissues.

Serum sickness, which was common previously when horse serum was used extensively for passive immunization against tetanus, is the prototype of type III hypersensitivity (Figure 3-10). A few days after the injection of the serum, foreign proteins appear in the circulation. As the titer of antibodies rises, the concentration of antigen decreases until all of it is completely complexed with antibodies and eliminated from circulation. Initially, the antigen-antibody complexes are small and sparse, but with time the antibody excess becomes overwhelming and the antigen is completely bound into large complexes. During the time of equilibrium or mild antibody excess, antigen-antibody complexes form that are rather soluble and not large enough to be phagocytized by macrophages. Such soluble antigen-antibody complexes remain in circulation and are filtered through the basement membranes of glomeruli and other sites where the plasma is ultrafiltered to produce body fluids. Such anatomic sites include the anterior chamber of the eye; the choroid plexus of the brain; and the serosal surface covering the pleura, pericardium, and the peritoneal cavity. Immune complexes that are trapped in these semipermeable membranes activate complement, which attracts PMNs and results in acute inflammation.

Localized immune complex formation occurs typically in various forms of vasculitis, such as *polyarteritis nodosa*. This disease can be reproduced experimentally in the form of the so-called **Arthus phenomenon.** The antigen is injected subcutaneously to produce sensitization and to stimulate antibody production. Upon rechallenge with the same antigen injected into another site, the antibodies from the circulation

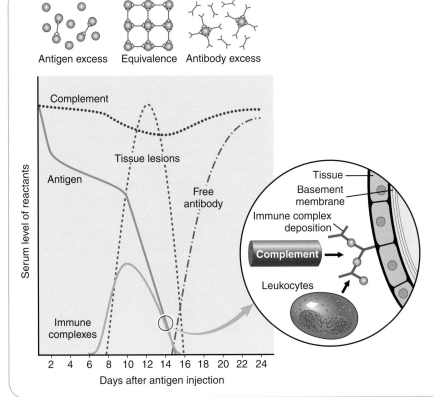

Figure 3-10 Serum sickness. This type III hypersensitivity reaction is mediated by formation of circulating immune complexes. Pathogenic immune complexes are formed only during the phase of antigen excess. The tissue lesions are caused by activated complement and leukocytes attracted to the site of antigen-antibody complex deposition.

diffuse toward the antigen in the tissue and react with it at the site of contact. Antigen-antibody complexes precipitate at the site of equilibrium, and this occurs typically in the vessel wall (Figure 3-11). Antigen-antibody complexes formed in the vessel wall activate complement, which attracts leukocytes. A localized acute inflammation develops, characterized by fibrinoid necrosis. Fibrinoid necrosis reflects the influx of plasma proteins that permeate the site of injury. Fibrinogen, which is also present, undergoes polymerization into fibrin, leading to localized clotting in the vessel walls.

The most important clinical entities mediated by type III hypersensitivity reactions are as follows:

- Systemic lupus erythematosus
- Poststreptococcal glomerulonephritis
- Polyarteritis nodosa

Systemic Lupus Erythematosus

Systemic lupus erythematosus (SLE) is an autoimmune disease of unknown origin, which is discussed in greater detail later in this chapter. Here it should be mentioned that patients with SLE have circulating immune complexes formed between various autoantigens and equivalent antibodies. Although it is unclear what elicits the autoimmune reaction, the consequences of immune complex deposition in tissues are well known. These include kidney disease, arthritis, skin disease, and a variety of other diseases.

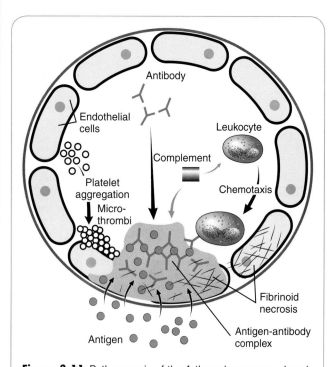

Figure 3-11 Pathogenesis of the Arthus phenomenon. Localized formation of antigen-antibody complexes results in complement activation and leukocytic inflammation. Necrosis of the vessel wall is accompanied by an influx of plasma proteins. Deposits of fibrin formed from its soluble precursor protein fibrinogen are prominent, accounting for the term *fibrinoid necrosis,* used to describe such lesions.

Poststreptococcal Glomerulonephritis

Poststreptococcal glomerulonephritis is an acute renal disease that typically follows an upper respiratory tract infection caused by certain nephritogenic (i.e., capable of inducing nephritis) strains of streptococci. Persons sensitized to streptococcal antigens during acute infection produce antibodies that react with soluble streptococcal antigens "planted" onto the glomerular basement membranes during filtration from the plasma. Antibodies may also react with the streptococcal antigens found in the circulation and thus form circulating immune complexes. Such antigen-antibody complexes are deposited in the glomerular basement membrane, evoking a complement-mediated inflammatory response.

Polyarteritis Nodosa

Polyarteritis nodosa, which is the clinical equivalent of the Arthus phenomenon, is an antigen-antibody–mediated inflammatory disease that typically involves small to medium-sized arteries. In the early stage the affected vessels show focal fibrinoid necrosis and acute inflammation. In the chronic stage the disease is marked by destruction of the vessel wall. Damaged vessels tend to thrombose and become occluded, causing tissue ischemia and infarcts.

TYPE IV HYPERSENSITIVITY

Type IV hypersensitivity is also known as *cell-mediated* or *delayed-type immune reaction.* It involves T lymphocytes and macrophages, which typically aggregate at the site of injury to form *granulomas.*

Type IV hypersensitivity reaction is initiated by complex antigens that are taken up by macrophages or equivalent APCs, such as Langerhans' cells of the epidermis. The antigen is processed and presented to T lymphocytes. Helper T lymphocytes that are exposed to the antigen and the cytokines produced by the APCs become primed and activated. This leads to formation of immune memory, which is important for subsequent exposure and the recruitment of other cells, most notably macrophages, and additional helper T and suppressor/cytotoxic T lymphocytes. Under the influence of cytokines, the macrophages transform into epithelioid cells, which produce even more varied mediators of inflammation than their predecessors, further promoting the formation of granulomas. IFN-γ, considered the most important cytokine responsible for the formation of granulomas, acts on epithelioid cells by augmenting their phagocytic activity and their ability to kill antigen-bearing cells and bacteria (e.g., *Mycobacterium tuberculosis* or tumor cells). IFN-γ also promotes the fusion of epithelioid cells into giant cells. Hence, fully formed granulomas consist of epithelioid cells, giant cells, and lymphocytes (Figure 3-12). Traditionally the giant cells in tuberculous granulomas have been called *Langerhans' giant cells;* however, today we know that these cells are not diagnostic of tuberculosis but can occur in other granulomas as well.

Type IV hypersensitivity reaction occurs in response to complex antigens of *M. tuberculosis, Mycobacterium leprae,*

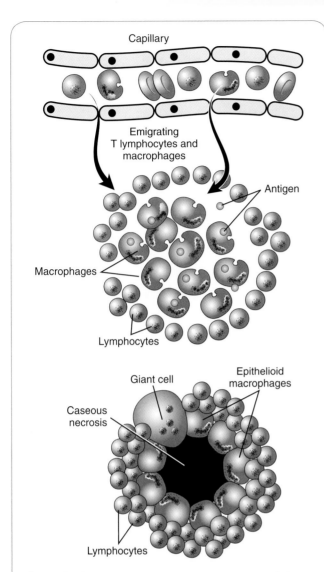

Capillary

Emigrating
T lymphocytes and
macrophages

Antigen

Macrophages

Lymphocytes

Giant cell

Epithelioid
macrophages

Caseous
necrosis

Lymphocytes

Figure 3-12 Granulomas, which are typical of type IV hypersensitivity, consist of lymphocytes and macrophages transformed into epithelioid cells and giant cells.

and various fungi. In addition to infectious granulomas, type IV hypersensitivity reaction accounts for granulomas that develop in response to tumors and for idiopathic granulomatous diseases, such as *sarcoidosis.*

Granulomas can be induced by injecting humans or animals with the antigen. For example, tuberculin, prepared from *M. tuberculosis,* may induce delayed hypersensitivity reactions. Thus it is possible to test whether somebody was exposed to tuberculosis by injecting purified tuberculin into the skin. If the tested person develops localized induration of the skin within 48 hours, the test is considered positive and the person is assumed to have been exposed to tuberculosis (or to have persistent disease).

Contact dermatitis, the most common clinical form of type IV hypersensitivity, also does not present with granulomas. In this disease, which may be caused by allergy to a variety of allergens (e.g., latex gloves, gold rings, or poison ivy), the skin usually contains infiltrates of T lymphocytes and macrophages but no granulomas. The inflammatory cells typically show perivascular cuffing, which correlates with altered vascular permeability, wheal formation, and edema of the affected skin.

The best example of contact dermatitis is the so-called poison ivy reaction, a hypersensitivity reaction to plant antigens. Surgeons may become allergic to latex gloves. Hypersensitivity reactions can occur to essentially any antigen in the environment, including antiperspirants, medical ointments, or laundry detergent (Figure 3-13).

TRANSPLANTATION

Solid tissues can be transplanted successfully from one individual to another, but the graft will be viable only if the donor and the recipient are immunologically similar enough to avoid immunologic rejection. Alternatively, the graft will "take" only if the immune system of the recipient is unable to react against foreign antigens. This is the case in congenitally immunodeficient children born without a thymus or in nude

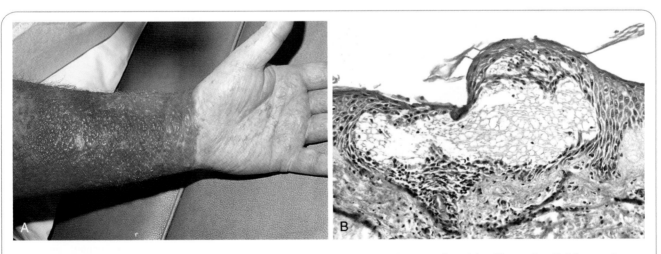

Figure 3-13 Acute contact dermatitis caused by laundry detergent. **A:** Clinical presentation of the skin reaction. **B:** Microscopic examination of the biopsy shows an intradermal vesicle filled with proteinaceous fluid and a few lymphocytes. (From Kumar V, Abbas AK, Fausto N, Aster JC, eds: Robbins and Cotran Pathologic Basis of Disease, 8th ed, Philadelphia, 2010, Saunders.)

athymic mice, which represent an animal model of this human immunodeficiency. The immune system can be partially inactivated with various *immunosuppressive* drugs, which are used in clinical medicine to facilitate the acceptance of transplants.

In the clinical setting, there are several forms of transplantation, which include the following:

- Autografts
- Isografts
- Homografts (allografts)
- Xenografts

If the patient is serving as both donor and recipient, the transplant is called an **autograft.** Such grafts are typically used for skin grafts, hair transplantation, and replacement of blood vessels of the heart with leg veins.

Tissue transplantation between genetically identical individuals of the same species, as in genetically syngeneic mouse strains or identical twins, is called an *isograft.* Such ideal grafts do not elicit a transplant reaction because the recipient does not recognize the tissue as foreign. Transplants between individuals of the same species who are not genetically identical are called **homografts** or **allografts.** In clinical practice, homografted tissues are accepted only if the donor and the recipient are matched at several major histocompatibility loci (HLAs) and have the same blood group. Best results are obtained with transplantation between relatives or siblings. However, to avoid immune reaction against foreign antigens, the recipients routinely receive immunosuppressive therapy before transplantation. **Xenografts**—tissue transplants between animals of different species (as in liver transplantation between monkeys and humans)—are poorly tolerated. However, avascular tissues, such as the cornea or heart valves, can be used for xenografting. Porcine heart valves are used to replace damaged human heart leaflets.

Before transplantation, the donor's tissue must be matched with that of the recipient. This is done by crossmatching the peripheral blood lymphocytes, because the lymphocytes carry the same major histocompatibility antigens as the cells of the solid organs. This test provides basic information on the similarities and disparities of the two individuals and makes it possible to determine to what extent they are *histocompatible.* The histocompatibility antigens form four major loci (HLA-A, HLA-B, HLA-C, and HLA-D). Together with a closely related antigen called *HLA-DR,* these antigens are inherited as a single unit of five loci known as the *haplotype.* Because haplotypes are inherited as single alleles, each of us has a 1 in 4 chance that a brother or sister has a haplotype that is identical to ours. Thus siblings are ideal tissue donor–recipient pairs. If an ideal match cannot be arranged, however, tissues from the patient's closest relatives or from unrelated donors may be used.

TRANSPLANT REJECTION

All homografts invariably evoke some **transplant rejection,** which is mediated by antibodies and a delayed cellular immune reaction. Several clinically distinct forms of transplant rejection are recognized (Figure 3-14). As an example,

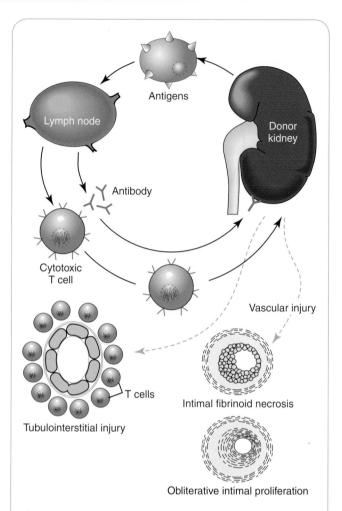

Figure 3-14 Transplant rejection is antibody mediated, cell mediated, or both. Antibodies bind to endothelial cells of the transplanted kidney and cause fibrinoid necrosis and thrombosis typical of hyperacute rejection. Chronic vascular rejection is characterized by obliterative endarteritis. Cell-mediated transplant rejection, typical of chronic transplant rejection, is characterized by chronic tubulointerstitial inflammation.

we shall describe the reaction to homotransplanted kidneys, which can occur in three forms:

- Hyperacute reaction
- Acute reaction
- Chronic reaction

Hyperacute Reaction

Hyperacute reaction typically occurs because the recipient has preformed antibodies to the donor's antigens. Typically the reactions occur during the operation. When the surgeon connects the donor's and recipient's blood vessels and the recipient's blood enters the graft, the preformed circulating antibodies react with the endothelial cells. Damage to the endothelial cells leads to thrombosis, and the graft cannot perfuse normally. Such transplants must be removed immediately to prevent even more serious and inevitable complications.

Acute Rejection

Acute rejection occurs most often within the first few weeks of transplantation but may also evolve later when the immunosuppressive treatment becomes ineffectual. It involves both antibody-mediated and cell-mediated immune reaction. Antibodies tend to damage the blood vessels, which show signs of vasculitis. The inflammatory reaction is most evident in the intima of medium-sized arteries. Cell-mediated immune rejection presents in the form of tissue infiltrates that consist of helper T and suppressor/cytotoxic T lymphocytes and macrophages. B lymphocytes and plasma cells are also present, indicating that this is a mixed reaction.

Chronic Reaction

Chronic transplant rejection evolves slowly over a period of several months or years. It also involves both antibody- and cell-mediated responses. Vascular changes cause obliteration of the arterial lumen (endarteritis), which in turn leads to hypoperfusion of tissues and chronic ischemia. Interstitial tissue inflammation contributes to the destruction of parenchymal cells and the ultimate deterioration of the function of the transplanted organ.

CLINICAL USE OF TRANSPLANTATION

Transplants are used extensively in clinical practice. Kidney transplants have been performed with considerable success for more than 30 years. Skin transplants are used for the treatment of burns. Livers, hearts, lungs, or pancreases that have been terminally damaged also can be replaced successfully with transplants.

Bone marrow transplantation is used to treat aplastic anemia and bone marrow failure. This procedure is also used in the treatment of leukemia, a neoplastic disease of the bone marrow. In such cases the bone marrow of the leukemic patient is irradiated to kill all the tumor cells and the bone marrow is then replenished with the stem cells removed from the bone marrow of a histocompatible donor.

The best way to prevent transplant rejection is to match the donor and recipient carefully. Because an ideal match is not always possible, recipients must be prepared for transplantation with adequate immunosuppression. This is accomplished by administering drugs, such as cyclosporine, which inhibits IL-2 production and thus impairs T cell response, or cyclophosphamide, which inhibits proliferation of lymphocytes. Antibodies to T-cell antigens are also used to reduce the number of these cells. However, immunosuppression is not an innocuous procedure, and it predisposes the patient to infections. Some drugs, such as cyclosporine, may have significant side effects and are nephrotoxic. Immunosuppressed patients are at increased risk for the development of infections with ubiquitous bacteria and fungi, which are then difficult to eradicate.

GRAFT-VERSUS-HOST REACTION

An important complication of transplantation, especially that of bone marrow, is the **graft-versus-host (GVH) reaction,** which develops as a result of the transfer of a donor's immunocompetent lymphocytes. In response to antigens on the recipient's tissues, the donor's lymphocytes initiate a cell-mediated type IV immune reaction. Because the host is usually immunosuppressed, the transplanted immunocompetent cells cannot be rejected; as a result, these cells proliferate and overwhelm the host's body. The donor's lymphocytes attack various tissues in the host, especially the epithelial cells of the gastrointestinal tract, the skin, and the liver. Severe dermatitis develops, with scaling of the epidermis. Diarrhea and fever are typical signs of gastrointestinal GVH reaction. Jaundice is the most prominent sign of liver involvement. GVH reaction may be difficult to treat, and the patient usually dies as a result of overwhelming infection.

BLOOD TRANSFUSION

Transfusion of blood from one person to another is a form of transplantation. In contrast to solid organs, however, blood is a tissue that is composed of dissociated cells circulating inside the vessels. Because RBCs outnumber white blood cells by an order of magnitude, the success or failure of blood transfusions depends primarily on the compatibility of the donor and the recipient with regard to their RBC blood group antigens.

Every RBC carries a set of surface antigens, which can be divided into three groups: major blood group antigens, minor blood group antigens, and Rh blood antigens.

Major blood group antigens (ABO) are encoded by three genes that can give the following six genotypes: AA, AB, AO, BO, BB, and OO. The A and B gene are dominant over the O gene, so there are only four blood groups: A (AA, AO), B (BB, BO), AB, and O.

ABO antigens have corresponding natural antibodies: group A blood contains anti-B antibodies, group B blood contains anti-A antibodies, and the O group contains both anti-A and anti-B antibodies (Figure 3-15). Group AB blood does not contain natural antibodies to A or B antigen. Thus A blood can be given to group A and group AB recipients, because the blood of these recipients does not contain antibodies to group A antigen. Group AB blood can be given only to AB group recipients, because all other groups persons contain antibodies to A or B or both. O group blood can be given to recipients of all blood groups. Accordingly, individuals with AB blood are called *universal recipients* and those with O blood are considered *universal donors.*

If the blood of an A group donor is infused into a B group recipient, the natural antibodies to A in the recipient will react with the donor's RBCs and cause their hemolysis. This transfusion reaction presents clinically with chills, shivering, and even mild fever. In most instances transfusion reaction is readily recognized and the transfusion is discontinued. If the

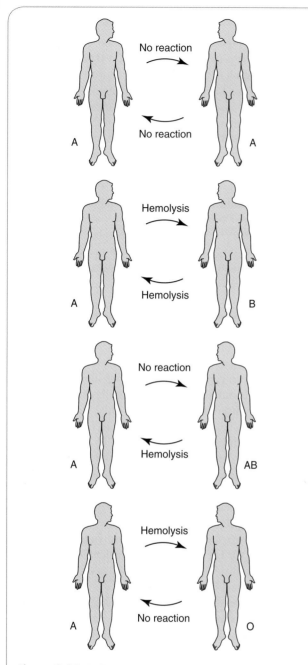

Figure 3-15 ABO blood groups. There are three genes—A, B, and O—that can yield six combinations. Because A and B are dominant over O, there are only four blood groups: A, B, AB, and O. Blood transfusion is well accepted between persons of the same group (A to A). The transfusion of A blood to a donor with group B blood causes hemolysis. A person with group AB blood can receive blood of all groups ("universal recipient"). A person with group O blood can give blood to all other groups ("universal donor").

To avoid transfusion reaction, the donor's blood must be crossmatched with the blood of the recipient. This is done before the transfusion by mixing the serum of the donor with the RBCs of the recipient and vice versa. The RBCs are incubated at body temperature in a test tube. The RBCs that are compatible with the serum will remain suspended in the fluid. However, if there are antibodies in the serum, these will attach to the RBCs and agglutinate them. Blood that agglutinates in the crossmatch is not suitable for transfusion.

Crossmatching of donor and recipient blood is essential to avoid transfusion reactions caused by ABO incompatibility. In addition, this procedure can also detect significant incompatibilities of minor blood group antigens. In most instances, incompatibility at these loci has no consequence, but occasionally it may cause a significant hemolytic reaction.

Rh FACTOR INCOMPATIBILITY

The Rh blood group system consists of a group of antigens expressed normally on the surface of human RBCs. Only three antigens, known as *cde/CDE,* are strong antigens, and of these only the d/D antigen is of practical significance. Persons who have the dominant allele D are Rh positive (Rh$^+$), and those who have two recessive d/d alleles are Rh negative (Rh$^-$). Approximately 15% of whites and 5% of African Americans are Rh$^-$, whereas most others, including Native Americans and Asians, are Rh$^+$.

In contrast to the ABO antigens, which are complemented with natural antibodies, Rh antigens do not have natural antibodies. Thus antibodies to dominant Rh antigens will be formed in Rh$^-$ persons who are transfused with Rh$^+$ blood. Furthermore, it is important to note that the antibodies to the ABO antigens are of the IgM class, whereas the newly generated anti-Rh antibodies are of the IgG class. As mentioned previously, the IgG antibodies can cross the placenta, which is an important consideration in maternofetal Rh factor incompatibility.

Maternofetal RH incompatibility involving the Rh antigen D has until recently been the most important cause of neonatal *hemolytic disease* and several syndromes known as *icterus gravis neonatorum,* **hydrops fetalis,** and *erythroblastosis fetalis.* These conditions, which involve Rh$^-$ women with Rh$^+$ mates, are all caused by the same mechanism; the different names for the syndromes merely reflect the extent of injury and its timing. If the child is Rh$^+$ because he or she has inherited the paternal D allele, the child's Rh$^+$ blood could sensitize the mother. During the first pregnancy, the Rh$^+$ child will not be affected because the mother does not have natural antibodies to the Rh antigen D (Figure 3-16). However, the mixing of fetal and maternal blood at the time of delivery may expose the Rh$^-$ mother to the dominant D antigen on fetal RBCs. This will immunize the mother and cause her to produce IgG-type anti-Rh antibodies. If the fetus in the subsequent pregnancy is again Rh$^+$ (i.e., d/D), the antibodies to D will cross the placenta and affect the fetal Rh$^+$ RBCs. Hemolysis will ensue in the fetal circulation, and the fetus may die *in utero* showing signs of severe *hydrops fetalis* (Figure 3-17).

reaction is not diagnosed, massive hemolysis may cause shock, with microthrombi and disseminated intravascular coagulation (DIC). Some patients may even die. Jaundice, from the bilirubin released from hemolyzed RBCs, develops in those who survive. Acute renal failure is a common complication.

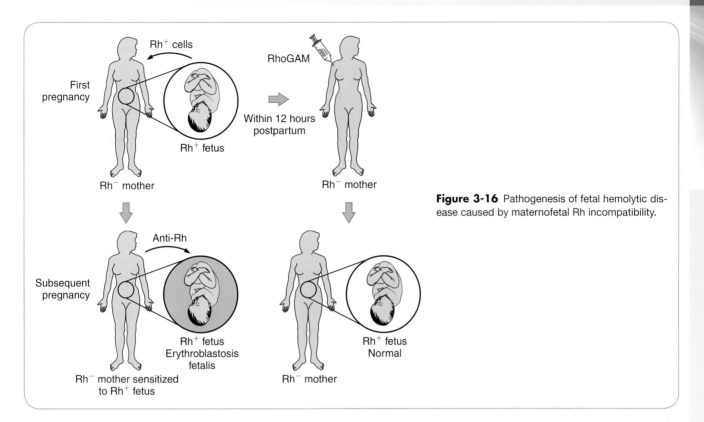

Figure 3-16 Pathogenesis of fetal hemolytic disease caused by maternofetal Rh incompatibility.

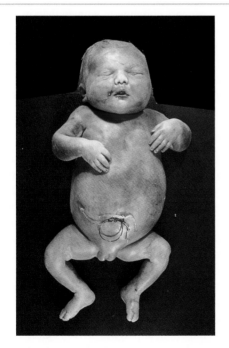

Figure 3-17 Hydrops fetalis caused by maternofetal incompatibility.

Essentially the hemolysis destroys fetal RBCs. The fetus becomes anemic and develops severe hypoxia and congestive heart failure. The term *erythroblastosis fetalis,* used as a synonym, indicates that the fetal bone marrow is maximally stimulated by the loss of RBCs and is trying to compensate for the loss. There is marked extramedullary hematopoiesis in the liver, spleen, and lymph nodes. The fetus is also jaundiced as a result of bilirubin released from the hemolyzed RBCs.

In milder cases, there is comparatively less hemolysis and massive edema does not develop. The newborn child does not show signs of massive edema, and the only external evidence of hemolysis is marked jaundice *(icterus gravis).* The major danger associated with icterus gravis is *kernicterus (kern* meaning "nucleus" in German) or jaundice of the basal ganglia (nuclei) of the brain. The massive elevation of serum bilirubin breaches the blood–brain barrier, and the bilirubin that normally does not cross into the brain is deposited preferentially in the basal ganglia. This bilirubin is toxic and may cause permanent neural damage.

Clearly, maternofetal Rh incompatibility has serious repercussions, and once the disease develops, it cannot be treated efficiently. Fortunately, this disease can be prevented by proper treatment of Rh⁻ pregnant women at risk. At the time that an Rh⁻ mother first delivers an Rh⁺ child, it is possible to prevent Rh immunization of the mother by injecting her with anti-D immunoglobulin (RhoGAM). This procedure, if performed during the first 72 hours postpartum, prevents maternal immunization and erythroblastosis fetalis in subsequent pregnancies. Unfortunately, if a pregnant Rh⁻ woman becomes immunized to the D antigen during pregnancy or abortion, treatment with RhoGAM is of no avail.

Immunoprophylaxis of maternofetal Rh incompatibility has almost completely eliminated this medical problem in the United States. Hemolytic disease of the neonate still occurs, albeit rarely, as a result of the incompatibility of the fetal and maternal major blood groups or some minor blood group antigens. In practice, this is usually encountered in fetuses of the A₁ subtype born to group O mothers who have acquired IgG antibodies to the A₁ antigen. Fortunately, this incompatibility results only in mild hemolysis and the newborn child usually shows only anemia and jaundice. There is no prophylactic measure that could be applied to prevent the consequences of maternofetal incompatibility in ABO or minor blood group antigens.

AUTOIMMUNE DISEASES

As stated previously, immune response is based on the ability of cells of the immune system to distinguish between self and non-self. The body is generally tolerant to antigens expressed on its own cells. Numerous control mechanisms have been devised in nature to suppress the response against self-antigens. Breakdown of autotolerance results in **autoimmune diseases.**

The diagnosis of autoimmune disorder is made when (1) the existence of autoantibodies can be documented, (2) there is evidence that the immune mechanisms are pathogenetically important and have caused the pathologic lesions, and (3) there is direct or indirect evidence of the immune nature of the disorder. For example, a disease is presumably autoimmune if it shows a favorable response to treatment with immunosuppressive drugs or if it can be diagnosed by immunologic techniques. The existence of autoantibodies cannot always be demonstrated, and their pathogenicity is often even more difficult to prove.

Autoimmune disorders occur with increased frequency in some families, suggesting that *genetic* factors have an important pathogenetic role. The genetic basis of these disorders has been best documented by studying the linkage of autoimmune disorders and certain HLA haplotypes. For example, HLA-B27 is strongly associated with ankylosing spondylitis. More than 90% of all patients with this spine disease, which causes extreme stiffness of the body with progressive forward bending of the spine, have this particular major histocompatibility antigen.

Most autoimmune diseases are more common in women than in men. The preponderance of women among the population affected by SLE, rheumatoid arthritis, or autoimmune thyroiditis suggests that *nongenetic* factors are also important and could influence the predisposition to these diseases.

Autoimmune diseases may present in two forms:
- Systemic, multiorgan disease
- Organ-specific disease limited to a single organ

Box 3-1 lists some of the more common autoimmune diseases. It is worth mentioning that many of these diseases were previously classified as collagen-vascular disorders or "collagenoses." Although many of these diseases adversely affect collagen and other components of the connective tissue, it would be incorrect to consider them primarily as connective tissue disorders. It has been conclusively shown that the

> **BOX 3-1   Autoimmune Diseases**
>
> **Systemic Diseases**
> Systemic lupus erythematosus
> Rheumatic fever
> Rheumatoid arthritis
> Systemic sclerosis
> Polyarteritis nodosa
>
> **Organ-Specific Diseases**
> Brain: multiple sclerosis
> Thyroid: Hashimoto's thyroiditis
> Blood: autoimmune hemolytic anemia
> Kidney: glomerulonephritis
> Liver: primary biliary cirrhosis
> Skin: pemphigus vulgaris
> Muscle: myasthenia gravis

primary defect for almost all these disorders is the dysregulation of the immune response and that this, rather than the connective tissue lesions themselves, is the most important unifying aspect for the entire group of diseases.

SYSTEMIC LUPUS ERYTHEMATOSUS

SLE is a prototype of an autoimmune disorder characterized by multisystemic involvement. It affects 1 in 2500 persons and is 10 times more common in women than in men. It may occur at any age but most often affects young adults. The disease, which is most severe among African Americans, shows a familial preponderance. There is a 30% concordance among identical twins. Collectively, these facts show that both genetic and nongenetic factors play important pathogenetic roles.

Pathogenesis

The etiology and pathogenesis of SLE are poorly understood. Generally it is believed that the basic defect is a malfunction of suppressor T cells, which allows polyclonal activation of B cells. Plasma cells derived from these uncontrolled B-cell clones secrete antibodies of variable specificity against both autoantigens and foreign antigens. A variety of antigens can be detected in the serum of patients with SLE, but it is unknown to what extent these antigens elicit noxious antibodies. Some authorities even believe it possible that the tissue lesions could be primarily inflicted by a virus, but this theory has not been proven.

The most important antibodies are to nuclear components: DNA, RNA, and nuclear proteins. Therefore these are called antinuclear antibodies (ANAs) and are best detected by using indirect immunofluorescence microscopy titration. The concentration of antibodies—that is, their titer—is determined by serially diluting the serum and testing it on cells until no more staining occurs. For example, a titer of 1:256 means that this dilution still yields a positive result but that the next dilution (1:512) produced no staining.

Virtually all patients with SLE have a positive ANA test. This test is good for screening, but it has low specificity for SLE and therefore one must use additional tests that have less sensitivity but more specificity. These include the tests for double-stranded DNA and the so-called Sm antigen (named after the patient Smith in whom it was first discovered), which are more reliable for diagnosing SLE. Unfortunately the anti–double-stranded DNA test is positive only in about 50% of SLE patients and the anti-Sm test is positive in only 25%. In practice, then, one must compromise between sensitivity and specificity of a given test and use all laboratory data in the proper clinical context.

Pathology

Antibodies of patients with SLE react not only with antigens in tissues but also with those released from cells damaged by other means. Skin exposed to sunlight is often affected. One hypothesis is that the damaged cells release their nuclear content, which then diffuses toward the antibodies, permeating the tissues. Antigen-antibody complexes form in the skin along the epidermodermal junction.

If the antigens reach the circulation, they form complexes with the antibodies in the serum. Such circulating antigen-antibody complexes are usually deposited in semipermeable membranes, such as the glomerular basement membranes. Other sites at which the deposits are seen include the synovial membrane of the joints, the serous membranes of the pleura and peritoneum, the endocardium of the heart valves, the choroid plexus in the ventricles of the brain, and the anterior eye chamber. In all these sites, the plasma is filtered across a membrane into a body cavity (e.g., joint space) or it penetrates into the tissue by diffusion (e.g., endocardium). The immune complexes are relatively large and are retained during this ultrafiltration. At the site of deposition, the immune complexes activate complement; this in turn elicits an inflammatory reaction, resulting in a number of organ-specific inflammatory diseases, such as glomerulonephritis, dermatitis, arthritis, and others (Figure 3-18).

Clinical Features

The symptoms of SLE are highly variable. The organs, tissues, and systems most often involved include the skin, joints, kidneys, and blood. Skin typically shows changes on sun-exposed surfaces such as the face. Inflammation of the joints (arthritis) is manifested by swelling, redness, and painful movement. The kidneys are involved in 75% of affected patients. Kidney symptoms may be mild, with renal involvement sometimes causing only minor urinary abnormalities, such as hematuria or proteinuria. Nevertheless, glomerulonephritis is common, and renal problems are among the most important manifestations of SLE. Previously patients used to die of SLE kidney disease, but today renal failure can be prevented by timely treatment with corticosteroids and other drugs that suppress the immune reactions.

? Did You Know?

The term *butterfly rash* is used for the facial rash of systemic lupus erythematosus because it involves both sides of the face. Imagine the nose as the body of the butterfly and the red rash as its wings.

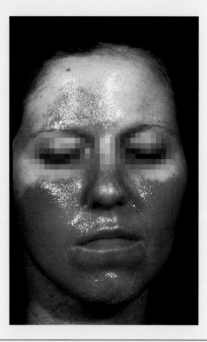

(From Damjanov I, Linder J: Pathology: A Color Atlas, St. Louis, 2000, Mosby.)

Circulatory antibodies damage the RBCs and cause anemia, a common sequela of the disease. The polyclonal activation of lymphocytes is usually associated with enlargement of the lymph nodes and spleen. Other organs, such as the heart, brain, and lungs, and skeletal muscles are less commonly involved.

The course of SLE is highly variable. Immunotherapy has achieved considerable success; indeed, more than 75% of treated patients are alive 10 years after the onset of disease. Kidney failure is still the most common serious complication of SLE. If all other treatment options fail, end-stage kidney disease can be treated by renal transplantation.

IMMUNODEFICIENCY DISEASES

Immunodeficiency diseases may be *congenital (primary),* or they may be *secondary,* occurring as a result of infections, metabolic diseases, cancer, or treatment. Secondary immunodeficiency is more common than primary immunodeficiency. AIDS, the most prevalent disease in this group, is one of the most important human diseases today.

Immunodeficiency, whether primary or secondary, may involve primarily B cells or subsets of T cells or may be generalized and involve the entire immune system. All

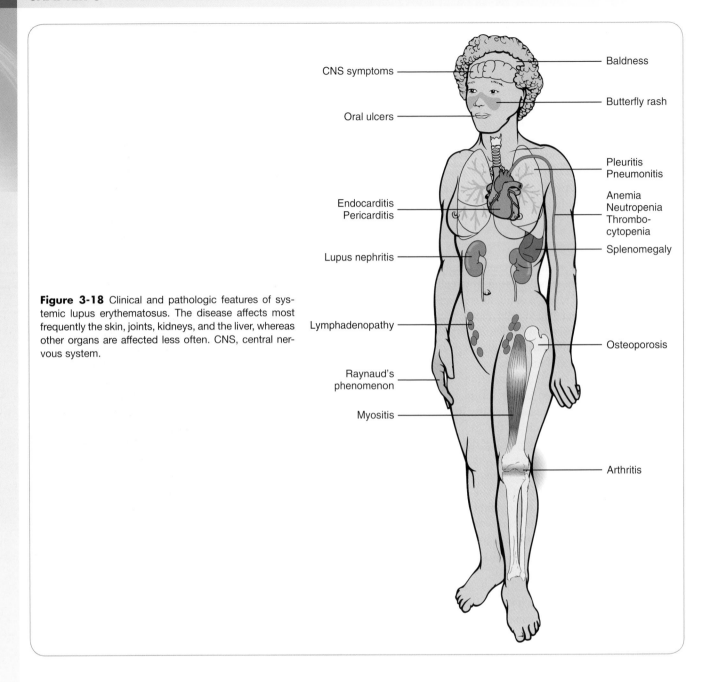

CNS symptoms

Oral ulcers

Endocarditis
Pericarditis

Lupus nephritis

Lymphadenopathy

Raynaud's
phenomenon

Myositis

Baldness

Butterfly rash

Pleuritis
Pneumonitis

Anemia
Neutropenia
Thrombo-
cytopenia

Splenomegaly

Osteoporosis

Arthritis

Figure 3-18 Clinical and pathologic features of systemic lupus erythematosus. The disease affects most frequently the skin, joints, kidneys, and the liver, whereas other organs are affected less often. CNS, central nervous system.

immunodeficiencies are characterized by *lymphopenia,* a low lymphocyte count in the peripheral blood. B-cell deficiencies are associated with low levels of serum immunoglobulins. Defective or inadequate function of T cells may be detected with immunologic tests for cell-mediated immunity (e.g., a patch test or tuberculin test). All immunodeficiencies cause reduced resistance to infections.

PRIMARY IMMUNODEFICIENCY DISEASES

Primary **immunodeficiency (congenital)** diseases are a heterogeneous group of inborn disorders affecting differentiation and maturation of the T and B lymphocytes. The block in differentiation can occur at any step in the developmental sequence that leads from the lymphoid stem cell to T cells on

one side and B cells on the other side of the developmental pathway. Many immunodeficiencies exist, but only three examples are presented here.

Severe combined immunodeficiency (Swiss-type agammaglobulinemia) is related to a defect of lymphoid stem cells, also known as *pre-B, pre-T cells.* Affected children lack both T and B cells. The thymus is hypoplastic, and the lymph nodes are small and lack germinal centers. Unless placed in strict isolation, these children succumb to infections and die early in infancy.

Isolated **IgA deficiency** is the most common congenital immunodeficiency, affecting 1 in 700 persons. The affected person cannot produce IgA, apparently as a result of a block in the terminal differentiation of B cells to IgA-producing plasma cells. Affected persons have a reduced resistance to intestinal infections, but many are otherwise asymptomatic.

DiGeorge syndrome is a deficiency of T cells related to a developmental block in the formation of the thymus. The thymus develops from the branchial clefts, fetal structures that also give rise to the parathyroid glands. Children born without a thymus are unable to mount a cell-mediated immune response and usually die of infection. As a result of congenital hypoparathyroidism, hypocalcemia also develops and these children experience severe spastic convulsions.

There are numerous other congenital immunodeficiencies that are beyond the scope of this discussion. Although these are generally not as common as the three described, it is important to keep them in mind. From time to time, an infant or young child will present with a history of recurrent infections and retarded development. In such cases, it is worth remembering that the child may have a congenital defect of the immune system. There are already encouraging experimental data that indicate that some of these children may be saved by genetic engineering. "Bubble children" (so called because they must be placed in strict isolation from all environmental pathogens) have already received transplants of genetically modified lymphoid cells. Transplanted cells have successfully repopulated the bone marrow of these immunodeficient children and colonized the secondary lymph organs. The immune defect has been completely corrected by this procedure in a dozen children.

ACQUIRED IMMUNODEFICIENCY SYNDROME

AIDS, as the name implies, is a syndrome (i.e., a complex of symptoms) that develops as a consequence of a severe acquired immunodepression caused by the **human immunodeficiency viruses (HIVs).**

Etiology and Epidemiology

HIVs are small RNA viruses that belong to the lentivirus family of viruses. This human virus is related to but distinct from immunodeficiency viruses that affect monkeys, called *simian immunodeficiency viruses* (SIVs), and other lentiviruses that infect horses, sheep, and many other animals. Clinical AIDS is most often caused by HIV-1, although HIV-2 is an important cause of AIDS in Africa.

The medical world became aware of AIDS in the early 1980s, after a series of reports about this new disease appeared. Initially, the reports concentrated on homosexual men who developed repeated bouts of pneumonia and various other **opportunistic infections** and who usually died, completely exhausted by disease and in a state of profound immunosuppression. Subsequently it became apparent that the disease could occur in other populations as well and that it could be transmitted in several ways. Ultimately this led to the discovery of the virus. Serologic tests were developed for the detection of the virus and the antibodies to the virus, which appear in essentially all infected persons. All these scientific advances made it possible not only to diagnose the viral infection but

also to study its spread and define the risk factors that allow the virus to spread from one person to another.

AIDS has a worldwide distribution. In 1994 the World Health Organization (WHO) reported that for the first time the number of recorded cases of AIDS had surpassed 1 million. By the year 2000, 22 million people had died of AIDS. The estimates are that at least 35 million people are infected with HIV worldwide.

The highest prevalence of AIDS has been reported in Africa, where the disease is still spreading at an alarming pace. In the United States the number of new cases has leveled off, but more than 100,000 new cases are still reported every year. Reports indicate that 1% of all college-age people (18 to 25 years of age) have serologic evidence of HIV infection.

Pathogenesis

HIV is an RNA retrovirus that cannot survive outside of human cells. Humans are the only source of infection. The virus is transmitted from one person to another by close contact that facilitates the transfer of body fluids. Intravenous drug abuse is an important mode of transmission because drug users often share the same blood-contaminated paraphernalia. Sexual secretions and sperm also contain HIV; thus sexual contact—homosexual or heterosexual—is an important mode of transmission of AIDS. In addition to bloodborne and sexually transmitted HIV infections, AIDS can also be acquired by maternofetal, transplacental transmission of the virus. Screening of blood donors has reduced the number of transfusion-related cases of AIDS.

From time to time there are news reports that AIDS has been acquired by casual contact and without exposure to infected blood or body fluids. There is no scientific evidence that AIDS can be acquired through casual contact. Minor open wounds, an accidental prick with an infected needle, or a minor incision during surgery in an HIV-infected person may serve as an entry point for HIV and constitute a risk for health professionals. Nevertheless, with appropriate precautions, the risk is very small. Only a few health professionals have died of AIDS acquired in the professional setting.

 Did You Know?

Misconceptions about acquired immunodeficiency syndrome (AIDS) are rampant, as demonstrated by the results of a recent survey:

- 25% of Americans believed human immunodeficiency virus (HIV) was transmitted by coughing, spitting, and sneezing.
- 20% believed HIV infection could occur from contact via a drinking fountain or toilet seat.
- 10% believed touching an HIV-infected person or a person with AIDS was dangerous.
- 25% refused to work with an HIV-infected person.

Such prejudices must be dispelled by informing the public about the nature of AIDS. To quote C. Everett Koop, the former U.S. Surgeon General: "I said education was our 'basic weapon.' Actually it's our only weapon. We've got to educate everyone about the disease so that each person can take responsibility for seeing that it is spread no further."

HIV infection is accompanied by a series of events that can be explained by two factors: selective affinity of HIV for certain human cells and the effects of the virus on the immune system. In the blood, HIV has an affinity for helper T lymphocytes (CD4-positive lymphocytes) and monocytes. Macrophages, which are the tissue-derived descendants of monocytes, can also become infected. Furthermore, fixed tissue phagocytic cells, such as the follicular dendritic cells in the lymph nodes and the microglia of the nervous system (which are also derived from monocytes), are also sites of infection. All these cells can serve as reservoirs for the virus.

Helper T lymphocytes, macrophages, and their fixed tissue equivalents are essential components of the immune system. HIV is cytotoxic, so a depletion of helper T lymphocytes and other infected cells is typical of AIDS.

Initial infection of an immunologically competent organism stimulates B cells to produce antibodies, which appear in the circulation within weeks of exposure. These antibodies are important for the diagnosis of HIV infection. However, serologic positivity alone (i.e., the presence of antibodies) does not mean that the person has AIDS. Actually, most infected persons enter a latent phase of infection and are asymptomatic for prolonged periods. As the virus replicates and destroys more and more helper T lymphocytes, the symptoms

of AIDS begin appearing. Cell-mediated and B-cell–mediated immunity ultimately become depressed, and the immunosuppressed organism cannot then defend itself from infection. Death usually occurs because of overwhelming infection. A small number of patients develop tumors that are the cause of death. These tumors can be of any kind, but most commonly they are lymphomas or a peculiar tumor of the blood vessels called **Kaposi's sarcoma.**

Clinical Features

According to the Centers for Disease Control and Prevention (CDC) in Atlanta, Georgia, HIV-infected persons belong to one of four groups, corresponding to four phases of the disease:

- Phase of acute illness (group I)
- Phase of asymptomatic infection (group II)
- Phase of generalized lymphadenopathy (group III)
- AIDS phase characterized by superimposed infections and complications (group IV)

These groups correspond clinically to the early acute, chronic, and crisis phases of the disease (Figure 3-19).

Acute illness occurs in approximately 50% of HIV-infected persons, usually 3 to 6 weeks after exposure. Typical symptoms are nonspecific and may include fever, night sweats, nausea, myalgia, headache, sore throat, skin rash, and mild

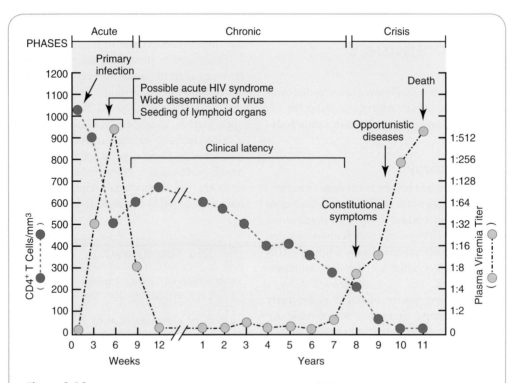

Figure 3-19 Typical course of human immunodeficiency virus (HIV) infection. During the early period after primary infection, there is widespread dissemination of virus and a sharp decrease in the number of CD4+ T cells in peripheral blood. An immune response to HIV ensues, with a decrease in detectable viremia followed by a prolonged period of clinical latency. The CD4+ T-cell count continues to decrease during the following years, until it reaches a critical level below which there is substantial risk of opportunistic diseases. (Redrawn with permission from Pantaleo G, Graziosi C, Fauci, AS: The immunopathogenesis of human immunodeficiency virus infection. The New England Journal of Medicine 328:327, 1993. Copyright © 1993 Massachusetts Medical Society)

lymph node enlargement. These symptoms last 2 to 3 weeks and then disappear spontaneously. During this period, some patients develop antibodies to HIV.

The phase of *asymptomatic infection* is of variable duration, lasting from a few months to a few years. The patient is asymptomatic but carries the virus and is infectious. Approximately 50% of HIV-infected patients develop AIDS within 10 years of initial diagnosis.

Persistent *generalized lymphadenopathy* may develop in patients who are initially asymptomatic. Alternatively, the lymphadenopathy may develop early in the course of infection and persist for months or years.

Group IV symptoms are categorized, according to CDC recommendations, into several subgroups. These patients show signs of AIDS, the most important of which reflect opportunistic infections, gastrointestinal disorders, central nervous system involvement, and neoplasia.

The diagnosis of HIV infection and AIDS is based on clinical findings and laboratory data. The most important laboratory tests are the test for antibodies to HIV and the lymphocyte count. The antibodies to HIV appear at a variable rate, 2 to 10 weeks after infection. The presence of the virus in the body can be confirmed by additional tests, which are often used to avoid false-positive results.

The lymphocyte count is very important for the evaluation of immunocompetence. In practice, it is used to determine the ratio of helper T to suppressor/cytotoxic T cells. Normally, this ratio is greater than 2 and reflects an absolute number of helper T (CD4-positive) cells that exceeds 500 per μL. During the early phases of the disease and during the chronic phase, the CD4-positive cell count exceeds 500. As the disease progresses, helper T cell counts decrease; once the number of CD4-positive cells falls below 200, the *crisis phase* ensues. In the last stages of disease, almost no CD4 cells are present in the circulation.

Pathology

The morphologic changes induced in the human organism by HIV are relatively nonspecific (Figure 3-20). These changes vary with time, the extent of viremia, and the degree of immunosuppression. For example, the lymph nodes initially enlarge and show hyperplasia of the follicles, reflecting the B-cell response to viral antigens that leads to the appearance of antiviral antibodies. After some time, the lymph nodes involute and become depleted of lymphocytes, especially in the T-cell–dependent parafollicular zones. In the last stages of AIDS, the lymph nodes may be infected with fungi or mycobacteria, which usually do not provoke an inflammatory response and almost never contain granulomas.

The brain is the only organ that shows HIV-specific changes. In the brain, HIV evokes a response of brain macrophages called microglia cells. Such a microglial response results in the formation of microglial nodules with multinucleated giant cells in the gray matter and subcortical gray matter of the cerebrum. Overshadowing these changes are lesions caused by opportunistic infections, which give rise to meningitis or encephalitis. Of the pathogens affecting the brain, the most important are viruses, such as herpesvirus and cytomegalovirus; fungi, such as *Cryptococcus neoformans;* and protozoa, such as *Toxoplasma gondii.* These infections may destroy parts of the brain directly or by occluding blood vessels and causing ischemic infarct.

The respiratory tract is a common site of infection in patients with AIDS. In the initial stages of the disease, the infections are typically localized to the upper respiratory tract and present as nasal infection (rhinitis) or throat infection (pharyngitis). Advanced immunosuppression predisposes the individual to pneumonia, which is often caused by fungi, such as *Pneumocystis jiroveci, Aspergillus fumigatus,* or *Candida albicans.* Mixed bacterial infections are also common. Pulmonary tuberculosis develops in a significant number of patients.

The gastrointestinal tract is also often infected, usually by the same pathogens that infect the lungs. Infections with pathogens that are rarely found in otherwise healthy people are also common. Protozoa, such as *Cryptosporidium;* worms, such as *Strongyloides;* and uncommon forms of tuberculosis, such as *Mycobacterium avium intracellulare* (MAI), may be identified in many patients. The diarrhea and malabsorption of nutrients caused by such infections are important cofactors in the pathogenesis of wasting that typically occur in AIDS.

Skin lesions are common in HIV-infected persons. The skin changes may present as mild seborrheic dermatitis (itching skin rash) or persistent infections with various viruses (herpesvirus), fungi (dermatomycoses), and bacteria (streptococcal folliculitis).

Tumors that develop in AIDS are important causes of mortality. Patients with AIDS show an increased incidence of all tumors. The most important among the malignant neoplasms occurring in patients with AIDS are lymphomas and Kaposi's sarcoma. Common cancers, such as squamous cell carcinoma of the skin or uterine cervix, occur also at an increased frequency and tend to grow more rapidly than in people who are not infected with HIV.

Lymphomas most frequently involve lymph nodes, which appear enlarged, but malignant lymphoid cells may involve the spleen, liver, and many extranodal sites as well. Brain lymphomas are more common than in persons who are not infected with HIV. Histologically, AIDS-related lymphomas do not differ from other lymphomas. Cytologically, they are often found to be of high grade, which correlates with their rapid proliferation and poor prognosis. Lymphoma can be treated with cytotoxic drugs, but the results are not optimal and those involving the CNS have especially high mortality.

Kaposi's sarcoma is a malignant disease that involves endothelial cells. It is caused by herpesvirus type 8 infection. It often occurs in the skin but may involve internal organs as well. For unknown reasons, it has an especially high prevalence among male homosexuals. On gross examination, it presents in the form of bluish red nodules. Histologically, these nodules are composed of anastomosing vascular spaces filled with blood. Kaposi's sarcoma grows slower than lymphoma. Nevertheless, it may cause extensive bleeding, and

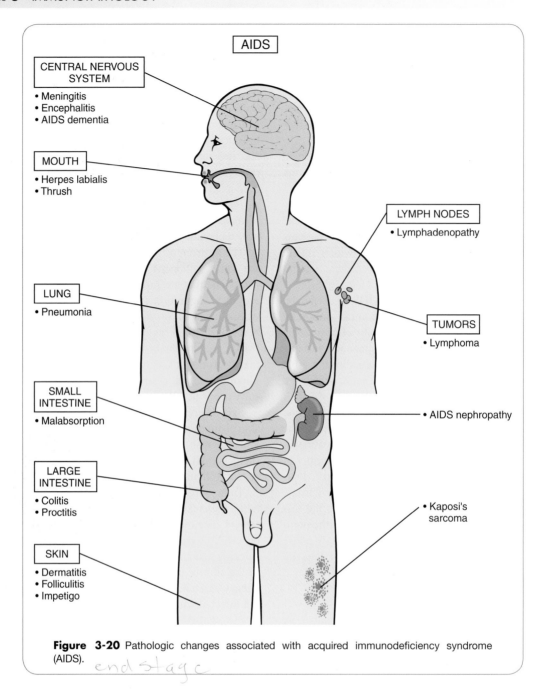

AIDS

CENTRAL NERVOUS SYSTEM
• Meningitis
• Encephalitis
• AIDS dementia

MOUTH
• Herpes labialis
• Thrush

LUNG
• Pneumonia

SMALL INTESTINE
• Malabsorption

LARGE INTESTINE
• Colitis
• Proctitis

SKIN
• Dermatitis
• Folliculitis
• Impetigo

LYMPH NODES
• Lymphadenopathy

TUMORS
• Lymphoma

• AIDS nephropathy

• Kaposi's sarcoma

Figure 3-20 Pathologic changes associated with acquired immunodeficiency syndrome (AIDS). *end stage*

the mass lesions may compress vital organs and cause death.

Treatment

New drugs that inhibit replication of viruses have improved the chances for survival of most HIV-infected patients. However, such drugs are expensive and are not readily available to the citizens of poor countries in Africa and Asia, who need them the most. Efforts to produce a vaccine against HIV have been unsuccessful so far. Once AIDS develops, the disease becomes essentially incurable. However, death can be postponed through vigorous treatment of opportunistic infections and general support of vital functions.

AMYLOIDOSIS

Amyloidosis is caused by deposition of a fibrillar substance called *amyloid*. Because amyloidosis is a multifactorial disease that is often related to abnormalities of the immune system or an abnormal response to chronic infection, it is reviewed in this chapter.

Amyloid was originally named so because it was thought to resemble starch (the meaning of the Greek term *amylon*). In routine microscopy slides it appears as an amorphous pink (eosinophilic) material called hyalin. With additional studies it can be distinguished from other substances that also appear like hyalin, such as condensed collagen or basement membrane.

Pathogenesis

Amyloid is not a chemically distinct entity. Instead it is defined in terms of its physical properties: fibers that are 7.5-nm thick and arranged into a beta-pleated sheet. Thus any fibrillar protein that forms a beta-pleated sheet is called *amyloid*. This conformational state can be recognized with radiographic crystallography. In histologic sections this would be impractical. Instead, amyloid is detected with Congo red, a dye that has the capacity to intercalate into beta-pleated sheets in a peculiar manner. Congo red, when bound to amyloid, is red. However, when examined under polarizing light, it becomes apple green. Amyloid fibrils also have a distinct appearance on electron microscopy.

Biochemically, there are several forms of amyloids that are all derived from distinct precursors. On the basis of the biochemical structure of the major fibrillar protein, amyloids are divided into several groups, the most important of which are the following:

- *AL amyloid,* derived from the light chain of the immunoglobulins. This is typically formed by neoplastic B cells, as seen in malignant lymphoma and plasmacytoma.
- *AA amyloid,* derived from serum amyloid A (SAA) protein. SAA is an acute-phase reactant that is produced by the liver in response to various stimuli, most notably infection (Figure 3-21).

Pathology

Deposits of amyloid in various organs change the function of tissues and cells. The deposits in the basement membranes of the blood vessels change their permeability. In the glomeruli, amyloid thus leads to proteinuria. The sinusoids of the liver and adrenal gland, which are normally fenestrated, transform into solid, tubelike, impermeable vessels. Furthermore, the deposits of amyloid compress the parenchymal cells, which together with ischemia causes atrophy and loss of cell function. Hepatic and adrenal insufficiency develop. Deposits of amyloid in the heart weaken myocardial contractions.

Two forms of amyloidosis account for most clinical forms of systemic amyloidosis: deposition of AL amyloid and deposition of AA amyloid. The *AL amyloid* of multiple myeloma, also called *primary amyloidosis,* is deposited in the kidneys but also in blood vessels of many other organs. *AA amyloid* is typically found in association with chronic inflammation (e.g., chronic tuberculosis of the lungs, suppurative bronchiectasis, and chronic osteomyelitis) and is therefore called secondary amyloidosis. *Secondary amyloidosis* typically affects the kidneys, liver, adrenals, and spleen and blood vessels in many other organs and tissue.

Clinical Features

Amyloidosis presents clinically in many forms, and the symptoms depend predominantly on the organ system involved. The definitive diagnosis can be made only by demonstrating

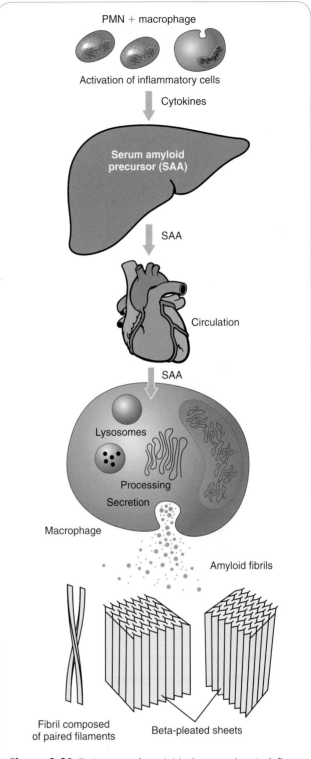

Figure 3-21 Pathogens of amyloidosis secondary to inflammation. Cytokines released from inflammatory cells stimulate the liver, which secretes serum amyloid A (SAA). This soluble precursor of amyloid is processed by macrophages and laid down in tissues in the form of fibrils that have a beta-pleated structure. PMN, polymorphonuclear neutrophils.

amyloid in tissues, Because amyloid deposit may be seen in many small blood vessels, it is customary to take a biopsy sample from the subcutaneous fat, gingival, or rectum, and examine it microscopically for deposits of amyloid. Kidney or liver biopsy may be performed as well. Kidney or liver tissue that is infiltrated with amyloid is brittle, so the biopsy must be done with extreme care to avoid uncontrollable bleeding. Amyloidosis cannot be treated efficiently.

REVIEW QUESTIONS

1. What is the main difference between natural and acquired immunity?

2. What are the functions of properdin and lysozyme?

3. What are antigens?

4. What are the main differences between T and B lymphocytes?

5. What is the difference between CD4- and CD8-positive lymphocytes?

6. How are plasma cells related to lymphocytes?

7. What are the most important common features of IgG, IgM, IgA, IgE, and IgD, and what features distinguish them from one another?

8. How do antigens induce production of antibodies?

9. How do antibodies react with antigens?

10. What is the role of the major histocompatibility complex and cytokines in the response of the body to foreign antigens?

11. Compare immune-mediated hemolysis with agglutination of red blood cells.

12. What is the mechanism of type I hypersensitivity?

13. Which diseases are caused by type I hypersensitivity reactions?

14. Correlate the pathologic findings and clinical features of respiratory, ocular, and skin manifestations of type I hypersensitivity reactions.

15. What is the pathogenesis of anaphylactic shock?

16. What are the two basic mechanisms of type II hypersensitivity?

17. Which diseases are caused by type II hypersensitivity reaction?

18. Compare the role of type II hypersensitivity in hemolytic anemia, Graves' disease, and myasthenia gravis.

19. Which diseases are caused by type III hypersensitivity reaction?

20. Compare Arthus phenomenon with systemic lupus erythematosus.

21. What is the mechanism of type IV hypersensitivity?

22. Which diseases are caused by type IV hypersensitivity reaction?

23. What is the difference among autografts, isografts, homografts, allografts, and xenografts?

24. What is the significance of haplotypes for transplantation of human organs?

25. What is the difference among hyperacute, acute, and chronic transplant rejection?

26. What is the pathogenesis and what are the clinical features of graft-versus-host reaction?

27. How could one determine whether a unit of donated blood could safely be transfused into a person in need of blood transfusion?

28. What is the cause of transfusion reaction, and how does it present clinically?

29. What happens if an Rh⁻ person receives a blood transfusion from an Rh⁺ donor?

30. What is the pathogenesis of erythroblastosis fetalis resulting from maternofetal Rh incompatibility?

31. What is kernicterus?

32. What clinicopathologic and laboratory findings must be present to allow the diagnosis of an autoimmune disorder?

33. What are the most common autoimmune diseases?

34. What are the pathogenesis and clinical and pathologic findings in systemic lupus erythematosus?

35. Describe common features of some primary immunodeficiency diseases.

36. How prevalent is HIV infection worldwide?

37. How is HIV transmitted from one person to another?

38. How does HIV spread in the human body, and what changes does it induce?

39. What are the clinical phases of HIV infection?

40. What are the pathologic manifestations of AIDS?

41. Which pathogens cause infections at an increased rate in patients with AIDS?

42. Which tumors typically occur in AIDS patients?

43. What is amyloid?

44. What are the most important forms of amyloid, and how are the amyloid deposits formed?

45. Which organs are most often involved in amyloidosis?

Neoplasia

4

Chapter Outline

Terminology
Classification of Tumors
  Benign and Malignant Tumors
  Metastasis
  Histologic Classification of Tumors
  Tumor Staging and Grading
Biology of Tumor Cells
  Biochemistry of Cancer Cells
  Growth Properties in Cell Culture
Causes of Cancer
  Identification of Human Carcinogens
  Chemical Carcinogens
  Physical Carcinogens

Natural Biologic Carcinogens
Viral Carcinogens
Human Oncogenes
Tumor Suppressor Genes
Hereditary Cancer
Immune Response to Tumors
Clinical Manifestations of Neoplasia
  Local Symptoms
  Systemic Symptoms
Cancer Epidemiology
  Incidence
  Prevalence
  Mortality

Key Terms and Concepts

Adenocarcinomas
Adenomas
Alpha-fetoprotein (AFP)
Anaplasia
Angiogenesis
Autocrine stimulation
Benign tumors
Burkitt's lymphoma
Cachexia
Cancer
Cancerogenic factors
Carcinoembryonic antigen (CEA)
Carcinogens
Carcinoma
Chondroma/chondrosarcoma
Clonal expansion
Contact inhibition
Cystadenoma/cystadenocarcinoma
Epstein-Barr virus (EBV)
Ewing's sarcoma
Familial adenomatous polyposis coli

Fibroma/fibrosarcoma
Glioma
Grading of tumors
Hepatitis B virus
Hodgkin's lymphoma
Human papillomaviruses (HPVs)
Human T-cell lymphoma/leukemia virus (HTLV-1)
Incidence
Kaposi's sarcoma
Leiomyoma/leiomyosarcoma
Lipoma/liposarcoma
Lymphoma
Malignant tumors
Metastasis
Mixed tumor
Mortality
Neoplasia
Neuroblastoma
Neurofibromatosis
Oncogenes

Oncogenic viruses
Oncology
Osteosarcoma
Papillomas
Paraneoplastic syndromes
Pleomorphism
Polycyclic aromatic hydrocarbons
Procarcinogen
Retinoblastomas
Rhabdomyoma/rhabdomyosarcoma
Sarcoma
Seminoma
Staging of tumors
Tumor antigens
Tumor suppressor genes
UV light
Warning signs of cancer
Wilms' tumor
Xeroderma pigmentosum
X-rays

After reading this chapter, the student should be able to:

1. Define neoplasia and its related terms: tumor, cancer, and oncology.
2. Classify tumors on the basis of their clinical behavior and histopathologic features.
3. Describe typical features of benign and malignant tumors.
4. Define metastasis and explain its pathogenesis.
5. List the common forms of carcinoma and sarcoma and their tissues of origin and describe their benign equivalents.
6. Explain the principles of tumor staging and grading and the TNM system.
7. Describe the various approaches to studying the etiology and pathogenesis of cancer.
8. Discuss environmental carcinogens that could affect humans.
9. Describe the evidence for viral carcinogenesis in humans, with special emphasis on human papillomavirus, Epstein-Barr virus, and hepatitis B virus.
10. Define oncogenes and tumor suppressor genes and explain their clinical significance.
11. Describe the host's immune response to neoplasia.
12. Describe the significance and the clinical value of tumor-associated antigens.
13. Describe five local and five systemic adverse effects of tumors on the host.
14. Discuss the changes in cancer incidence that have occurred over the last 100 years and list the three most common forms of cancer in men and women previously and now.
15. Describe the geographic differences in the incidence of the main forms of cancer.
16. Describe the main contributions of cancer epidemiology to our understanding of neoplasia.

Neoplasia, literally meaning "new growth", is a term derived from the Greek words *neos* ("new") and *plasia* ("growth"). It is used to denote uncontrolled growth of cells whose proliferation cannot be adequately controlled by normal regulatory mechanisms operating in normal tissues.

The proliferation of normal cells is regulated internally by (1) the genetic program of each cell, (2) signals transmitted from one cell to another through direct contact, and (3) various soluble substances that have growth-promoting or growth-inhibiting effects. Once the cells stop proliferating, they assume specialized functions by activating a set of genes specific for each cell type. This selective activation of genes, typically associated with the suppression of other genes, is called *differentiation.* Tumor cells differ from normal cells in that they usually do not achieve the same level of differentiation.

In contrast to the tightly regulated growth of normal cells, the proliferation of neoplastic cells is as follows:

- *Autonomous*—independent of growth factors and stimuli that promote the growth of normal cells
- *Excessive*—unceasing in response to normal regulators of cellular proliferation
- *Disorganized*—not given to following the rules governing formation of normal tissues and organs

TERMINOLOGY

The proliferation of neoplastic cells leads to the formation of masses called *tumors.* This term is derived from the Latin word *tumor,* which means "swelling." The Greek term for a "swelling," *onkos,* has been used to construct the term **oncology,** which is the most widely used name for the scientific discipline concerned with *cancer. Clinical oncologists* deal with neoplastic diseases in the clinical setting, primarily from a diagnostic and therapeutic point of view. *Experimental oncologists* work in the laboratory and study the etiology, pathogenesis, and cellular and molecular biology of neoplasms. *Cancer epidemiologists* deal with neoplasia in human populations and also study the environmental causes of tumors.

The terms *neoplasm* and *tumor* are used synonymously. However, it is very important to note that not all neoplasms form tumors. For example, leukemia is a malignant disease of the bone marrow, but the malignant cells are in the blood circulation and thus do not form distinct masses. In addition, not all swellings are neoplasms, as mentioned in the chapter on inflammation in which the Latin term *tumor* was listed as one of the cardinal signs of inflammation. It is also important to note that there are many forms of tumors and that neoplastic disease is not a single clinical or pathologic entity but rather a broad spectrum of pathologic processes.

A final note should be added regarding the term *cancer,* which is the most widely used synonym for *neoplasms.* **Cancer** is a Latin word, closely related to the Greek term *karkinos,* which means "crab." It was introduced into the medical terminology by ancient Latin and Greek physicians who observed that tumors invaded tissues like crawling crabs. The term *cancer* came to be widely accepted and even today is used as a collective designation for all tumors.

CLASSIFICATION OF TUMORS

Tumors can be classified according to many criteria, none of which are generally valid or universally accepted. The most important classifications are as follows:

- *Clinical classification*—This classification takes into account the clinical presentation and outcome of neoplastic diseases.
- *Histologic classification*—This classification is based on histologic examination of tumors. On the basis of histologic features, pathologists can determine whether the tumor is composed of epithelial cells, mesenchymal (connective tissue) cells, lymphoid cells, or other cell types. For many years, pathologists have been correlating the clinical course of various neoplastic diseases with the histologic characteristics of tumors. On the basis of this correlation of clinical and pathologic data, criteria for *benign* tumors and *malignant* tumors have been established. The histologic classification of tumors thus correlates very well with the clinical classification. In practice, these classifications are used interchangeably and complement one another.

BENIGN AND MALIGNANT TUMORS

Most tumors can be classified clinically as either benign or malignant. **Benign tumors** have a limited growth potential and a good outcome, whereas **malignant tumors** grow uncontrollably and eventually kill the host. As with anything else in nature, though, there are many exceptions to this simple rule.

The clinical behavior of neoplasms—that is, whether a tumor is benign—can be predicted from a pathologic examination. Typically, such an examination includes naked eye (macroscopic) inspection supplemented by microscopic examination of histologic sections of the tumor. Additional data may be obtained with various ancillary techniques, such as electron microscopy, immunohistochemistry, chromosomal analysis, and molecular biologic studies of tumoral DNA.

Macroscopic Features

On gross or naked eye examination, benign tumors are sharply demarcated from normal tissue and are often encapsulated (Figure 4-1). The capsule is usually composed of connective tissue. Benign tumors have an expansive growth and compress the adjacent normal tissue, which undergoes atrophy and fibrosis, often forming a pseudocapsule. The distinction between a capsule and a pseudocapsule is not important, because in both cases these structures provide a sharp border between the tumor and normal tissue, allowing the surgeon to easily remove ("shell out") the tumor.

Malignant tumors lack a capsule and are not as clearly separated from normal tissue as benign tumors are. In contrast to the expansive growth of benign tumors, malignant tumors invade the surrounding tissue by infiltrating normal tissue just as the roots of a tree penetrate the soil. Because of their infiltrative growth and lack of sharp borders, malignant tumors cannot be removed as easily as benign ones.

Microscopic Features

On histologic examination, benign tumors are composed of cells that resemble the tissue from which they have arisen. By contrast, the cells of malignant tumors may differ considerably from cells in normal tissues. It is said that malignant cells show prominent **anaplasia;** that is, they exhibit new features not inherent to the tissue of their origin. In contrast to benign tumors, which show high degrees of differentiation, malignant tumors are *undifferentiated* (Figure 4-2).

Cellular Features

The differences between benign and malignant tumors also can be appreciated at the level of individual cells. Benign tumors are composed of a uniform cell population in which all

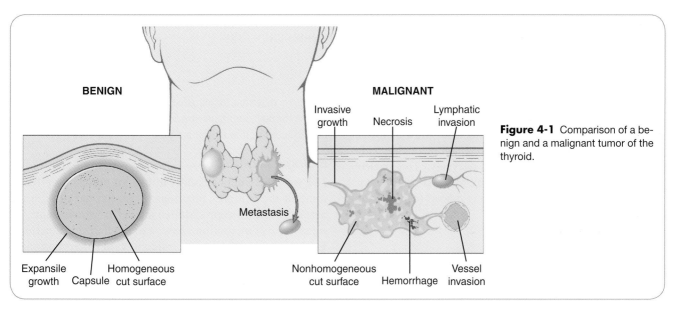

Figure 4-1 Comparison of a benign and a malignant tumor of the thyroid.

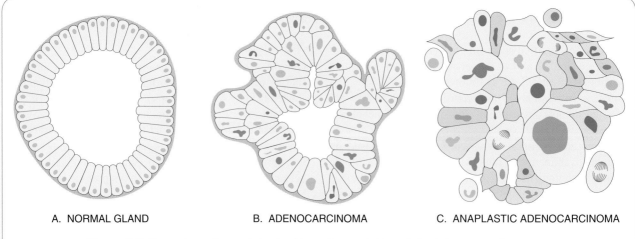

A. NORMAL GLAND   B. ADENOCARCINOMA   C. ANAPLASTIC ADENOCARCINOMA

Figure 4-2 Comparison of normal glands with carcinoma. *A,* Normal glands have smooth contours and uniform nuclei. *B,* Adenocarcinoma is composed of irregular glands. *C,* Anaplastic or undifferentiated carcinoma forms cell groups that show little resemblance to glands.

cells have approximately the same features. By contrast, malignant tumors consist of heterogeneous cell populations that often show marked nuclear **pleomorphism,** meaning variation in size and shape and staining properties of tumor cell nuclei.

Benign tumor cells have regularly shaped nuclei that may be round, oval, or elongated but that are usually of the same size. Malignant cell nuclei are pleomorphic. Benign cells have a well-developed cytoplasm, with well-developed cytoplasmic organelles, enabling them to perform complex functions. Like the rapidly proliferating undifferentiated embryonic cells that have no specialized cytoplasmic functions, undifferentiated tumor cells often have very little cytoplasm and contain a reduced number of cytoplasmic organelles. In well-differentiated normal and benign tumor cells, the nucleus accounts for a small part of the total cell volume, whereas in malignant cells, the nucleus is relatively larger. Typically, malignant cells have a high *nuclear-to-cytoplasmic (N/C) ratio.* This is best seen in cytologic smears, such as the vaginal Papanicolaou (Pap) smear. In contrast to benign cells, which have a small nucleus and abundant cytoplasm, malignant cells have a larger nucleus surrounded by a narrow rim of cytoplasm (Figure 4-3).

The nuclei of benign cells exhibit a regular, even distribution of chromatin. The nucleoli are not overly prominent. In comparison with normal cells, the nuclei of most malignant cells are hyperchromatic (i.e., they contain more chromatin) and the chromatin is distributed unevenly. The nucleoli are often prominent and may be multiple. Malignant tumors contain more cells that are undergoing mitosis (cell division) than do benign tumors.

Chromosomal Studies

Benign tumors usually have a normal number of chromosomes. By contrast, malignant cells are often *aneuploid,* which means they do not have a normal diploid (46,XX or 46,XY) number of chromosomes. The chromosomes may be structurally abnormal

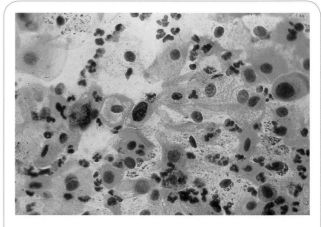

Figure 4-3 Cytologic features of malignant disease detected by a vaginal Papanicolaou smear. Malignant cells have enlarged hyperchromatic nuclei in contrast to the small nuclei of normal cells.

owing to deletions or translocations of parts of their arms or newly formed fragments formed during the disorderly mitoses that are common in malignant tumors (Figure 4-4).

Biologic Features

The well-differentiated cells of benign tumors may retain some of the complex functions of the normal cells in the tissue of their origin. Malignant cells, which show no signs of differentiation, have no specialized functions. Their entire metabolism is geared toward supporting rapid growth and replication. To this end, the cells have a modified basic metabolism and function that gives them a growth advantage and allows them to outpace normal cells.

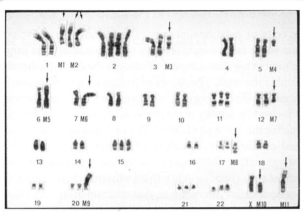

Figure 4-4 Abnormal chromosomes in a cancer cell. The cell is polyploid; that is, it contains more than two sets of 23 chromosomes. Many abnormal chromosomes (M1 to M5) are marked by arrows.

Metastasis involves a spread of tumor cells from a primary location to some other site in the body. The spread can occur through three main pathways:

- Through the lymphatics
- Via blood, also known as *hematogenous spread*
- By seeding of the surface of body cavities

Regardless of the pathway for dissemination of tumor cells, the sequence of events leading to metastasis is essentially the same and includes several distinct steps, collectively known as the *metastatic cascade* (Figure 4-5).

Not all malignant cells are capable of metastasis. The first step, then, is acquisition of a capacity to metastasize. Cells that have acquired the capacity to metastasize expand clonally, forming a distinct subpopulation. As this clone expands by successive divisions, its cells reach the lymphatics or the blood vessels or enter a body cavity. The fluid in these spaces (i.e., the lymph in the lymphatics, the blood in the blood vessels, or the pleural and peritoneal fluid) carries the cells from

The most important differences between benign and malignant tumors are listed in Table 4-1.

METASTASIS

Metastasis denotes a process in which cells move from one site to another in the body. Only malignant tumor cells have the capacity to metastasize. Benign tumors never metastasize and always remain localized.

TABLE 4-1 Comparison of Benign and Malignant Tumors

Feature	Benign	Malignant
Growth	Slow Expansive	Fast Invasive
Metastases	No	Yes
Gross Appearance		
External surface	Smooth	Irregular
Capsule	Yes	No
Necrosis	No	Yes
Hemorrhage	No	Yes
Microscopic Appearance		
Architecture	Resembles that of tissues of origin	Does not resemble that of tissues of origin
Cells	Well differentiated	Poorly differentiated
Nuclei	Normal size and shape	Pleomorphic
Mitoses	Few	Many irregular

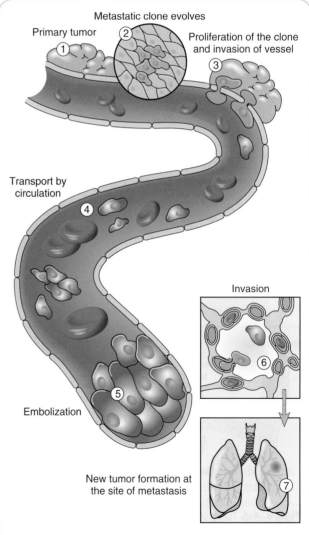

Figure 4-5 Metastatic cascade occurs in several steps, marked 1 through 7.

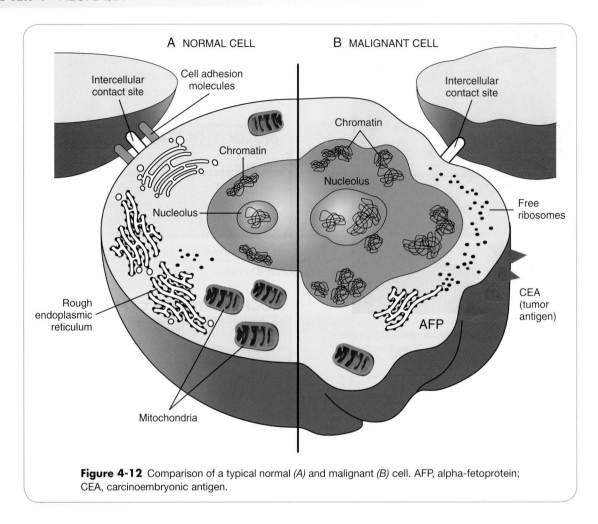

Figure 4-12 Comparison of a typical normal *(A)* and malignant *(B)* cell. AFP, alpha-fetoprotein; CEA, carcinoembryonic antigen.

new, atypical features is called *anaplasia.* Anaplastic cells are larger than normal and often show nuclear irregularity. Tumor cells may also "regress" and assume fetal features. For example, liver cancer cells secrete **alpha-fetoprotein (AFP),** a major secretory product of fetal liver cells that is not synthesized by normal adult cells. Similar changes occur in intestinal carcinoma cells, which produce **carcinoembryonic antigen (CEA),** a glycoprotein normally found only on embryonic intestinal cells.

GROWTH PROPERTIES IN CELL CULTURE

Tumor cells have less stringent requirements for nutrients and can survive on their own outside the body. Cell growth in test tubes is called *in vitro* cell culture because the first dishes used for these experiments were made of glass (*vitrum,* meaning "glass" in Latin). Most differentiated normal cells require complex growth media and survive for only a limited time *in vitro.* Primitive cells, such as fibroblasts, can survive longer *in vitro.* Nevertheless, even these cells pass through only a limited number of mitoses and then die. In contrast to normal cells, cancer cells survive much more easily because they require only simple growth media containing carbohydrates, proteins, vitamins, and essential minerals. Many malignant

cells are actually *"immortal"* (i.e., they can be kept in cell culture indefinitely).

Normal cells that are explanted *in vitro* grow in an orderly manner, and when the bottom of the culture flask is completely covered, the cells stop dividing. This phenomenon is called **contact inhibition.** The malignant cells show no such contact inhibition and tend to pile up, forming aggregates and nodules. Cancer cells lack the adhesiveness of normal cells, in part as a result of a loss of cell surface adhesion molecules. Malignant cells tend to detach from the bottom of the culture flasks and float in the culture medium. All normal cells except the hematopoietic cells require firm support for growth (so-called *anchorage-dependent growth*). Malignant cells do not require such support and can be grown even in "roller bottles"—vessels that are constantly rotated to prevent cell attachment to the vessel wall. Cancer cells can be explanted into soft agar, in which they float suspended, forming round colonies. By contrast, normal cells, including the relatively sturdy fibroblasts, die if the agar prevents them from attaching to the surface of the dish.

The growth of tumor cells *in vitro* mimics tumor cell growth *in vivo* (i.e., in the body). *In vitro* tumor cell growth is *autonomous* and does not depend on exogenous growth stimuli. Many tumor cells secrete their own growth factors (**autocrine stimulation**) or express growth factor receptors that are amplified and respond to minimal external stimulation. The growth of tumor cells is *excessive* and unregulated because the neoplastic cells do not respond to the normal inhibitory influences of adjacent cells. Inappropriate cell-to-cell adhesion results in a lack of cohesion and detachment of cells, allowing cells to survive in anchorage-independent conditions. The lack of contact inhibition that normally prevents cellular overgrowth results in piling of cells and exuberant proliferation. As in the body, the growth of tumor cells *in vitro* is irregular and disorganized.

CAUSES OF CANCER

The cause of most human cancers is unknown. Nevertheless, many potential **carcinogens** have been identified, and the pathogenesis of many tumors has been elucidated (Figure 4-13). Because cancer is a multifactorial disease with numerous forms,

there are no general rules; for teaching purposes, however, it is convenient to divide the causes of cancer that have been identified thus far into two major groups: *exogenous* causes and *endogenous* causes. Exogenous causes of cancer include a number of **cancerogenic factors** (cancer-forming factors) that can be classified as follows:

- Chemicals
- Physical agents
- Viruses

Endogenous causes of cancer reside in the genome of cells and are, like other genetic traits, heritable. However, as we shall see, exogenous carcinogens cause changes in the genome of the target cells that are similar to those caused by endogenous factors. The distinction of exogenous and endogenous factors has become even more difficult since the discovery that some human cancer genes, so-called **oncogenes,** are identical to exogenous viral genes. Cellular oncogenes can be isolated and used like viruses to infect normal cells. This procedure, called *transfection,* results in malignant transformation of previously normal cells.

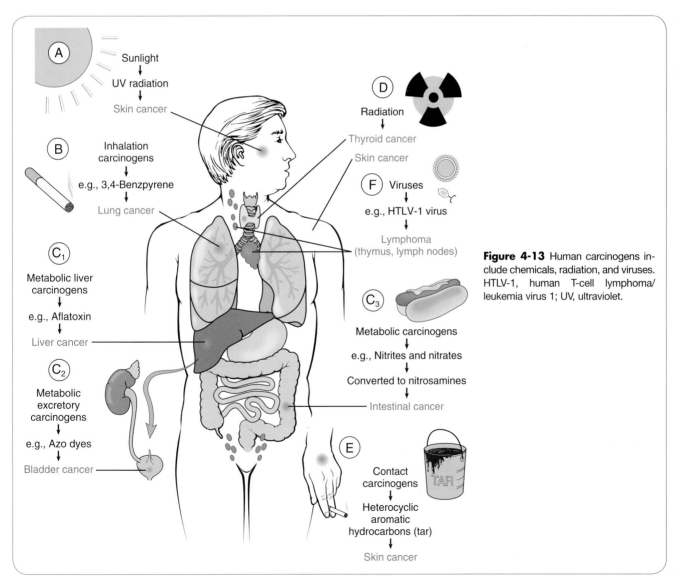

Figure 4-13 Human carcinogens include chemicals, radiation, and viruses. HTLV-1, human T-cell lymphoma/leukemia virus 1; UV, ultraviolet.

IDENTIFICATION OF HUMAN CARCINOGENS

The search for causes of cancer is usually based on a three-pronged approach that includes the following:

- Clinical studies
- Epidemiologic studies
- Experimental studies

Clinical studies include data gathered by practicing physicians observing cancer patients (Figure 4-14). Some of these clinical observations are reported in the medical literature as *case reports*. Other data are culled retrospectively into a large series that is then analyzed to provide guidance for future medical practice. Still other data are collected prospectively in carefully planned clinical trials. Knowledge about most human cancers is primarily derived from clinical studies.

Epidemiologic studies concentrate on identifying the exogenous causes of cancer in the environment and the endogenous (genetic) factors in the human population (see Figure 4-14). For example, epidemiologic studies have pointed out that lung cancer is caused by tobacco smoking. Asbestos-related lung cancer and pleural mesotheliomas were first identified by epidemiologic studies. Some familial forms of breast cancer and colon cancer were also identified by cancer epidemiologists.

Experimental studies can be performed on animals or cells and tissues removed from the clinically identified tumors (see Figure 4-14). Tumors removed by surgeons can be explanted *in vitro* and studied under controlled conditions. Many cancer cell lines have been established in such studies.

? Did You Know?

Did you ever hear about the cancer cell line **HeLa,** used in many research laboratories worldwide? This best known human cancer cell line was isolated in 1941 from a cancer patient at Johns Hopkins University in Baltimore, Maryland. HeLa stands for the first two letters of the name Henrietta Lacks, the woman from whose tumor the cell line was derived. Although Henrietta died, her cells are still alive in many research laboratories.

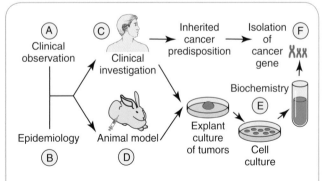

Figure 4-14 Study of the etiology of human cancer begins with clinical observations *(A)*, which are amplified by data obtained by epidemiologic study *(B)*, additional clinical studies *(C)*, experimental studies in animals *(D)*, and *in vitro* studies *(E)*. The final goal is identification and isolation of cancer genes *(F)*.

Experimental studies of cancer performed on animals may serve as models for human tumors. The presumptive carcinogens in the environment, such as various chemicals and viruses, are given to animals to produce tumors or simply to study the adverse effects of a potential carcinogenic agent. For example, rabbits were taught to smoke, which enabled scientists to study the adverse effects of tobacco smoke on lungs. Human genes isolated from tumors may be inserted into mice and studied further *in vivo*. Such transgenic animals, so called because they carry genes of another species, are excellent models for the study of human oncogenes.

The search for causes of a particular cancer usually begins with clinical observation. Any clues about the causation of that cancer based on clinical reasoning must be validated with epidemiologic studies. The suspected causative agent must be identified biochemically. The carcinogenic potential of the putative carcinogen may be tested *in vitro* and *in vivo*. The final proof is at hand when the cancer can be reproduced in animals injected with the carcinogen.

The classic story of such a search for causes of common cancer began in 1775, when the British physician Sir Percival Pott reported that the chimney sweeps in England often developed carcinoma of the scrotum. He hypothesized that scrotal cancer developed because of the adverse effects of soot that was rubbed into the scrotal skin when chimney sweeps straddled the chimneys. This observation was received with incredulity and remained forgotten for many years. In 1875, German epidemiologists noted an increased incidence of skin cancer in chemical industry workers who handled tar, which apparently contains the same possible carcinogens as soot. The German study was amplified in 1915 by Yamagiwa and Ishikawa. These Japanese scientists painted tar on the ears of rabbits and induced tumors, thus proving that the tar contained carcinogens. The tumors produced in rabbits were linked to dibenzanthracene, a chemical carcinogen isolated in 1929 from tar. Dibenzanthracene was identified in the soot as well. In the 1960s, it was shown that tobacco smoke also contains dibenzanthracene and related polycyclic hydrocarbons, which are all capable of inducing cancer in animals. These chemicals were applied to normal human cells in culture and were found to interact with DNA and cause genetic mutations that transform normal cells into malignant cells. More than 200 years after the initial observation, the pathogenesis of scrotal cancer in chimney sweeps was explained as a consequence of a chemical injury of the DNA in cells exposed to the adverse effects of polycyclic hydrocarbons.

Industrial Carcinogens

Humans are exposed to chemical carcinogens in many situations. The most important exposure is in the workplace because it can be prevented and the risk of cancer can be minimized through proper industrial hygiene. For example, exposure to asbestos, common in the ship-building industry during World War II, has been identified as a cause of lung cancer and asbestos is no longer used. Naphthylamine, found in aniline dyes, has been found to cause bladder cancer. Mining of nickel ore has been found to be associated with nasal cancer. Vintners using arsenic as an insecticide have developed skin cancer. All these forms of cancer can be prevented through proper protection and precautionary measures.

Drugs as Carcinogens

Many drugs successfully used in cancer treatment are also carcinogenic. Secondary cancer that develops in patients treated with alkylating agents, such as nitrogen mustard or cyclophosphamide, is an unfortunate complication of such treatment. However, the risk of developing cancer caused by drugs is low, so it is still better to try to cure a potentially lethal cancer, even if there is a slight chance that another will develop many years after. For example, Hodgkin's lymphoma has become a treatable disease, and most patients are cured with chemotherapy. Nevertheless, a secondary, treatment-related cancer develops in 1% to 3% of patients so treated.

CHEMICAL CARCINOGENS

Chemical carcinogens abound in our environment, and it is almost impossible to live without being exposed to some chemical carcinogen. Such carcinogens can be classified according to origin, chemical composition, or their mode of action, as listed in Table 4-3.

Chemical carcinogens can be classified as natural or as human-made. In the most important group of carcinogens, the so-called **polycyclic aromatic hydrocarbons,** one may find representatives of both (Figure 4-15). Aflatoxin B_1 is, for example, a very potent natural liver carcinogen produced by the fungus *Aspergillus flavus.* Polycyclic hydrocarbons, such as 3,4-benzpyrene, are important components of tobacco smoke. Tar and fossil fuels used in the manufacturing of gasoline contain the same polycyclic hydrocarbons. It should be noted that steroid and sex hormones also have a polycyclic structure. Sex hormones, especially estrogens, may also induce tumors in sensitive tissues. Estrogens produced in excess endogenously by the ovary and adrenals can cause cancer of the breast and uterus. Exogenous estrogens are also manufactured and administered as drugs. Many postmenopausal women who take estrogens must weigh the benefits of these hormones against their possible harmful effects.

Action of Chemical Carcinogens

The chemicals entering the body may act in several ways, as follows:

- *Locally.* Skin carcinogens, for example, act at the site of contact. Pulmonary carcinogens inhaled as smoke act on the bronchial mucosa.
- *At the site of digestion in the intestines.* This type of activation of carcinogens is typically mediated by intestinal bacteria. For example, nitrites and nitrates that are ingested in food are converted into nitrosamines, which may have a carcinogenic effect on the large intestine.
- *At the site of metabolic activation in the liver.* The liver is the primary organ involved in the degradation or alteration of carcinogens and other chemicals into other compounds. Aflatoxin is thus activated into a most potent liver carcinogen.
- *At the site of excretion in urine.* Aromatic amines derived from azo dyes are metabolized in the body and converted into potential carcinogens that are excreted in urine. These carcinogens act on the urinary bladder.

Chemical carcinogenesis is a multistep process. The initial step is the conversion of the potentially harmful substance—the **procarcinogen**—into a carcinogen. This conversion is mediated by enzymes locally active in the exposed cells or in the liver, which acts as the major conversion site for most exogenous chemicals. The carcinogens formed from procarcinogens act on the DNA of the exposed cells. This event, characterized by an induction of irreversible genetic changes in the exposed cells, is called *initiation* (Figure 4-16). In the second step, called *promotion,* the initiated cells can be stimulated to proliferate. Promotion can be achieved through continuous exposure to the carcinogen or to another substance that is not carcinogenic in itself but that can promote the growth of initiated cells. These substances are called *promoters.* The promoters must be applied until the cells acquire an ability to proliferate on their own and convert to a new cell type *(conversion). Progression,* the next phase in cancer development, is marked by an acquisition of new genetic features and expansion of cell clones that do not regress after the carcinogen or the promoter has been removed. These cells grow rapidly and give rise to identical daughter cells called *clones* **(clonal expansion).** Proliferation of divergent clones

TABLE 4-3 Examples of Chemical Carcinogens

Category of Chemical	Compound	Source	Mode of Action	Tumor Induced
Polycyclic aromatic hydrocarbons	3,4-Benzpyrene	Tobacco tar	Inhalation Skin contact	Carcinoma of lung Skin cancer
	Aflatoxin B_1	Fungi	Metabolic	Liver cancer
Aromatic amines	β-Naphthylamine	Dye and rubber industry	Excretion in urine	Bladder cancer
Nitrosamines	Nitrates	Food additives	Bacterial conversion in the gut	Intestinal cancer
Steroid hormones	Estrogens	Ovary/adrenal or injection	Stimulation of endometrium	Endometrial carcinoma
Metals and inorganic compounds	Arsenic sulfate Nickel sulfate	Pesticides Ore	Skin contact Inhalation	Skin cancer Nasal cancer

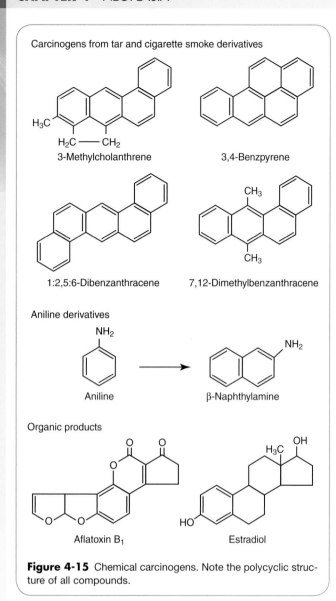

Carcinogens from tar and cigarette smoke derivatives

3-Methylcholanthrene

3,4-Benzpyrene

1:2,5:6-Dibenzanthracene

7,12-Dimethylbenzanthracene

Aniline derivatives

Aniline → β-Naphthylamine

Organic products

Aflatoxin B₁

Estradiol

Figure 4-15 Chemical carcinogens. Note the polycyclic structure of all compounds.

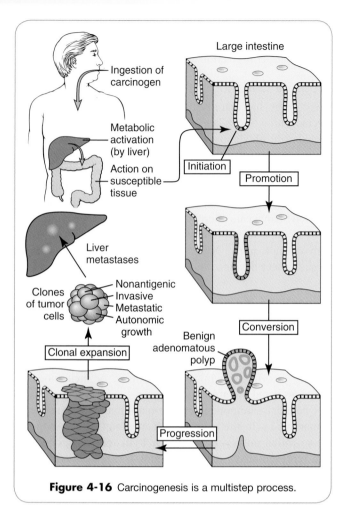

Ingestion of carcinogen

Metabolic activation (by liver)

Action on susceptible tissue

Liver metastases

Clones of tumor cells

Nonantigenic
Invasive
Metastatic
Autonomic growth

Clonal expansion

Large intestine

Initiation

Promotion

Conversion

Benign adenomatous polyp

Progression

Figure 4-16 Carcinogenesis is a multistep process.

that arise by mutation of unstable tumor cell genome leads to tumor cell heterogeneity. Some clones are invasive; others are capable of metastasizing, and others become dormant; still others differentiate along the same lines as the normal cells from which they have arisen. Diversification of tumor cell populations is unpredictable. Nevertheless, a *selection* takes place in favor of the most vital clones and cells that have adapted best to adverse conditions. Ultimately these clones outgrow all others.

PHYSICAL CARCINOGENS

The most important among the various physical agents that cause cancer is radiation (see Figure 4-13). Radiation may originate from several sources, such as the following:

- Ultraviolet (UV) light
- X-rays
- Radioactive isotopes
- Atomic bombs

UV light is a potent skin carcinogen. Long-term exposure to UV light in sunlight causes several forms of skin cancer, such as basal cell carcinoma, squamous cell carcinoma, and melanoma. Persons working in the sun, such as fishermen or farmers, are at increased risk. Skin cancer is most prevalent in the southern United States and is especially common in Australia. Light-skinned persons are at increased risk because they lack the protective effects of melanin. Skin cancer is uncommon among African Americans.

It is thought that UV light damages the DNA of skin, thus causing mutations that lead to malignant transformation. Incidental UV-induced DNA damage is enzymatically repaired in the damaged cells (Figure 4-17). Individuals lacking these enzymes, such as those with congenital **xeroderma pigmentosum,** a genetic defect, are particularly sensitive. Affected persons develop skin lesions early in life and must avoid sun exposure. They tend to develop skin cancer in childhood and puberty.

X-rays have been used extensively in medicine ever since their discovery by Konrad Roentgen in 1895. The pioneers of roentgenology were unaware of the carcinogenic effects of x-rays, and many of them developed cancer. X-rays have been considered a professional risk for radiologists, but with adequate protection this risk can be reduced to a minimum.

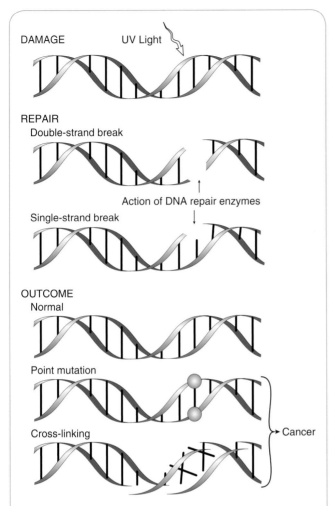

DAMAGE — UV Light

REPAIR
Double-strand break

Action of DNA repair enzymes

Single-strand break

OUTCOME
Normal

Point mutation

Cross-linking → Cancer

Figure 4-17 Repair of DNA damaged by ultraviolet (UV) light. Patients also have xeroderma pigmentosum and lack DNA repair enzymes. Abnormal DNA repair results in mutations that may lead to cancer.

Conventional hospital x-ray instruments pose almost no risk if properly used.

X-rays are also used for treatment of malignant tumors. Such radiation carries a definitive risk. Secondary tumors may develop but usually after a long latent period, sometimes 20 to 25 years after exposure. The benefits of radiation therapy outweigh the risk of secondary cancer.

Radioactive materials occur in the environment and are also human-made for use in research and for medical purposes. Alpha, beta, and especially gamma rays emitted by these radioactive substances have potential carcinogenic effects. For example, many miners in Joachimsthal, a Polish uranium mine established at the beginning of the twentieth century, have developed lung cancer from inhaling the radioactive ore. In those days the dangers of radioactivity were unknown and workers were not protected adequately. Factory workers who painted early phosphorescent watch dials with radioactive phosphorus in the U.S. plant that was operational after World War I developed bone cancer. Today we

are aware of these risks. The use of radioactive isotopes is tightly regulated, and the risk to fully protected laboratory workers is minimal. Similarly, the radioactive material used in atomic power plants poses very little, if any, danger. However, should a mishap occur, as was the case with the Ukrainian power station at Chernobyl in 1986, the emitted radioactive fumes may pose a serious health problem to the exposed populations.

The *atomic bomb* is a powerful source of radioactive material. The first atomic bombs dropped on Hiroshima and Nagasaki in 1945 caused not only immediate massive devastation but also long-term effects, including an increased occurrence of cancer. The most prominent among these neoplasms were leukemia and carcinoma of the thyroid. The incidence of the more common cancers, such as those of the breast and lung, also increased.

> **? Did You Know?**
>
> An increased incidence of thyroid cancer among children was noticed after the meltdown of the Chernobyl atomic power station. Most of the affected children lived many miles away, but all of them were west of the place of the accident. The prevailing east-west winds had obviously carried the radioactive fumes to places initially thought to be safe.

NATURAL BIOLOGIC CARCINOGENS

Some fungi produce potent carcinogens; for example, the fungus *A. flavus* produces aflatoxin. *Aflatoxin* was discovered when liver cancer began appearing in flocks of turkeys in England; the turkeys were fed peanuts imported from Brazil that were contaminated with the fungus. Aflatoxin is considered an important cause of liver cancer in subtropical and tropical parts of Africa and Asia.

Various parasites have been associated with an increased incidence of cancer and are thought to be involved in carcinogenesis. For example, infection of the urinary bladder with *Schistosoma haematobium,* a parasitic infection common in Egypt, is associated with an increased incidence of bladder cancer. Infection with the fluke *Opistorchis sinensis* is associated with an increased incidence of liver cancer in China. However, in the Western world such infections are uncommon, and the most important biologic causes of cancer are thought to be viruses.

VIRAL CARCINOGENS

It has been known for many years that certain animal tumors can be transmitted by cell-free extracts prepared from such tumors and injected into a new host. This was first shown by Whipple Rous, who studied chicken sarcoma and in 1910 induced the same tumor by injecting a cell-free extract of the original tumor into a new host.

Many years later the cause of these tumors was identified as an RNA virus known today as *Rous sarcoma.* Numerous other tumor viruses have been isolated from animal tumors since then. Depending on their structure, tumor viruses are classified as DNA or RNA viruses (Figure 4-18). The oncogenic DNA viruses become directly integrated into the genome of the infected cells. RNA viruses have an enzyme called *reverse transcriptase,* which uses the message encoded in the viral RNA to synthesize fragments of DNA. This DNA is incorporated into the cellular genome.

RNA tumor viruses are of two kinds: acute-transforming and slow-transforming RNA viruses. *Acute-transforming RNA viruses* direct the formation of a cellular oncogene that is the exact copy of the viral oncogene. This process is called *transduction. Slow-transforming oncogenic RNA viruses* do not produce a cellular oncogene. Instead, such viruses form a replica of their own RNA, which is inserted into the cellular genome at a point where it activates a latent cellular proto-oncogene into an active oncogene. The transformation of an infected normal cell into a tumor cell occurs only if this insertional mutagenesis occurs at a locus that activates an oncogene capable of transforming the cell. Because the insertion is random, numerous insertions must occur before a cell is transformed; therefore, such **oncogenic viruses** are called *slow-transforming RNA viruses.*

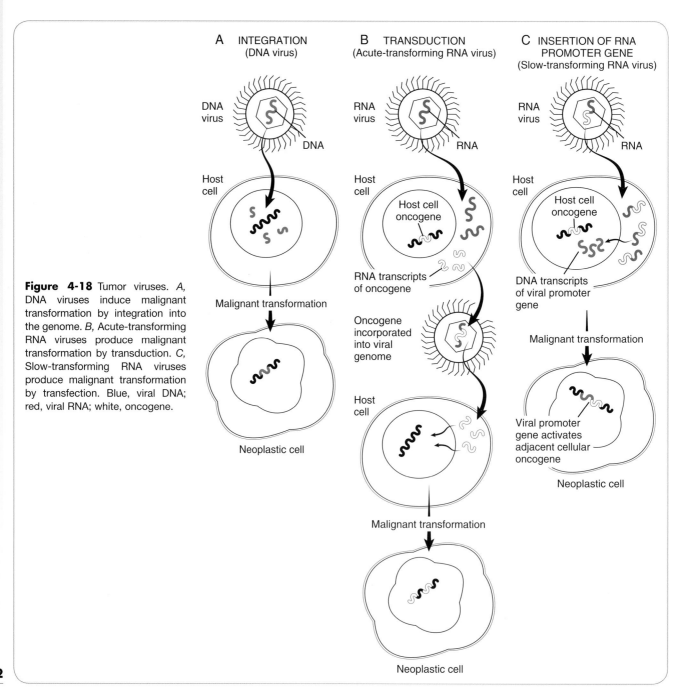

Figure 4-18 Tumor viruses. *A,* DNA viruses induce malignant transformation by integration into the genome. *B,* Acute-transforming RNA viruses produce malignant transformation by transduction. *C,* Slow-transforming RNA viruses produce malignant transformation by transfection. Blue, viral DNA; red, viral RNA; white, oncogene.

Human DNA Viruses

Several human DNA viruses have been linked to cancer. The most compelling evidence implicates the following viruses:

- Human papillomaviruses
- Epstein-Barr virus
- Hepatitis B virus
- Human T-cell lymphoma/leukemia virus 1

HUMAN PAPILLOMAVIRUSES

Human papillomaviruses (HPVs) are classified into more than 70 subtypes, several of which have been linked to human lesions, such as common warts, genital warts, laryngeal papillomas, dysplasia of the cervical epithelium, and cervical carcinoma. Some types of HPV cause benign lesions, whereas others cause malignant tumors. In the cervix of the human uterus, HPV types 6 and 11 cause lesions that are always benign. However, the lesions caused by HPV types 16, 18, and several other "unfavorable" types of HPVs have a propensity for progressing to cancer. HPV type 16 can be identified in 60% of human cervical carcinoma, and another 10% contain HPV type 18.

EPSTEIN-BARR VIRUS

Epstein-Barr virus (EBV) is a human *herpesvirus* that has a predilection for B lymphocytes. This virus is extremely prevalent. More than 90% of adults in the United States have antibodies to it, indicating that they have been infected with it at some point during their life. The infection may pass unnoticed, or it can produce infectious mononucleosis (the so-called kissing disease). EBV seems to be related to several forms of cancer, most notably Burkitt's lymphoma and nasopharyngeal carcinoma. **Burkitt's lymphoma** is a B-cell neoplasia that occurs most often in sub-Saharan Africa and typically affects children. Nasopharyngeal carcinoma related to EBV is most prevalent in China but may occur in other parts of the world as well. As shown later in this chapter, EBV causes chromosomal breaks that result in activation of endogenous cancer genes (oncogenes).

HEPATITIS B VIRUS

Hepatitis B virus (HBV) is a double-stranded DNA virus that is transmitted from one person to another by blood. Epidemiologists have noted that the high incidence of viral hepatitis in Japan, China, and Southeast Asia is associated with a high incidence of liver cancer. Numerous studies have revealed that the HBV is integrated into the DNA of neoplastic cells. The pathogenesis of HBV-related liver cancer is not understood because the virus does not contain any known oncogenic sequences. Experimentally, HBV cannot transform normal liver cells in culture into malignant cells. However, liver cell tumors that contain HBV develop in transgenic mice.

HUMAN T-CELL LYMPHOMA/LEUKEMIA VIRUS 1

Human T-cell lymphoma/leukemia virus 1 (HTLV-1) is an RNA virus that belongs to the same group of retroviruses as human immunodeficiency virus (HIV), the well-known cause of acquired immunodeficiency syndrome (AIDS). Fortunately, HTLV-1 does not represent such a public health problem as HIV does. This virus was originally isolated in southern Japan, where it caused a rare form of adult T-cell leukemia. Subsequently HTLV-1 has been identified in Africa, the Caribbean islands, and the United States. HTLV-1 can infect human T lymphocytes *in vitro* and transform them into malignant cells, which is definitive proof that the virus is carcinogenic.

HUMAN ONCOGENES

Studies of viral carcinogenesis led to the discovery of cellular genes that have the same structure and nucleotide composition as the viral oncogenes. In contrast to viral oncogenes *(v-onc),* these cellular genes were named cellular oncogenes *(c-onc).* It was shown that *c-oncs* are mutated normal cellular genes, called *proto-oncogenes.* Proto-oncogenes encode for proteins important for basic cell functions. Proto-oncogenes can be transformed into oncogenes by four basic mechanisms (Figure 4-19):

1. Point mutation
2. Gene amplification
3. Chromosomal rearrangement
4. Insertion of the viral genome

Point Mutation

Point mutation includes a single base substitution in the DNA chain, resulting in a miscoded protein that has an amino acid substituted for another amino acid. Point mutations have been observed in a number of human tumors carrying a mutated *ras* gene.

Gene Amplification

In the case of *gene amplification,* the cell acquires an increased number of copies of the proto-oncogene. For example, in widespread *neuroblastoma* of childhood, the tumor cells contain multiple copies of the *N-myc* gene. The more copies of the oncogene the cell contains, the more malignant is the tumor.

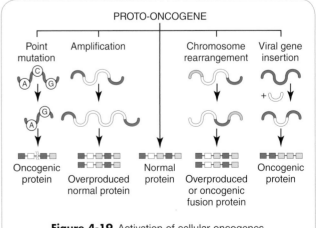

Figure 4-19 Activation of cellular oncogenes.

Chromosomal Rearrangements

In chromosomal rearrangements, translocations of one chromosomal fragment onto another, or deletion of a fragment of the chromosome, leads to juxtapositioning of genes that are normally distant from one another. Such gene complexes may result in overactivation of proto-oncogenes, stimulated by an adjacent gene that acts as a promoter. For example, *c-myc*, which is normally located on chromosome 8, is positioned next to the immunoglobulin gene in *Burkitt's lymphoma* because of the translocation of a piece of chromosome 8 to chromosome 14 (Figure 4-20). This immunoglobulin gene promotes the activity of *c-myc*, which ultimately results in tumor formation.

Insertion of Viral Genome

Insertion of the viral genome, an insertional mutagenesis typical of slow-transforming viruses, results in the disruption of normal chromosomal architecture and genetic dysregulation. HBV is found incorporated into the genome of liver cancer cells.

Proto-oncogenes have numerous functions in normal cells. Proto-oncogenes encode proteins that function as growth factors, growth factor receptors, and intracellular signal molecules. All of these proteins are important for cell growth, and their dysregulation can cause neoplastic transformation.

TUMOR SUPPRESSOR GENES

Normal cells have regulatory genetic mechanisms that protect them against activated or newly acquired oncogenes. Such genes are called **tumor suppressor genes.** For example, if a malignant cell is fused with a normal cell, the resultant hybrid cell will be benign because the tumor suppressor genes of the normal cell suppress the oncogenes contributed to the hybrid by the malignant cell.

The two best-known tumor suppressor genes are the *retinoblastoma gene (Rb-1)* and *tumor protein p53 (Tp53).* Several other tumor suppressor genes are listed in Table 4-4.

The *retinoblastoma gene* was isolated in studies involving a malignant eye tumor known as *retinoblastoma.* This tumor occurs in a *hereditary* and *sporadic* form and becomes clinically evident in early life. The *hereditary form* of retinoblastoma, which is often bilateral, shows a deletion of a segment of the long arm of chromosome 13 that carries the *Rb-1* tumor suppressor gene. If the remaining allele of *Rb-1* is mutated or lost in any of the retinal cells, such cells will not be able to control the expression of oncogenes. Accordingly, a tumor will develop in the retina. Other malignant tumors may develop in these children, albeit at an older age. Some patients with hereditary retinoblastoma have been cured of eye tumors but have succumbed to **osteosarcoma** that developed in their bones at puberty. This shows that the *Rb-1* gene has a general tumor suppressor function that is not limited to the eye (Figure 4-21).

In *sporadic retinoblastoma,* the child is born with two normal alleles of the *RB1* gene. However, if these alleles are mutated as a result of some exogenous factor and both *RB1* genes are inactivated or lost, eye tumors will develop. Such tumors are usually one sided.

Gene TP53, named after the molecular weight of the protein it encodes, is unique in that it acts both as a tumor suppressor gene and an oncogene. It may transform normal cells into neoplastic cells by transfection. A loss of *TP53* or its mutation leads to tumor formation. It has been implicated in the pathogenesis of numerous human cancers, most importantly carcinoma of the colon and breast.

HEREDITARY CANCER

It has been known for many years that certain human cancers occur more often in certain families. These observations have led to an intensive search for possible cancer genes. The *RB1*

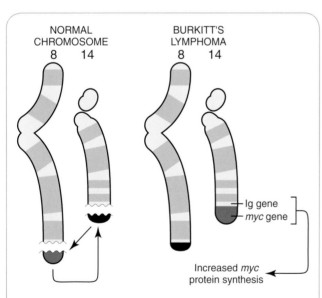

Figure 4-20 Chromosomal translocation in Burkitt's lymphoma leads to the activation of *myc* oncogene. The immunoglobulin *(IG)* gene juxtaposed to the oncogene acts as a promoter. Tumors are lymphomas because the immunoglobulin gene is active in lymphocytes. (Adapted from Kumar V, Abbas AK, Fausto N, Aster, JC: Robbins and Cotran Pathologic Basis of Disease, 8th ed, Philadelphia, 2010, Saunders.)

TABLE 4-4 Tumor Suppressor Genes	
Suppressor Gene	**Tumor Related to This Gene**
Rb-1	Retinoblastoma (eye)
TP53	Numerous cancers (e.g., breast and colon cancer)
NF-1	Neurofibromatosis 1 (peripheral nerves)
WT-1	Wilms' tumor (kidney)
APC	Familial adenomatous polyposis coli (large intestine)
BRCA1 and *BRCA2*	Breast carcinoma and ovarian carcinoma

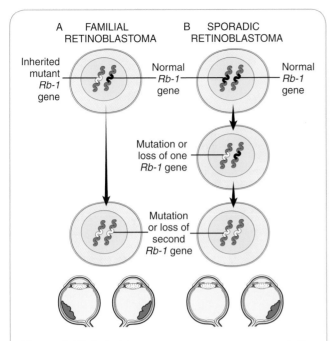

Figure 4-21 Retinoblastoma tumor suppressor gene. *A,* Patients with hereditary retinoblastoma are born with only one *Rb-1* gene; the other one is deleted. Mutation of the remaining *Rb-1* gene makes cells of the retina susceptible to cancer because such cells do not have any normally functioning *Rb-1*. *B,* Sporadic retinoblastoma occurs in persons who are born with two *RB1* alleles. For the tumor to develop, both alleles must be either inactivated or mutated.

tumor suppressor gene was identified through such a search, and many other tumor suppressor genes have been discovered in families with hereditary tumors.

Neurofibromatosis type I is the most common autosomal dominant disease in humans. The disease, which affects more than 3 million Americans, presents with numerous subcutaneous neural sheath tumors *(neurofibromas).* Affected patients also have pigmented lesions of the skin, called *café au lait spots,* and often have other tumors, such as intracranial *meningiomas* and adrenal pheochromocytomas. These lesions have

been linked to the mutations or loss of function of the *NF1* tumor suppressor gene. The *NF1* gene product is a protein that inactivates a cytoplasmic signal transduction protein encoded by the *ras* oncogene. If the *NF1* gene is defective or missing, the *ras* protein remains active all the time, leading to tumor formation.

Several other neoplastic syndromes are also inherited as autosomal dominant traits. The most important of these are *familial adenomatous polyposis coli* and *Wilms' tumor.*

In **familial adenomatous polyposis coli,** the large intestine contains numerous polyps that start appearing in childhood and are fully established in most affected family members by the age of 20 years (Figure 4-22). Over time many of these polyps undergo malignant transformation. **Wilms' tumor** *(nephroblastoma)* is a renal malignant tumor of infancy and childhood. Each of these diseases has been linked to a specific tumor suppressor gene (see Table 4-4).

The incidence of cancer is increased in families affected by certain inborn errors of metabolism. Among this group of diseases, which are usually inherited as autosomal recessive traits, is *xeroderma pigmentosum,* which, as already mentioned, is an inborn deficiency of DNA repair enzymes. Affected patients cannot repair the DNA damage induced by UV light and are prone to the development of skin cancer. *Chromosomal fragility syndromes,* such as Bloom's syndrome and Fanconi's syndrome, also show a predisposition to cancer. Inborn immunodeficiency syndromes also predispose individuals to neoplasia, especially malignant lymphomas.

Most common cancers are not inherited as Mendelian traits. Nevertheless, it is known that the incidence of breast cancer and colon cancer is increased in some families. Any woman whose mother or sisters had or have breast cancer has a five to six times greater risk of developing breast cancer than other women. The tendency for such persons to develop cancer is apparently polygenic and, like other polygenic diseases, is strongly influenced by exogenous factors. Recent discovery of a breast cancer gene is the first step toward elucidating the genetic aspects of this important human disease.

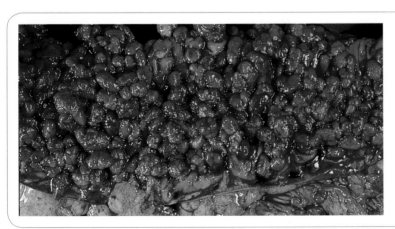

Figure 4-22 Familial adenomatous polyposis coli. Numerous polyps cover the mucosa of the large intestine. (From Damjanov I, Linder J: Pathology: A Color Atlas, St. Louis, 2000, Mosby.)

IMMUNE RESPONSE TO TUMORS

Benign tumor cells may resemble the cells in the tissue of their origin, whereas malignant tumor cells differ from their normal ancestors. Malignancy may alter tumor cells so much that they become "foreign" to the body's own immune system. **Tumor antigens** that are perceived as foreign to the body will induce antibody production and a cell-mediated immune response. Ultimately this immune response can limit the growth of the tumor. It is believed that many small tumors that form during the human life span are eliminated by the immune system. Many of the tumor cells that have entered into the blood circulation from established tumors are destroyed by the immune system. Some clinically apparent tumors that "heal spontaneously" also are most likely destroyed by the immune system. There is clinical evidence that some tumors may regress if treated by immunotherapy. All these facts point to antitumoral immunity as an important byproduct of the interaction between the tumor and the host.

Antigenic changes that occur during malignant transformation also have diagnostic value in the clinical laboratory. Among the tumor-associated antigens, the best known is CEA, a glycoprotein normally found on the surface of fetal intestinal cells but also expressed on adenocarcinoma of the colon. The measurement of CEA in the serum is valuable for monitoring tumor growth in patients with colon carcinoma. AFP, the major product of fetal liver cells, is also produced by liver cell carcinoma and is the most useful marker for this cancer.

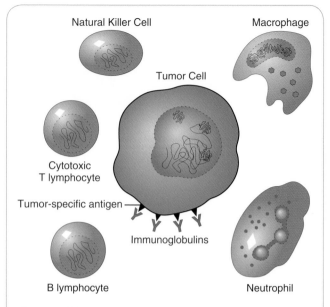

Figure 4-23 Host response to tumor cells is mediated by lymphocytes (T, B, and natural killer [NK] cells), macrophages, and neutrophils.

 Did You Know?

Cancer can heal spontaneously. Although this occurs infrequently, the medical literature contains many reports of spontaneous cancer cure. Scientists have been intrigued with such cases. Among these spontaneously healing tumors, the most common are melanoma, a pigmented skin tumor, and neuroblastoma, a tumor of malignant immature neural cells (neuroblasts). The cause of cure in such cases can only be surmised. It seems that the cure of melanoma is related to an immune response of the body. It is known that the immune cells can destroy malignant melanoma cells, and there are documented cases of regression of such tumors. Attacked by immune cells, melanomas lose their pigmentation and ultimately disappear. Neuroblastomas have been shown to undergo a peculiar form of maturation. During this process, the malignant neuroblasts transform into nonproliferating mature neural cells. In other words, in this respect, the malignant cells resemble maturing embryonic neuroblasts. Spontaneous maturation of neuroblastomas has spurred scientists to look for maturation-inducing factors as possible remedies for cancer.

The immune response of the host to tumor cells may be augmented for therapeutic purposes. The host response is mounted by NK cells, macrophages, cytotoxic lymphocytes, and, to a lesser extent, antibody-producing cells (Figure 4-23). The tumor cells that are highly immunogenic are the best targets for immunotherapy. Such tumors are typically infiltrated with lymphocytes, many of which belong to the NK cell sub-

set. The lymph nodes draining a tumor-infiltrated area may contain granulomas, which represent a cell-mediated immune response to the tumor.

Immunotherapy of tumors has achieved best results in the treatment of melanomas. These skin tumors evoke a strong lymphocytic response and may even regress spontaneously. Some of the fetal tumors, such as **neuroblastoma,** also may heal spontaneously by transforming into ganglioneuroma, a tumor composed of mature ganglion and glial cells. It is assumed that the immature tumor cells express the fetal antigens that are recognized as foreign by the adult host's immune system; immune response then modifies the growth or maturation of these tumor cells. Excellent results have been achieved in bladder cancer treatment by injecting attenuated tuberculosis bacillus, known as *bacille Calmette-Guérin (BCG),* into the urinary bladder. This nonspecific stimulus evokes an influx of macrophages, which destroy tumor cells. Unfortunately, most human tumors do not respond to any type of immunotherapy.

The important function of the immune system in controlling tumor growth is evident in the frequent occurrence of tumors in immunosuppressed hosts. People with AIDS typically develop lymphomas and Kaposi's sarcoma and other forms of cancer.

CLINICAL MANIFESTATIONS OF NEOPLASIA

Clinical manifestations of neoplasia are highly variable because cancer is not a single disease. Cancer may present in various forms; thus it is prudent to think of cancer whenever some unusual symptoms of disease occur. The seven **warning signs of cancer** listed under the mnemonic CAUTION are listed in Box 4-1.

The clinical features of tumors depend on the following:

- Type of tumor
- Location of the tumor
- Histologic grade of the tumor
- Clinical stage of the tumor
- Immune status of the host
- Sensitivity of the tumor cells to therapy

LOCAL SYMPTOMS

As tumors grow, they compress adjacent normal tissues. The symptoms depend primarily on the location of the tumors (Figure 4-24). For example, compression of the brain can cause epileptic seizures. Tumor of the lungs may compress

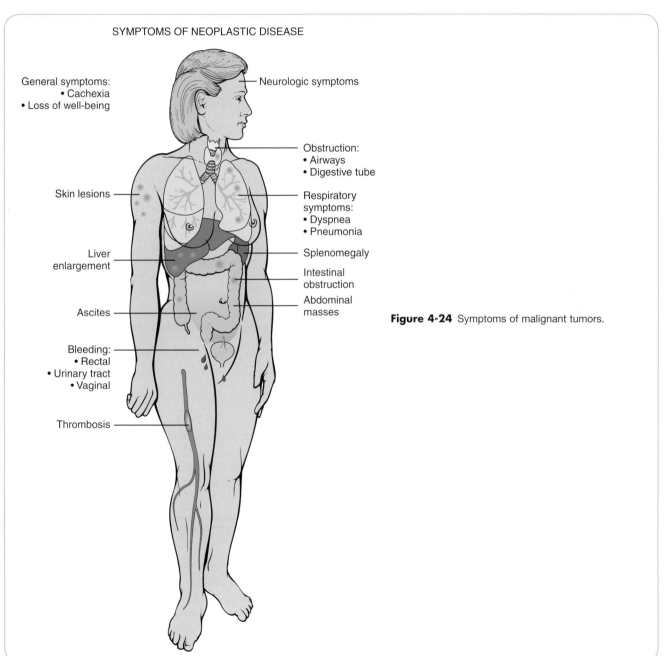

SYMPTOMS OF NEOPLASTIC DISEASE

General symptoms:
• Cachexia
• Loss of well-being

Neurologic symptoms

Skin lesions

Obstruction:
• Airways
• Digestive tube

Respiratory symptoms:
• Dyspnea
• Pneumonia

Liver enlargement

Splenomegaly

Intestinal obstruction

Abdominal masses

Ascites

Bleeding:
• Rectal
• Urinary tract
• Vaginal

Thrombosis

Figure 4-24 Symptoms of malignant tumors.

the bronchi and cause coughing. Persistent compression of normal tissues may cause atrophy, as is commonly seen in benign tumors adjacent to bones. Malignant tumors invade the tissues and also cause destruction of normal organs. Invasion of blood vessels and erosion of normal tissues by tumors often result in hemorrhage. Hemorrhage is actually the most common presenting sign of tumors of the large intestine, kidneys, and urinary bladder.

Tumors growing into the lumen of hollow organs, such as the intestines, may cause narrowing of the lumen or obstruction. In the large intestine the stools passing through a narrowed segment appear pencil-like. Ultimately, the intestinal passage could be blocked completely. Bronchial obstruction by lung cancer causes stagnation of mucus in the bronchus and coughing.

SYSTEMIC SYMPTOMS

Cancers cause a variety of systemic symptoms. These symptoms include **cachexia** or generalized weakness, weight loss, loss of appetite (anorexia), and a variety of *paraneoplastic syndromes.* Cachexia is caused by wasting secondary to the adverse effects of cancer on the body. Cancer can be considered a parasite that drains the energy from the body and also competes for nutrients. Cancers of the gastrointestinal tract may interfere with nutrition. For example, cancer of the esophagus may impede swallowing. Carcinoma of the pancreas may impede the entry of pancreatic juices into the intestine, which may lead to malabsorption of nutrients, minerals, and vitamins.

Paraneoplastic syndromes are caused by various substances secreted by cancer cells. Paraneoplastic syndromes include various endocrine, hematologic, neuromuscular, cardiovascular, and other changes. For example, carcinoma of the lung may secrete adrenocorticotropic hormone (ACTH) and produce hyperstimulation of the adrenals (Cushing's syndrome). Tumor-derived parathyroid hormone–related polypeptide (PTrP) may cause demineralization of bone and fractures. Bone demineralization is a common feature of breast cancer and is typically associated with hypercalcemia.

Many patients with cancer have hypercoagulable blood and develop thrombosis. This hypercoagulability results from the entry of tumor degradation products or secretions (e.g., pancreatic enzymes) into the circulation. In pancreatic cancer, thrombosis is often described as migratory; that is, it sequentially affects different veins without apparent order or regularity. Thrombosis is often associated with inflammation of occluded veins (thrombophlebitis). Migratory thrombophlebitis is known as *Trousseau's syndrome,* named after the doctor who first described it. Although it is most often associated with pancreatic cancer, it may be caused by other cancers as well.

An understanding of clinical symptoms of cancer is most important for the diagnosis and early detection of neoplasia. The most important cancer risk factors and presenting signs are listed in Table 4-5. However, it should be noted that cancer may present with many other symptoms. There are no symptoms specific to cancer; therefore the best way to diagnose this disease is to consider it in almost any clinical setting. Because most cancers remain incurable if diagnosed

TABLE 4-5 Risk Factors and Presenting Signs of Common Cancers

Cancer Type	Most Important Risk Factors	Most Common Initial Symptoms
Lung	Smoking	Cough
Breast	Family history of cancer	Lump
Colon	Family history of colonic polyps	Blood in stool
Cervix	Promiscuity	Vaginal bleeding ("spotting")
Uterus	Hormonal imbalance and treatment	Vaginal bleeding
Skin	Sun exposure, fair skin	Skin lesion
Prostate	Old age	Dysuria

BOX 4-2 Seven Safeguards against Cancer

Breast: Beginning at age 40, annual mammogram and breast exam by doctor or nurse; report any breast changes to your doctor or nurse

Lung: Reduction and ultimate elimination of cigarette smoking; avoidance of smoke-filled environments

Colon-rectum: Beginning at age 50, regular colorectal testing; talk to your doctor about the test that is best for you

Cervix: Beginning 3 years after becoming sexually active or no later than age 21, regular Pap tests every 1 to 2 years; beginning at age 30 may have Pap test every 2 to 3 years if a woman has had 3 normal Pap tests in a row

Prostate: Beginning at age 50, talk to doctor about risks and potential benefits of testing so you can decide if testing is the right choice for you

Skin: Avoidance of excessive exposure to sun or tanning beds

Oral: examination of oral cavity as part of periodic health checkup

Basic: Routine periodic physical examination for all adults

From the American Cancer Society, 2010.

in an advanced stage, the best hope of conquering cancer lies in its early detection and regular preventive examinations. Seven safeguards against cancer recommended by the American Cancer Society are listed in Box 4-2.

CANCER EPIDEMIOLOGY

Epidemiology of neoplasia is concerned with the study of cancer in human populations. Epidemiologic studies are based on data gathered from cancer registries and clinical records or by active inquiry. In prospective studies, epidemiologic data are used for vital statistics and for planning of health policies. The most important epidemiologic data relate to cancer incidence, prevalence, and mortality.

INCIDENCE

Incidence of cancer is the number of new cases that have been registered over a specific period in a defined population. It has been shown that the incidence of cancer varies geographically. For example, gastric cancer is common in Japan and Iceland and is less common in Western Europe and the United States. This discrepancy is thought to be attributable to different dietary habits and the high consumption of raw and smoked fish in the former countries. Indeed, the descendants of Japanese immigrants in the United States have less cancer of the stomach than their relatives who are still living in Japan.

The incidence of cancer in the United States has changed over the past 50 years. Gastric cancer, which was prevalent in earlier years, has become less common than colon cancer. The incidence of lung carcinoma has been rising. This form of cancer was uncommon among women, but today it is as common in women as in men. These changes in the incidence of cancer reflect changes in living conditions, habits, and diet. For example, the increased incidence of lung cancer in women is directly related to an increase in smoking that occurred when women joined the work force during World War II. The most common sites of cancer in males and females and the mortality associated with neoplasms are shown in Figure 4-25.

PREVALENCE

Prevalence of cancer is the number of all cases of cancer—new and old—within a defined population at a defined time. The prevalence of cancer has increased over the years. This is in

Males			Females		
Estimated New Cases					
Colon and rectum	75,590	10%	Breast	192,370	27%
Kidney and renal pelvis	35,430	5%	Colon and rectum	71,380	10%
Leukemia	25,630	3%	Kidney and renal pelvis	22,330	3%
Lung and bronchus	116,090	15%	Lung and bronchus	103,350	14%
Melanoma of the skin	39,080	5%	Melanoma of the skin	29,640	4%
Non-Hodgkin lymphoma	35,990	5%	Non-Hodgkin lymphoma	29,990	4%
Oral cavity and pharynx	25,240	3%	Ovary	21,550	3%
Pancreas	21,050	3%	Pancreas	21,420	3%
Prostate	192,280	25%	Thyroid	27,200	4%
Urinary bladder	52,810	7%	Uterine corpus	42,160	6%
All sites	766,130	100%	All sites	713,220	100%
Estimated Deaths					
Colon and rectum	25,240	9%	Brain and other nervous system	5,590	2%
Esophagus	11,490	4%	Breast	40,170	15%
Kidney and renal pelvis	8,160	3%	Colon and rectum	24,680	9%
Leukemia	12,590	4%	Leukemia	9,280	3%
Liver and intrahepatic bile duct	12,090	4%	Liver and intrahepatic bile duct	6,070	2%
Lung and bronchus	88,900	30%	Lung and bronchus	70,490	26%
Non-Hodgkin lymphoma	9,830	3%	Non-Hodgkin lymphoma	9,670	4%
Pancreas	18,030	6%	Ovary	14,600	5%
Prostate	27,360	9%	Pancreas	17,210	6%
Urinary bladder	10,180	3%	Uterine corpus	7,780	3%
All sites	292,540	100%	All sites	269,800	100%

Figure 4-25 Leading sites of new cancer cases and deaths—2009 estimates. (Source: Estimated new cases are based on 1995–2005 incidence rates from 41 states and the District of Columbia as reported by the North American Association of Central Cancer Registries (NAACCR), representing about 85% of the U.S. population. Estimated deaths are based on data from *U.S. Mortality Data, 1969–2006,* National Center for Health Statistics, Centers for Disease Control and Prevention, 2009, compiled by American Cancer Society, Inc., Surveillance and Health Policy Research, 2009. *Cancer Facts and Figures, Estimated New Cancer Cases and Deaths by Sex, U.S., 2009,* accessed at www. Cancer.org, February, 2010. Rounded to the nearest 10; estimated new cases exclude basal and squamous cell skin cancers and *in situ* carcinomas except urinary bladder. About 62,280 female carcinoma *in situ* of the breast and 53,120 melanoma *in situ* will be newly diagnosed in 2009.)

part attributable to improved diagnostic methods and life-prolonging treatment, but it may also be the result of increased exposure to environmental carcinogens. Prevalence of skin cancer is directly correlated with sun exposure. Thus it is no wonder that skin cancer is more prevalent in the southern United States than in the north. Prostate cancer is more prevalent in the elderly population. The increased prevalence of prostate cancer correlates with the generally increased longevity of human populations, especially in the Western world.

MORTALITY

Mortality of cancer is the number of deaths attributed to cancer during a specified period in a defined population. For example, the mortality of patients with testicular cancer has decreased dramatically since the 1970s. However, the mortality from lung cancer has remained the same over the past 30 years.

The study of epidemiology has provided new insights into the endogenous and exogenous causes of cancer. Among the most important exogenous cancer-provoking agents identified in these studies are the following:

- Smoking, as the major cause of lung cancer
- Sunlight, as the major cause of skin cancer
- Dietary fats, as the possible cause of colon cancer

In the industrial setting, epidemiologic studies have identified such carcinogens as asbestos (as a cause of lung cancer and mesothelioma) and aniline dyes (as a cause of bladder cancer). However, the cause of most human cancers remains unknown.

 Did You Know?

The overall incidence of cancer is on the increase. However, cancer is not a new disease. Archeologists have found bone tumors in Egyptian mummies and even in cavemen. Because cancer occurs most often in older people, and there are more older men and women than ever before in history, the increased incidence of cancer in our times is not unexpected.

 Did You Know?

Cancer is the second most common cause of death in the United States, eclipsed only by cardiovascular disease. More than 500,000 persons die of cancer every year.

REVIEW QUESTIONS

1. What are neoplasms?
2. How are human tumors classified?
3. What are the main differences between benign and malignant tumors?
4. How do tumors metastasize?
5. List a few benign mesenchymal tumors and their malignant equivalents.
6. List a few benign epithelial tumors and their malignant equivalents.
7. How do carcinomas differ from sarcomas?
8. Define lymphoma, glioma, seminoma, and teratoma.
9. List three eponymic tumors.
10. What is the difference between tumor staging and grading?
11. Compare normal and malignant cells, taking into account their morphology, some basic biologic functions, and biochemical properties.
12. How do tumor cells grow *in vitro*?
13. What are the most important exogenous and endogenous causes of cancer?
14. How do scientists identify potential human carcinogens?
15. List some chemical carcinogens and explain how they cause cancer.
16. How does ultraviolet light cause cancer?
17. Compare the carcinogenic action of oncogenic RNA and DNA viruses.
18. Which human DNA viruses have been linked to cancer?
19. How do proto-oncogenes transform into oncogenes?
20. What are tumor suppressor genes, and how do they cause cancer?
21. Explain the role of heredity in the pathogenesis of cancer.
22. Describe the immune response to tumors and explain its clinical significance.
23. What are the common warning signs of neoplasia?
24. Explain the pathogenesis of common local symptoms of neoplasia.
25. What is the pathogenesis of tumor-induced cachexia and hypercoagulability of blood?
26. Define paraneoplastic syndrome and provide specific examples of syndromes dominated by endocrine, hematologic, or neuromuscular changes.
27. List some risk factors for common cancers.
28. What is the difference between incidence and prevalence of cancer?
29. The incidence of which cancers has increased or decreased over the past 60 years?
30. Discuss important safeguards against cancer.

Genetic and Developmental Diseases

5

Chapter Outline

NORMAL EMBRYONIC DEVELOPMENT
DEVELOPMENTAL MALFORMATIONS
  Genetic Factors
  Exogenous Teratogens
    Physical Teratogens
    Chemical Teratogens
    Microbial Teratogens
  Chromosomal Abnormalities
    Structural Chromosomal Abnormalities
    Numerical Chromosomal Abnormalities
    Abnormalities of Sex Chromosomes
  Single-Gene Disorders
    Autosomal Dominant Disorders
    Autosomal Recessive Disorders
    X-Linked Recessive Disorders

Multifactorial Inheritance
  Anencephaly
  Diabetes Mellitus
Prenatal Diagnosis
Prematurity
  Neonatal Respiratory Distress Syndrome
Birth Injury
Sudden Infant Death Syndrome

Key Terms and Concepts

Anencephaly
Autosomal dominant inheritance
Autosomal recessive inheritance
Birth injury
Chorionic villus biopsy
Chromosomal abnormalities, numerical and structural
Cystic fibrosis
Cytogenetics
Down's syndrome
Dysraphic anomaly

Fetal alcohol syndrome (FAS)
Fragile X syndrome
Hemophilia
Klinefelter's syndrome
Lysosomal storage diseases
Marfan's syndrome
Mendelian genetics
Multifactorial inheritance
Muscular dystrophies
Neonatal respiratory distress syndrome

Phenylketonuria (PKU)
Prematurity
Prenatal diagnosis
Spina bifida
Sudden infant death syndrome (SIDS)
Tay-Sachs disease
Teratogens
TORCH syndrome
Turner's syndrome

Learning Objectives

After reading this chapter, the student should be able to:

1. Define and describe the following: gamete, zygote, cleavage-stage embryo, blastocyst, germ layers, organ primordia (anlagen), and organogenesis.
2. Define developmental malformations (birth defects).
3. Explain teratogenesis and list the five most common identifiable causes of birth defects in humans.
4. Describe TORCH syndrome and list the four most common causes of this set of malformations.
5. Define the structural chromosomal abnormalities of deletion and translocation and explain their significance.
6. Define chromosomal monosomy and trisomy and give appropriate examples.
7. Describe three possible functional consequences of single-gene mutations.
8. Explain the principles of Mendelian inheritance.
9. List three important autosomal dominant disorders.
10. List three important autosomal recessive disorders.
11. Explain the pathogenesis of lysosomal storage diseases and give three specific examples of prototypic disorders.
12. List three important X-linked recessive disorders.
13. List the cardinal features of multifactorial inheritance and list three important diseases that are inherited in such a way.
14. Describe prenatal diagnosis of genetic and developmental disorders.
15. Define prematurity and list three of its causes.
16. Define fetal pulmonary maturity and describe how immaturity of the lungs causes neonatal respiratory distress syndrome.
17. List three lesions induced by birth injury and explain their pathogenesis.
18. Discuss sudden infant death syndrome.

The beginning of human life cannot be scientifically defined. Without fertilization, there is no human life. For practical purposes, we shall assume that life begins at the moment of fertilization—that is, the meeting of the female germ cell, or ovum, and the male gamete, or sperm. However, this is an arbitrary definition because the concepts of life and death are socially determined. These concepts have changed through history and will most likely change in the future as advancing technology inevitably expands our capacity to influence basic events of human life. For the purpose of this discussion, consider the following:

- Human life is just the continuation of the life of two living cells. Both sperm and ovum are living cells. One cannot produce living humans from dead germ cells.
- Germ cells ensure the continuity of life from one generation to another. However, technology has made it possible to modify or temporarily interrupt this sequence. For example, the sperm or ova can be frozen and stored in freezers at very low temperature (70°C). Frozen cells can be kept indefinitely and then used for *in vitro* fertilization. Even early embryos can be frozen and stored for indefinite periods. Such frozen embryos retain viability and can subsequently be defrosted and implanted into hormonally induced surrogate mothers in whom they develop into normal human beings.
- Human life develops only from cells that carry human genetic material. However, human genes can be isolated and transferred to animal germ cells. Such *transgenic animals* may express human genetic traits. In other words, some aspects of human life can be perpetuated outside the human organism.
- Human life cannot be generated from nonliving material. At this time we do not know how to produce life from inorganic chemicals. However, this does not preclude the possibility that one day new life will be generated in the test tube.

NORMAL EMBRYONIC DEVELOPMENT

Following fertilization, the newly formed *zygote* (fertilized ovum) divides into two and then into four and eight cells, reaching the stage of *morula* within 3 to 4 days (Figure 5-1). A central cavity is formed inside the morula as it transforms into a *blastocyst*. Early *cleavage-stage embryos* consist of cells whose developmental potential has not been firmly programmed. Loss of single cells at the two-, four-, and eight-cell stages can easily be compensated for without any adverse consequences. However, at the blastocyst stage, the fate of embryonic cells has been determined: Cells of the inner cell mass will give rise to the embryo proper, whereas the outer layer, called the *trophoblast,* will give rise to the placenta. After this stage of development, any cell loss in the inner cell mass will result in embryonic defects because such cell losses cannot be replaced.

The inner cell mass gives rise to the primordial *germ layers:* ectoderm, mesoderm, and endoderm. These germ layers produce the *primordia* of fetal organs (in German, *anlagen*). For example, the skin and the nervous system develop from the ectoderm, the intestines develop from the endoderm, and the bones and muscle arise from the mesoderm. The development of organs is tightly regulated by special master genes, called *homeobox genes,* which regulate and coordinate the expression of other genes in the developing tissues. As the genes are turned on and off, each organ goes through a specific organogenetic period. During the *critical stages* of *organogenesis,* which are those characterized by extensive cell division, migration, and cell-to-cell interaction, the developing organs are very sensitive to adverse external influences. Chemical, physical, and viral agents are most prone to induce developmental defects during these developmental stages. Generally speaking, the critical period for most organs is in the first trimester of pregnancy.

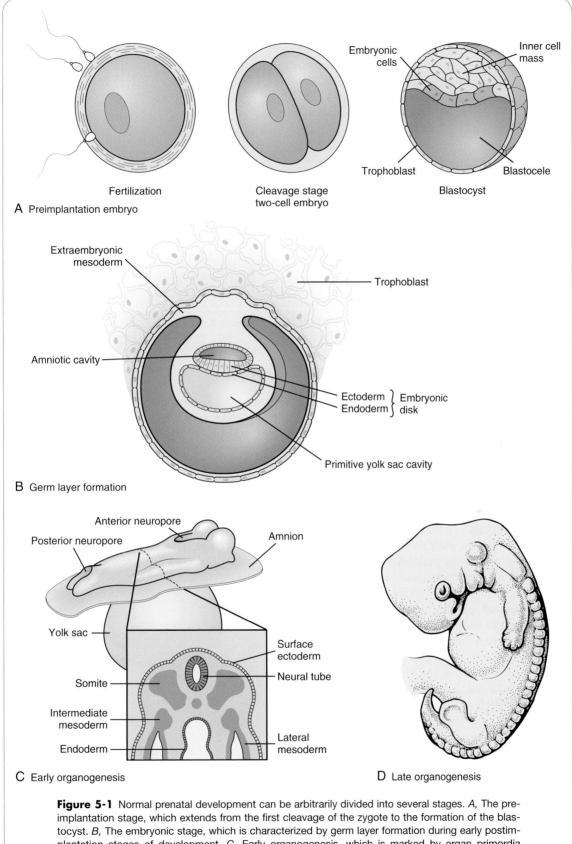

Figure 5-1 Normal prenatal development can be arbitrarily divided into several stages. *A,* The pre-implantation stage, which extends from the first cleavage of the zygote to the formation of the blastocyst. *B,* The embryonic stage, which is characterized by germ layer formation during early postimplantation stages of development. *C,* Early organogenesis, which is marked by organ primordia formation. *D,* Late organogenesis, during which the anatomic and functional maturation of organs occurs.

However, some organs, such as the brain, do not complete development during intrauterine life and are therefore susceptible to adverse influences for several months after birth.

In humans, the period of organogenesis that is conventionally called *fetal life* lasts approximately 9 months. During this period, the organs become anatomically recognizable; they assume specific histologic features and become functionally active. Anatomically defined fetal organs can be seen with ultrasonography. For example, by 10 to 12 weeks' gestation, one can recognize the fetal penis and determine the sex of the fetus. It is also possible to see whether the kidneys have been formed and to examine many other organs to determine whether they are developing normally.

Fetal organs have a "fetal histology," being composed of cells that have functions different from those of normal adult organs. For example, the red blood cells (RBCs) contain fetal hemoglobin, which at birth is replaced by adult hemoglobin. Likewise, fetal liver cells produce alpha-fetoprotein (AFP) as the major plasma protein, in contrast to adult liver cells, which secrete albumin. Fetal lungs are functionally immature because they secrete a different form of surfactant than the adult lung and therefore are incompetent for respiration. Functional maturation occurs generally at a slower rate than anatomic maturation. Many organs acquire full functional competence only at puberty, and some need special stimuli to mature. For example, female breast acini develop fully only after pregnancy and during lactation.

DEVELOPMENTAL MALFORMATIONS

Disturbances of development are the subject of a science called *teratology* (from the Greek *teraton,* meaning "monster," and *logos,* meaning "study"). The agents that cause fetal abnormalities (malformations) are thus called **teratogens.** The cause of most malformations (approximately 75%) is never established (Figure 5-2). Among the identifiable causes of developmental malformations, the most prominent are genetic factors (20%). Various exogenous teratogens, such as drugs, alcohol, or x-ray exposure, account for a small number of human malformations. Such chemical, physical, and microbial agents are nevertheless important to know. By avoiding exposure to potential teratogens, pregnant women can protect their unborn babies and prevent the development of some malformations.

GENETIC FACTORS

Genes inherited from the parents control not only specific traits, such as height or skin color, but also development *in utero.* The lack of certain essential genes or their mutation (lethal mutations) results in abnormal development. Such embryos and fetuses are not viable beyond a certain stage of development and are usually aborted spontaneously. Numerous studies performed on spontaneously aborted fetuses have shown that most of them had genetic defects and that many had abnormal chromosomes.

The genetic basis of malformations has been documented for a number of human congenital defects. For example, the incidence of cleft lip (commonly known as *harelip*) is

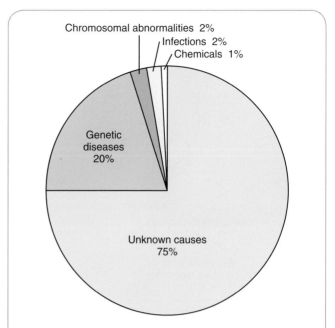

Figure 5-2 Causes of congenital defects in humans. The etiology of most defects is not known. Among the causes identified, genetic and chromosomal abnormalities are the most common.

increased in some families and is inherited as a multifactorial trait. *Dwarfism,* which is characterized by short arms and legs *(achondroplastic dwarfism),* is inherited as an autosomal dominant *Mendelian trait.*

? Did You Know?

This child was born with two heads that are incompletely separated from each other. The cause of this congenital malformation, like most others, remains unknown.

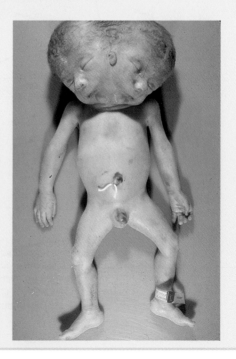

EXOGENOUS TERATOGENS

Exogenous teratogens are classified as physical, chemical, and microbial. Some of the most common of these are presented in the following sections.

PHYSICAL TERATOGENS

The best-known physical teratogens are x-rays and other forms of corpuscular radiation (alpha, beta, and gamma rays). Exposure to radioactive radiation during pregnancy thus poses a definite risk. For example, an increased incidence of malformations was noted among Japanese children born to mothers exposed during pregnancy to the atomic bomb explosions in Hiroshima and Nagasaki in 1945. Modern x-ray procedures require small amounts of x-rays and are considered safe. Nevertheless, unnecessary exposure to x-rays during pregnancy should be avoided.

CHEMICAL TERATOGENS

Many chemical teratogens exist in nature, and even more of them are human-made. These agents are often used in industry or are ingested as drugs. The most important set of preventable fetal malformations related to the maternal ingestion of a chemical is **fetal alcohol syndrome (FAS).** Alcohol abuse during pregnancy causes intrauterine growth retardation. It also affects the development of the fetal brain. Children who are born with the full-blown syndrome have typical facial features, such as a small cranium and jaws, a thin upper lip, and palpebral abnormalities (Figure 5-3). Most important, they

have reduced mental processes and lower-than-normal IQs. Other internal organs may be affected as well. Mental retardation can occur, even without these external signs of FAS.

> ### ? Did You Know?
>
> The cause of most human birth defects is not known. From time to time, however, we become aware of a substance that can produce birth defects.
>
> The story of thalidomide is a good example. It has taught us an important lesson. This sleeping pill was introduced for medicinal use in the late 1950s. Because nobody suspected that it could have any adverse effects, it was given to many sleepless pregnant women. First reports indicating that thalidomide caused birth defects were ignored. Subsequently, over a period of 5 years, more than 3000 abnormal children were born to women who took thalidomide during pregnancy. The children were born with malformed and shortened limbs resembling the flippers of a seal. (This malformation is called *phocomelia,* a term derived from the Greek words *phoca,* meaning "seal," and *melos,* meaning "limb.") Tragedies like this could have been prevented by proper drug testing. U.S. rules and regulations now require that every new drug be tested on pregnant animals to determine whether the drug is safe for use during pregnancy.

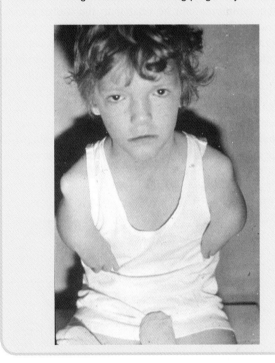

MICROBIAL TERATOGENS

Various infections during pregnancy may affect the fetus directly or indirectly. Indirect effects, which result from the weakening or physical exhaustion of the mother, typically cause fetal weight reduction, growth retardation, or premature birth. Direct effects, secondary to the transplacental passage of microbes and subsequent infection of fetal organs, are more serious and have consequences that are more deleterious.

Several human pathogens have been identified as especially noxious to the fetus. These infectious pathogens cause

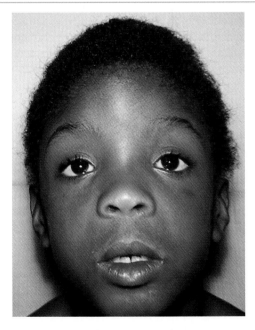

Figure 5-3 Fetal alcohol syndrome (FAS). Note the short palpebral fissure, length, mild ptosis, and long simple philtrum. (From Zitelli BJ, Davis HW: Atlas of Pediatric Diagnosis, ed 5, Philadelphia, 2007, Mosby.)

a syndrome of fetal defects known by the acronym **TORCH.** The name is derived from the first letters of the pathogens that cause it: *t*oxoplasma, *r*ubella, *c*ytomegalovirus (CMV), and *h*erpesvirus. The letter *O* stands for *o*ther less common infectious agents, such as Epstein-Barr virus, varicella virus, *Listeria monocytogenes, Leptospira,* and several other bacteria.

The syndrome is marked by the involvement of several internal organs. The brain is most often affected, and mental retardation, often combined with neurologic symptoms, dominates the clinical presentation. In children born with congenital rubella, the brain is small *(microcephaly)* and often structurally abnormal. In those exposed to toxoplasmosis and CMV infection, the brain shows *microcalcifications* of the basal ganglia and dilation of the lateral ventricles *(hydrocephalus).* Small eyes *(microphthalmia),* inflammation of the inside layers of the eye with calcifications *(chorioretinitis),* and clouding of the lens *(cataract)* are common. Heart defects are most common in those with congenital rubella infection. Inflammations of the liver and lung and reactive enlargement of the lymph nodes and the spleen are common. Skin lesions, such as *petechial hemorrhages and vesicles,* are also present, especially after herpesvirus infection.

All the symptoms can be related to the transplacental passage of infectious agents during the critical stages of organogenesis. For example, the triad of microcephaly, microphthalmia, and congenital heart disease, which is typical of congenital rubella, occurs only if an unimmunized mother is infected with rubella virus during the first trimester (Figure 5-4). Central nervous system defects, typical of toxoplasma, CMV, or herpes infection, can result even when the infection occurs during the later stages of pregnancy. Congenital rubella syndrome can be prevented completely by maternal immunization, but there are no vaccines against toxoplasma, herpesvirus, or CMV.

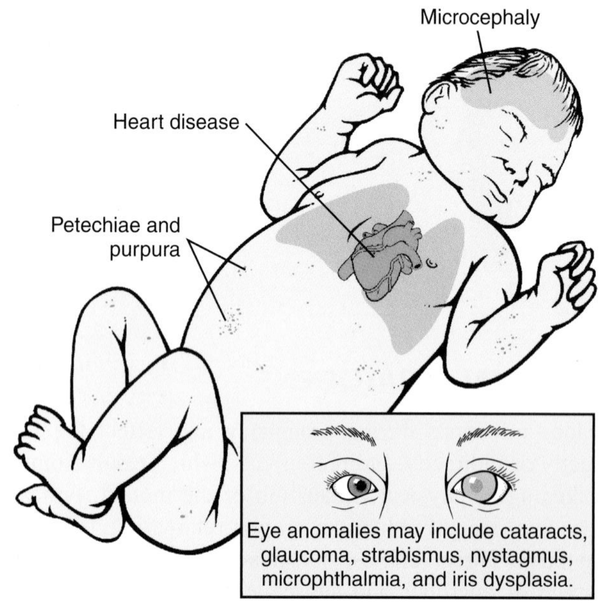

CHROMOSOMAL ABNORMALITIES

Human genes are encoded by triplets of *nucleotides.* Double-helix DNA is strung into *nucleosomes,* which in turn are arranged into larger units called *chromatin fibers.* During mitosis, the chromatin fibers condense into chromosomes, which can be seen on light microscopy.

Normal human cells contain two sets of 23 chromosomes. Twenty-two of these are in identical pairs, numbered 1 through 22 according to their unique features, and are called *autosomes.* The remaining chromosome, called the *sex chromosome,* may be either X or Y. Females have two X chromosomes and a 46,XX karyotype, whereas males have an X and a Y chromosome and a 46,XY karyotype. One set of 23 chromosomes is inherited from the mother and the other from the father. Because all female cells, including the maternal ovum, contain only X chromosomes, it is the paternal sperm (which may carry either the X or Y sex chromosome) that determines the sex of the child.

Chromosomal abnormalities can be classified as either structural or numerical and can involve abnormalities either of the autosomes or of the sex chromosomes.

STRUCTURAL CHROMOSOMAL ABNORMALITIES

Structural chromosomal abnormalities occur in many forms. The most important of these are *deletion* of a portion of the chromosomal arms and *translocation* of a portion of one chromosome to another chromosome (Figure 5-5).

Deletions of a portion of a short arm of chromosome 11 are associated with a complex syndrome characterized by congenital *W*ilms' tumor of the kidney, *a*niridia (lack of iris), *g*enital malformations, and mental *r*etardation (WAGR syndrome). Apparently, the lost, deleted part of the chromosome contains several genes that are important for normal development, as well as a tumor suppressor gene (Wilms' tumor [*WT*] gene). Children born with deletions of a segment of the long arm of chromosome 13 develop retinoblastomas, which are eye tumors originating in the retina. This segment of the chromosome contains the retinoblastoma *(RB)* suppressor gene.

Translocations are often associated with infertility, or congenital malformation syndromes. For example, some cases of Down's syndrome are associated with translocation of chromosome 21 to chromosome 14.

NUMERICAL CHROMOSOMAL ABNORMALITIES

Numerical chromosomal abnormalities involve a loss or a gain of chromosomes, resulting in a karyotype known as *aneuploidy.* Instead of the normal diploid number of chromosomes,

Figure 5-4 Congenital rubella syndrome is marked by a triad that includes microcephaly, microphthalmia, and congenital heart disease.

(Figure labels: Microcephaly; Heart disease; Petechiae and purpura; Eye anomalies may include cataracts, glaucoma, strabismus, nystagmus, microphthalmia, and iris dysplasia.)

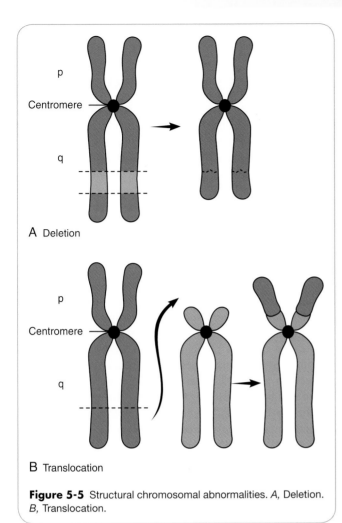

Figure 5-5 Structural chromosomal abnormalities. *A,* Deletion. *B,* Translocation.

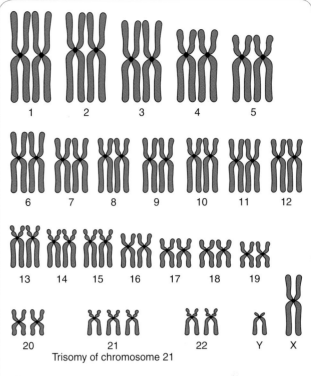

Trisomy of chromosome 21

Figure 5-6 The karyotype of Down's syndrome consists of 47 chromosomes and shows trisomy 21.

it may be hyperdiploid (46 + 1, 46 + 2, etc.) or hypodiploid (46 − 1, 46 − 2, etc.). The loss of one chromosome is called *monosomy,* whereas the gain of an additional chromosome is called *trisomy.* Autosomal monosomy—loss of an autosome—is not compatible with life. Similarly the embryo that has only a Y chromosome and no X chromosome usually dies early in pregnancy. On the other hand, embryos with a 45,XO karyotype are viable. Trisomies of sex chromosomes also are compatible with life. Trisomies of autosomes 13, 18, or 21 result in malformations and are often lethal. Most abnormal fetuses are spontaneously aborted or stillborn. Nevertheless, approximately 1 in 1000 neonates has an autosomal trisomy and is severely malformed.

Trisomy 21 (Down's Syndrome)

Trisomy 21 is the most common numerical abnormality involving an autosome (Figure 5-6). It is diagnosed in 1 of 800 neonates. It is clinically recognizable as a constellation of characteristic physical and mental abnormalities known as **Down's syndrome.**

The pathogenesis of Down's syndrome is not fully understood. It is known that trisomy of chromosome 21 is mostly of maternal origin and is a consequence of "nondisjunction"

during the meiotic (reduction) division of a maturing oocyte. Abnormal meiosis allocates an extra chromosome 21 to the ovum; if this ovum is fertilized, the zygote and all cells that develop from it in the embryo will have 47 chromosomes. In the notation of **cytogenetics** (the study of cellular constituents concerned with heredity), this is registered as 47,XX + 21 or 47,XY + 21, because the baby may be either male or female. The reasons for nondisjunction are not known, but it appears that this mishap occurs more often in older women, suggesting that the final stages of meiotic division are affected by advanced maternal age.

The symptoms of Down's syndrome include the following (Figure 5-7):
- Mental retardation.
- Typical facial features, including a wide face, a *low-bridged nose,* and *closely set, slanted eyes* with epicanthus. *Epicanthus* is a medial fold of the upper lid that gives the eyes an East Asian appearance. There is also *macroglossia* (large tongue), and the tongue often protrudes through the gaping mouth.
- Abnormal extremities. The legs and arms of affected individuals are usually short. The hands are wide and show a "simian crease" extending across the entire width of the palms. The fifth finger is shorter than normal and crooked.
- Congenital defects of internal organs, which may include heart defects, gastrointestinal atresia or stenosis, and infertility. Men are invariably sterile, but some women with Down's syndrome are fertile.

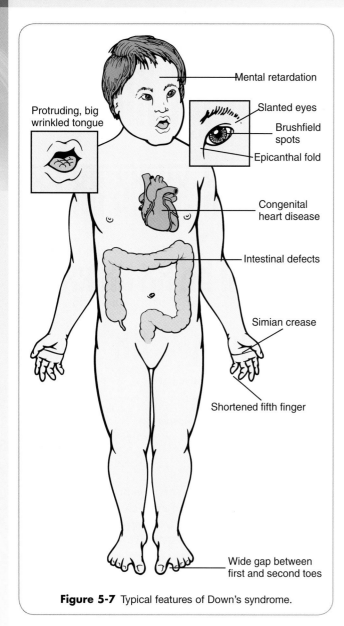

Figure 5-7 Typical features of Down's syndrome.

- Hematologic abnormalities. These abnormalities may be mild, such as anemia, but it is also known that Down's syndrome predisposes individuals to development of leukemia. Some patients also suffer from immune deficiencies and are susceptible to infections.

Down's syndrome represents a severe handicap, primarily because of the incapacitating mental retardation. Furthermore, there is increased mortality related to congenital heart disease and increased susceptibility to infections. With proper care, the life expectancy of affected persons can be prolonged, and the average age at death of these patients is 55 years.

Down's syndrome cannot be cured, but it can be prevented by timely cytogenetic studies in early pregnancy by *chorionic villus biopsy* or *amniocentesis* of material obtained from women at high risk. Because the nondisjunction of chromosomes occurs most often in oocytes of older women, who are thus at increased

risk of giving birth to children with Down's syndrome, prenatal diagnosis is offered to them on a regular basis.

ABNORMALITIES OF SEX CHROMOSOMES

Numerical abnormalities of X and Y chromosomes are more common in clinical practice than those involving the autosomes, and the karyotypic abnormalities of sex chromosomes are less lethal and cause less fetal wastage. The most important of these are monosomy X (45,X, or **Turner's syndrome**), which affects 1 in 3000 neonates, and trisomy of sex chromosomes (47,XXY, or **Klinefelter's syndrome**), which occurs in 1 in 700 newborn infants.

Turner's and Klinefelter's syndromes can be related to abnormal segregation of X or Y chromosomes during meiosis in the female or male gonads (Figure 5-8). If the sperm does not receive an X or Y and such a defective sperm fertilizes the normal ovum, the zygote and the embryo that develops from it will lack one sex chromosome. Clearly this could occur during female meiosis as well, and a zygote resulting from the fertilization of an X chromosome-deficient ovum will also contain only 45 chromosomes. If the sex chromosome in such a zygote is an X (45,X), a viable child with Turner's syndrome will be born. However, if the fertilizing sperm carries a Y chromosome, a 45,Y zygote will be formed; this zygote is not viable and will be aborted spontaneously.

Trisomy of sex chromosomes results also from abnormal segregation of chromosomes in meiosis. If the ovum retains both X chromosomes (24,X + X) and is fertilized with a Y sperm, the zygote will have 47,XXY karyotype. The same could result from the fertilization of a normal ovum with a 24,X + Y sperm.

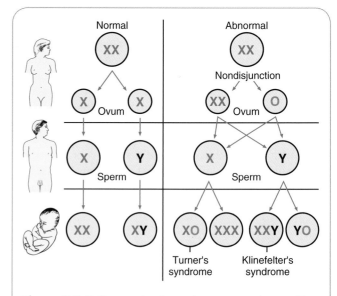

Figure 5-8 Pathogenesis of sex chromosome abnormalities. Because of abnormal disjunction during meiotic division, the ovum or the sperm may contain more than one sex chromosome or no sex chromosomes at all. Such gametes, when fertilized with a normal gamete of the opposite sex, will give rise to zygotes that are trisomic or monosomic for sex chromosomes.

Turner's Syndrome

Turner's syndrome is clinically recognizable by features that include short stature, webbing of the neck, abnormal extremities, a broad chest, and often, congenital heart disease (Figure 5-9). Patients with Turner's syndrome have normal female genital organs except for the ovaries, which do not develop normally. Ovaries in these patients are unable to nurture germ cells, which disappear early in infancy. The ovaries then transform into streak gonads—that is, fibrous strands devoid of oocytes and specific ovarian stromal cells. These women never experience puberty and do not develop secondary sex characteristics. Infertility is the norm. Sex hormone therapy may improve the individual's body image, but it will not cure the infertility.

Klinefelter's Syndrome

Patients with Klinefelter's syndrome are phenotypical males but are infertile. The testes of 47,XXY men are atrophic and are unable to produce sperm (Figure 5-10). Secondary sex characteristics in affected males do not develop at puberty.

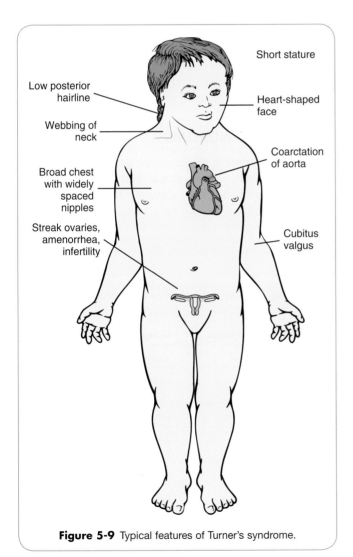

Figure 5-9 Typical features of Turner's syndrome.

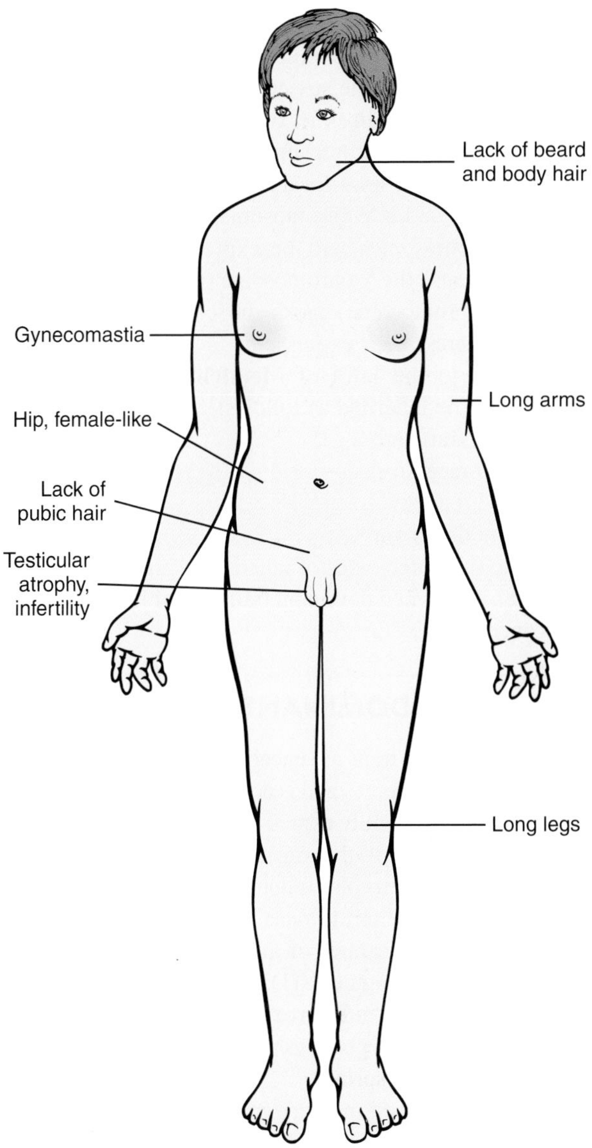

Lack of beard and body hair
Gynecomastia
Long arms
Hip, female-like
Lack of pubic hair
Testicular atrophy, infertility
Long legs

Figure 5-10 Typical features of Klinefelter's syndrome.

The penis is small and the pubic hair is scant. Typically these patients are tall and effeminate, with eunuchoid proportions and often *gynecomastia* (enlargement of the breasts).

SINGLE-GENE DISORDERS

Single genes are encoded by nucleotide triplets that occupy defined loci on the chromosomes. Genes located on the autosomes are all expressed in duplicate and are known as *alleles,* each of which is found on the same site of the two homologous chromosomes. In relationship to each other, these genes can be either *dominant* or *recessive.* Dominant genes overshadow the recessive ones. Persons with one dominant and one recessive gene express the trait encoded by the dominant

Short stature
Low posterior hairline
Heart-shaped face
Webbing of neck
Coarctation of aorta
Broad chest with widely spaced nipples
Streak ovaries, amenorrhea, infertility
Cubitus valgus

gene and are called *heterozygotes.* Recessive genes are expressed only if they are paired with another recessive allele—that is, if they are expressed in a *homozygous* state. In contrast to autosomes, the sex chromosomes X and Y do not represent identical replicas of one another. In females who have two identical X chromosomes, the rules of gene expression are the same as those for autosomes. However, in males who have an X and a Y chromosome, many recessive genes of the X chromosomes will be expressed as if they were dominant, because the Y chromosome (which is much shorter than the X chromosome) lacks the complementary alleles needed to suppress their expression.

According to the laws of **Mendelian genetics,** human traits can thus be inherited as follows:

- Autosomal dominant
- Autosomal recessive
- Sex-linked recessive
- Sex-linked dominant

Only the first three types of inheritance are discussed here, because the sex-linked dominant traits are of limited practical significance.

AUTOSOMAL DOMINANT DISORDERS

Autosomal dominant traits are encoded by a gene that is located on one of the 22 autosomes and is dominant in relationship to its allele. Thus the trait is fully expressed in heterozygotes (i.e., the trait is expressed even if only one copy of the gene is present). For example, black skin color is dominant over white skin color; therefore all children born to racially mixed couples will have dark skin. The basic features of **autosomal dominant inheritance** are as follows (Figure 5-11):

- The trait is apparent in heterozygotes.
- The affected heterozygote has a 50% chance of transmitting the gene to each offspring.
- The trait is expressed in every generation.
- The unaffected offspring of the symptomatic carrier do not transmit the trait.

These are general rules, and in reality some additional facts must be taken into consideration. For example, if a dominant trait becomes apparent in a child, one would expect that one of the parents has the trait. Sometimes a defective

gene is present in one of the parents, but the expression of the parental gene might have been hindered. This is explained in terms of *low penetrance* of that gene. If neither of the parents has the gene for the abnormal trait, one must assume that the child is affected by a *new mutation.* Finally, some children of affected parents inherit the abnormal gene but do not show the trait. It is assumed that such a gene has low penetrance.

For example, neurofibromatosis, a disease characterized by numerous peripheral nerve tumors *(neurofibromas)* and pigmented light-brown skin lesions *(café au lait spots),* is inherited as an autosomal dominant trait. However, in more than 50% of cases the parents of the affected person do not have the abnormal gene and the disease represents a new mutation. The children of some patients have full-blown syndromes associated with numerous tumors, whereas others develop only a few lesions, presumably because of low expressivity of the gene.

There are more than 1000 autosomal disorders; a few of the most important are listed in Table 5-1. From this table it is clear that any of the major organ systems may be affected, either directly or indirectly. Predisposition to several tumors is inherited as an autosomal dominant trait. The disease is often multisystemic. For example, the defective gene for collagen type I causes *osteogenesis imperfecta,* a disease marked by numerous bone fractures. However, many other organs in the body are also affected because collagen type I is present in almost all tissues. For example, affected children have blue sclerae because of the abnormal refraction of light through the eye, which is composed of abnormal connective tissue.

MARFAN'S SYNDROME

Marfan's syndrome is an autosomal dominant disease that affects 1 in 5,000 persons. It has been hypothesized that President Lincoln had this disease, because he had a "Marfanoid habitus." This disease is included here to illustrate how a structural protein defect can affect multiple organs.

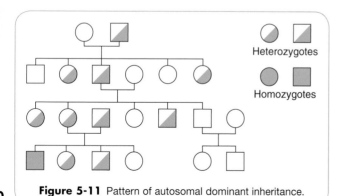

Figure 5-11 Pattern of autosomal dominant inheritance.

Heterozygotes

Homozygotes

TABLE 5-1	Representative Autosomal Dominant Diseases
Affected Organ/Tissue	**Disease**
Connective tissue	Marfan's syndrome
Bones	Achondroplastic dwarfism Osteogenesis imperfecta
Cardiovascular system	Familial hypercholesterolemia
Kidney	Adult polycystic kidney disease Wilms' tumor
Hematopoietic system	Spherocytosis
Gastrointestinal system	Familial polyposis coli
Nervous system	Huntington's disease Neurofibromatosis

Marfan's syndrome is a multisystemic disease (Figure 5-12). The most important features are as follows:

- *Skeletal changes.* The skeleton is slender and the affected person is tall. The head is elongated *(dolichocephalic)* with prominent frontal bosselation. The joints are loose and the ligaments are weak, resulting in frequent luxations and spinal deformities *(kyphoscoliosis).*
- *Cardiovascular changes.* The connective tissue of the large vessels is weak, resulting in dilation of the aorta *(aortic aneurysm),* fraying of tissue, and weakening of the vessel wall. The blood separates the layers of the weakened aorta, ultimately producing dissecting aneurysms, which are prone to rupture. The cardiac valves are also loosely structured (so-called floppy valves) and tend to malfunction, leading to heart failure.
- *Ocular changes.* The loosening of the ocular connective tissue causes deformities of the eye. The lens may be displaced *(subluxation of lens),* and cataracts, retinal detachment, and blindness are common.

The pathogenesis of Marfan's syndrome is related to the dysfunction of the gene that codes for fibrillin. This connective tissue protein is essential for the maintenance of tissue structure of various organs but most notably for tendons and other connective tissue-rich structures, such as heart valves or blood vessels. Tendons and vessel walls that are devoid of normal fibrillin become loose and cannot support normal body functions. Death is most often caused by heart failure secondary to valvular dysfunction or rupture of aortic aneurysms. *Exsanguination* from ruptured aortic aneurysms is a well-known complication of Marfan's syndrome.

FAMILIAL HYPERCHOLESTEROLEMIA

Familial hypercholesterolemia is probably the most important autosomal dominant disease. It affects 1 in 500 Americans and is a common cause of cardiovascular disease in the United States.

Familial hypercholesterolemia is caused by a mutation in the gene encoding the receptor for low-density lipoprotein (LDL). LDLs transport approximately 70% of the total blood cholesterol and are the principal carriers for the removal of cholesterol from the blood (Figure 5-13). This occurs through a high-affinity liver receptor that mediates the entry of lipids into the liver cells. In patients with a receptor deficiency, LDL cholesterol is removed from the blood only by a less efficient, receptor-independent mechanism. Inefficient cholesterol removal results in hypercholesterolemia and the deposition of lipids in various tissues, the most important of which are the arteries. This deposition results in accelerated atherosclerosis and an increased incidence of coronary heart disease. Deposition of cholesterol in connective tissue of the skin leads to formation of lipid-rich yellow nodules called *xanthomas.*

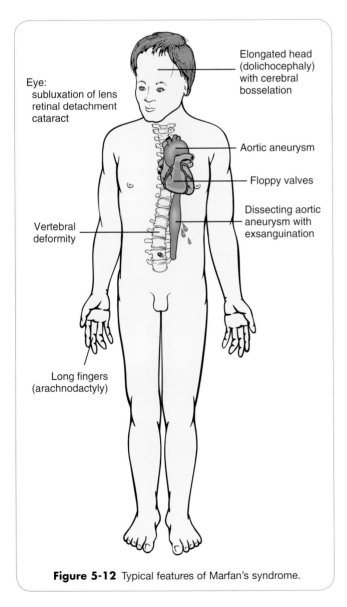

Figure 5-12 Typical features of Marfan's syndrome.

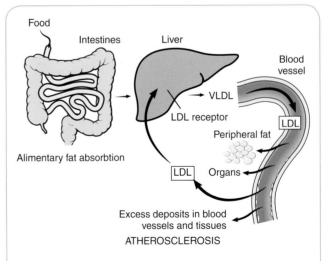

Figure 5-13 Familial hypercholesterolemia. The lack of a normal low-density lipoprotein (LDL) receptor results in hyperlipidemia and the deposition of cholesterol in the vessel wall, which leads to accelerated atherosclerosis. VLDL, very low density lipoprotein.

Xanthomas consist of macrophages that have phagocytized cholesterol (Figure 5-14).

Familial hypercholesterolemia cannot be cured. However, the progression of the disease can be retarded by dietary measures (low-fat diet) and even natural medicinal plant products that can block uptake of cholesterol in blood vessels. New cholesterol-lowering drugs, known as *statins,* can prevent atherosclerosis in these patients.

AUTOSOMAL RECESSIVE DISORDERS

Autosomal recessive traits are encoded by genes located on one of the 22 autosomes. These genes are expressed only under homozygous conditions—that is, only if paired with an identical allele. The basic features of **autosomal recessive inheritance** are as follows (Figure 5-15):

- The gene effect is apparent only in homozygotes who have inherited one allele of the mutated gene from each parent.
- The parents of the affected homozygote are usually asymptomatic carriers of the trait.
- The children of the affected homozygote and a normal spouse are not symptomatic, but 50% of the children carry the gene for the trait.
- Among the siblings of the affected homozygote, 25% are symptomatic homozygotes, 50% are asymptomatic carriers of the gene for the trait, and 25% are unaffected and do not carry the gene for the trait.

Diseases inherited as autosomal recessive traits are more common than diseases inherited as autosomal dominant traits. Nevertheless, because the symptoms occur only in homozygotes, the overall incidence of such diseases is lower. However, these autosomal recessive diseases are important causes of morbidity in certain populations. For example, sickle cell anemia affects 1 in 600 newborn African Americans. The

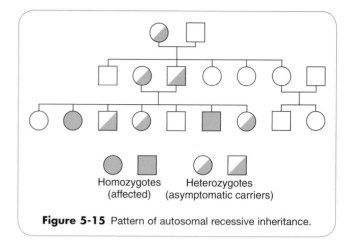

Homozygotes (affected)   Heterozygotes (asymptomatic carriers)

Figure 5-15 Pattern of autosomal recessive inheritance.

heterozygous carrier rate of the mutated gene for the *Tay-Sachs disease* is as high as 1 in 30 among Ashkenazi Jews in the United States. Representative autosomal recessive diseases are listed in Box 5-1.

CYSTIC FIBROSIS

Overall, **cystic fibrosis** is the most common autosomal recessive lethal disease, affecting 1 in 2500 neonates in the United States. It has been estimated that 1 in 25 persons is an asymptomatic carrier of the cystic fibrosis gene. The disease is almost entirely limited to whites and is extremely rare in other races.

The gene responsible for cystic fibrosis codes for the protein called *cystic fibrosis conductance regulator* (CFTR), which is the critical part of the chloride transport channel in the cell membrane. The defect in the transport of chloride across the cell membrane results in a lack of sodium chloride in the glandular secretions of all exocrine glands, most importantly the pancreas, intestine, and the bronchi (Figure 5-16). Because sodium chloride has an osmotic effect, those secretions contain less water and are viscid. The viscid mucus accounts for the synonym *mucoviscidosis,* another name for

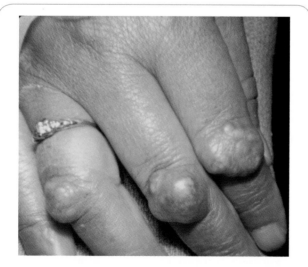

Figure 5-14 Familial hypercholesterolemia. Subcutaneous nodules formed from the accumulation of cholesterol-filled macrophages.

BOX 5-1   Representative Autosomal Recessive Diseases

- Cystic fibrosis
- Anemias
  - Sickle cell anemia
  - Thalassemia
- Lipidoses
  - Tay-Sachs disease
  - Niemann-Pick disease
- Mucopolysaccharidoses
  - Hurler's syndrome
  - Hunter's syndrome
- Amino acid disorders
  - Phenylketonuria
  - Albinism

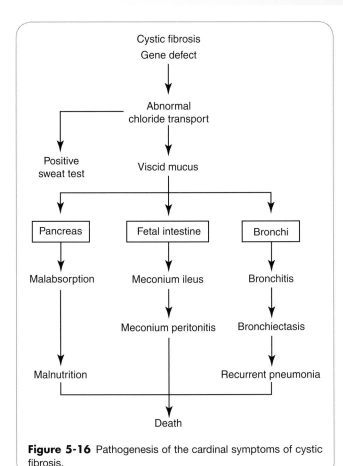

Figure 5-16 Pathogenesis of the cardinal symptoms of cystic fibrosis.

cystic fibrosis. Viscid mucus leads to the obstruction of the lumen of these organs (Figure 5-17). The obstruction of the fetal intestine by dehydrated meconium (the content of fetal intestines) may cause intestinal rupture and dissipation of intestinal contents throughout the abdominal cavity *(meconium peritonitis)*. The obstruction of pancreatic ducts with viscid mucus prevents the flow of pancreatic juices into the intestine. Because the pancreatic enzymes are essential for the digestion of food, *malabsorption* ensues. The stools contain undigested food and are bulky, greasy, and foul smelling *(steatorrhea)*. Affected children have *malnutrition* and typically show *growth retardation*.

The most important complication of cystic fibrosis pertains to the hyperviscosity of bronchial mucus. Bronchial mucus transforms into viscous plugs that prevent normal respiration. At the same time, the mucus provides a fertile ground for bacterial growth, predisposing the individual to recurrent bacterial infections. As a consequence of bacterial infections, patients with cystic fibrosis often have chronic bronchitis and bouts of recurrent pneumonia. Continuous infections cause dilation of bronchi *(bronchiectasis)* and pulmonary fibrosis *("honeycomb lung")*.

Other exocrine glands are also affected by this disease. From a diagnostic point of view, abnormalities of the sweat glands are the most important. Because the sweat glands cannot reabsorb chloride once it has entered their lumina, the sweat contains increased amounts of salt. This can be measured biochemically by collecting sweat or by stimulating sweating with drugs (the pilocarpine test).

Cystic fibrosis is an incurable disease, and most affected individuals die in their 20s as a result of pulmonary infections. However, prevention and prompt antibiotic treatment of

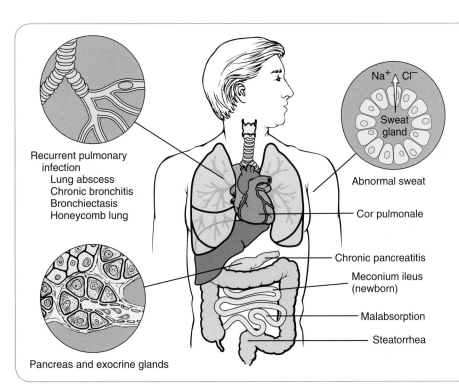

Figure 5-17 The abnormal chloride transport associated with cystic fibrosis results in a lack of sodium chloride in the secretions of all exocrine glands, especially the pancreas, intestine, and bronchi.

infections and correction of nutritional deficiencies may prolong the life of these patients.

LYSOSOMAL STORAGE DISEASES

Autosomal recessive diseases are often related to a deficiency of enzymes involved in intermediary metabolism. The metabolites that cannot be fully degraded, digested, or incorporated into other molecules accumulate inside the affected cells and are most often stored in lysosomes. These **lysosomal storage diseases** are classified, depending on the primary metabolic pathway affected, as lipidoses, glycogenoses, mucopolysaccharidoses, and so on. Furthermore, they are also known by eponyms relating to the names of the physicians who discovered them, such as Tay-Sachs disease, Niemann-Pick disease, Gaucher's disease, and so forth. These eponyms are still in clinical use, although many have been renamed according to the basic biochemical defect or the missing enzyme. For example, **Tay-Sachs disease** is a defect in the function of hexosaminidase A, which leads to the accumulation of GM$_2$ ganglioside. Thus it is referred to as *hexosaminidase A deficiency* or *gangliosidosis GM$_2$*.

All lysosomal storage diseases are characterized by the accumulation of metabolites that cannot be processed because of an inborn enzyme deficiency (Figure 5-18). These metabolites stored in the lysosomes can be recognized by electron microscopy as amorphous granules or concentric whorls of membranes (myelin figures). By light microscopy, such cells appear to be swollen and granular or vacuolated, especially if the material that fills the lysosomes is lipid (Figure 5-19). The final diagnosis is usually made on the basis of biochemical tests that demonstrate the specific enzyme.

The symptoms of lysosomal storage diseases are extremely variable. Some of these diseases are lethal in early childhood. Tay-Sachs disease affects the brain and eyes and causes death, usually during the first 3 to 5 years of life. On the other hand, some forms of Gaucher's disease cause only enlargement of the spleen and mild anemia but do not affect life expectancy. *Mucopolysaccharidoses,* such as Hunter's or Hurler's syndrome, typically involve the skeletal and the central nervous system and cause gross body deformities ("gargoylism," so called because the body resembles the gargoyle sculptures on Gothic cathedrals), neurologic symptoms, and mental retardation.

At present there is no cure for lysosomal storage diseases. However, most of these diseases can be diagnosed *in utero* and the affected fetus can be aborted.

PHENYLKETONURIA

Phenylketonuria (PKU), an inborn error of protein metabolism, is included here to show that enzyme deficiencies do not all result in lysosomal storage diseases. It is also included to show that the consequences of this enzyme defect can be counterbalanced and its deleterious effects prevented.

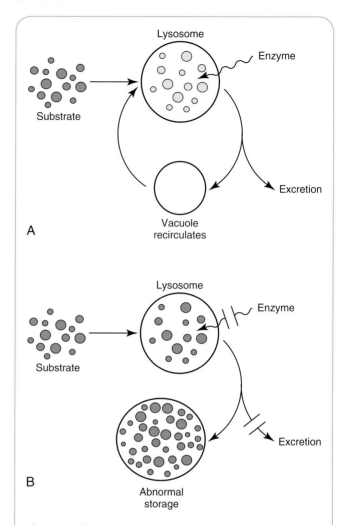

Figure 5-18 Pathogenesis of lysosomal storage disease. *A,* Normal lysosomes digest the material included within the lytic bodies. *B,* Lack of degradation enzymes leads to the accumulation of metabolic residues inside the lysosomes.

Phenylketonuria is a congenital deficiency of phenylalanine hydroxylase (PAH), an enzyme that metabolizes phenylalanine into tyrosine (Figure 5-20). Phenylalanine ingested in the food cannot be metabolized in affected individuals and accumulates in their blood and tissues. There is also a shifting of its catabolism into another pathway, resulting in the formation of phenylpyruvic acid and related phenylketones, which are excreted in urine. Phenylketones were originally detected in urine, hence the name PKU.

Infants born with PKU are initially healthy. Typical features of the disease include a lack of pigmentation secondary to inadequate melanin synthesis, which is inhibited by an excess of phenylalanine in blood. Therefore the children are fair-haired and fair-skinned and have blue eyes. They also have a mousy odor attributable to the accumulation of intermediary metabolites of phenylalanine.

The diagnosis of PKU is made at the time of birth, usually by routine screening, which is mandatory in the

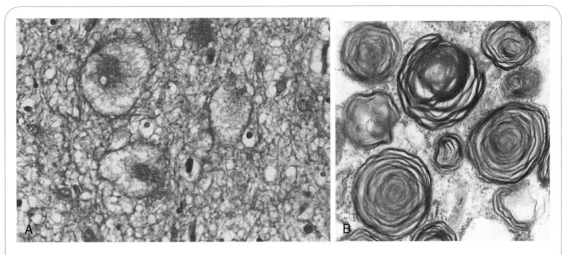

Figure 5-19 Tay-Sachs disease. *A*, On light microscopy the neural system cells appear to be swollen and vacuolated because their cytoplasm contains an increased number of lipid-rich lysosomes. *B*, On electron microscopy the cells are seen to contain myelin figures composed of concentric membranes.

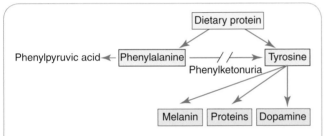

Figure 5-20 Phenylketonuria. Lack of phenylalanine hydroxylase blocks the transformation of phenylalanine into tyrosine. Unmetabolized phenylalanine is shunted into the pathway that leads to the formation of phenylketones. Excess phenylalanine also inhibits formation of melanin from tyrosine.

speaking, heterozygous for it express the gene in a "dominant" manner because the Y chromosome does not have the corresponding alleles to overshadow its expression. Because of their recessive nature, the X-linked genes are not expressed in females unless the person is homozygous, which is extremely rare.

The basic features of X-linked recessive inheritance are as follows (Figure 5-21):

- The gene effect is usually evident only in males and only rarely in females.
- The gene is transmitted from an asymptomatic mother.
- Sisters of an affected male are all asymptomatic. They could be carriers of the trait but may not be. Unaffected brothers do not carry the gene and do not transmit the trait.

United States. A special phenylalanine-deficient diet is prescribed for affected infants. This ensures normal psychoneural development. However, if the infant receives a normal diet that contains phenylalanine, the resulting hyperphenylalaninemia will adversely affect the developing central nervous system, causing slow but progressive and irreversible mental retardation.

X-LINKED RECESSIVE DISORDERS

X-linked recessive traits are encoded by recessive genes that are located on the X chromosome but that are not found on the Y chromosome. Because they are recessive, these traits are rarely expressed in females, who are usually heterozygous and have a dominant allele for this trait on the other X chromosome. However, males who carry the gene on their X chromosome and who are, technically

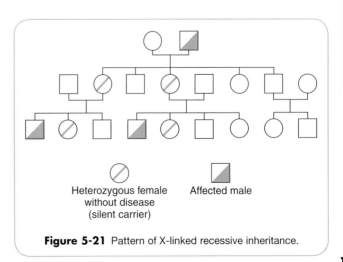

Heterozygous female without disease (silent carrier)   Affected male

Figure 5-21 Pattern of X-linked recessive inheritance.

- Each son of a carrier female has a 50% chance of being affected. Affected males do not transmit the gene to their sons, but all their daughters are asymptomatic carriers.
- The disease presents rarely in females, who are homozygous. These women have inherited one abnormal allele from the affected father and one from the asymptomatic carrier mother.

More than 100 genes have been identified on the X chromosome, and many of these are linked to important diseases (Figure 5-22). The most common of these diseases are listed in Box 5-2.

HEMOPHILIA

Hemophilia, a hereditary bleeding disorder, is linked to mutations of the genes that code for the coagulation factor VIII or IX. Factor VIII deficiency is the underlying cause of the common disorder, hemophilia A, whereas factor IX deficiency accounts for hemophilia B. Hemophilia A affects 1 in 5000 boys, whereas hemophilia B affects 1 in 30,000. The gene for factor VIII is located on the terminal portion of the long arm of chromosome X. It is a very long gene that accounts for 0.1% of the total genome of the X chromosomes. Such a long gene is subject to point mutations, deletions, or insertions that alter its expression. This is reflected in the frequent occurrence of new mutations, evidenced by the fact that 50% of all patients have the inherited form of the disease, whereas the others have a new mutation. The gene for factor IX is much shorter and less prone to mutations. Thus hemophilia B is less common.

Hemophilia A can occur in a severe, moderately severe, or mild form. The severity of the disease depends on the extent of the gene defect; more severe defects cause severe bleeding problems, whereas minor defects may prove to be asymptomatic or may cause only minor bleeding episodes. Hemophilia B is unfortunately always a severe bleeding disorder. Hemorrhage in the hemophiliac may be spontaneous, or it may follow minor trauma. Internal hemorrhage, especially into the joints *(hemarthrosis),* is common (Figure 5-23). Deformity of the joints resulting from hemarthrosis remains a common complication. Cerebral hemorrhage, previously a common cause of death, is rare today, because the course of the disease can be ameliorated through the administration of the deficient clotting factors and through blood transfusions. The genes for factors VIII and IX have been cloned, and the recombinant clotting factors produced in the laboratory are available for treatment of hemophilia.

MUSCULAR DYSTROPHY

Muscular dystrophies are diseases of unknown etiology marked by progressive wasting of muscles. In this group of diseases, two specific forms—known as *Duchenne-type* and *Becker's muscular dystrophy* (DBMD)—are linked to a single gene. This disorder, which affects males and is only rarely found in females, is inherited as an X-linked recessive trait.

The gene for DBMD, which has been localized to the midportion of the short arm of the X chromosome, codes for *dystrophin,* a structural cell protein forming a network beneath the plasma membrane that interacts with other cytoskeletal and contractile proteins. Without dystrophin, the cells cannot retain their proper form or adapt to stress and therefore tend to disintegrate. Although dystrophin is a widespread protein, the consequences related to its abnormality are most prominent in the skeletal muscles. The dystrophin gene is one of the largest human genes. The size of the gene defect may vary from one patient to another. This may result in either

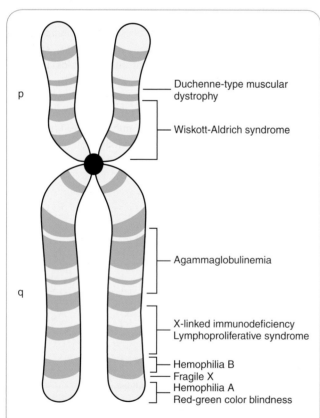

Figure 5-22 Representative genes encoding clinically important diseases mapped to the short *(p)* and long *(q)* arms of the X chromosome.

p — Duchenne-type muscular dystrophy
— Wiskott-Aldrich syndrome
— Agammaglobulinemia
q — X-linked immunodeficiency Lymphoproliferative syndrome
— Hemophilia B
— Fragile X
— Hemophilia A
— Red-green color blindness

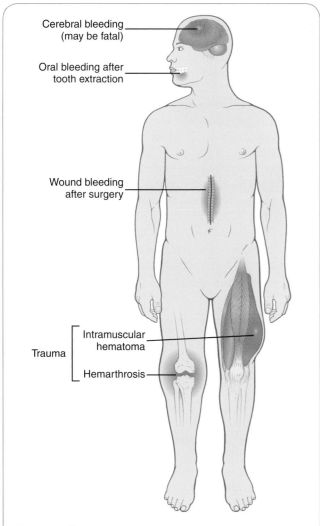

Figure 5-23 Hemophilia. Bleeding may occur as a result of minimal trauma. Hemarthrosis (accumulation of blood in the joint) is a common symptom.

severe muscular disease, which is clinically known as *Duchenne-type dystrophy,* or a less severe disease, known as *Becker's dystrophy.*

Duchenne-type dystrophy affects 1 in 3300 males, most of whom are born to asymptomatic parents. In two-thirds of cases, the mother is the carrier of the gene. It has been estimated that the spontaneous mutation rate of the DBMD gene is approximately 1 in 10,000. One-third of all affected persons have a nonfamilial disease related to new mutations. Becker's dystrophy is less common, affecting 1 in 20,000 males. Clinical features of muscular dystrophies are discussed in Chapter 20.

FRAGILE X SYNDROME

Fragile X syndrome is a form of mental retardation linked to increased fragility of the subterminal portion of the long arm of the X chromosome. In affected persons this chromosomal region, known as *Xq27,* consists of an amplified number of repeats of three nucleotides: cytosine, guanine, and guanine (termed the *CGG triplet repeat*). The chromosomal site occupied by an amplified number of triplet repeats appears to be more fragile than normal and can be detected by special cytogenetic techniques. It has been shown that 80% of males with this chromosomal abnormality have mental deficiency. Mental retardation can also occur in females with fragile X chromosome but less often than in males.

Children born to mentally normal carriers of the fragile X can be mentally retarded. This underscores the peculiar features of inheritance of trinucleotide repeats. These genetic anomalies seem not to follow all the rules of Mendelian genetics, and the symptoms related to the abnormal gene tend to become more prominent in each subsequent generation. One could predict that the incidence of mental retardation related to fragile X chromosome might increase in the future from the current rate of 1 in 1250 males and 1 in 2500 females. Even now it is already the most common form of hereditary mental deficiency in males.

MULTIFACTORIAL INHERITANCE

Familial diseases that are not inherited according to the rules of Mendelian genetics are considered the result of **multifactorial inheritance** patterns. Such diseases are the product of several genes that interact with each other and are also influenced by exogenous *(epigenetic)* factors. Most human traits and diseases are the end products of a complex interaction of genes and environment. The risk for developing multifactorial disorders can be estimated only approximately, and it is usually in the range of 5% to 10%. This risk varies from one trait to another and also can be altered by lifestyle, environmental influences, or other diseases. Representative multifactorial traits and disease are listed in Table 5-2.

Multifactorial inheritance has the following features:

- The trait or the disease is the product of several genes. The inheritance cannot be explained in terms of Mendelian single-gene inheritance.
- Exogenous and endogenous factors influence the expression of the trait and determine the severity of the disease.

TABLE 5-2 Multifactorial Traits and Diseases

Traits/Process	Diseases
Height	Dwarfism
Intelligence	Mental retardation
Blood pressure	Hypertension
Metabolism	
Carbohydrates	Diabetes mellitus
Uric acid	Gout
Development	Anencephaly Cleft lip or palate

- The genes encoding the trait or the disease show a dose effect, which determines the severity of the disease. Persons affected by a more severe form of the disease have an increased chance of transmitting it to their offspring.
- The risk of disease in siblings can be estimated on the basis of family data, the severity of the disease, and the sex of the affected individuals.

ANENCEPHALY

Anencephaly is a good example of a multifactorial developmental defect (Figure 5-24). This disorder occurs because of incomplete fusion of the midline structures covering the brain: the meninges, the bones of the calvarium, and the overlying skin of the convexity of the head. This type of midline fusion anomaly is termed a **dysraphic anomaly** (in Greek, *raphe* is the "midline seam"). The development of the brain and spinal cord, which depends on the protective covering, is severely disturbed. If the calvarium does not form, the child is born severely malformed, without a brain or with only a rudimentary basal part of the brain. It is clear that numerous genes regulate the development of the brain and that the dysfunction or inappropriate activation of even a single gene can lead to an abnormal developmental cascade. The outcome of altered activity of several genes may result in major defects, such as anencephaly, or a minor defect of the vertebral bones **(spina bifida).** A whole spectrum of pathologic changes has been recorded. For example, if incomplete fusion of the vertebral bodies and the meninges *(meningocele)* is accompanied by a posterior protrusion of the spinal cord, the lesion is called a *meningomyelocele.*

The predilection for developmental gene malfunction is heritable. If one child has anencephaly or related malformations, there is a 5% chance that a subsequent sibling will be born with the same defect. If two children are born with these defects, the third child has a 20% chance of being born with the defect.

The interplay of genetic and environmental factors in anencephaly is best illustrated by epidemiologic data. The highest occurrence of anencephaly was noticed in Ireland, probably because of the high prevalence of abnormal genes in that population. The risk of anencephaly among Irish living in the United States was five times higher than that among African Americans. Nevertheless, the risk among the Irish in the United States is only one half of the risk of those living in Ireland. This illustrates further the complex interaction of genetic predisposition and environmental factors. Recent data indicate that folic acid administration during pregnancy may prevent anencephaly in high-risk populations.

DIABETES MELLITUS

Diabetes mellitus, a disturbance of intermediate metabolism resulting in hyperglycemia, occurs more often in some families than in others. The adult-onset disease, called *type 2* or *non–insulin-dependent diabetes mellitus* (NIDDM), is a good example of multifactorial disease with genetic and epigenetic determinants.

The evidence for the genetic basis of this disease includes the following:

- Familial incidence. Almost 50% of affected patients have a relative who also has NIDDM.

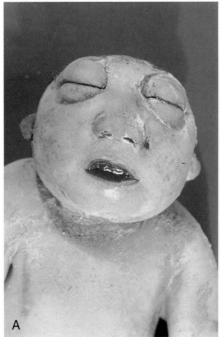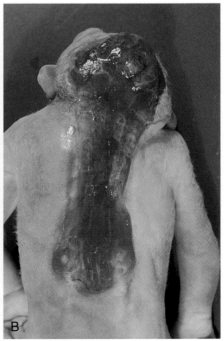

Figure 5-24 Anencephaly and craniorachischisis. *A,* Frontal view. The entire cranium is missing and the foreshortened face appears froglike. *B,* Posterior view. The brain is missing and the spinal canal is open.

A

B

- High incidence of the disease in some populations with a high rate of intermarriage. A high incidence has been noted, for example, in the Pima Indians in Arizona.
- High concordance of disease among monozygotic (identical) twins. If one twin has NIDDM, the other twin has nearly a 100% chance of developing the disease.

Nevertheless, transmission of the disease from an affected parent occurs only in about 15% of offspring. The siblings of affected persons have only a 10% to 15% chance of becoming diabetic. The development of symptoms also depends on environmental factors. The most important adverse epigenetic factors include diet, obesity, and a sedentary lifestyle (i.e., lack of exercise). However, NIDDM can develop in nonobese persons, and not all obese persons in affected families have the symptoms of diabetes. The interaction in this disease between genetic predisposition and environment is apparently too complex to be explained on the basis of current medical knowledge.

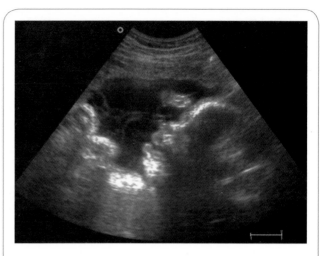

Figure 5-25 Ultrasound of a normal intrauterine pregnancy.

PRENATAL DIAGNOSIS

Most genetic and developmental disorders represent complex therapeutic problems, and many of the disorders are incurable. Such diseases cause considerable human suffering and expenditure of health resources, and adequate prevention and early diagnosis can help alleviate some of the suffering and health resource expenditure. Gene therapy will likely become available in the not-so-distant future, but for now it is applicable only to a few diseases and is still considered an experimental procedure.

Prevention of genetic and developmental diseases is a complex issue. Common preventive measures, such as rubella immunization, have prevented some forms of prenatally acquired diseases, but many others remain. The best example of the latter is acquired immunodeficiency syndrome (AIDS), which is readily transmitted from an infected mother to her fetus across the placenta *in utero*. Alcohol is also one of the known causes of human malformations and thus should be avoided in pregnancy. A healthful lifestyle, safer sex practices, and avoidance of substance abuse should be encouraged. Persons with known hereditary disorders should be counseled, and the risk of congenital malformations in their offspring should be weighed against their wish for parenting children.

Prenatal diagnosis is one of the most important elements of genetic counseling. Many genetic diseases and chromosomal abnormalities can be diagnosed while the fetus is in the early stages of development. Such abnormal fetuses can be aborted early in pregnancy, sparing the parents the suffering and the cost of caring for an incurable child.

Prenatal diagnosis is based on the following:

- *Ultrasonographic examination* of the fetus and placenta (Figure 5-25). Ultrasonograms can detect malformations of the head, extremities, and internal organs and abnormal development and positioning of the placenta.
- **Chorionic villus biopsy.** Placental biopsy during early pregnancy is a safe procedure that can provide fetal cells for chromosomal analysis or for biochemical testing for enzyme deficiencies typical of single-gene defects (Figure 5-26).

Genetic analysis, using techniques of molecular biology, can also be performed to demonstrate mutant genes.

- *Amniotic fluid analysis.* Fluid aspirated from the amniotic sac during the twelfth to eighteenth week of pregnancy is suitable for biochemical analysis. It also contains fetal cells that can be submitted for chemical, molecular genetic, or chromosomal analysis.
- *Maternal blood analysis.* Certain substances produced by the fetus enter the maternal circulation and can be measured biochemically. For example, AFP produced by the fetus is readily detectable in the mother's serum. High levels of AFP are common in pregnancies involving a fetus with anencephaly or congenital kidney malformations. Triple-screen marker test, encompassing the measurement of the maternal blood AFP, human chorionic gonadotropin, and unconjugated estriol, can detect intrauterine Down's syndrome in 65% of cases in which the fetus has this disease.

Prenatal diagnosis is based on rather complex procedures. Because of the high cost, such procedures cannot be performed during every pregnancy and are presently limited to those women considered to have a high-risk pregnancy. Because older women have an increased likelihood of bearing a child with Down's syndrome, prenatal chromosomal examination is routinely recommended in women older than 35 years. Prenatal diagnosis is also recommended for families known to be affected by Mendelian traits.

PREMATURITY

The normal pregnancy lasts 40 weeks, by which time the fetus attains viability and an average weight of 3500 g. Children born before the thirty-seventh week of pregnancy and those who weigh less than 2500 g are considered *premature*. Those weighing less than 1500 g are labeled as *immature*. Such neonates are not only anatomically immature but also functionally immature and cannot survive without medical assistance and treatment in special neonatal intensive care units.

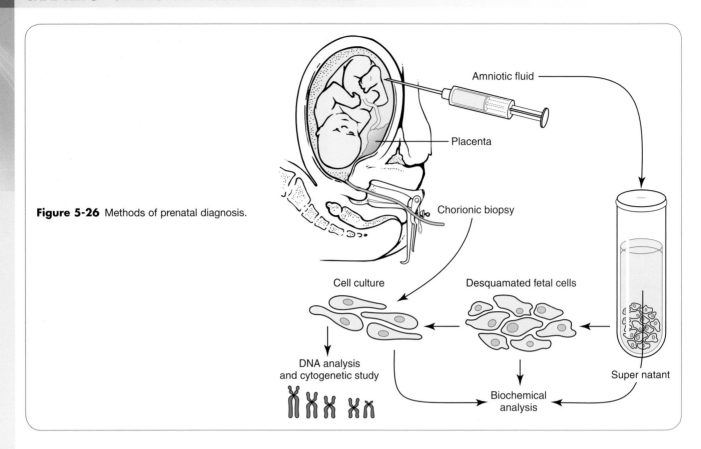

Figure 5-26 Methods of prenatal diagnosis.

Amniotic fluid

Placenta

Chorionic biopsy

Cell culture

Desquamated fetal cells

Super natant

DNA analysis
and cytogenetic study

Biochemical
analysis

Approximately 5% to 10% of all pregnancies terminate prematurely. There are many causes of **prematurity.** These causes can be categorized into three groups as follows:

- Maternal factors
- Fetal factors
- Placental factors

Unfortunately, in most cases the cause of premature birth remains unknown. The most important risk factor is premature rupture of amniotic membranes, which may occur because of trauma or infection but is usually not linked to any identifiable cause. Among the maternal factors, the best known are malnutrition, smoking, and substance abuse. Various infections affecting the mother, or both the mother and the fetus, are also well-known causes of prematurity. Fetal malformations and genetic diseases also predispose the individual to premature birth. Placental insufficiency is often postulated, but it remains poorly documented.

Premature infants show signs of anatomic and functional immaturity of their vital organs, most notably the lungs and the brain. As a consequence of pulmonary immaturity, these children tend to develop **neonatal respiratory distress syndrome,** also known as *pulmonary hyaline membrane disease.*

NEONATAL RESPIRATORY DISTRESS SYNDROME

The maturation of the fetal lungs occurs rapidly during the last 3 months of pregnancy. During this time, the lungs expand and the principal components of the respiratory units of alveoli are formed. In preparation for their respiratory function after birth, the alveolar pneumocytes type II begin secreting a surfactant rich in lecithin. Lecithin is the surface active substance that keeps the pulmonary alveoli open and prevents their collapse. During fetal life, the surfactant is released into the amniotic fluid that fills the fetal lungs. Because there is no need for prenatal respiration as a result of the oxygen being delivered via the placenta from the mother, the surfactant produced by the fetal lungs is not required for pulmonary function *in utero.* However, if the fetus is born prematurely, the functionally immature lungs cannot sustain normal respiration. The alveoli in such premature infants tend to collapse (Figure 5-27). The oxygen from the inspired air cannot diffuse into the pulmonary circulation because the respiratory surface has been reduced by the collapse of alveoli (atelectasis). Oxygen can reach the blood only through the wall of the alveolar ducts and terminal bronchioles. Because these anatomic structures are not suitable for oxygen transport, their surface epithelium is easily damaged. The necrotic cells are sloughed off, and the epithelial defects of the alveolar ducts and terminal bronchioles are covered with proteinaceous material derived from the plasma. The plasma proteins coagulate and form sheets of fibrin known as *hyaline membranes* (Figure 5-28). These impede gas exchange further, and unless the alveolar spaces open up, the infant will die of severe anoxia within the first 48 hours after birth. Those infants who do survive may have respiratory problems for the rest of their lives.

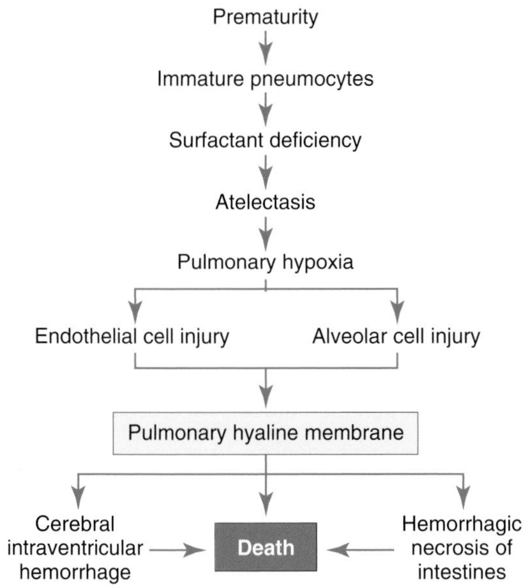

Prematurity
↓
Immature pneumocytes
↓
Surfactant deficiency
↓
Atelectasis
↓
Pulmonary hypoxia
↓
Endothelial cell injury   Alveolar cell injury
↓
Pulmonary hyaline membrane
↓
Cerebral intraventricular hemorrhage → **Death** ← Hemorrhagic necrosis of intestines

Figure 5-27 Pathogenesis of neonatal respiratory distress syndrome.

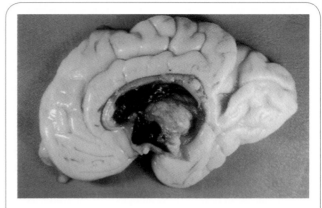

Figure 5-29 Intraventricular hemorrhage in a premature neonate affected by respiratory distress syndrome.

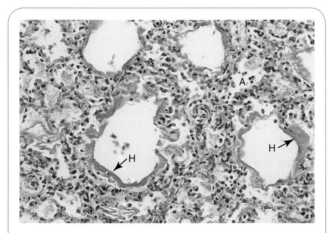

Figure 5-28 The appearance of the hyaline membranes in neonatal respiratory distress syndrome. Pink, fibrin-rich membranes *(H)* line the respiratory bronchioli and alveolar ducts, whereas the alveoli *(A)* are atelectatic.

Although anoxia caused by the neonatal respiratory distress syndrome affects the entire organism, it most prominently affects the immature brain, which is prone to *periventricular hemorrhage* (Figure 5-29). This hemorrhage occurs in the periventricular matrix, the part of the brain that is occupied by the developing neural cells destined to migrate to the surface of the brain in the last few weeks of intrauterine life. Because these cells are metabolically active, they require a copious supply of blood and oxygen. The blood is supplied by temporary, makeshift vessels that have thin walls. Anoxia at this critical stage of development leads to necrosis of the cerebral germinal matrix and the thin-walled blood vessels. Cerebral bleeding from thin-walled vessels may spill into the ventricles, causing hematocephalus—that is, accumulation of blood in the ventricles.

BIRTH INJURY

The term **birth injury** is used for various lesions caused by mechanical trauma during delivery. Such lesions occur rarely today and are registered in 1 of 5000 deliveries. Trauma occurs most often during the delivery of very large fetuses or abnormally positioned fetuses or in cases in which there is a disproportion between the fetus and the birth canal. Most common are lesions of the head and extremities. Rupture of internal organs, such as the liver, spleen, or intestines, has been reported in severe injury.

The minor hemorrhages or edema of the head that normally occur in most children during birth should not be considered birth injuries.

Skull fractures may be induced by forcing the infant's head through a narrow pelvis or by applying external pressure with forceps. Minor linear fractures heal without treatment. However, fragmentation of the cranial bones and depressed fractures, which compress the brain and can cause neurologic symptoms, require surgical correction.

Intracranial hemorrhage is caused by the same mechanisms as skull fractures; indeed, skull fracture may be complicated by intracranial hemorrhage. The hemorrhage is typically located between the dura and arachnoid *(subdural hemorrhage)* and is the result of tearing of the major cerebral veins traversing this space. Minor hemorrhages resolve without serious consequences. Massive hemorrhage is usually lethal. Neurologic symptoms are common in children who have survived large intracranial hemorrhages.

Peripheral nerve injury results from severance or avulsion of nerves of the extremities (e.g., *brachial plexus palsy*) or the cranial nerves (e.g., *facial nerve palsy*).

111

Long-bone fractures may occur if the fetus is extracted from the uterus by force or if the fetal position is unusual and incompatible with spontaneous delivery. The clavicle and humerus are most often affected.

SUDDEN INFANT DEATH SYNDROME

Sudden unexpected death in infants older than 2 months and younger than 9 months is called **sudden infant death syndrome (SIDS),** or "crib death." The death of these otherwise healthy infants usually occurs during sleep. No obvious cause of death can be determined on autopsy. SIDS, which is the most common cause of death in infants beyond the immediate neonatal period, has an incidence of 1 in 500. The cause of SIDS is unknown, but it appears to be associated with a set of maternal and infant risk factors. SIDS is most common in children born to young mothers, women of low socioeconomic status and education, and those who are smokers and substance abusers. SIDS occurs more often in families that have already experienced such an accident. Premature infants and those who have had a previous gastrointestinal disease are at an increased risk. The pathogenesis of SIDS remains unknown. It has been postulated that these children are prone to apnea and stop breathing without any obvious reason. At autopsy there are signs of anoxia, but otherwise the morphologic findings are unremarkable.

REVIEW QUESTIONS

1. How do germ cells ensure the continuity of life from one generation to another?

2. What is the difference between developmentally pluripotent cells in cleavage-stage embryos and those forming the primordial germ layers?

3. How do fetal cells differ from those in the adult organism?

4. What are the main causes of congenital defects in humans?

5. Which physical, chemical, and microbial teratogens have been proved to cause malformations in humans?

6. What is TORCH syndrome?

7. List common structural chromosomal abnormalities and relate them to the congenital defects they cause.

8. List common numerical chromosomal abnormalities and relate them to the clinical syndromes they cause.

9. What are the most common clinical and pathologic findings in Down's syndrome?

10. Compare Turner's syndrome with Klinefelter's syndrome.

11. What is the difference between autosomal dominant and autosomal recessive alleles?

12. List the basic features of autosomal dominant inheritance.

13. List the most common autosomal dominant diseases.

14. Describe the pathogenesis and the pathology of Marfan's syndrome and familial hypercholesterolemia.

15. List the basic features of autosomal recessive inheritance.

16. List the most common autosomal recessive diseases.

17. Describe the pathogenesis and pathology of cystic fibrosis.

18. Explain the concept of lysosomal storage diseases and give specific examples.

19. Explain the pathogenesis and pathology of phenylketonuria.

20. List the basic features of X-linked recessive inheritance.

21. Describe the pathogenesis and pathology of hemophilia.

22. Describe the pathogenesis and pathology of muscular dystrophy.

23. How is fragile X syndrome related to triple nucleotide repeats?

24. List the main features of multifactorial inheritance and the most common diseases in this category.

25. Explain the pathogenesis of anencephaly and related dysraphic disorders and describe the main pathologic findings in these conditions.

26. What is the evidence that adult-onset diabetes mellitus has a genetic basis?

27. Describe the principles of prenatal diagnosis.

28. Define prematurity and list the most important causes of premature termination of pregnancy.

29. Explain the pathogenesis of neonatal distress syndrome and describe the main pathologic findings in this condition.

30. List the most important pathologic changes related to birth injury.

31. Define sudden infant death syndrome and discuss its possible causes.

Fluid and Hemodynamic Disorders

6

Chapter Outline

Edema
Forms of Edema
Hyperemia
Active Hyperemia
Passive Hyperemia
Hemorrhage
Cardiac Hemorrhage
Aortic Hemorrhage
Arterial Hemorrhage
Capillary Hemorrhage
Venous Hemorrhage

Thrombosis
Embolism
Infarction
White or Pale Infarcts
Red Infarcts
Shock
Cardiogenic Shock
Hypovolemic Shock
Hypotonic Shock

Key Terms and Concepts

Acute respiratory distress syndrome
(ARDS)
Congestion
Disseminated intravascular
coagulation (DIC)
Edema
Embolism
Embolus

Exudate
Hematemesis
Hematochezia
Hematoma
Hematuria
Hemoptysis
Hemorrhage
Hyperemia

Hypoalbuminemia
Infarction
Melena
Metrorrhagia
Shock
Thrombosis
Transudate

Learning Objectives

After reading this chapter, the student should be able to:

1. Describe the distribution of fluid between the intracellular and extracellular compartments and identify the basic aspects of normal circulation.
2. Define edema and give five clinical examples.
3. Explain the pathogenesis of edema caused by increased intravascular hydrostatic pressure, a reduction in colloid osmotic pressure of the plasma, and increased retrograde pressure in the veins and lymphatics.
4. Explain active hyperemia and congestion and give clinically important examples of each process.
5. Define hemorrhage and give clinically important examples of this pathologic process.
6. Explain normal hemostasis and the role of endothelial cells, platelets, and the coagulation proteins in this process.

7. Describe the role of endothelial injury in thrombogenesis.
8. Define and explain hypercoagulability.
9. Describe the morphology of thrombi and explain mural thrombi, occlusive thrombi, and thrombophlebitis.
10. Describe the fate of thrombi with special emphasis on their organization, recanalization, and embolization.
11. Describe the clinical consequences of venous and arterial thrombi.
12. List five conditions that predispose an individual to arterial thrombi.
13. Define emboli and give five clinically important examples.
14. Define infarction and explain its pathogenesis.
15. Define shock and explain its pathogenesis.

Water accounts for approximately 60% of the total body weight. Two-thirds of the body fluid water is intracellular, whereas the remaining one-third occupies the interstitial space in the tissues or circulates in the blood (Figure 6-1). Plasma—the fluid portion of blood that can be separated from blood cells by centrifugation—accounts for approximately 5% of the total body weight in healthy adults; for a 70-kg man, this amounts to 3.5 L. Plasma volume can be expanded or reduced, but only within narrow physiologic

limits and only in counterbalance with other body fluid compartments. When these boundaries of normal physiologic variation are exceeded, pathologic overhydration or dehydration ensues. Other derangements include the following:

- Redistribution of body fluids
- Loss of fluids secondary to bleeding, sweating, or diarrhea
- Retention of fluids because of inadequate renal excretion
- Disruption of the circulation of fluids in tissues and vessels

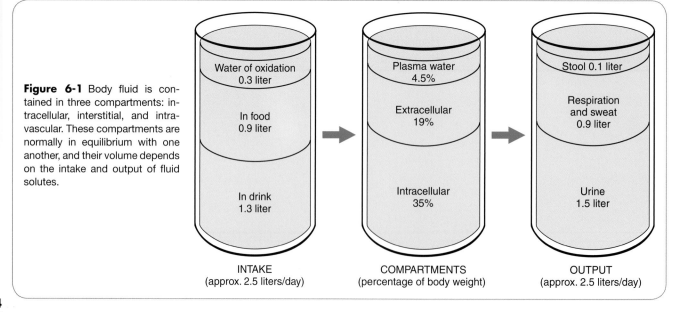

Figure 6-1 Body fluid is contained in three compartments: intracellular, interstitial, and intravascular. These compartments are normally in equilibrium with one another, and their volume depends on the intake and output of fluid solutes.

INTAKE
(approx. 2.5 liters/day)

Water of oxidation 0.3 liter

In food 0.9 liter

In drink 1.3 liter

COMPARTMENTS
(percentage of body weight)

Plasma water 4.5%

Extracellular 19%

Intracellular 35%

OUTPUT
(approx. 2.5 liters/day)

Stool 0.1 liter

Respiration and sweat 0.9 liter

Urine 1.5 liter

EDEMA

Edema is an excess of fluid in the interstitial spaces and/or the body cavities. It can be localized or generalized. Localized edema may involve any tissue or organ and is then designated descriptively as, for example, cerebral edema, pulmonary edema, or periorbital edema. Accumulation of edematous fluid in the abdominal cavity is called *ascites* or *hydroperitoneum;* in the pleural cavity, it is termed *hydrothorax* and in the pericardial cavity, *hydropericardium.* Generalized edema is called *anasarca.*

The fluid accumulating in edematous tissues can be classified as an *exudate* or a *transudate.* **Exudate** is rich in protein and blood cells and is typical of inflammation. Indeed, edema is one of the first manifestations of inflammation and is one of its cardinal signs ("tumor" or tissue swelling). Inflammatory edema is primarily related to the increased permeability of the blood vessels but is also attributable to complex hydrodynamic changes in the peripheral circulation, discussed in Chapter 2, that promote the passage of fluids from the blood vessels into the interstitial spaces.

Transudate contains less protein and fewer cells than exudate. This edema is in essence an ultrafiltrate of plasma fluid that may accumulate in tissues because of several factors, including the following:

- Increased hydrostatic pressure inside the blood vessels
- Decreased oncotic pressure of the plasma
- Lymphatic obstruction of the interstitial fluid drainage
- Increased tissue hydration because of sodium retention

The fluid in the circulating blood is separated from the interstitial fluid by the vessel wall, which serves as a semipermeable filtration barrier. The movement of fluids across the vessel wall of capillaries is determined by several factors that maintain the typical gradients holding the fluid in circulation or promoting its passage into the extravascular compartment.

Most of the exchange of fluids occurs in the capillaries. As shown in Figure 6-2, the arterial blood enters the capillaries under pressure that is counterbalanced by the oncotic pressure of the plasma. This oncotic (colloid osmotic) pressure is primarily a function of osmotically active proteins, such as albumin. At the arterial end of capillaries the hydrostatic pressure exceeds the oncotic pressure of plasma, whereas at the venous end the oncotic pressure is higher than the hydrostatic pressure, causing the flow of fluids to be redirected from the interstitium into the capillary lumen. The excess of interstitial fluid that is not returned into the capillaries is normally drained from the tissue through the lymphatics.

FORMS OF EDEMA

In general terms edema occurs as a result of an imbalance between the forces that keep the fluid in the vessels and those that promote its exit into the interstitial spaces (Table 6-1). The most important forms of edema are discussed here.

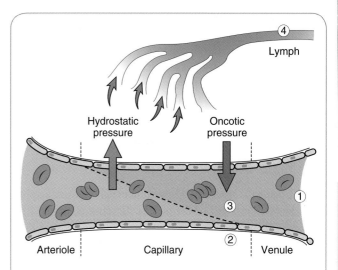

Figure 6-2 Pathogenesis of edema. The most important pathogenetic factors are increased venous pressure *(1)*, increased permeability of the vessel wall *(2)*, decreased oncotic pressure of plasma resulting from low albumin concentration *(3)*, and obstruction of lymphatics *(4)*.

TABLE 6-1   Forms of Edema

Form of Edema	Mechanism	Example(s)
Inflammatory	Vessel permeability Hyperemia	Acute inflammation
Hydrostatic	Increased arterial pressure Increased venous backpressure	Hypertension Heart failure
Oncotic	Hypoproteinemia Increased protein loss	Nephrotic syndrome
	Decreased protein synthesis	Cirrhosis of the liver
Obstructive	Lymphatic obstruction	Lymphatic blockade (e.g., tumor)
Hypervolemic	Retention of sodium	Hyperaldosteronism

INFLAMMATORY EDEMA

In inflamed tissues the fluid leaks through the vessel wall, which has been made more permeable by the mediators of inflammation and increased blood flow due to the dilation of precapillary arterioles. The edema fluid is initially a transudate but soon transforms into a protein-rich exudate containing numerous inflammatory cells.

HYDROSTATIC EDEMA

Increased pressure inside the blood vessels may be encountered in persons who have arterial hypertension. Increased intravascular pressure promotes the transmembranous passage of fluids. The intravascular pressure in the capillaries can be increased in a retrograde fashion by venous pressure. Venous stagnation is actually the most common cause of hydrostatic edema and is typically found in individuals with congestive heart failure (so-called backward heart failure). In either case increased pressure will promote transmembranous passage of fluids from the intravascular to the interstitial space.

ONCOTIC EDEMA

Oncotic edema is caused by a reduction in colloid osmotic pressure (oncotic pressure) of the plasma. Because albumin is the most active osmotic plasma protein, oncotic edema is, in clinical practice, a consequence of *hypoalbuminemia*. **Hypoalbuminemia** may be caused by increased loss of protein in the urine *(proteinuria),* as seen in nephrotic syndrome, or decreased protein synthesis, as seen in end-stage liver disease *(cirrhosis).*

Oncotic edema is usually generalized but shows a predilection for loosely textured tissues. Therefore it is prominent in the face ("puffiness"), especially around the eyes (periorbital edema).

LYMPHEDEMA

Obstruction of the lymphatics resulting in decreased drainage of interstitial fluid is a rare cause of edema. Normally lymphatics serve as a route for the removal of interstitial tissue fluid that has not been resorbed at the venous end of the capillaries. Thus any obstruction of these thin-walled vessels will produce edema. The lymphatics are most often occluded by tumor cells or chronic inflammation. In parts of Africa infested with parasites, lymphatic edema may be caused by worms, such as filaria, which can produce massive swelling of the legs. This is referred to as *elephantiasis* because the legs resemble those of elephants.

HYPERVOLEMIC EDEMA

Hypervolemic edema is typically caused by retention of sodium and water in the kidneys. The excretion of sodium and water is controlled by a complex system of regulators and depends on the normal structure and function of the kidneys and on the action of renin, angiotensinogen, and aldosterone. Kidney disease promotes the release of renin, which stimulates the formation of angiotensin. Angiotensin acts on the adrenal cortex, which releases aldosterone. Aldosterone promotes renal sodium retention, which is accompanied by retention of water.

COMPLEX FORMS OF EDEMA

In clinical practice, edema is often multifactorial. For example, edema caused by chronic heart failure is usually a combination of hydrostatic and hypervolemic edema (Figure 6-3). As a result of heart failure, the kidney is hypoperfused with blood, which stimulates the release of renin and renal retention of fluid. Increased venous backpressure resulting from pump

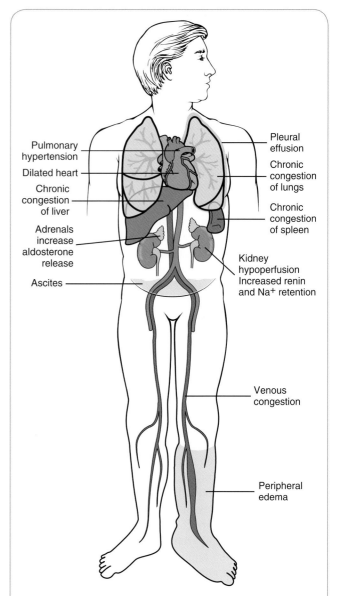

Figure 6-3 Edema of heart failure. Left-sided heart failure leads to pulmonary congestion, edema, and pleural effusion. Right-sided heart failure leads to chronic congestion of the liver and spleen, formation of ascites, venous congestion of lower extremities, and edema. Hypoperfusion of the kidneys leads to increased secretion of renin, which acts on the adrenals, stimulating the release of aldosterone. These hormonal changes contribute to renal retention of sodium and water, which aggravates heart failure and contributes to generalized edema.

failure of the heart further promotes edema. Edema of heart failure is most prominent in the lower extremities because it is gravity dependent. It is also referred to as *pitting edema,* because the compressed subcutaneous tissue rebounds slowly and shows finger marks after compression.

Clinicopathologic Correlations

Edema is a very important clinical symptom that indicates dysfunction of major organs, such as the heart, kidneys, or liver. The distribution of edema depends on its cause. As mentioned earlier, edema of the lower extremities is typical of heart failure. Because edema secondary to heart failure is gravity dependent, in patients confined to bed it becomes redistributed and is most prominent on the back. Cardiac edema, caused by left ventricular failure and consequent pulmonary hypertension, is most prominent in the lungs. This pulmonary edema is characterized by an accumulation of proteinaceous fluid in the lungs. By contrast, edema associated with renal failure or with nephrotic syndrome is typically diffuse. Patients with liver cirrhosis accumulate fluid in the abdominal cavity *(ascites);* this is attributable partially to hypoalbuminemia and partially to hydrostatic pressure because of the increased portal venous pressure caused by the deformed and heavily scarred liver.

Edema is not only a symptom of a major disease, but it may often be a cause of clinical problems. For example, pulmonary edema fills the alveolar spaces, thus preventing the normal entry of oxygen from the inhaled air into the blood. Therefore shortness of breath *(dyspnea)* is a typical consequence. Brain edema causes an expansion of the brain. Because the brain is enclosed in a rigid, bony structure (the skull), intracranial hypertension results. If the increased pressure is not relieved, the compression of vital centers of the brain will cause death.

HYPEREMIA

Hyperemia, a Greek term meaning "too much blood," denotes accumulation of blood in the peripheral circulation. Hyperemia can be either active or passive and acute or chronic.

ACTIVE HYPEREMIA

Active hyperemia is a consequence of dilation of arterioles (i.e., precapillary sphincters) and the resultant influx of blood into the capillaries. This typically occurs during blushing or exercise and is mediated by neural signals that lead to the relaxation of the arteriolar smooth muscles. Hyperemia is also a feature of acute inflammation.

PASSIVE HYPEREMIA

Passive hyperemia, or **congestion,** is caused by increased venous backpressure. Typically it is a consequence of heart failure and most often occurs in a chronic form. The stagnation of venous deoxygenated blood contributes to a bluish discoloration of the tissue *(cyanosis)* and is often associated with hydrostatic edema. Chronic passive congestion in the lungs leads to the formation of edema and also to extravasation of blood into the alveoli (Figure 6-4). Disintegrated red blood cells (RBCs) are taken up by alveolar macrophages. The hemoglobin of the RBCs is degraded into brown pigment (hemosiderin), which accumulates in the lysosomes of the macrophages. These macrophages, called *heart failure cells,* can be recognized in histologic sections of lung tissue and in cytologic smears of expectorated mucus. Chronic passive

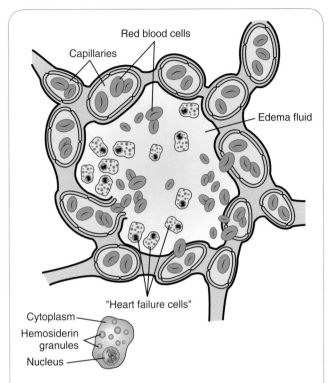

Figure 6-4 Chronic passive congestion of the lungs. Increased venous pressure leads to extravasation of red blood cells into the alveoli and alveolar edema. The hemosiderin formed from hemoglobin released from hemolyzed red blood cells is taken up by intraalveolar macrophages ("heart failure cells").

congestion is accompanied by anoxia and often results in pulmonary fibrosis.

HEMORRHAGE

Hemorrhage, or extravasation of blood, refers to passage of blood outside of the cardiovascular system. Depending on the source, hemorrhage may be classified as *cardiac, aortic, arterial, capillary,* or *venous.* Clinically it may be of sudden onset (acute), long standing (chronic), or recurrent and marked by repeated episodes of blood loss (Figure 6-5).

CARDIAC HEMORRHAGE

Cardiac hemorrhage may result from a gunshot or stabbing wound and is often fatal. In addition, a softening of the heart muscle caused by a myocardial infarct can result in ventricular rupture and lethal cardiac hemorrhage.

AORTIC HEMORRHAGE

Aortic hemorrhage is often caused by trauma, such as that sustained in a car accident. Aortic wall weakening and dilation *(aortic aneurysm)* also may occur, resulting in aortic rupture and massive hemorrhage and death.

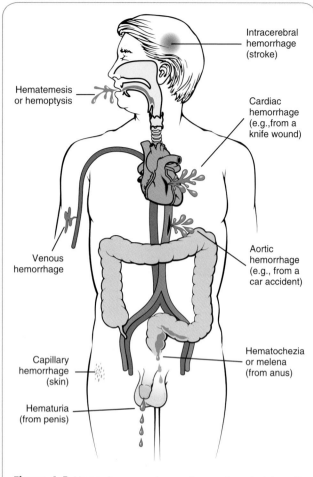

Figure 6-5 Hemorrhage may be cardiac, aortic, arterial, capillary, or venous.

ARTERIAL HEMORRHAGE

Arterial hemorrhage is most often caused by penetrating wounds inflicted by bullets or a knife. Fractured bone may also tear arteries and cause hemorrhage. All these mechanisms of hemorrhage involve arterial blood, which is oxygenated and therefore bright red. The blood squirts out of the arteries under pressure, and its flow is usually pulsating. Unless stopped, these hemorrhages are usually lethal.

CAPILLARY HEMORRHAGE

Capillary hemorrhage is marked by pinpoint droplets of blood appearing on the surface of the skin or mucosa or in various tissues. This form of hemorrhage may be related to trauma, increased venous pressure, or weakening of the capillary walls, as may occur in vitamin C deficiency *(scurvy).*

VENOUS HEMORRHAGE

Venous hemorrhage is usually traumatic. Venous blood is deoxygenated and dark red or bluish; it does not have the pulsatile flow characteristic of arterial blood.

Hemorrhages can be classified as external or internal. During external hemorrhage, the blood flows out of the body, which may result in exsanguination and death or a marked reduction in blood volume *(hypovolemia).* Blood released by internal hemorrhage may fill various body cavities (e.g., causing *hemothorax, hemoperitoneum,* or *hemopericardium*) and form **hematomas** (literally, a blood-filled swelling or tumor [-oma]). Small hemorrhages into the skin and mucosa that are less than 1 mm in diameter are called *petechiae;* those that measure 1 mm to 1 cm in diameter are termed *purpura,* and larger, blotchy bruises are called *ecchymoses.*

Several clinical terms denoting various forms of hemorrhage are worth noting:

Hemoptysis: Respiratory tract bleeding with expectoration.
Hematemesis: Vomiting of blood.
Hematochezia: Anorectal bleeding.
Melena: Passage of black, discolored blood in the stool. This represents upper gastrointestinal tract bleeding in which the blood is exposed to gastric hydrochloric acid, which produces the color change.
Hematuria: Blood in urine.
Metrorrhagia: Uterovaginal bleeding. In contrast to profound menstrual bleeding, which is called *menorrhagia.* Metrorrhagia is unrelated to the normal monthly bleeding of menstruation.

Both hematomas and small-tissue hemorrhages contain RBCs and plasma. The clotting factors of plasma are activated on contact with tissue, which leads to coagulation of the extravasated blood. The clot, or *thrombus,* that forms usually occludes the tear in the vessel wall, thus contributing to cessation of the hemorrhage. The clot in the tissue has essentially the same fate as intravascular thrombi, which are described later.

Clinicopathologic Correlations

The clinical consequences of hemorrhage depend on the amount of blood loss, the site of hemorrhage, its duration, and many other factors. For instance, a healthy young person will tolerate a massive hemorrhage much better than will a chronically ill older person. Moreover, a single episode of hemorrhage has fewer consequences than do repeated hemorrhages.

Massive acute hemorrhage should be treated as a potentially life-endangering event. Most adults can lose 500 mL of blood without any adverse consequences. This is the amount of blood routinely removed from blood donors for transfusion. However, loss of 1000 to 1500 mL of blood may result in profound circulatory shock, and loss of blood in excess of 1500 mL is usually lethal.

Chronic hemorrhages, such as those from a bleeding gastric ulcer, usually result in anemia. Anemia can result even from heavy menstruation. Normal menstrual hemorrhage contains about 70 mL of blood; if the lost hemoglobin iron is not replenished in adequate amounts, iron deficiency anemia will ensue.

The extravasated blood may damage tissues. For example, bleeding into the brain ("stroke") is usually associated with loss of neurons and paralysis caused by the destruction of motor centers. Large hematomas are space-occupying lesions in any site, and these may compress normal structures, cause pain, or irritate tissue by the substances released from the disintegrated blood cells. The release of hemoglobin-derived bilirubin in large hematomas may even cause jaundice.

THROMBOSIS

Thrombosis, or clotting, is transformation of the fluid blood into a solid aggregate encompassing blood cells and fibrin. *Fibrin* is polymerized fibrinogen; it forms a meshwork of thin filaments that binds together the cellular elements of the blood, forming a *thrombus,* or hemostatic plug.

Pathogenesis

Thrombi form only in living organisms. This distinguishes thrombi from postmortem clots or coagulated blood in a test tube. Thrombi are the end products of the coagulation sequence, which is normally activated to prevent blood loss from disrupted vessels. When the same coagulation sequence is activated in intact vessels, pathologic intravascular thrombosis develops.

The normal blood consists of a protein-rich fluid, called *plasma,* and blood cells. To circulate, the blood must be fluid and the blood cells must be freely suspended in the plasma. The fluidity of plasma is the product of interaction between factors that promote coagulation and those that inhibit it. Under normal conditions, the clotting and anticlotting factors are in balance (homeostasis). Clotting factors and platelets promote thrombosis, whereas endothelial cells and plasmin counteract it.

Intravascular coagulation is the result of the interaction of three factors:

- Coagulation proteins
- Endothelial cells
- Platelets

COAGULATION PROTEINS

The coagulation of blood depends on the proper activation of the coagulation cascade, which includes a dozen plasma proteins. This process may be activated through an endogenous or exogenous pathway. In the sequence of events that follows activation, the coagulation factors act on each other and finally form thrombin (Figure 6-6). Thrombin acts as a catalyst, promoting the polymerization of fibrinogen into fibrin. The meshwork of fibrin represents the framework for the clot, which includes all the blood cells and many plasma proteins.

ENDOTHELIAL CELLS

Endothelial cells normally secrete substances that prevent coagulation of the blood. Injured vessels switch from an anticoagulant to a procoagulant state, allowing them to bind coagulation proteins and promote thrombus formation. This usually occurs in inflammation or because of mechanical or chemical injury. Mediators of inflammation, such as interleukin-1 (IL-1) or tumor necrosis factor (TNF), activate the endothelial cells, which then lose their negative

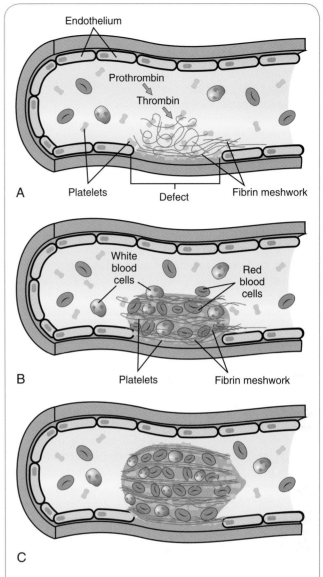

Figure 6-6 The formation of thrombi involves platelets, coagulation proteins, and endothelial cells and occurs in several sequences. *A,* An endothelial cell defect is covered with fibrin and platelets. *B,* Fibrin forms a meshwork that anchors the blood cells into the nascent thrombus. *C,* The fully formed thrombus consists of layers of fibrin and blood cells.

charge and antithrombogenic properties; thereafter they can become initiators of thrombosis.

PLATELETS

Platelets circulating in peripheral blood are the third component of normal thrombogenesis. Platelets participate in blood clotting in several ways, the most important being their ability to neutralize heparin and other anticoagulation factors and to secrete thromboxane, which directly stimulates the coagulation process. Thrombi formed under normal circumstances are typically small and short lived. Small thrombi are easily washed away by the circulating blood or degraded by thrombolytic substances, such as *plasmin.* Pathologic thrombi disrupt the circulation and can have serious functional consequences for the organs in which they have been formed.

The formation of pathologic thrombi can be traced to one of three predisposing conditions known as *Virchow's triad:*

- Endothelial cell injury
- Hemodynamic changes
- Hypercoagulability of the blood

Endothelial Cell Injury

As mentioned earlier, the intact endothelium has distinct anticoagulant properties. Under the influence of mediators of inflammation, however, the endothelium loses its anticoagulant properties and becomes thrombogenic. For example, stimulated endothelial cells release *von Willebrand factor,* which is important for the activation of coagulation factor VIII and the adhesion of platelets. More severe injury—for example, necrosis of endothelial cells and their loss—exposes the blood to connective tissue of the blood vessels and perivascular collagen, which serve as strong activators of the extrinsic coagulation pathway.

Hemodynamic Changes

Factors that promote coagulation are of two kinds: those that *disturb* the normal laminar flow of blood, causing turbulence, and those that *slow* the blood flow. Under both conditions, there is separation of blood elements that allows the platelets to be exposed to the blood vessel wall and to discharge their granules as a result of mechanical stimulation. Slow blood flow promotes sedimentation of blood cells and formation of blood eddies. The resulting turbulence in the blood flow promotes coagulation and also damages the endothelial cells. The slow fluid flow is less efficient in washing away small thrombi than the normal, more vigorous blood flow. Small thrombi that are not dissolved by antithrombolytic substances tend to persist and even grow in the sluggish bloodstream.

Hypercoagulability of Blood

Hypercoagulability of blood is, to a great extent, a function of platelets and the soluble coagulation factors of the plasma. Hypercoagulability of blood is usually hard to document, although there is ample evidence that this occurs in pregnancy, in cancer, and even in chronic cardiac failure. The blood is hypercoagulable in severely burned persons, probably because of fluid loss and hemoconcentration. *Disseminated intravascular coagulation (DIC)*, a feature of *shock*, is discussed later.

Pathology

Thrombi are classified on the basis of their location as follows (Figure 6-7):

- *Intramural thrombi* are attached to the mural endocardium of the heart chambers and are commonly found overlying a myocardial infarct.
- *Valvular thrombi* appear as small, fibrinous excrescences in debilitated persons and cause changes that mimic those of

endocarditis. Accordingly, these lesions are called *nonbacterial (marantic)* or *sterile thrombotic endocarditis.*

- *Arterial thrombi* are attached to the arterial wall and typically cover ulcerated atheromas in an atherosclerotic aorta or the coronary arteries. Aortic *aneurysms* also contain thrombi.
- *Venous thrombi* are usually found in dilated veins *(varicose veins).* Long-standing venous thrombi are organized by granulation tissue that grows into them from the vessel wall, thus giving an impression of inflammation *(thrombophlebitis).*
- *Microvascular thrombi,* so called because they involve small blood vessels in the peripheral portion of the circulation, are found in arterioles, capillaries, and venules and are typical of DIC.

On the basis of gross features, thrombi are classified as either *red (conglutination) thrombi,* which are composed of tightly intermixed RBCs and fibrin, or *layered (sedimentation) thrombi,* which show distinct layering of cellular elements and fibrin (Figure 6-8). The white layers in these thrombi are called the *lines of Zahn.* Thrombi in small vessels tend to be red. Thrombi in large arteries and veins, as well as mural thrombi, tend to be layered. Histologically, all thrombi consist of RBCs, which appear dark red, and fibrin, which appears as lighter red strands. Nucleated cells and platelets are intermixed with the fibrin and RBCs.

Outcome

The fate of thrombi depends on their size, location, and the general state of hemodynamics in the vessels. Most small thrombi are *lysed* with no consequences (Figure 6-9). Larger thrombi remain attached to the surface of the vessel wall or endocardium. Initially this attachment is mediated by the action of adhesion molecules, such as fibronectin or fibrin. With time the thrombus stimulates the ingrowth of inflammatory cells and vessels. This granulation tissue provides a much firmer anchorage. This process is called *organization.* The inflammatory cells of the granulation tissue dissolve the thrombus. Ultimately the thrombus is replaced by collagenous fibrous tissue that develops from granulation tissue. Occlusive thrombi may also be recanalized, and blood could flow again through the previously unpassable lumen with reestablishment of the circulation from the coalescence of anastomosing blood vessels. However, if the thrombus cannot be organized and firmly attached or dissolved, it may break off from the anchoring surface, giving rise to *emboli.* Thromboemboli are carried by the circulating blood to another anatomic site, and if they occlude other blood vessels, they may cause an ischemic infarction.

Clinicopathologic Correlations

The clinical significance of thrombi cannot be overemphasized. Thrombotic occlusions of cardiac and cerebral arteries are major causes of death in the United States. Pulmonary emboli are associated with significant mortality, but the exact prevalence of this complication of thrombosis is not known because

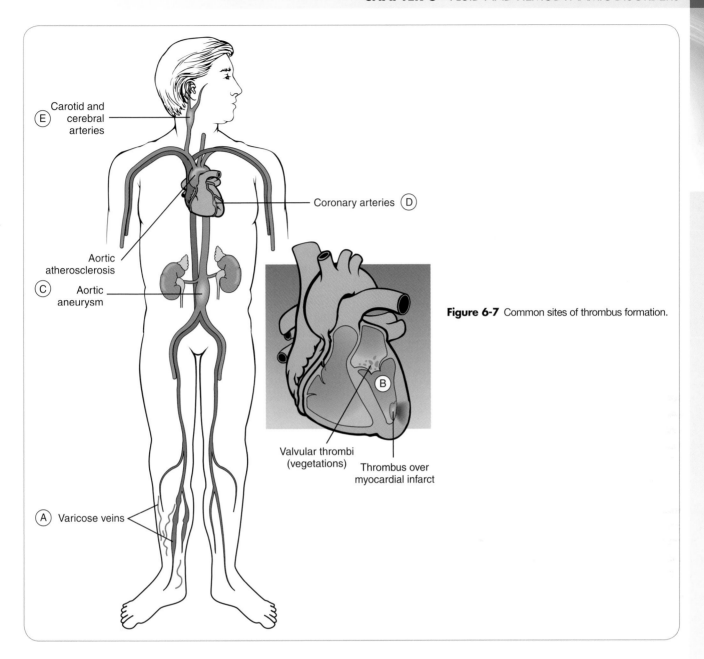

Carotid and cerebral arteries Ⓔ

Coronary arteries Ⓓ

Aortic atherosclerosis Ⓒ

Aortic aneurysm

Valvular thrombi (vegetations)

Thrombus over myocardial infarct

Ⓑ

Ⓐ Varicose veins

Figure 6-7 Common sites of thrombus formation.

pulmonary **embolism** is often not recognized clinically. The autopsy data indicate that at least one-third of all patients with pulmonary embolisms are not diagnosed correctly before death.

The clinical symptoms of thrombosis depend on the site, the extent of thrombi, the rapidity with which they are formed, the duration of thrombosis, and the widespread nature of the disease and its distant complications. Thrombi may do the following:

- *Occlude the lumen of the blood vessel.* Arterial occlusion typically causes ischemia. Thrombotic occlusion of the coronary arteries is the most common cause of myocardial infarction.

- *Narrow the lumen of blood vessels and reduce blood flow.* This results in hypoxia and reduced function of the affected organ. Chronic heart failure is often caused by such narrowing, which is mostly a combination of atherosclerosis and thrombosis.

- *Serve as a source of emboli.* Detached thromboemboli carried by blood cause infarcts. Pulmonary emboli stem from venous thrombi in the legs. Cerebral infarct, caused by thromboemboli that become detached from the myocardial chambers overlying the infarct, is one of the most serious late complications of myocardial infarction.

In addition to these three major complications, thrombosis plays a major role in the pathogenesis of atherosclerosis, as

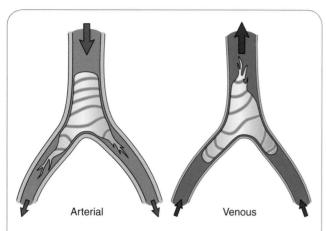

Figure 6-8 Diagram showing the gross appearance of a thrombus, depending on its site of origin. Note the lines of Zahn, which are composed of fibrin and platelets.

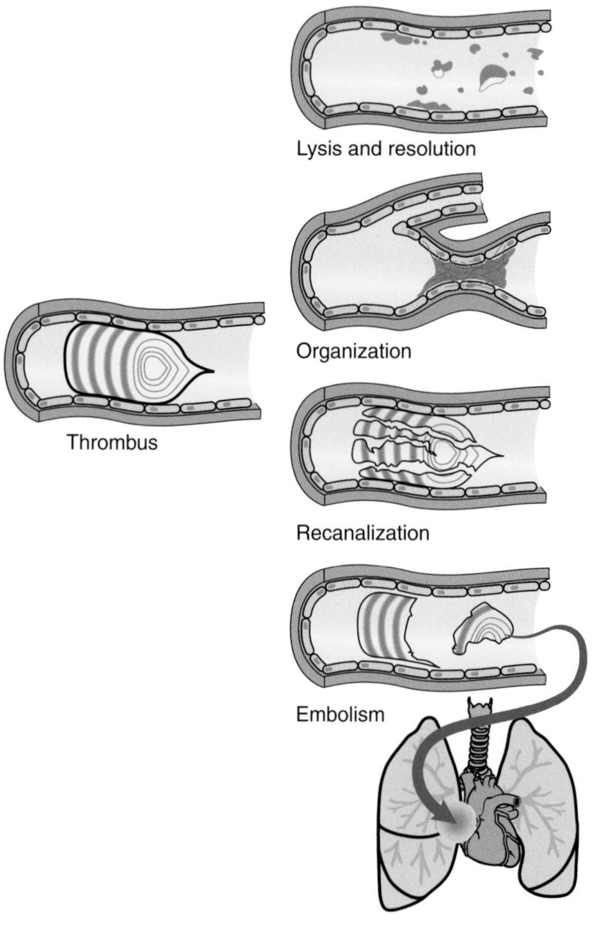

Lysis and resolution

Organization

Thrombus

Recanalization

Embolism

Figure 6-9 The fate of thrombi.

discussed in Chapter 7. Thrombi are also fertile grounds for bacterial growth and are prone to infection. These infected thrombi give rise to *septic emboli.*

EMBOLISM

An **embolus** is a freely movable, intravascular mass that is carried from one anatomic site to another by blood. There are several forms of emboli, including the following:

- *Thromboemboli.* These represent fragments of thrombi carried by venous or arterial blood. Infected thrombi give rise to septic emboli.
- *Liquid emboli.* These may include fat emboli that occur after bone fracture and amniotic fluid emboli caused by the entry of amniotic fluid into uterine veins during delivery.
- *Gaseous emboli.* Air embolism can be produced by injecting air into veins. Air that is liberated under decreased pressure (causing caisson disease or decompression sickness) is another form of embolism.
- *Solid particle emboli.* Cholesterol crystals that detach from atheromatous plaques, tumor cells, or bone marrow can also embolize. Cholesterol emboli may cause occlusive symptoms. Bone marrow emboli (i.e., fragments of bone marrow forcibly pressed into the circulation after bone fracture) are usually of no clinical significance and may be found coincidentally at autopsy after rib fractures caused by energetic cardiac resuscitation. *Tumor emboli* formed from detached fragments of solid neoplasms or cells that have actively entered the blood vessels are important for metastasis.

Clinicopathologic Correlations

The clinical significance of emboli lies in the fact that all emboli can occlude blood vessels (embolism), thus interrupting the blood supply to an organ. Thromboemboli account for most of the emboli in clinical practice and thus deserve particular emphasis.

Thromboemboli are classified on the basis of the vessels through which they are carried in the blood (Figure 6-10).

VENOUS EMBOLI

As the name implies, these emboli originate in veins and are carried by the venous circulation. They typically lodge in the pulmonary artery and its branches, causing pulmonary embolism. *Arterial emboli* originate in the left atrium or ventricle, aorta, and major arteries. They are carried by arterial blood and are an important cause of infarction resulting from the occlusion of peripheral arteries. Venous emboli that reach the arterial circulation through the foramen ovale or an interventricular septal defect or some other anastomoses are called *paradoxical emboli.* These emboli are by origin venous, but they can travel by both venous and arterial blood and cause symptoms similar to those of arterial emboli.

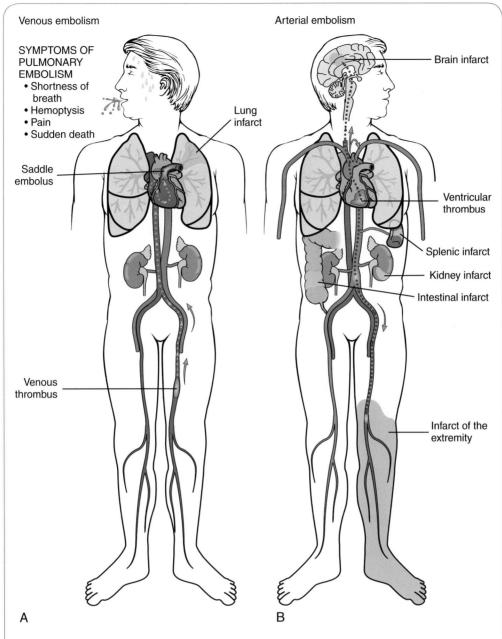

Figure 6-10 Venous and arterial emboli. *A,* Venous emboli can lodge in the lung, causing a variety of symptoms and conditions. *B,* Arterial emboli may occlude arteries in many organs.

? Did You Know?

Hospital records show that pulmonary thromboemboli cause more than 50,000 deaths every year in the United States. The number of people dying of pulmonary embolism outside of hospitals is probably even higher.

The symptoms of pulmonary embolism are often nonspecific. Autopsy studies show that 30% to 40% of all pulmonary emboli discovered postmortem were not even suspected while the patient was alive.

Pulmonary embolism is the most important complication of venous emboli. These emboli typically originate in the veins of the lower extremities and are carried by venous blood to the vena cava and then through the right atrium and ventricle into the pulmonary artery. A massive thromboembolus may occlude the pulmonary artery or its main branches. Such *saddle emboli* are often lethal (Figure 6-11) because they prevent the entry of blood into the lung and cause acute anoxia. Smaller emboli lodge in the minor branches of the pulmonary vascular tree and cause pulmonary infarcts. Pulmonary infarcts are triangular, corresponding to the area

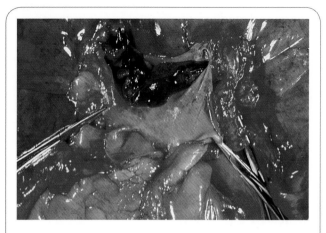

Figure 6-11 Saddle embolus of the pulmonary artery.

supplied by the occluded branch, and are often subpleural. These infarcts cause irritation of the pleura, which is associated with typical "pleuritic pain." Pleuritic pain is sharp, its location can be pinpointed by the patient, and it is accentuated by inspiration.

ARTERIAL EMBOLI

Most arterial emboli originate from cardiac mural or valvular thrombi. In cases of bacterial endocarditis, the emboli may be infected. Other sources of arterial emboli are the thrombi on ulcerated atherosclerotic plaques of the aorta and its major branches. Moreover, aortic aneurysms often contain thrombi, which may give rise to emboli.

Arterial emboli are mechanically fragmented inside the vessels because arterial blood flows fast and disrupts them. Thus they tend to lodge in medium-sized and small arteries. The greatest risk is associated with emboli of the cerebral circulation, which typically lodge in the middle cerebral artery and cause infarcts of the basal ganglia. Cerebral embolization is associated with high mortality, and patients who do survive often have residual neurologic defects.

Other organs commonly affected by arterial emboli are the spleen, kidneys, and intestines. Infarcts that develop from splenic emboli are functionally unimportant. The only symptom is usually a sharp, subcostal pain. Renal infarcts may also be painful and are often associated with hematuria. Intestinal infarcts often represent major medical emergencies. If an embolus lodges in one of the major intestinal arteries and if this happens in an elderly person who already has compromised circulation through the intestinal blood vessels, the embolus may cause gangrene of large segments of the intestine.

INFARCTION

Infarction is an insufficiency of blood supply of sudden onset that results in an area of ischemic necrosis. The terms for the process *(infarction)* and the anatomic lesion *(infarct)* are often used synonymously. Most infarcts are caused by thrombi or emboli. Depending on the site of vascular occlusion, infarcts may be arterial or venous.

On the basis of their gross appearance, infarcts may be classified as either red or white.

WHITE OR PALE INFARCTS

White infarcts are pale because of arterial occlusion, which prevents the entry of blood into the infarcted area. It is typically found in solid organs, such as the heart, kidney, or spleen (Figure 6-12). The area of ischemic necrosis caused by the obstruction of the arteries is typically paler than the surrounding tissue. It is often rimmed by a thin red zone containing extravasated blood that was destined to reach the ischemic zone from surrounding anastomotic blood vessels.

Because the heart and kidney have functionally terminal arteries that do not form large anastomoses among themselves, these abortive attempts to resupply the area with blood from another source are inefficient. If blood from collateral blood vessels ultimately reaches the infarcted area within a few days after the occlusion, the pale infarct will become mottled. In recurrent infarct of the heart, the tissue may exhibit several colors: brown, indicating a normal heart that has survived ischemia; pale brown muscle that is ischemic; yellow necrotic tissue, often infiltrated with polymorphonuclear scavenger leukocytes; RBCs extravasated into the tissue; and white or gray fibrous tissue indicative of connective tissue repair.

RED INFARCTS

These infarcts are typical of venous obstruction involving the intestines or testis. In these sites the venous circulation may be interrupted as a result of twisting of the organ around its supporting structure. Twisting of the sigmoid colon *(volvulus)* causes compression of the blood vessels in the mesentery. Because the veins have thin walls, they are compressed much

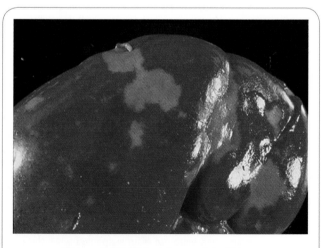

Figure 6-12 White infarcts of the kidney.

more easily than the arteries. This leads to sudden onset of venous congestion, local ischemia, and necrosis (i.e., hemorrhagic infarction) (Figure 6-13). Similar changes result from torsion of the testis, a fairly common sport-related lesion in children and adolescents. Thrombosis of the major veins has the same effect.

Red infarcts are also typically found in organs that have a dual blood supply, such as the lung or liver. To understand the pathogenesis of red lung infarcts let us remember that the venous blood reaches the lung parenchyma through the branches of the pulmonary artery. The branches of the bronchial arteries, originating from the aorta, provide the nutrient arterial blood. These two circulatory systems communicate through small anastomoses that are not functional under normal circumstances. If the thromboemboli occlude the branches of the pulmonary artery, the infarcted lung and its blood vessels undergo necrosis. In time the blood from the small bronchial arteries reaches the infarcted area and through the anastomoses enters the branches of the pulmonary artery behind the embolic occlusion. Because these vessels have been damaged or are completely necrotic, this pulmonary artery blood leaks into the tissue and floods the infarcted area of the lung. Such infarcts are thus red.

Outcome

The fate of infarcts depends on many factors, such as their anatomic site, the general circulatory status of the affected person, and the body's capacity to repair the area of infarction. Ischemic necrosis in organs composed of postmitotic cells, such as the heart, cannot be repaired except by replacement of damaged cells with fibrous tissue. This results in myocardial fibrosis, or scarring. Necrotic brain cells cannot be replaced by regeneration either. Fibrous scars do not form, and the liquefied necrotic brain tissue is ultimately resorbed, leaving behind a cyst filled with clear fluid.

Infarcts involving tissues composed of mitotic or facultative mitotic cells, such as the liver, heal with relatively few residual effects. Small infarcts of the intestine or mucosa also may be repaired by regeneration. However, larger infarcts usually result in defects that cannot be replaced and result in scarring.

SHOCK

Shock is a state of hypoperfusion of tissues with blood. It is caused by one of three possible mechanisms:
- Pump failure of the heart (cardiogenic shock)
- Loss of fluid from the circulation (hypovolemic shock)
- Loss of peripheral vascular tone resulting in overexpansion of the peripheral vascular space and redistribution of fluids (hypotonic shock)

Common to all these conditions are a collapse of circulation and a disproportion between the circulating blood volume and the vascular space. The resulting hypoperfusion of tissues produces tissue anoxia and multiple organ failure. Anoxia potentiates the loss of vascular tone, which ultimately leads to death as a result of cardiorespiratory failure (Figure 6-14).

CARDIOGENIC SHOCK

Cardiogenic shock results from pump failure of the heart. Most often it is secondary to an infarction that destroys a large part of the functioning myocardium. Loss of contractile elements dramatically decreases the ability of the heart to pump blood. Similar consequences may result from myocarditis or valvular heart disease, such as endocarditis. Sudden heart stoppage secondary to cardiac conduction block or arrhythmia also may result in cardiogenic shock.

HYPOVOLEMIC SHOCK

Hypovolemic shock results from a loss of circulatory volume. This may be attributable to massive hemorrhage as seen after major trauma and wounding or during surgery. Shock may also complicate fluid loss related to burns, vomiting, or diarrhea.

HYPOTONIC SHOCK

Hypotonic shock, also called *distributive shock,* results from dilation of blood vessels and the pooling of blood in dilated peripheral blood vessels. This typically occurs in individuals with anaphylactic shock caused by exposure to an allergen (e.g., a bee sting) and vasodilatory effects of histamine and similar vasoactive mediators of inflammation; adverse neurogenic stimuli (e.g., a spinal cord injury or pain caused by trauma); or bacterial endotoxins that directly act on blood vessels (e.g., sepsis).

Pathogenesis

Shock represents a series of events that, if uninterrupted, act synergistically to produce vicious cycles that ultimately result in death. Early stages of shock are reversible and treatable. However, once serious organ failure ensues, the

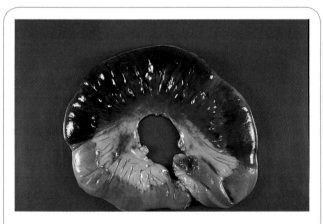

Figure 6-13 Red infarct of the intestine.

16. Compare pale (white) and red infarcts and explain their pathogenesis.

17. What is the fate of infarcts?

18. Compare the pathogenesis of cardiogenic and hypovolemic shock.

19. List the most important pathologic findings associated with shock.

20. Compare the clinical features of compensated and decompensated shock with those of irreversible shock.

The Cardiovascular System

7

Chapter Outline

NORMAL ANATOMY AND PHYSIOLOGY
  Heart
  Blood Vessels
  Lymphatics
OVERVIEW OF MAJOR DISEASES
  Congenital Heart Disease
    Septal Defects
    Tetralogy of Fallot
  Atherosclerosis
    Atherosclerosis of the Aorta
    Peripheral Vascular Disease
    Coronary Heart Disease
  Hypertension and Hypertensive Heart Disease

Rheumatic Heart Disease
Infectious Diseases of the Heart
  Endocarditis
  Myocarditis
  Pericarditis
Cardiomyopathy
Cardiac Tumors
Iatrogenic Heart Lesions
Arterial Diseases
  Polyarteritis Nodosa
  Giant Cell Arteritis
  Raynaud's Disease
Diseases of the Veins
Lymphatic Diseases

Key Terms and Concepts

Adrenaline
Aldosterone
Aneurysms
Angina pectoris
Angiotensin
Arrhythmia
Atheromas
Atherosclerosis
Atrial myxoma
Atrial septal defect
Cardiac tamponade
Cardiac transplantations
Cardiomyopathy
Congenital heart disease

Congestive heart failure
Coronary heart disease
Cor pulmonale
Diabetic microangiopathy
Endocardial mural thrombus
Endocarditis
Giant cell arteritis
Hemopericardium
Hyperlipidemia
Hypertension
Hypertensive stroke
Ischemic
Lymphangitis
Myocardial infarct

Myocarditis
Pericarditis
Polyarteritis nodosa
Raynaud's disease
Renin
Septic emboli
Tetralogy of Fallot
Thrombophlebitis
Troponin
Vasculitis
Ventricular aneurysm
Ventricular rupture
Ventricular septal defect

Learning Objectives

After reading this chapter, the student should be able to:

1. Describe the normal components of the cardiovascular system and their function.
2. List the five most common forms of heart disease in the United States.
3. List the three most common congenital heart diseases and describe the pathogenesis of each.
4. Discuss the pathogenesis and risk factors of atherosclerosis.
5. Describe the major pathologic lesions of atherosclerosis and list three major complications.
6. Describe the gross and microscopic features and complications of myocardial infarct and correlate these pathologic findings with site and clinical symptoms.
7. Discuss the pathogenesis of hypertension and compare primary and secondary hypertension.
8. Describe the typical gross and microscopic lesions of endocarditis, myocarditis, and pericarditis and correlate the pathologic findings with the clinical findings.
9. Discuss the pathogenesis of rheumatic heart disease and describe the typical cardiac lesions of rheumatic fever.
10. List three causes of cardiomyopathy and describe the pathologic findings in this disease.
11. Describe two surgical operations performed on the heart and their consequences or complications.
12. Discuss the pathogenesis of arteritis and relate it to its pathologic and clinical features.
13. Describe varicose veins and list the possible causes and consequences of this disease.
14. Describe lymphangitis.

NORMAL ANATOMY AND PHYSIOLOGY

The cardiovascular system, as the name implies, comprises the heart (the Greek term *cardia* means "heart") and vessels. The primary function of this system is circulation of the blood; therefore it is also called the *circulatory system.* The heart is the centerpiece of the circulatory system; through its incessant rhythmic action, it pumps the blood and keeps it flowing. The vessels represent the venues through which the blood circulates. However, blood vessels also regulate the blood flow and thus actively participate in the circulation.

HEART

The heart weighs approximately 250 to 350 g and is the size of a person's fist. The heart is located in the pericardial sac. The inside of the pericardial sac is lined with a smooth surface epithelium that also covers the opposing external surface of the heart, the epicardium. When these two surfaces slide over each other during heart movements, they are separated only by a few drops of clear pericardial fluid that keep the surface moist and prevent friction.

The heart consists of four chambers: two upper chambers called *atria* and two lower chambers called *ventricles* (Figure 7-1). The right atrium is separated from the left atrium by an interatrial septum composed of connective tissue. By comparison, the interventricular septum is much thicker and is composed of cardiac muscle cells. The atria are separated from the ventricles by *atrioventricular valves* that regulate the proper inflow and outflow of blood from each chamber during heart contractions. The outflow tract

of each ventricle also has a valve, known as the *semilunar valve,* so named because its cusp is half-moon–shaped.

The wall of the ventricles (myocardium) is formed by striated muscle cells that resemble skeletal muscle cells. In contrast to skeletal muscle fibers, which contract only when stimulated with nerve impulses, the myocardial fibers contract rhythmically on their own. However, these muscle fibers also respond to the electrophysiologic impulses of the cardiac conduction system and can be influenced by various chemicals, transmitters, and drugs. The internal surface of the heart chambers is covered by endocardium, whereas on the outside, the heart is covered by epicardium. The epicardium is continuous with the pericardium.

Blood is supplied to the heart by two coronary arteries. These arteries originate from the proximal aorta, just above the aortic semilunar valve. The left coronary artery usually bifurcates into two major branches, the anterior descending and the left circumflex arteries, which provide most of the blood for the anterior and lateral side of the left ventricle and the anterior portion of the interventricular septum. The right coronary artery does not bifurcate but forms a single major trunk from which several major branches originate. The right coronary artery provides the blood for the right ventricle and the posterior wall of the left ventricle and the posterior portion of the interventricular septum.

Normally the heart contracts rhythmically at a rate of 60 to 80 times per minute. The contraction of the heart is called *systole,* whereas the relaxation of the myocardium that results in dilation of the cardiac chambers is called *diastole.*

In diastole the heart chambers dilate, which allows filling of the right side of the heart with peripheral venous blood while the left side of the heart is filled with oxygenated pulmonary venous blood. During diastole, the ventricles and

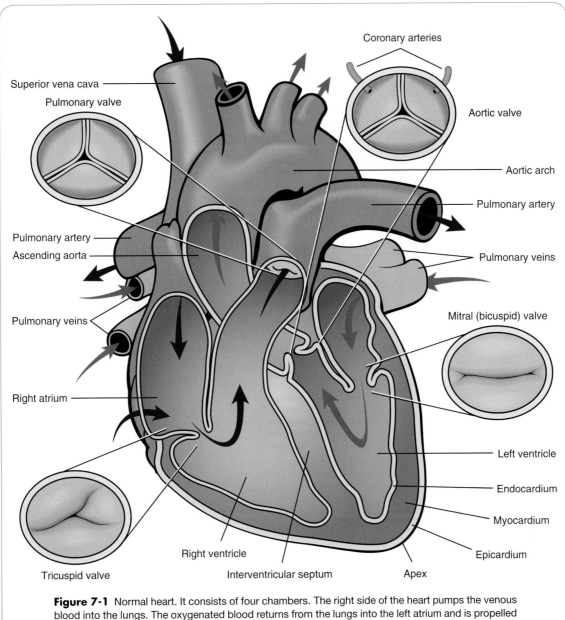

Figure 7-1 Normal heart. It consists of four chambers. The right side of the heart pumps the venous blood into the lungs. The oxygenated blood returns from the lungs into the left atrium and is propelled by the left ventricle into the aorta. The insets show closed valves; the tricuspid valve has three leaflets, whereas the mitral valve has two leaflets. The aortic and pulmonary artery valves have three leaflets and resemble one another except for the fact that the coronary arteries originate from behind the cusps in the aorta.

atria are dilated and the semilunar pulmonary and aortic valves are closed to prevent regurgitation of blood from the large vessels across these orifices. At the same time, the mitral and tricuspid valves are opened to allow inflow of blood into the dilated ventricles from the atria.

Contraction of the heart and the closing and opening of the valves generate *sounds* and *murmurs* stemming from the flow of blood through the cardiac chambers and across the valves. Various pathologic lesions are associated with distinct auscultatory findings, and an experienced cardiologist can diagnose many important cardiac diseases, especially those involving the valves, by auscultation.

BLOOD VESSELS

The blood vessels form the second major compartment of the cardiovascular system (Figure 7-2). These include arteries, veins, and capillaries that are sealed into a closed system through which the blood circulates back and forth from the heart to the peripheral tissues. All blood vessels are lined by endothelial cells, which form the innermost layer of the arteries and veins. The endothelium is the only cell layer of the capillaries. Overall, the arteries are thicker than the veins, and although both consist of several concentric tissue layers, the

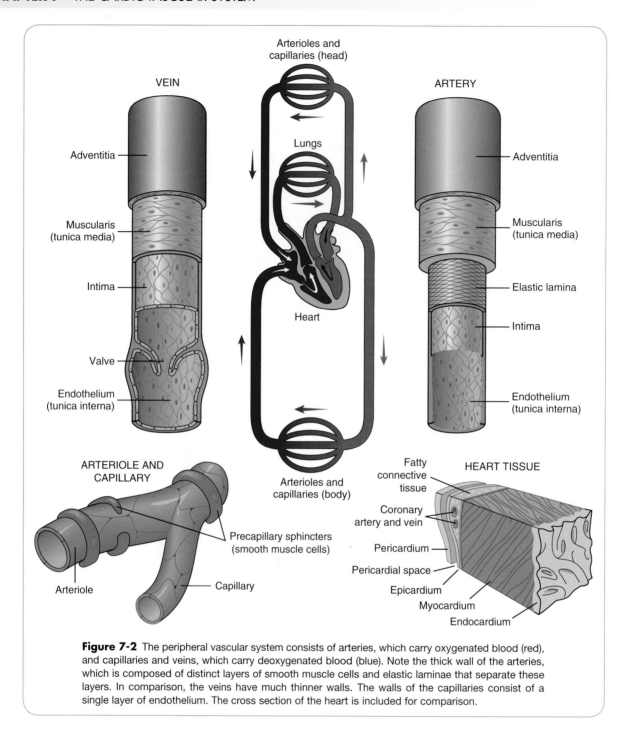

Figure 7-2 The peripheral vascular system consists of arteries, which carry oxygenated blood (red), and capillaries and veins, which carry deoxygenated blood (blue). Note the thick wall of the arteries, which is composed of distinct layers of smooth muscle cells and elastic laminae that separate these layers. In comparison, the veins have much thinner walls. The walls of the capillaries consist of a single layer of endothelium. The cross section of the heart is included for comparison.

tissues forming the arteries are generally more cellular and contain more extracellular matrix than those forming the veins. Therefore the arteries have thicker walls than veins.

The arteries are of two types. The larger arteries, including the aorta, are classified as *elastic,* whereas the smaller arteries are called *muscular.* The elastic arteries expand with the internal pressure generated by blood flow during systole and then recoil during diastole. The muscular arteries and their smaller branches, *arterioles,* contract or dilate to accommodate the blood volume in their lumen, the tissue requirements for blood, and the velocity of circulation.

The veins have thinner walls than do the arteries and generally do not have the elasticity or the contractile capacity of the arteries. Thick walls and elasticity are not essential properties for venous function because the venous blood flow is less pulsatile and is under less pressure than the flow in the arteries. To prevent backflow of blood, the veins have *valves* that hinder the retrograde blood flow that could easily develop in this low-pressure system.

The capillaries are the primary sites at which oxygen is transferred from blood into the tissues and metabolites are exchanged. To this end, the capillaries have a thin wall composed of a single endothelial cell layer. Capillaries and venules are also the primary sites at which the blood cells exit into the interstitial spaces and through which fluids enter the interstitial spaces or reenter the circulation from the peripheral tissues.

LYMPHATICS

The lymphatic vessels form the third component of the circulatory system. The primary function of the lymphatic system is to facilitate and enable the centripetal flow of lymph from the peripheral tissues toward the heart. Lymph is similar to blood but differs from it in that it does not contain red blood cells or clotting factors (i.e., it will not coagulate). This fluid is formed in the peripheral tissues and various organs from serum and other extracellular fluids. The lymph enters the open-ended, thin, capillary-like lymphatics and is then transported to the central lymphatic vessels under pressure generated in the peripheral tissues. These vessels converge into the main lymphatic vessels and the thoracic duct, which empty their contents into the large veins in the neck. The lymph that enters the venous circulation does not recirculate like the blood.

In contrast to blood circulation, which occurs through continuous channels, flow through the lymphatic channels is interrupted by lymph nodes. These lymph nodes serve as barriers or large filters that clear from the lymph bacteria and other noxious substances. At the same time, lymph nodes contain white blood cells, primarily lymphocytes, which enter the lymph and are transported into the central circulation. Many lymphocytes recirculate, returning to the lymph nodes from which they originated or reaching some other tissue to which they are transported for special functions, as in inflammation.

OVERVIEW OF *MAJOR DISEASES*

The most important diseases of the cardiovascular system can be classified into the following categories:
- Congenital heart disease
- Ischemic vascular disease
- Hypertension-related disease
- Inflammatory disease (infectious and autoimmune disorders)
- Metabolic disease

Two major arterial diseases are presented: atherosclerosis and arteritis. Among the diseases involving the veins, discussion is limited to varicose veins and the complications of venous thrombosis. Diseases involving the lymphatics are not discussed in detail except for lymphangitis, an acute inflammatory condition involving the small lymph vessels.

Several facts important to an understanding of cardiovascular pathology are presented here, before a discussion of specific pathologic entities:
1. Cardiovascular diseases account for more than one half of all mortality in industrialized countries. The most common among these diseases are atherosclerosis and hypertension.

Atherosclerosis, along with its major manifestations, is the cause of death in more than 50% of all adults who die in the United States and the industrialized countries of the West (Figure 7-3). Atherosclerosis of the coronary arteries, the aorta and its main branches, or the cerebral blood vessels accounts for most of the related morbidity.

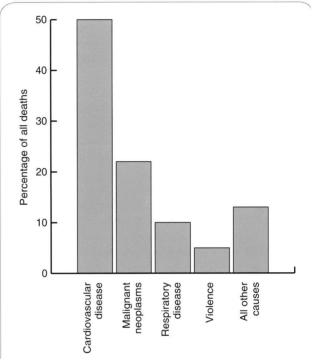

A Mortality due to all causes

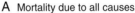

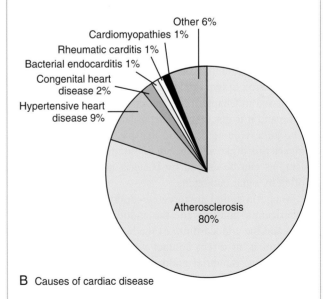

B Causes of cardiac disease

Figure 7-3 Incidence of cardiovascular diseases. *A,* Note that cardiovascular diseases are more common than any other disease. *B,* Atherosclerosis accounts for 80% of the total mortality from cardiovascular diseases.

Hypertension is an important complication of atherosclerosis. It contributes to the severity of the disease and aggravates its symptoms. However, hypertension can occur independent of atherosclerosis and may even precede it. Hypertension accounts for approximately 10% of all heart diseases.

2. Abnormal development of the heart during fetal life is a significant cause of heart disease. The development of the heart, most of which is completed during the first 2 months of fetal intrauterine life, involves complex embryologic processes (e.g., induction, resorption, inversion, rotation, etc.). It is important to recognize that, with such a complex morphogenesis, much can go wrong. **Congenital heart disease,** resulting from abnormal fetal heart development, is therefore very common. At least 1 in 100 of all neonates has a minor cardiac abnormality. Luckily, most such defects produce no symptoms or heal on their own.

3. Heart action is critically dependent on a constant supply of nutrients and oxygen. Occlusion of the arteries or reduction of the lumen secondary to narrowing impedes blood supply and causes ischemia. Sudden occlusion of the arterial blood flow causes an infarct, whereas chronic ischemia leads to pump failure of the heart, which is typical of chronic **coronary heart disease.** This may be associated with bouts of chest pain known as **angina pectoris.** Total occlusion of coronary arteries may cause a **myocardial infarct.**

4. Arterial blood pressure, which primarily depends on heart action and the elastic and contractile properties of arteries and arterioles, is regulated by hormones and biogenic amines. Blood flow depends on pressure gradients generated by the action of the heart and the peripheral resistance of arteries and arterioles. The smooth muscle cells in the muscular arteries and arterioles contract under the influence of adrenergic nerves, which release the catecholamines epinephrine and norepinephrine. These biogenic amines are also produced by adrenal medullary cells and released into the circulation. Other humoral regulators of blood pressure include renin, angiotensin, and aldosterone. Abnormalities in the regulation of blood pressure result in hypotension or hypertension. Hypotension was previously discussed in Chapter 6. Hypertension is an important disease, and it is discussed in detail later in this chapter.

5. The large volume of blood that passes through the heart makes this organ susceptible to bloodborne infections. Infections can be caused by bacteria and viruses and less often by other pathogens.

Bacteria found in infected blood during bacteremia (septicemia) may invade the endothelium of blood vessels and the endocardium of the heart. Because the endocardium is in direct contact with blood, it is involved most often. Bacterial endocarditis is therefore the most common infectious lesion of the heart. Preexisting lesions, such as congenital heart defects, deformities of the valves, or mural thrombi, predispose individuals to cardiac infections. Such lesions facilitate the penetration of bacteria into the tissues and their local growth. Clotted blood seems to be the most suitable growth medium for bacteria; therefore clots in the ventricles (mural thrombi) or those attached to the valves (endocardial vegetations) often become infected. Infected thrombi may give rise to emboli **(septic emboli)** and bacterial aneurysms in the small arteries (mycotic aneurysms). Infection of venous thrombi may lead to inflammation of the vessel wall **(thrombophlebitis).**

Viruses can also infect the heart and typically cause myocarditis or pericarditis. Viral myocarditis is thought to be one of the common causes of dilated cardiomyopathy, an incurable disease that can be treated adequately only by cardiac transplantation.

Fungi and other pathogens infect the heart less often, except in immunosuppressed persons. Protozoal infections of the heart are distinctly rare in the United States, but in Brazil infectious myocarditis caused by the parasite *Trypanosoma cruzi* affects approximately 10 million people.

6. Immunoglobulins in the blood and circulating immune complexes may be deposited in the heart and blood vessels and may cause inflammatory and destructive lesions. Normal blood contains immunoglobulins, which are normal components of the serum. These immunoglobulins have no adverse influences on the heart and blood vessels. When circulating immunoglobulins are complexed with antigen into immune complexes (as in systemic lupus erythematosus), they may become pathogenic and cause vasculitis or endocarditis. Immune complexes may also form locally in the vessel wall, as in various forms of **vasculitis.** Hypersensitivity reactions that elicit formation of autoantibodies—that is, antibodies to the body's own tissues—can damage the heart and blood vessels, as in rheumatic fever.

7. Systemic metabolic diseases often affect the heart and the blood vessels. The most important metabolic disease affecting the cardiovascular system is diabetes mellitus. This systemic disorder of intermediary metabolism, caused by a relative or absolute deficiency of insulin or a resistance of tissues to insulin, primarily affects small blood vessels **(diabetic microangiopathy).** It also represents an important risk factor for atherosclerosis. Diabetes is discussed in detail in Chapter 12.

8. The cardiovascular system rarely gives rise to malignant tumors. Malignant tumors of the heart, which by their mesenchymal origin are classified as sarcomas, are extremely rare. Hemangiosarcomas, the malignant tumors of blood vessels, are somewhat more common but still rare overall. On the other hand, hemangiomas, which are small benign tumors, are very common but of limited clinical significance. Benign tumors of the heart (rhabdomyomas) and atrial myxomas are also rare.

CONGENITAL HEART DISEASE

Any defect involving the heart or the large arteries and veins that is present at birth is considered a congenital heart disease. Approximately 25,000 babies with heart defects are born annually in the United States.

The symptoms of congenital heart disease may be evident at birth or during early infancy, or they may become evident only later in life. These defects may be classified as either *minor* (those that are either asymptomatic or produce only negligent symptoms) or *major* (those that cause serious problems and may be lethal if not treated adequately).

Etiology and Pathogenesis

The causes and the pathogenesis of most congenital heart defects are not known. Because the heart develops early in embryonic life and is completely formed and functioning by 10 weeks, all congenital heart defects develop before the tenth week of pregnancy. This is important to know because some of these defects can be prevented by avoiding toxic substances, viral infections, and x-ray exposure during the early critical stages of pregnancy.

The fetal heart develops like a tube, being subdivided by a septum that grows from one end while the tube undergoes twisting and segmentation by the primordia of the future valves. If the left side of the heart is not completely separated from the right side, arterial septal defects or ventricular septal defects develop. If the twisting of the heart and its subdivision into the four chambers does not occur normally, complex anomalies such as tetralogy of Fallot form. In that anomaly, the base of the heart seems to be twisted too much to the right, causing the aorta to be displaced to the right *(dextroposition of the aorta)*. The malpositioned aorta causes narrowing of the adjacent pulmonary artery, which results in *pulmonary stenosis*. There are many other examples of abnormal positioning of the large vessels, but these are relatively uncommon.

The causes of congenital heart diseases can theoretically be classified as either exogenous or endogenous. Among the former, the most important are viruses and alcohol, whereas chromosomal abnormalities are among the most important endogenous causes.

- *Viruses.* The best-known cause of a congenital heart defect is the *rubella virus,* the cause of German measles. Infection of the mother during the first 3 months of pregnancy is associated with a high incidence of congenital heart disease in offspring. Apparently the virus crosses the placenta, enters the fetal circulation, and damages the developing heart. Rubella can be prevented by immunization. Widespread immunization against rubella in the United States has decreased the incidence of heart defects caused by this virus.
- *Alcohol.* The complex syndrome of fetal anomalies called *fetal alcohol syndrome* is often associated with heart defects. Alcohol affects the fetal heart directly and interferes with its development. It has been proposed that alcohol is toxic to fetal heart cells and destroys them, but the exact teratogenic mechanism of alcohol remains unknown.
- *Chromosomal abnormalities.* Chromosomal abnormalities are associated with several developmental syndromes, many of which include congenital heart disease. The best known example is Down's syndrome or trisomy 21, which often is associated with heart defects.

Pathology

Pediatric cardiologists have recognized more than 50 congenital heart defects, the diagnosis and treatment of which are usually coordinated by highly specialized teams that include a pediatric cardiologist, radiologist, and cardiac surgeon. Only three examples are presented: two simple septal defects and one complex congenital heart defect *(tetralogy of Fallot).*

SEPTAL DEFECTS

The left side of the heart is separated from the right side by a septum. This septum may be defective—that is, it may have a hole in it that, according to its location, may be called either *atrial* or *ventricular.* They may occur as isolated defects, which is most often the case, or they may be part of complex malformation syndromes. Of the two abnormalities, interventricular septal defect is the more serious condition. Septal defects represent the most common form of congenital heart disease, accounting for 30% to 40% of all clinically recognized cases.

ATRIAL SEPTAL DEFECT

Atrial septal defect most often results from incomplete or defective closure of the foramen ovale and the formation of adjacent connective tissue part of the interatrial septum. Other forms of atrial septal defect, which may also involve the lower part of the septum and thus may affect the formation of mitral and tricuspid valves (called *endocardial cushion defect*) or other parts of the septum are less common.

Atrial septal defects are recognized clinically by the murmur caused by the passage of blood from the left to the right atrium during systole. Most often this left-to-right shunt has only minor functional consequences, until it becomes more prominent or becomes complicated by endocardial infection. Atrial septal defects can be easily closed by surgical intervention.

VENTRICULAR SEPTAL DEFECT

Ventricular septal defect is the most common congenital heart defect recognized in clinical practice. The symptoms of this condition result from the mixing of blood in the left and right heart chambers as a consequence of the septal defect (Figure 7-4). Because pressure within the left heart chamber generally exceeds the pressure in the right chamber, the arterial blood from the left ventricle or atrium will flow to the right side of the heart, resulting in a left-to-right shunt. As a result of the increased backflow of blood, this left-to-right shunt overburdens the right ventricle, causing it to work twice as hard as normal and resulting in right ventricular hypertrophy. The increased flow of blood through the pulmonary arteries leads to pulmonary hypertension, which is usually accompanied by anatomic changes in the pulmonary artery and its branches. The rising pulmonary hypertension and the narrowing of pulmonary artery branches finally reaches a point at which the pressure in the right ventricle exceeds the pressure in the left ventricle. This reverses the blood flow.

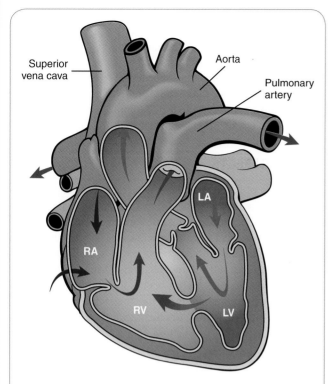

Figure 7-4 Ventricular septal defect. In the early stages of this disease, the blood flows from left to right. Once pulmonary hypertension develops, the direction of the blood flow through the shunt reverses, and the venous blood from the right ventricle (RV) enters the left ventricle (LV), where it mixes with the arterial blood. This dilution of arterial blood with unoxygenated venous blood leads to cyanosis ("late cyanosis"). LA, left atrium; RA, right atrium.

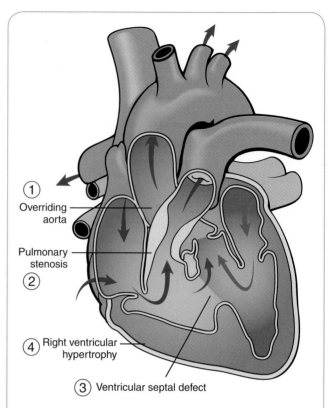

Figure 7-5 Tetralogy of Fallot. The heart shows dextroposition of the aorta, which is overriding a ventricular septal defect and is associated with pulmonary stenosis. Because of the congenital stenosis of the pulmonary artery, which prevents the outflow of blood from the right ventricle, there is right-to-left shunting of the blood and early cyanosis.

A right-to-left shunt ensues, at which point the unoxygenated venous blood from the right ventricle and atrium enters the systemic circulation. The venous blood dilutes the arterial blood and reduces its oxygen content, resulting in *cyanosis,* or a bluish discoloration of the skin (in Greek, *kyanos* means "blue").

Septal defects produce distinct high-pitched systolic heart murmurs. Most patients have no symptoms. Some of the small defects close spontaneously. However, the larger ones require surgical intervention, whereby a patch of Dacron or some similar artificial material is sutured over the defect. A patient's own connective tissue, removed from other parts of the body, may also be used to patch up the septal defect. The results usually are excellent.

TETRALOGY OF FALLOT

Tetralogy of Fallot, a complex congenital defect of the heart and the major vessels, is the most common cause of cardiac cyanosis in newborn children, accounting for 10% of all congenital heart defects. The pathologic changes associated with this condition, first described by the French physician Fallot, include four typical lesions (Figure 7-5):

- Valvular stenosis (narrowing) of the pulmonary artery
- Ventricular septal defect involving the uppermost membranous part of the septum

- Dextroposition of the aorta whereby the aorta is moved to the right of its normal position and overrides the septum, thus receiving blood from both the left and the right ventricles
- Hypertrophy of the right ventricle, which is adaptive in nature and develops as a result of the increased workload of the right ventricle

Infants affected by this defect develop cyanosis early after birth and present as "blue babies." The skin turns bluish, most notably over the fingers and toes, lips, cheeks, and earlobes.

The reason for the cyanosis can be deduced from Figure 7-5. Note that the pulmonary artery is narrowed, which limits the amount of blood that can enter the lungs to become oxygenated. The right ventricle attempts to overcome this obstacle at its own outflow tract by pumping more blood. This additional effort causes hypertrophy of the right ventricle. The venous blood in the right ventricle that cannot enter the narrowed pulmonary artery is shunted through the septal defect into the aorta. The mixing of blood from the right and left ventricle is facilitated by the abnormal position of the aorta, which overrides the septum. Thus the aorta can be filled with blood from both ventricles and will contain both venous and arterial blood.

Without surgical repair, most children born with this defect die before puberty. Surgical correction of the defect provides some hope, but the outcome depends on the severity of the defect and other extenuating circumstances.

ATHEROSCLEROSIS

Atherosclerosis is a systemic disease affecting the arteries. The term—derived from the Greek word *athere,* meaning "gruel" or "porridge," and *scleros,* meaning "hard"—describes the simultaneous hardening and softening of the arteries that occur in this disease.

Although atherosclerosis may affect all arteries in the body, in clinical practice it is common to encounter patients in whom the symptoms of a single organ predominate. Thus in addition to the generalized form, it is customary to recognize four major localized forms of atherosclerosis (Figure 7-6):

- Atherosclerosis of the coronary arteries, known as **coronary heart disease**
- Atherosclerosis of the brain arteries, known as cerebrovascular disease or, more commonly, as a cause of cerebrovascular accidents (CVAs)
- Atherosclerosis of the aorta, which usually presents in the form of aortic calcifications and aortic aneurysms
- Atherosclerosis of the arteries in the extremities, known as *peripheral vascular disease*

Etiology and Pathogenesis

Atherosclerosis is, in general, a disease of old age. However, the earliest arterial lesions usually develop long before they become symptomatic and clinically apparent. It is believed that the first damage occurs at the interface between the blood and the arterial wall. This endothelial cell injury, which may be a consequence of metabolic derangements or physical force (e.g., hypertension), is accompanied by the deposition of blood platelets and serum lipoproteins. Growth factors released from platelets stimulate the proliferation of smooth muscle cells in the wall of the artery (Figure 7-7). The altered environment and the changes in the internal metabolism of smooth muscle cells promote the accumulation of cholesterol and other lipids in their cytoplasm. Typically the smooth muscle cells transform into foam cells. Some of the lipid-laden smooth muscle cells die, releasing lipid into the interstitial spaces; this is either oxidized, degraded, or deposited in the form of cholesterol crystals. These lesions then attract macrophages, which act as scavengers. Macrophages take up cell remnants and the lipid released from dying or injured smooth muscle cells and also transform into foam cells. Macrophages secrete cytokines and biologically active substances, such as tumor necrosis factor (TNF), transforming growth factor beta (TGF-beta), and others, that affect other cells in the atheroma, causing more damage. Collagen deposition within atheromas leads to hardening of the arteries *(sclerosis).*

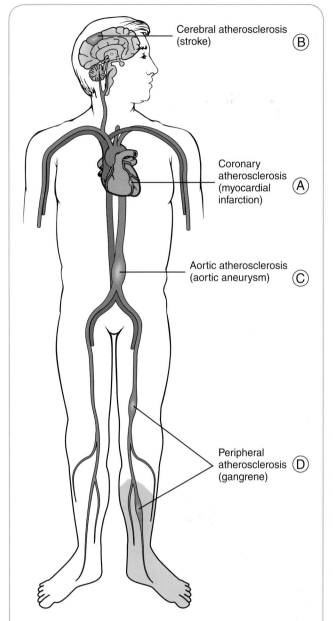

Figure 7-6 The four major forms of atherosclerosis are classified as coronary *(A),* cerebral *(B),* aortic *(C),* and peripheral vascular *(D).*

Atheromas are the prototypical lesions of atherosclerosis. As shown in Figure 7-8, atheromas bulge into the lumen of the artery. The central part of the atheroma is soft and consists of lipids and cellular debris. This soft core is covered on the surface by fibrous tissue that forms a *surface cap* on such lesions. However, even this reinforcement is not adequate to preserve the integrity of the vessel wall. The pressure of the liquefied porridge-like material may cause rupture of the surface cap, leading to intimal ulceration. The content of the atheroma entering into the lumen of the artery is highly thrombogenic, and it initiates formation of a blood clot that typically covers the rough base of the intimal ulcer (see Figure 7-8). In large arteries like the aorta, these

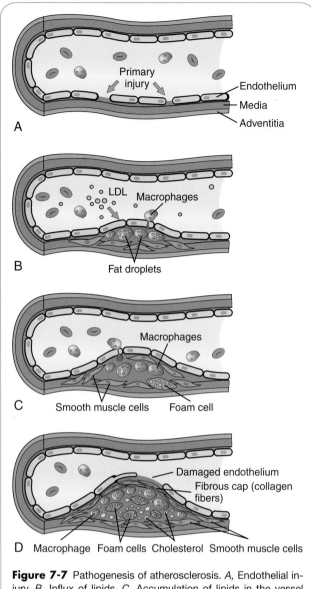

Figure 7-7 Pathogenesis of atherosclerosis. *A,* Endothelial injury. *B,* Influx of lipids. *C,* Accumulation of lipids in the vessel wall, proliferation of smooth muscle cells, and accumulation of macrophages. *D,* Atheromas consist of a lipid-rich soft part and a firm fibrous cap. LDL, low-density lipoprotein.

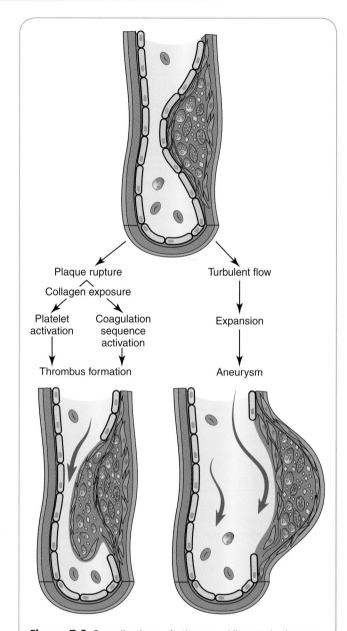

Figure 7-8 Complications of atheroma. Ulcerated atheromatous lesions are often sites of thrombosis. The weakened arterial wall may bulge outward, giving rise to an aneurysm.

thrombi do not cause immediate symptoms but eventually become organized, ultimately transforming into fibrous scars. In smaller arteries, such as the coronary or cerebral arteries, formation of the thrombus is usually accompanied by complete occlusion of the lumen of the vessel, with subsequent infarction.

The major complication of atherosclerosis is hardening of vessels, primarily a consequence of calcification of the vessel wall. In pathogenetic terms, this calcification is dystrophic (i.e., precipitated by local tissue degeneration). Lipids released from dead cells and abnormal extracellular matrix extract calcium salts. Calcium salts are thus deposited both in atheromas and in the fibrous tissue. Calcified arteries can be seen on radiographs because calcium salts are radiodense.

The atherosclerotic aorta tends to dilate and form **aneurysms** (from the Greek *aneurysma,* meaning "dilation"). Blood flow in the aneurysms is irregular. Eddies and whorls inside the aneurysm predispose the individual to thrombosis. Such thrombi can have a beneficial effect because they prevent further widening of the aneurysm. Nevertheless, most aneurysms dilate progressively as a result of internal pressure.

Risk Factors

Atherosclerosis is considered a multifactorial disease with many risk factors (Table 7-1). The exact role of these risk factors is unknown, but it is important to remember that the risks can be diminished by changing one's lifestyle. The beneficial

TABLE 7-1 Cardiovascular Risk Factors

Risk Factors That Cannot Be Changed	Risk Factors That Can Be Changed	Protective Factors
Age Gender Heredity	Lipid metabolism–related factors: Diet Hyperlipidemia Obesity Diabetes mellitus Hypertension Clotting factors Cigarette smoking Behavior	Exercise Estrogen

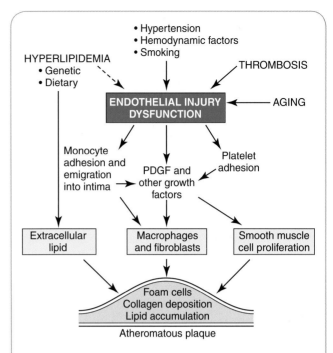

Figure 7-9 Endothelial cell injury plays a crucial role in atherosclerosis. Hyperlipidemia and thrombosis are major contributing factors. PDGF, platelet-derived growth factor.

effects of an atherosclerosis prevention program are evident from a review of public health records, which show a significant reduction in atherosclerotic heart disease and other forms of atherosclerosis in the United States. This reduced incidence of atherosclerosis is probably related to changes in the American diet, increased emphasis on exercise and physical fitness, and reduced smoking.

The following risk factors are clinically important:
- *Age.* Atherosclerosis is a disease of older age.
- *Sex.* Atherosclerosis affects more males than females. After menopause, the sex difference becomes less prominent. Apparently, the female sex hormones have a beneficial effect. In postmenopausal women, regular intake of estrogens may reduce the progression and extent of atherosclerosis.
- *Heredity.* It has been known for many years that atherosclerosis affects some families and spares others. However, even the hereditary forms of atherosclerosis have many causes, and the inheritance is considered *polygenic.*
- *Lipid metabolism–related factors.* Lipid accumulates in atheromas and is unquestionably one of the major pathogenetic factors in the formation of atherosclerotic lesions (Figure 7-9). Elevated serum levels of lipids—cholesterol, lipoproteins, and triglycerides—directly correlate with the extent and severity of atherosclerosis and, most importantly, with the early onset of clinical symptoms.

Hyperlipidemia can occur as a primary, familial, or secondary (externally induced) disease. Familial hyperlipidemias occur in several forms. In most instances, these polygenic diseases may be significantly modified by exogenous factors, most notably by the diet. Hyperlipidemias are aggravated by overeating and especially by a diet rich in unsaturated fats, such as animal fats or coconut oil. A high-fiber, low-fat diet and the use of vegetable oils, such as olive oil, in place of unsaturated fats have a favorable effect.

Secondary hyperlipidemia is most often encountered in obese people. Some of these persons have an underlying genetic predisposition that, combined with overeating, results in an overall increased deposition of fat in the body. Because the tissue fat is in equilibrium with the circulating lipids, the increased total body fat leads to hyperlipidemia.

Overall, obese people develop atherosclerosis at an earlier age and have more pronounced atherosclerotic lesions than do age-matched controls of normal habitus. Several disturbances of intermediate metabolism affect the metabolism of fats, but the most important disease in this category is diabetes mellitus. Diabetes predisposes individuals to atherosclerosis and also aggravates the course of the disease. Thus most people with diabetes whose disease is inadequately controlled develop arterial lesions early in life and have more prominent atherosclerosis than those whose diabetes is controlled with a strict diet or insulin.

- *Hypertension.* Clinical studies have shown that hypertension correlates with atherosclerosis. If the hypertension develops at an early age and is not properly controlled, it will accelerate the development of atherosclerosis. Medical control of hypertension has greatly contributed to the reduced incidence of atherosclerosis in the United States that has been observed during the past two decades. The exact role of hypertension in the development of atheromas is not fully understood. Hypothetically, it is possible that the elevated pressure of the blood compresses the intimal cells, making them **ischemic** or stimulating them to release some cytokines that promote atherosclerosis or initiate proliferation of smooth muscle cells. The jet stream of blood could also contribute to the insudation of lipids into the vessel wall, a process likened to forceful filtration of plasma across the intimal layer. Finally, hypertension may cause changes in the clotting system by damaging the platelets, causing their aggregation and the release of bioactive substances from their cytoplasm.

- *Clotting factors.* Soluble clotting factors, such as fibrin, thrombin, and platelets, play an important role in the initiation of atherosclerotic lesions. The exact mechanism of action of the clot on the endothelium and the underlying smooth muscle cells is poorly understood. However, it has been shown that aspirin, which prevents clotting, may reduce the incidence of atherosclerotic complications if given prophylactically.

- *Cigarette smoking.* Epidemiologic studies have implicated cigarette smoking as one of the most important risk factors of atherosclerosis. The adverse effects of cigarette smoke on blood vessels are not fully understood, but they are partially related to nicotine and partially related to tar and other harmful components of smoke. It is hoped that the campaign against smoking will contribute further to the decreased mortality from atherosclerosis. In Eastern European countries and the Far East, where smoking is still highly prevalent, the incidence of atherosclerosis is still on the rise.

- *Behavior.* Clinical studies indicate that constant stress may accelerate or aggravate atherosclerosis, but such claims are not fully documented and therefore are not generally accepted. It appears that individuals who are under constant pressure to perform develop atherosclerosis more often than relaxed phlegmatics. However, the lifestyle of the overachievers is so much different from those who "take it easy" that it is not possible to separate the consequences of "endogenous personality trait" from the influences of the environment in which they live. It is widely accepted that a healthful lifestyle—work accompanied by periodic relaxation and regular exercise—can reduce the risks of atherosclerosis.

ATHEROSCLEROSIS OF THE AORTA

Atherosclerosis of the aorta is a very common finding in older men. Almost all persons older than 50 years have atherosclerosis of the aorta of some degree. The lesions vary from mild to severe and may be focal to diffuse. Clinically such lesions may be symptomatic, but most often they are asymptomatic.

The mildest forms of atherosclerosis are found in young or middle-aged persons. Such individuals have fatty streaks, slightly raised fibrotic plaques, and only occasionally atheromas. As the disease progresses, the atheromas become more numerous and coalesce, occupying large surface areas. Atheromas may rupture, at which time they are covered with thrombi that narrow the lumen of the aorta or distort the blood flow. Calcifications of the atheromas and the fibrous tissues surrounding them reduce the elasticity of the blood vessel. In the final stages of the disease, the aorta transforms into a rigid, calcified tube that has a rugged, partially ulcerated, internal surface covered focally with thrombi (Figure 7-10).

The atherosclerotic aorta cannot adapt to the changes of blood pressure that occur during the normal cardiac contraction cycle. Because the aorta cannot expand during systole, hypertension develops as the same amount of blood now passes through a narrower blood vessel. The pressure from inside causes dilation of the inelastic aorta, which leads to the formation of an aneurysm.

Aneurysms are dilations of the aortic lumen that may occur in several forms. Most often they are spindle shaped *(fusiform)* or appear as eccentric dilations *(saccular)* (Figure 7-11). Aneurysms can occur in any part of the aorta. Atherosclerotic aneurysms are most often located in the abdominal aorta.

Aneurysms are often clinically silent, and many are discovered accidentally during a detailed medical examination. The major danger is that the aneurysm may rupture and cause death by exsanguination. In such cases the jet of blood may also dissect between the layers of the aortic wall, forming a second lumen, or through the wall of the aorta into the adjacent soft tissue. Such bulging lesions traditionally have been called *dissecting aneurysms,* even though they are actually intramural or periaortic hematomas. *Aortic dissection* is a much better name because it describes more accurately the pathogenesis of this lesion.

Aneurysms can be resected surgically and replaced by an artificial vessel made of Dacron or some similar plastic material. Rupture of aneurysms is associated with high mortality.

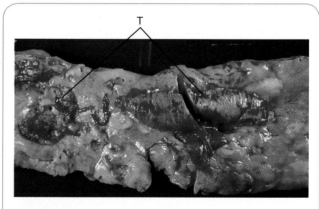

Figure 7-10 Gross appearance of an atherosclerotic aorta. The surface of the aorta is rugged and irregular. Organized thrombi (T), one of which was incised by the pathologist, are seen protruding from the endothelial surface.

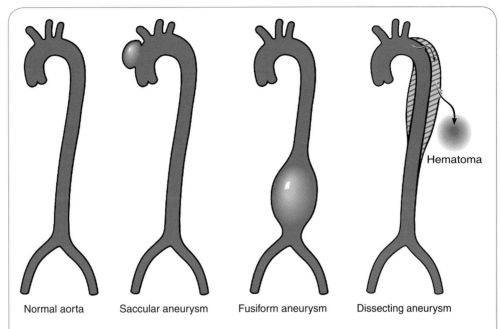

Hematoma

Normal aorta   Saccular aneurysm   Fusiform aneurysm   Dissecting aneurysm

Figure 7-11 Various forms of aneurysms. The so-called *dissecting aneurysm* is also included even though this lesion represents an actual intramural hematoma in the aortic wall or a soft tissue periaortic hematoma.

PERIPHERAL VASCULAR DISEASE

Peripheral vascular disease refers to atherosclerosis involving the arteries that supply the blood to the extremities and the major abdominal organs, such as the intestines and kidney. Atherosclerosis of the peripheral arteries is common in elderly people, persons with diabetes, and those who have hyperlipidemia and hypertension. It is often part of a generalized atherosclerosis and is associated with atherosclerosis of the aorta and coronary and cerebral arteries. From a clinical point of view, it is customary to distinguish between symptoms caused by ischemia of the major organs and those caused by ischemic changes in the extremities.

Atherosclerosis of the renal arteries is common in persons with atherosclerosis of the aorta. The renal arteries originate from the aorta and are relatively short. Thus aortic atherosclerosis easily spreads into the renal arteries. Because the renal arteries are much narrower than the aorta, symptoms caused by their occlusion are often more prominent. Reduced flow of blood through the renal arteries causes hypoperfusion of the kidneys, which results in reduced renal functional capacity. This renal dysfunction, combined with an increased release of renin (a hormone produced by the kidney in response to ischemia), leads to hypertension. Reduced excretion of urine and urinary sodium further aggravates hypertension, which in turn damages the kidneys. Atherosclerosis may thus cause irreversible (end-stage) kidney failure.

Atherosclerosis of the intestinal arteries causes ischemia in the small and large intestines. Such ischemia may be chronic or acute. Chronic ischemia caused by narrowing of the arteries

and partial occlusion of their lumina is the most common form. Chronic ischemia usually has a gradual onset and causes nonspecific gastrointestinal problems: constipation, poor digestion, intolerance of certain foods, and malabsorption. These symptoms may fluctuate, but generally they are progressive. Many older persons have chronic constipation and a variety of other intestinal ailments.

Acute occlusion of the intestinal arteries causes massive intestinal infarction. Usually it is a consequence of thrombotic or embolic occlusion of a major intestinal artery. Intestinal infarction is associated with high mortality.

Atherosclerosis of the extremities typically affects the legs more often than the arms. It may present as chronic ischemia or as acute occlusion of the blood flow.

Chronic ischemia of the lower limbs secondary to the progressive narrowing of the femoral artery or popliteal artery results in underperfusion of the leg muscles. When a person is at rest or moves around slowly, the blood supply is adequate and no symptoms are present. However, if the same person walks a long distance or tries to run, the blood supply becomes inadequate and the leg muscles develop cramps. This is called *intermittent claudication* (from the Latin term *claudicatio*, meaning "limping"). Surgical cleansing of the vessels *(endarterectomy)* or removal of the atheromas with catheters may improve the clinical picture.

Sudden occlusion of the arteries of the lower limb, usually at the level of one of the smaller branches, results in gangrene. The necrotic tissue, which is typically black and mummified *(dry gangrene),* may become infected and diffluent *(wet gangrene)*. Both forms of gangrene require surgical treatment, which usually entails resection of the extremity.

CORONARY HEART DISEASE

Atherosclerosis of the coronary arteries may present in several clinical forms, all of which have the same underlying pathogenetic mechanism: *myocardial ischemia* (Figure 7-12). The clinical presentation depends on several factors:

- Extent of the occlusion
- Rapidity with which the ischemia develops
- Extent of atherosclerosis in other branches of the coronary system
- Anatomic location of the occluding lesion
- Presence or absence of other changes and diseases, such as hypertension or hyperthyroidism, which may complicate the course of ischemia

Myocardial ischemia may develop as a result of a slowly progressive narrowing of the coronary arteries or a sudden occlusion. *Chronic progressive ischemia* results in hypoperfusion of the myocardium and slowly evolving pump failure. The patient may be asymptomatic or have precordial pain, known as angina pectoris. Ultimately, progressive ischemia leads to **congestive heart failure.** Coronary thrombosis is common in arteries narrowed by atherosclerosis.

Sudden occlusion of a major coronary artery results in an infarct in an anatomically defined area. Thus an anterior wall infarct is typically caused by occlusion of the descending branch of the left coronary artery, an infarct of the lateral wall of the left ventricle is usually the result of occlusion of the circumflex branch of the left coronary artery, and an infarct of the right ventricle and the posterior wall of the left ventricle is usually caused by occlusion of the right coronary artery (Figure 7-13). Occlusion of the anterior descending branch of the left coronary artery accounts for approximately 50% of all cases, whereas the right coronary artery is occluded in 30% to 40% of cases, and the remaining 15% to 20% of cases involve occlusion of the left circumflex artery.

Pathology

The coronary arteries affected by atherosclerosis are typically transformed into rigid, heavily calcified cylinders that can be palpated beneath the epicardium as thick nodular sinews. On cross sectioning, their lumina are narrowed because of prominent fibrotic plaques and atheromas. The wall of the coronary arteries contains deposits of calcium salts. In acute occlusion, the plaques rupture and the defect of the endothelium is covered with a clot occluding the narrowed lumen (Figure 7-14). In older lesions, such thrombi are partially organized by granulation tissue that has grown into them from the vessel wall. Some thrombi appear to be recanalized—that is, traversed by numerous small blood vessels that have reestablished blood flow across the occluded segment of the artery.

Sudden occlusion of a coronary artery leads to myocardial infarction. An infarct is characterized by ischemic cell death, which can be recognized morphologically first by typical microscopic changes and then by macroscopic changes in the heart.

The first light microscopic changes occur approximately 24 hours after the onset of occlusion. These include nuclear signs of cell death, such as pyknosis, karyorrhexis, and karyolysis; cytoplasmic signs of coagulation necrosis; and the appearance of the first inflammatory cells, polymorphonuclear neutrophils (PMNs). PMNs predominate during the next 2 to 3 days, and then on day 4 to 5 the infarcted area is gradually infiltrated with macrophages. Macrophages persist in the lesion for some time, during which they phagocytize and remove the necrotic myocardial cells and help in the formation of granulation tissue that begins appearing toward the end of the first week. As in wound healing, granulation tissue is composed of small blood vessels, myofibroblasts, and fibroblasts depositing extracellular matrix. In older infarcts, fibroblasts predominate, the collagenous matrix is more prominent, and small blood vessels are less prominent. Ultimately the necrotic myocardium is replaced by an acellular fibrous scar.

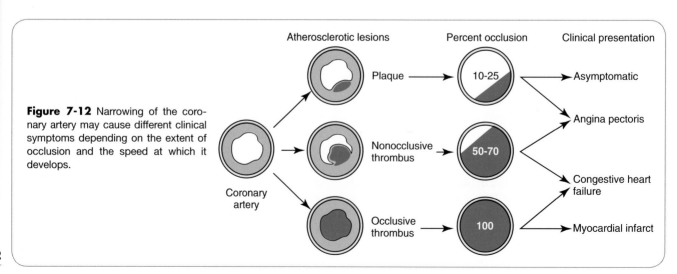

Figure 7-12 Narrowing of the coronary artery may cause different clinical symptoms depending on the extent of occlusion and the speed at which it develops.

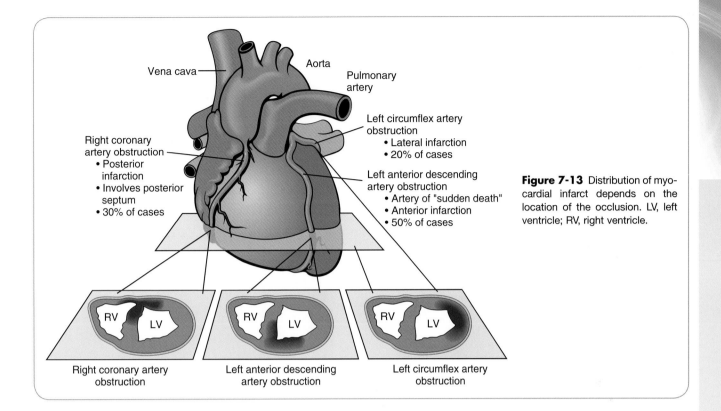

Figure 7-13 Distribution of myocardial infarct depends on the location of the occlusion. LV, left ventricle; RV, right ventricle.

Labels in figure:
- Vena cava
- Aorta
- Pulmonary artery
- Right coronary artery obstruction
  - Posterior infarction
  - Involves posterior septum
  - 30% of cases
- Left circumflex artery obstruction
  - Lateral infarction
  - 20% of cases
- Left anterior descending artery obstruction
  - Artery of "sudden death"
  - Anterior infarction
  - 50% of cases
- Right coronary artery obstruction
- Left anterior descending artery obstruction
- Left circumflex artery obstruction

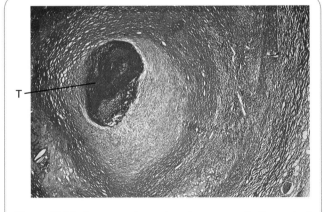

Figure 7-14 Coronary atherosclerosis accompanied by marked narrowing of the lumen of the coronary artery and an intraluminal thrombus (T).

These histologic changes correlate with the macroscopic findings. On gross examination, the infarcted area cannot be definitively identified during the first 1 to 2 days. There may be some pallor of the infarcted area, but this is not prominent. Approximately 3 to 5 days after the occlusion, the infarct becomes yellow and is surrounded by a hemorrhagic rim. The yellow infarcted myocardium is softened as a result of the action of hydrolytic enzymes released from the leukocytes. This softening is most prominent toward the end of the first week after occlusion. Softened myocardium may rupture,

causing sudden death as a result of the accumulation of blood into the pericardial sac **(hemopericardium).**

The ingrowth of granulation tissue, which brings into the infarcted area new blood and connective tissue, imparts to the infarct a grayish red and mottled appearance that persists for 1 to 2 weeks. Thereafter, cross sections of the heart show that fibrosis predominates; old infarcts appear as whitish gray, firm, and irregularly shaped scars that are slightly depressed and easily distinguishable from the brown color of normal myocardium.

Complications

Complications of myocardial infarction (Figure 7-15) may include the following:

- **Ventricular rupture.** Softened necrotic myocardium may rupture as a result of the increased pressure of the blood within the ventricle. The blood that penetrates through the ruptured left ventricle fills the pericardial sac, compressing the heart (hemopericardium).
- **Cardiac tamponade.** This compression of the heart by blood in the pericardial cavity typically occurs 5 to 7 days after infarction and usually is lethal (Figure 7-16).
- **Ventricular aneurysm.** Massive myocardial infarcts of the left ventricle, which are replaced by fibrous scars, bulge under the pressure of blood in the left ventricle, forming an aneurysm. The heart is dilated and contracts irregularly because the fibrous scar forming the wall of the aneurysm does not contain contractile elements.
- **Endocardial mural thrombus.** The endocardium overlying the infarcted myocardium is often damaged and disrupted.

143

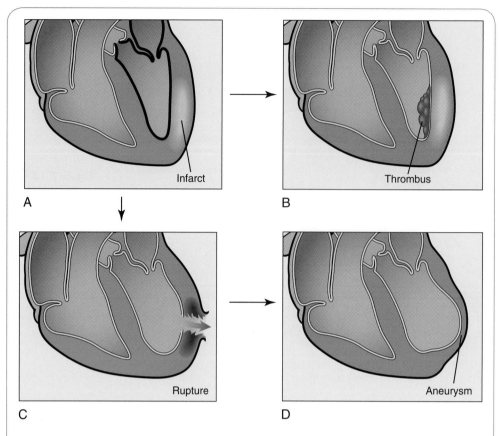

Figure 7-15 Complications of myocardial infarct. *A,* Myocardial infarct. *B,* Mural thrombus. *C,* Rupture. *D,* Aneurysm.

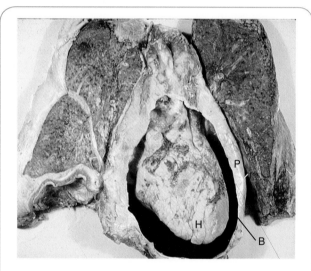

Figure 7-16 Hemopericardium caused by rupture of an infarct. The pericardial sac (P) is filled with blood (B) surrounding the heart (H).

The blood within the ventricle coagulates in contact with the necrotic endocardium or the exposed myocardium and forms a thrombus attached to the wall of the ventricle (the Latin term *mural* means "pertaining to the wall"). Such thrombi impede the blood flow and weaken the contraction of the ventricular myocardium, which may contribute to heart failure. Furthermore, fragments of the thrombus may detach, giving rise to *emboli,* which can cause infarcts in distant organs. Cerebral infarcts caused by such emboli are an important complication of myocardial infarcts.

Clinical Features

Coronary heart disease results from ischemia caused by atherosclerotic plaques and coronary thrombosis (Figure 7-17). The most important clinical presentations of coronary heart disease are the following:

- Congestive heart failure
- Angina pectoris
- Myocardial infarct

CONGESTIVE HEART FAILURE

Most of the symptoms of coronary heart disease are a consequence of hypoxia of the myocardium, which results in pump failure. Because the heart does not pump blood efficiently, backpressure from stagnant blood impedes the venous blood return to the heart. Right ventricular failure causes congestion of the peripheral organs and extremities (Figure 7-18). Typically the legs become swollen, especially toward the end of the day. The chronic passive congestion also causes enlargement of the liver. The enlarged liver stretches the capsule, and this stimulates the nerves in the capsule, causing pain below

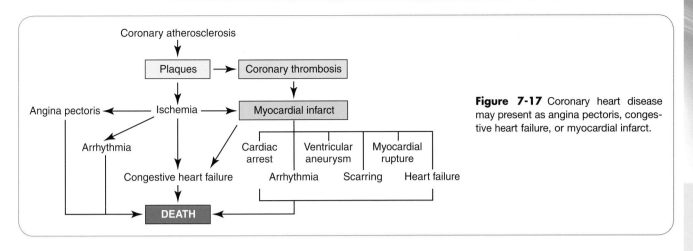

Figure 7-17 Coronary heart disease may present as angina pectoris, congestive heart failure, or myocardial infarct.

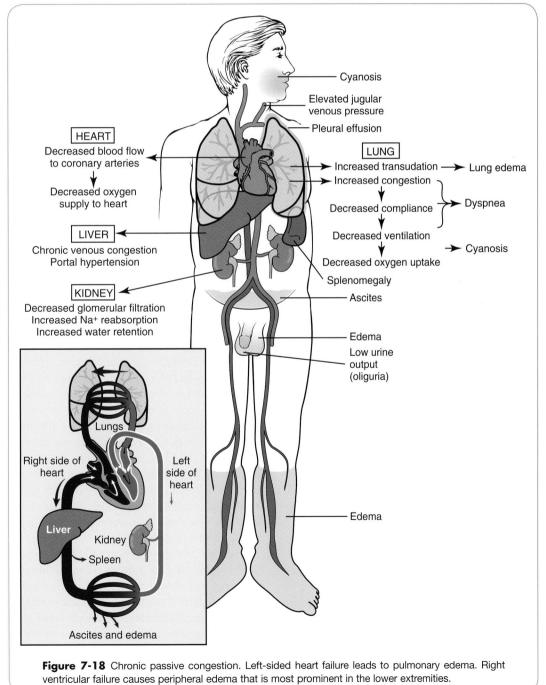

Figure 7-18 Chronic passive congestion. Left-sided heart failure leads to pulmonary edema. Right ventricular failure causes peripheral edema that is most prominent in the lower extremities.

the right costal margin. In addition, pressure in the abdominal veins may lead to the accumulation of fluid in the abdominal cavity (i.e., formation of *ascites*). These changes are schematically shown in Figure 7-18. Failure of the left ventricle leads to pulmonary congestion and pulmonary edema secondary to transudation of fluids into the alveoli. Pleural effusions also develop, and patients become short of breath (i.e., develop *dyspnea*). In severe heart failure, dyspnea is present at all times. In milder cases, dyspnea develops only when the patient exercises or works strenuously.

Hypoperfusion of the major organs impairs their functions. Because of a lack of oxygen, brain functions are slowed and patients become somnolent, cannot concentrate, and easily develop mental fatigue. Hypoperfusion of the kidneys results in a reduction in urine formation *(oliguria)*. Renal failure causes retention of sodium and water, which results in generalized edema, called *anasarca*. Affected patients die of progressive heart failure and multiple organ failure.

ANGINA PECTORIS

The myocardium that is inadequately perfused may function normally until additional demands are made by exercise, climbing of stairs, or running. This additional effort cannot be sustained because the narrowed blood vessels do not allow influx of blood into the myocardium. The resulting ischemia causes pain, which is called angina pectoris, the Latin term for "*chest pain.*" Attacks of angina pectoris are typically precipitated by exercise or strain and can be alleviated by nitroglycerin, a drug that dilates the vessels. However, as the atherosclerosis progresses, nitroglycerin becomes less and less efficient.

MYOCARDIAL INFARCT

Rapid, sudden occlusion of a coronary artery causes an infarct. Myocardial infarct is a serious condition. Sudden death occurs in approximately 25% of cases. In most cases this is a consequence of major **arrhythmia** *(ventricular fibrillation), heart block,* and subsequent pump failure, or *asystole* (cardiac arrest). Patients typically experience crushing precordial pain, often followed by loss of consciousness or fainting. By the time the infarct is recognized, the patient is prostrate, without a pulse, and in severe distress. Unless cardiothoracic resuscitation is initiated immediately, death occurs within minutes. Even with closed chest cardiac massage, mouth-to-mouth resuscitation, and electric shock treatment to restart the heart, the results are poor if the asystole has lasted a few minutes.

Among the 75% of patients who survive the onset of an acute myocardial infarct, most develop signs of heart failure and cardiogenic shock (Figure 7-19). Because of inadequate perfusion of tissues by blood from the failing heart, multisystemic major organ failure develops. Most dangerous are the consequences of cerebral ischemia, which may lead to permanent mental injury and loss of central nervous system functions. Any cerebral ischemia that lasts longer than a few minutes irreversibly damages the brain, resulting in an ischemic stroke with major neurologic deficits such as paralysis, loss of sensations, or loss of consciousness. Even if they

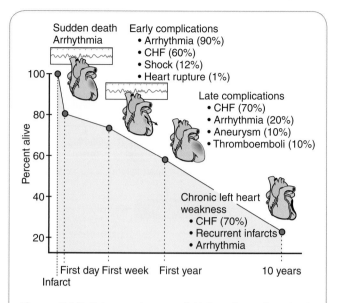

Figure 7-19 Outcome of myocardial infarct. Immediate death, early complications (first week), and later complications account for the 40% mortality rate during the first year after the infarct. The 10-year survival rate is approximately 25%. CHF, congestive heart failure.

recover, many patients have permanent neurologic or mental defects.

Many other organs may be affected, but the kidneys are the organs most often damaged. Typical signs of renal failure, such as oliguria and anuria, are common. Therefore it is important to monitor urine output in these patients. To this end, most patients in coronary intensive care units have an indwelling urinary catheter.

Diagnosis

The diagnosis of myocardial infarction is made on the basis of typical complaints (e.g., chest pain, shortness of breath, and fainting) and clinical and laboratory findings. Electrocardiography and the measurement of enzymes released from the damaged myocardium into the serum are most useful in this respect. The *electrocardiogram (ECG),* the precordial recording of heart action currents, shows typical changes such as elevation of the ST segment. Various disturbances of the cardiac conduction system resulting in arrhythmia or heart block are also common. Myocardial infarction is associated with distinct laboratory findings related to the release of proteins from the cytoplasm of damaged or dead cardiac myocytes into the blood (Figure 7-20).

The first protein to appear in blood is myoglobin, which can be detected 1 to 2 hours after the onset of infarction. However, the elevation of blood myoglobin should not be taken as a definitive sign of myocardial infarction, because myoglobin is often released from injured skeletal muscles and could appear in blood even after minor trauma. However, the appearance of cardiac proteins troponin I or troponin T in blood, which occurs 3 to 6 hours after infarction, is

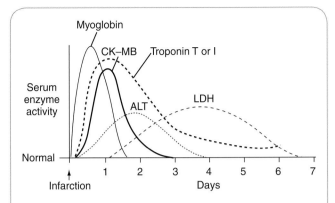

Figure 7-20 Enzymatic diagnosis of myocardial infarcts. Troponin T or I are currently the most important biochemical markers of myocardial infarction. Myoglobin may rise rapidly after myocardial infarction, but this finding is relatively nonspecific. Creatine kinase (CK-MB) is used less often. Alanine aminotransferase (ALT) and lactic dehydrogenase (LDH) rise in serum after myocardial infarction, but these findings are nonspecific.

highly specific and is currently the best laboratory marker of infarction. These changes are followed 1 to 2 hours later by an elevation of the MB fraction of creatine kinase (CK-MB), which is also specific. Other enzymes, such as alanine aminotransferase (ALT) and lactate dehydrogenase (LDH), become elevated after the second day and may remain elevated for some time. These nonspecific indicators of cell injury are less important in the diagnosis of myocardial infarction today.

Treatment

With modern therapy, the survival of patients with myocardial infarction has improved considerably. Nevertheless, 30% to 40% of all patients die during the first year. These statistics include acute mortality and death from various complications or the recurrence of infarcts. The remaining patients recover to a variable extent and lead a normal life. Most require periodic medical control and medication for the rest of their lives. Many undergo a coronary artery bypass to repair the sites of arterial occlusion. Unfortunately the damaged heart cannot be repaired, but in severe cases it can be replaced with a newly transplanted heart. Cardiac transplantation is currently reserved for younger persons.

HYPERTENSION AND HYPERTENSIVE HEART DISEASE

The pressure generated by the left ventricle for the ejection of blood into the aorta is called *arterial pressure*. It is measured with a sphygmomanometer placed on the cubital artery. Normal blood pressure is usually in the range of 120 mmHg during systole and 80 mmHg during diastole. During exercise, running, vigorous work, or excitement, the blood pressure rises but subsequently returns to normal values. Individuals with systolic pressures exceeding 160 mmHg or diastolic pressures greater than 90 mmHg have hypertension. Clinically, hypertension is classified as mild, moderate, or severe.

Etiology and Pathogenesis

In most hypertensive patients (approximately 90%), no specific cause for the elevated blood pressure can be found. These people have primary or essential hypertension. Although the pathogenesis of essential hypertension remains unknown, many contributing factors have been identified, including genetic determinants, occupation, lifestyle, and diet. Although the causes and mechanisms of essential hypertension are unknown, this disease can be treated successfully with modern drugs and appropriate changes in lifestyle and eating habits.

In approximately 10% of patients, the cause of hypertension is an underlying disease or medication or it is related to a physiologic event, such as pregnancy. These forms of hypertension are called *secondary*. Treatment of the underlying causative disease typically cures the hypertension. The most common causes of secondary hypertension are listed in Table 7-2.

The primary determinants of blood pressure are the *volume of circulating blood,* the *cardiac output,* and the *void space volume* of the cardiovascular system that has to be filled with the circulating blood (Figure 7-21). Each of these determinants can be modified upward or downward. Therefore normal blood pressure can be either decreased *(hypotension)* or increased *(hypertension)*. A *normotensive* state results from a balanced interaction of the physiologic determinants of blood pressure and their regulators.

BLOOD VOLUME

The blood volume is determined by many factors, such as age, body size, and sex. Seventy percent of the human body is made up of water, and the fluids in circulation are in

TABLE 7-2 Hypertension: Causes and Treatment

Form of Hypertension	Cause	Treatment
Essential	Unknown	Drugs
Secondary		
Renal	Kidney disease	Treatment of underlying kidney disease
Endocrine	Adrenocortical tumor Adrenomedullary tumor (pheochromocytoma)	Surgery Surgery
Neurogenic	Complex/psychological	Sedatives
Drugs	Examples: oral contraceptives, nasal decongestants, painkillers	Discontinue drug intake

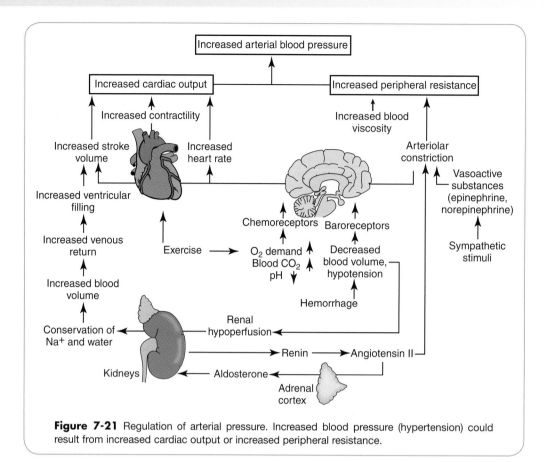

Figure 7-21 Regulation of arterial pressure. Increased blood pressure (hypertension) could result from increased cardiac output or increased peripheral resistance.

balance with those in the interstitial spaces in tissues and the intracellular fluids. Various physiologic factors regulate the passage of fluids from one body compartment to another and the accumulation of fluids in these compartments. The intake of fluids and the elimination of surplus fluids through the kidneys, intestines, sweat, excrement, and body secretions are all tightly regulated.

 Did You Know?

CABAGE is used for treatment of coronary atherosclerosis. This term does not refer to the leafy vegetable; it is the acronym for the surgical procedure used to revascularize the heart: coronary artery *bypass grafting.* More than 100,000 CABAGE procedures are performed every year in the United States.

Two examples of the importance of blood volume are presented here. A person with exsanguination secondary to a stab wound will become hypotensive. During such hypotensive shock, the kidneys stop producing urine to prevent fluid loss so that the perfusion of the vital organs can be maintained. Diametrically opposing events occur in kidney failure, when pathologically altered kidneys cannot eliminate fluid by excreting it in urine. In such instances, fluids overwhelm the body and overburden the circulation. To pump the extra fluid,

the heart must generate increased systolic pressure. When an overburdened heart fails, the diastolic pressure also rises because some blood that cannot be ejected remains in the cardiac chambers. This process causes hypertension, which can usually be treated successfully with diuretics (drugs that increase excretion of urine).

CARDIAC OUTPUT

Cardiac output can be calculated according to a formula that takes into account the capacity of the heart to pump blood, the amount of blood filling the chambers *(volume load),* and the resistance that it has to overcome in the aorta *(pressure load).* Any stimulus that increases the contractility of the heart, such as **adrenaline** (secreted from the adrenals in stress) or thyroid hormones (which increase the heart rate), can cause hypertension. Exercise and excitement, both of which are associated with the release of numerous vasoactive and cardiostimulatory substances, have a similar effect.

PERIPHERAL RESISTANCE

Peripheral resistance is regulated at many sites, but most importantly at the level of the arterioles. The walls of these precapillary vessels are composed of smooth muscle cells that can contract, thereby reducing the capillary blood flow. At the same time, the constricted arterioles increase resistance to the blood entering them from larger arteries, and this is transmitted backward to the aorta and the left ventricle.

The left ventricle, confronted with increased resistance in the arterial system, must increase pressure, which leads to hypertension.

The arterioles are critical for regulating blood pressure. The arterioles react to a number of humoral substances that cause their constriction or relaxation and dilation. Many neurotransmitters bind to the alpha- and beta-adrenergic receptors on the cell membrane of smooth muscle cells in arterioles. Thus hormonal and neural factors may directly affect this most important regulator of blood pressure in the arterial system.

The most important regulator of arteriolar tonus is the *renin-angiotensin system.* **Renin** is a hormone secreted by the juxtaglomerular apparatus in the kidney. Renin acts on a liver-derived plasma polypeptide called *angiotensinogen* to transform it into **angiotensin** I. *Angiotensin-converting enzyme (ACE)* found in the lungs converts angiotensin I to *angiotensin II,* which produces vasoconstriction of the arterioles and directly increases blood pressure. Angiotensin II also stimulates the adrenal cortex to release aldosterone. **Aldosterone** is a hormone that acts on the renal tubules to increase resorption of sodium. Sodium retention in the kidney is accompanied by retention of fluid, which also contributes to the elevation of blood pressure. Drugs, such as ACE inhibitors or antagonists of aldosterone, are used effectively in the treatment of hypertension. Diuretics that increase the excretion of sodium and water in urine are also widely used. Atrial natriuretic factor is a natural antagonist of renin and angiotensin, and it also lowers the blood pressure.

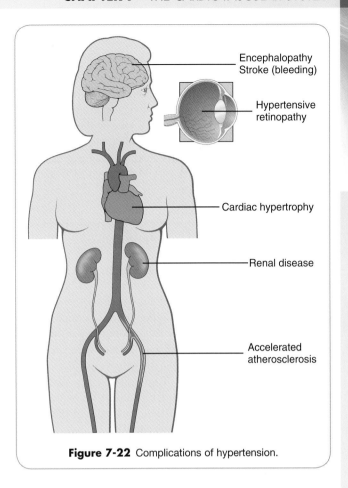

Figure 7-22 Complications of hypertension.

Pathology

The morphologic consequences of hypertension are seen in the heart and the peripheral vessels, especially in the kidney, brain, and eye (Figure 7-22).

CARDIOMEGALY

Enlargement of the heart, primarily as a consequence of the concentric hypertrophy of the left ventricle, is the principal consequence of hypertension. The thickness of the left ventricle increases from a normal thickness of 1.2 cm to 2.5 cm or more. Histologic examination reveals that all muscle fibers are thickened. Because the enlarged muscle cells need more blood than do normal cells, single cells often die as a result of ischemia and are replaced with fibrous tissue. Thus myocardial fibrosis is a common histologic finding in cardiomegaly.

Inefficient pumping of the blood from the left ventricle leads to backpressure, which increases pulmonary artery pressure. This in turn causes more work for the right ventricle and will eventually cause hypertrophy of the right ventricle. The hypertrophy of the left ventricle is the most common cause of right ventricular hypertrophy. Clinically the functional consequences of right ventricular hypertrophy and failure are called **cor pulmonale.**

VASCULAR PATHOLOGY

Hypertension damages the aorta, major and minor arteries, and arterioles. Hypertension accelerates the development of atherosclerosis. It is one of the major risk factors for ischemic heart disease. In the peripheral vascular system, hypertension-related changes are most prominent in the arterioles and small arteries.

Long-standing hypertension, also known as *benign hypertension,* causes hyalinization of the arterioles and fibrosis of the small arteries. *Malignant hypertension,* which is of sudden onset, may cause fibrinoid necrosis of these vessels and concentric proliferation of smooth muscle cells in arterioles *(proliferative endarteriolitis).* Renal ischemia caused by the narrowing of arterioles triggers the release of renin from the juxtaglomerular cells, aggravating the hypertension even more.

HYPERTENSIVE ENCEPHALOPATHY

Hypertensive encephalopathy refers to vascular changes in the brain that usually cause acute or chronic cerebral ischemia. Microscopic signs of chronic cerebral ischemia, such as focal nerve cell loss and microinfarcts, can be detected on histologic examination of the brain. Such patients may have only minor mental problems (e.g., forgetfulness), but often they are rather incapacitated. **Hypertensive stroke,** caused by sudden rupture of damaged brain arteries, presents as intracerebral hemorrhages that can be recognized by computed tomography (CT) scanning as well as during gross examination of the brain on autopsy. Hypertensive strokes produce major neurologic symptoms (e.g., paralysis) and are often lethal. Because of more efficient means of

149

treating hypertension, hypertensive strokes are less common today than 50 years ago.

HYPERTENSIVE RETINOPATHY

Retinal changes are an important complication of hypertension because they may impair vision and can eventually cause blindness. Retinal arteries are easily seen with the ophthalmoscope, and retinal changes are among the first signs of hypertension that can be clinically documented. The eye examination is therefore an important part of the physical workup of any patient with hypertension.

RHEUMATIC HEART DISEASE

Rheumatic fever (RF) is a systemic, immunologically mediated disease related to streptococcal infections. It affects not only the heart but also other organs and tissues such as the joints, the skin, and occasionally the brain. Rheumatic heart disease (RHD) was previously an important cause of morbidity and mortality. Although worldwide there are more than 15 million new cases diagnosed every year, in the United States, the incidence of this disease has decreased dramatically. This is primarily the result of the widespread use of antibiotics and more efficient treatment of the bacterial infections that invariably precede RF.

Etiology and Pathogenesis

RF typically occurs 2 weeks after an episode of "strep throat" (Figure 7-23). The immune response of the body elicited by the streptococcal antigens provides the body with a defense mechanism against the infection, which clearly is beneficial. It has been postulated that the antibodies against the streptococcal antigens cross-react with similar antigens found in the human heart and several other organs and tissues, such as the joints, skin, and brain. In addition to antibodies, a cell-mediated immune reaction develops and the suppressor/cytotoxic T lymphocytes and macrophages also may damage various tissues.

Pathology

RF affects all parts of the heart and is thus a pancarditis encompassing endocarditis, myocarditis, and pericarditis. **Endocarditis** is an inflammation of the internal surface lining of the heart chambers. The most prominent changes are seen on the endocardium covering the valves of the left side of the heart. This valvulitis begins with inflammation of the valvular surface, leading to an ulceration. Surface defects are covered with fibrin thrombi, which progressively grow and assume the form of larger vegetations or excrescences. Ongoing inflammation inside the valves leads to destruction of the valves, followed by fibrous scarring that causes valve deformities (Figure 7-24). The chordae tendineae inserting into the mitral valve are typically shortened and thickened and become fused to one another.

RHD affects the left side of the heart more than the right side. Because of the deformity of the leaflets and the changes in the chordae, the valves become incompetent and

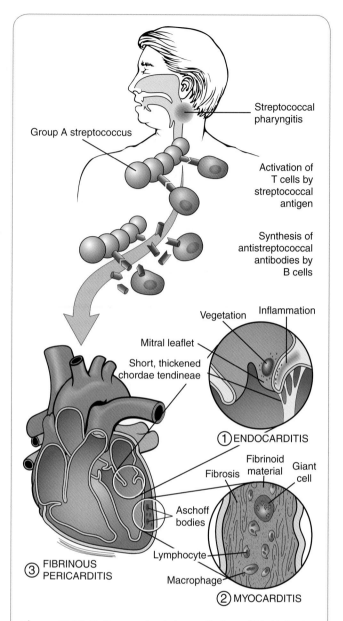

Figure 7-23 Pathogenesis of rheumatic fever (RF). Following infection ("strep throat"), an immune response elicited by the streptococci acts on the heart and several other organs, most notably the joints, skin, and central nervous system. In the heart it causes endocarditis, myocarditis, and pericarditis.

do not close completely during systole; alternatively, the orifice may become *stenotic* (from the Greek *stenosis*, meaning "narrowing"), preventing normal flow of blood from one chamber into another. Mitral valvular insufficiency causes reflux of blood across the mitral valve from the ventricle into the atrium during systole. In aortic insufficiency, the blood flows back from the aorta into the left ventricle during diastole. The ventricles of such hearts are dilated and hypertrophic.

Mitral stenosis causes stagnation of blood in the left atrium, which is transmitted into the pulmonary circulation and into the right ventricle. Therefore the typical consequences of

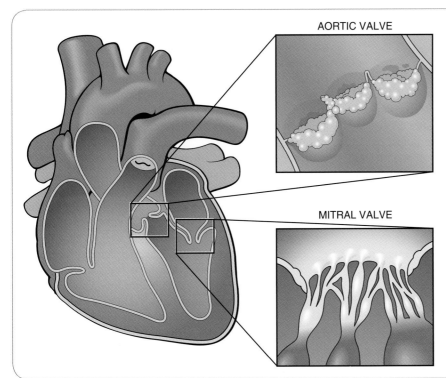

AORTIC VALVE

MITRAL VALVE

Figure 7-24 Chronic rheumatic endocarditis. Mitral and aortic valves are most often involved. The aortic valve leaflets are deformed as a result of nodularity, whereas the chordae tendineae of the mitral valve are thickened or fused and shortened.

mitral stenosis are left atrial, pulmonary, and right ventricular hypertension (cor pulmonale).

Aortic stenosis impedes the blood flow from the left ventricle into the aorta. To overcome the increased resistance at its outflow tract, the left ventricle increases the ejection pressure, causing left ventricular hypertrophy. As long as the left ventricle is compensated, there are no major clinical symptoms. However, when the hypertrophic heart fails, the backpressure of the blood is transmitted from the left ventricle into the left atrium and into the pulmonary circulation, again resulting in cor pulmonale.

Myocarditis is common in RHD. Its histologic hallmarks are *Aschoff bodies,* which consist of aggregates of lymphocytes and macrophages around a central zone of fibrinoid necrosis. Aschoff bodies destroy the myocardium (see Figure 7-23, inset 2). Such lesions are relatively small and rarely cause massive myocardial dysfunction. However, if the Aschoff bodies are in the area of the conduction system, they may cause arrhythmias or cardiac conduction problems.

Pericarditis is found only in severe cases of RHD. Typically it presents in the form of fibrinous exudate on the epicardium and pericardium and free fluid in the pericardial sac. Pericardial fibrosis and adhesions develop in chronic cases.

Clinical Features

RF affects children and young adults. The disease is multisystemic, and cardiac involvement is just one of its symptoms. The diagnosis of RF is based on Jones' criteria, which are subclassified as major and minor. Jones' major criteria are (1) polyarthritis (i.e., joint inflammation); (2) carditis (i.e., inflammation of the heart); (3) chorea, a neurologic disorder characterized by involuntary movements caused by brain lesions; (4) subcutaneous nodules; and (5) erythema marginatum, a peculiar skin disease that reflects the changes in the subcutaneous connective tissue. Jones' minor criteria include joint pain (arthralgia), fever, evidence of a group A streptococcal infection preceding the disease, a previous bout of RF, an elevated erythrocyte sedimentation rate, and ECG signs of heart damage. RF is diagnosed if two major criteria or one major and two minor criteria are fulfilled.

Complications of RHD are common. Bacterial endocarditis is the most prevalent complication because the thrombotic vegetations on the valves are readily infected. Valvular vegetations also give rise to emboli, which cause infarcts of the brain, kidney, or extremities.

Rheumatic carditis cannot be cured with drugs. Accordingly, most of the lesions that develop are irreversible and can be treated only by surgery. Calcified, deformed valves can be excised and replaced with artificial valves—made of metal and plastic or derived from animal (e.g., pig) valves—that are surgically implanted into the heart. Such interventions prolong the life of these patients who otherwise would die from heart failure.

INFECTIOUS DISEASES OF THE HEART

The heart is prone to infections, most of which originate from microbes carried by the blood. As a rule, bacterial and fungal infections affect the endocardium, causing endocarditis. Viral and parasitic infections affect the myocardium and cause myocarditis. Pericarditis may be caused by viruses or bacteria.

ENDOCARDITIS

Bacterial infections of the cardiac valves cause an erosion of the surface layers, allowing entry of the bacteria into the valves. Destruction of the connective tissue ensues because of the action of the bacterial lytic enzymes. The defect of the surface endocardium is soon covered with fibrin and platelet thrombi that serve as nidi to attract even more thrombogenic material. These small bumps on the valves grow rapidly and enlarge into wartlike structures—hence the term *verrucous endocarditis* (Figure 7-25). These vegetations or excrescences

are more abundant than in rheumatic endocarditis. In contrast to the valvular vegetations of rheumatic endocarditis, which represent sterile thrombi, the verrucae of infectious endocarditis are also composed of thrombi, but they contain bacteria. Bacteria invade the valves, causing intravalvular inflammation, which in turn destroys portions of the valves, thereby causing deformities (Figure 7-26). Surface defects (ulcers) are common. Severely inflamed valves may rupture.

Infected valvular vegetations may break off and give rise to septic emboli, most often involving the brain and kidneys and the tips of the extremities (Figure 7-27). Because these thromboemboli contain bacteria, they not only cause ischemic infarcts, such as the sterile vegetations of the rheumatic endocarditis, but also form new foci of infection. These *septic infarcts* transform into *microabscesses.*

Bacterial endocarditis may involve normal valves, but most often it affects valves that have been altered by some other pathologic process. Individuals with valves previously destroyed by rheumatic endocarditis and those with congenital valvular defects are especially prone to infection. Cardiac surgery, and even cardiac catheterization, also may damage the valves and predispose them to infection.

Endocarditis is most often caused by pyogenic bacteria, such as staphylococci and streptococci. Gram-negative bacteria and even fungi may be isolated from some patients, especially those who have been receiving anticancer therapy and are immunosuppressed and weakened by the disease and the chemotherapy. Mixed infections are a cause of endocarditis in drug addicts who inject themselves intravenously using nonsterile instruments.

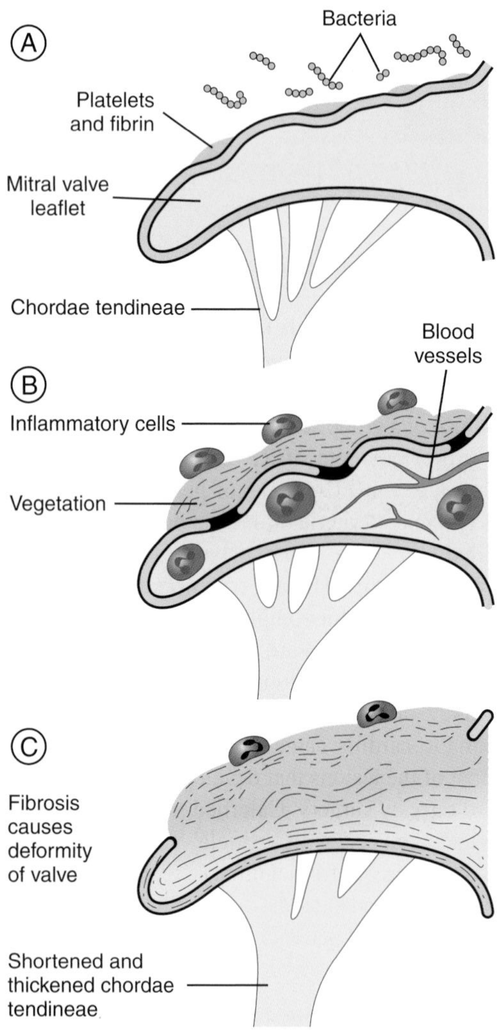

Figure 7-25 Bacterial endocarditis. *A,* The initial site of endothelial injury is covered with a fibrin clot, which is infected with bacteria. *B,* Inflammatory cells from the blood invade the thrombus. The valve is infiltrated with inflammatory cells and contains blood vessels. *C,* The inflammation heals by fibrosis, which causes deformity of the valve.

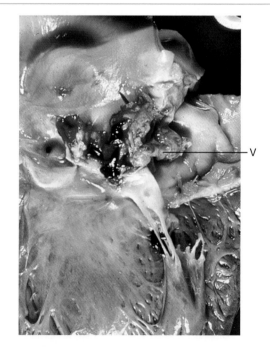

Figure 7-26 Bacterial endocarditis. The valves are covered with extensive vegetations (V).

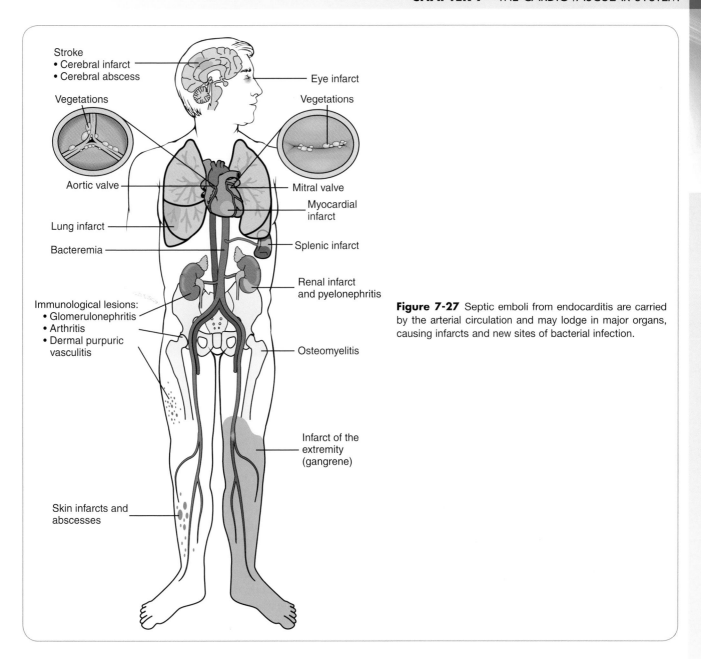

Stroke
• Cerebral infarct
• Cerebral abscess

Eye infarct

Vegetations

Vegetations

Aortic valve

Mitral valve

Myocardial infarct

Lung infarct

Bacteremia

Splenic infarct

Renal infarct and pyelonephritis

Immunological lesions:
• Glomerulonephritis
• Arthritis
• Dermal purpuric vasculitis

Osteomyelitis

Infarct of the extremity (gangrene)

Skin infarcts and abscesses

Figure 7-27 Septic emboli from endocarditis are carried by the arterial circulation and may lodge in major organs, causing infarcts and new sites of bacterial infection.

Clinical Features

The clinical features of bacterial endocarditis are variable. The disease may present as a febrile illness of sudden onset *(acute bacterial endocarditis)* or as a lingering weakness accompanied by mild temperature elevations that wax and wane over a prolonged period *(subacute bacterial endocarditis)*. The most characteristic findings are the numerous murmurs produced by the blood flowing over the deformed valves. Because the valves cannot close completely, valvular insufficiency develops and the blood regurgitates from the aorta into the left ventricle or from the left ventricle into the left atrium. All these abnormalities impose an increased workload on the heart, ultimately leading to heart failure.

Bacterial endocarditis is more common in the left side of the heart than in the right side. Detached vegetations give rise to arterial emboli. Symptoms of peripheral embolization and dissemination of infection through the septic thromboemboli produced "in showers" contribute further to the progression of the disease. The most dangerous are emboli of the central nervous system. Bacteremia with shaking chills is very common because bacteria are constantly released into the circulation from the infected valves. This may occur even without evidence of embolic phenomena. Endocarditis in drug addicts typically affects the tricuspid valve and causes pulmonary emboli and abscesses.

Bacterial endocarditis can be treated with antibiotics. Treatment may be prolonged until all the bacteria are eradicated. Dysfunctional, deformed, and defective valves remaining after the infection must be surgically replaced with artificial valves.

MYOCARDITIS

Myocarditis is most often caused by viruses. Coxsackievirus A and B and other enteroviruses account for most infections in the United States, but it may be caused by other viruses, most notably human immunodeficiency virus (HIV). *Trypanosoma cruzi*, the cause of Chagas's disease, which is endemic in Brazil and parts of South America, is a common cause of myocarditis in that area of the world. These intracellular viruses and intracellular parasites cannot survive outside the cells, so they must invade the myocardial cells to survive. In the myocardial cells they damage the vital organelles and cause cell death. This weakens the myocardium and contributes to heart failure. In addition, the myocardium is invaded by T lymphocytes that are attracted there by the virus or parasite. T lymphocytes secrete various biologically active substances (cytokines), such as TNF and interleukins, which are supposed to kill the virus or parasite. However, cytokines also kill virus- or parasite-infected myocardial cells and may have other untoward effects on the heart.

Clinical Features

The symptoms of myocarditis are vague, and the diagnosis of this disease cannot be made easily. Affected patients usually present with mild fever; shortness of breath; and other signs of heart failure, such as tachycardia, peripheral cyanosis, pulmonary edema, and precordial pressure pain. Severe myocarditis may be indistinguishable from acute myocardial infarction. Viral myocarditis may cause widespread interstitial fibrosis, which clinically presents as dilated cardiomyopathy and progressive heart failure that is resistant to conventional therapy.

PERICARDITIS

Pericarditis is a term used to describe inflammation of the pericardium and of the epicardium, because the inflammation of one of the layers lining the pericardial sac invariably causes changes in the other. Pericarditis may be isolated, but it is most often associated with other infections of the heart, such as myocarditis. In addition, infections involving the adjacent thoracic structures may spread to the pericardium. Tuberculous pericarditis secondary to lung tuberculosis was common previously but is rare today.

Pericarditis may be caused by bacteria, viruses, and, rarely, fungi. Rheumatic pericarditis is a part of pancarditis encountered in severe RHD. Some autoimmune disorders, such as systemic lupus erythematosus, may also affect the pericardium. Finally, inflammation of the pericardium and epicardium can be caused by metabolic waste products that accumulate in the blood in uremia. Trauma and radiation injury also may cause sterile inflammation. Open heart surgery usually causes sterile pericarditis.

Pathology

Pericarditis is always associated with exudation of fluid into the pericardial sac. The fluid is clear yellow in serous pericarditis, and such fluid usually accompanies viral infections.

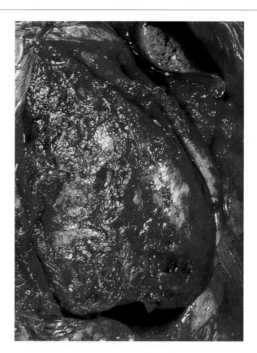

Figure 7-28 Pericarditis. The surface of the heart is covered with fibrin and blood and appears "shaggy."

Serofibrinous exudate is associated with more severe damage and is typically found in those with RF or early bacterial infection. Fibrinohemorrhagic pericarditis, found in more pronounced infection as well as in autoimmune diseases, will give the epicardial heart surface a "shaggy" red appearance (Figure 7-28). *Purulent exudate* is a hallmark of infections caused by pus-forming bacteria, such as staphylococci and streptococci. *Constrictive pericarditis* is characterized by fibrosis obliterating the pericardial cavity and thus preventing the diastolic dilation of the heart; it is usually a late complication of other forms of pericarditis.

CARDIOMYOPATHY

Cardiomyopathy, a relatively noncommittal term (literally meaning "an ailment of the heart"), is used to describe a group of diseases affecting the myocardium. In response to injury, the heart may undergo dilation or hypertrophy. Cardiomyopathy is divided into three forms:
- Dilated cardiomyopathy
- Hypertrophic cardiomyopathy
- Restrictive cardiomyopathy (Figure 7-29)

In dilated cardiomyopathy the ventricles are markedly dilated and the heart appears to have a myocardium that is either flabby or thinned and that has been partially replaced by fibrous tissue. Among the identifiable causes of this heart disease, alcohol figures highly. Some cases of dilated cardiomyopathy are precipitated by viral myocarditis, but in most instances the disease has no obvious causes. Anticancer drugs,

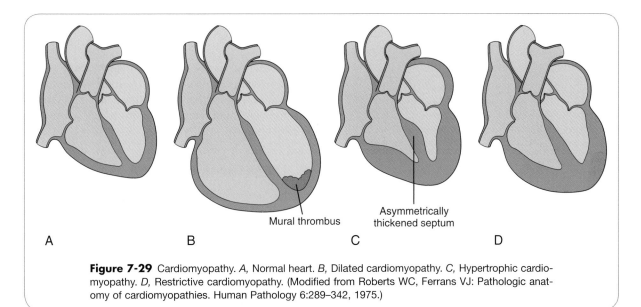

Figure 7-29 Cardiomyopathy. *A,* Normal heart. *B,* Dilated cardiomyopathy. *C,* Hypertrophic cardiomyopathy. *D,* Restrictive cardiomyopathy. (Modified from Roberts WC, Ferrans VJ: Pathologic anatomy of cardiomyopathies. Human Pathology 6:289–342, 1975.)

such as doxorubicin, may cause similar changes because of their cumulative cardiotoxicity.

Hypertrophic cardiomyopathy is marked by extensive thickening of the left ventricular myocardium. The disease is often familial and is inherited as an autosomal dominant trait. Specific mutations of several genes encoding myocardial contractile proteins, such as myoglobin, or proteins regulating the contraction of myocytes, such as **troponin** I and T, have been identified as the cause of cardiac hypertrophy in some cases.

The third form of cardiomyopathy is called *restrictive* because the heart cannot expand adequately to receive the inflowing blood. In most cases this occurs because the myocardium is infiltrated with some abnormal material, such as *amyloid.*

Cardiomyopathies are incurable diseases, and the only hope for the affected patients is heart transplantation.

 Did You Know?

The first successful transplantation of a heart was performed not in the United States but in South Africa. It was performed in 1967 by Dr. Christian Barnard, who instantly became an international celebrity. Today, 2000 to 3000 cardiac transplants are performed every year in this country and many more are performed abroad.

CARDIAC TUMORS

Primary tumors of the heart are extremely rare. The only benign tumor worth mentioning is **atrial myxoma.** This tumor, which is typically polypoid, attaches to the mitral valve and protrudes into the left atrium. It may occlude the mitral orifice.

Secondary tumors may involve the heart; most often these are spread to the pericardium and surface of the heart from the lung. The reasons for the rarity of cardiac metastases are not obvious; most likely the tumor cells do not enter readily into a constantly contracting heart, which also does not provide a fertile environment for growing tumor cells.

IATROGENIC HEART LESIONS

Iatrogenic (meaning "doctor-induced" in Greek) lesions of the heart are becoming increasingly prevalent. These include drug- and radiation-induced diseases and surgery-related cardiac changes. Drugs may affect the heart directly and/or indirectly. Many cardiac drugs used to enhance heart function, such as digitalis, are toxic in large doses. Several anticancer drugs, such as doxorubicin, are cardiotoxic.

Radiation therapy delivered to the chest area for the treatment of breast or lung cancer may damage the heart. This occurs only after long-term therapy and high-dose irradiation. The most prominent changes are seen in the epicardium and pericardium; these lead to obliterative fibrous changes *(constrictive pericarditis)* and may impair the function of the heart.

Cardiac surgery is performed often, mostly to repair occluded coronary arteries. Other cardiac operations, such as artificial valve insertion, are performed routinely with very low mortality rates (Figure 7-30). **Cardiac transplantations** are performed as the treatment of choice for many previously incurable diseases such as cardiomyopathies. In most instances these operations have few serious complications. Pericarditis may be caused by mesothelial cell reaction to the operative field blood that lies on the surface of the heart.

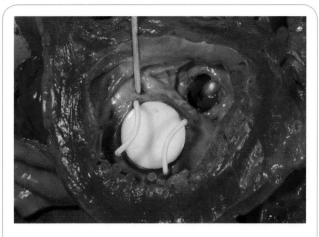

Figure 7-30 An artificial valve replacing the pathologically altered mitral valve.

Adhesions between the epicardium and pericardium, some postoperative pain, and minor discomfort may result. Functional consequences are rare. The intraoperative death rate is currently in the range of 1% to 2%.

Cardiac transplants are performed to replace hearts terminally damaged by myocarditis, cardiopathy of unknown origin, and genetic diseases. Younger persons are the prime candidates for such transplantations, which can prolong life considerably. Because hearts are transplanted from unrelated donors, the foreign heart almost invariably elicits an immune response in the host. Immunosuppressive drugs are given routinely during the postoperative period and sometimes for the rest of the patient's life. Cardiac biopsies are used to monitor the immune reaction against the grafted heart and to determine the appropriate dosage of immunosuppressive drugs. Overall, the results of cardiac transplantation have been most encouraging. The only reasons that more cardiac transplantations are not performed are the high costs and the insufficient supply of hearts for transplantation.

 Did You Know?

From time to time, the news media record the death of a young athlete who collapsed and died in the sports arena in front of thousands of spectators. The sudden death of a young person may be related to a preexisting, clinically unrecognized heart disease. The most important diseases in this category are congenital cardiomyopathies and myocarditis. In others, sudden death may be related to coronary spasm induced by cocaine. At autopsy the hearts of persons who died of cocaine abuse are normal, but chemical analysis of the blood will usually yield positive results. In some cases, however, sudden death cannot be explained. In such cases it is postulated that the heart arrest is caused by ventricular fibrillation, conduction block, or some other irregularity in the transmission of electric stimuli in the heart.

ARTERIAL DISEASES

Atherosclerosis is the most important disease affecting the blood vessels. All other diseases account for less than 1% of clinically recognized arterial lesions. Among these are various forms of autoimmune vasculitis which will be discussed here as follows:

POLYARTERITIS NODOSA

As the name implies, polyarteritis is an inflammation (hence the suffix -*itis*) that involves many vessels (*poly* meaning "many" in Greek). It is an autoimmune disorder affecting medium and small muscular arteries. The disease is thought to result from immune complexes formed between antibodies and an antigen, which may be either endogenous (autoantigen) or exogenous (e.g., a virus). The immune complexes are deposited in the wall of the arteries. In the vessel wall the immune complexes activate complement, which attracts neutrophils. These neutrophils then invade the artery, causing destruction of the vessel wall and fibrinoid necrosis (Figure 7-31). Damaged arteries often become completely occluded by thrombi that form at the site of injury. Local destruction of the vessel wall results in the formation of microaneurysms, which may become thrombosed. These can be palpated as small nodules in the tissues, accounting for the -*nodosa* part in the name of the disease.

Polyarteritis nodosa is a multisystemic disease. Symptoms affecting the heart, brain, and kidney predominate in severe cases, whereas nonspecific symptoms involving minor organs abound in other patients. Overall the clinical picture, the course of the disease, and its outcome are variable and unpredictable. The treatment of choice is the administration of immunosuppressive drugs, but this is often ineffectual.

GIANT CELL ARTERITIS

Giant cell arteritis, a disease of unknown etiology, is also known as *temporal arteritis.* On histologic examination, this disease is characterized by infiltrates of macrophages and giant cells in the media of medium-sized arteries, causing obliteration of their lumina. Temporary arteries on the lateral side of the head are most often involved, and these arteries resemble tortuous wires coursing beneath the skin. This is typically a disease of elderly persons, affecting an estimated 1% of all people older than age 80. Usually, giant cell arteritis produces no serious complications, but some patients have visual problems that result from ischemic changes in the eyes.

RAYNAUD'S DISEASE

Raynaud's disease is a functional disturbance causing contraction of smooth muscle cells in muscular arteries and arterioles. The cause of the disease is not known, but a similar contraction of vessels may occur in several autoimmune

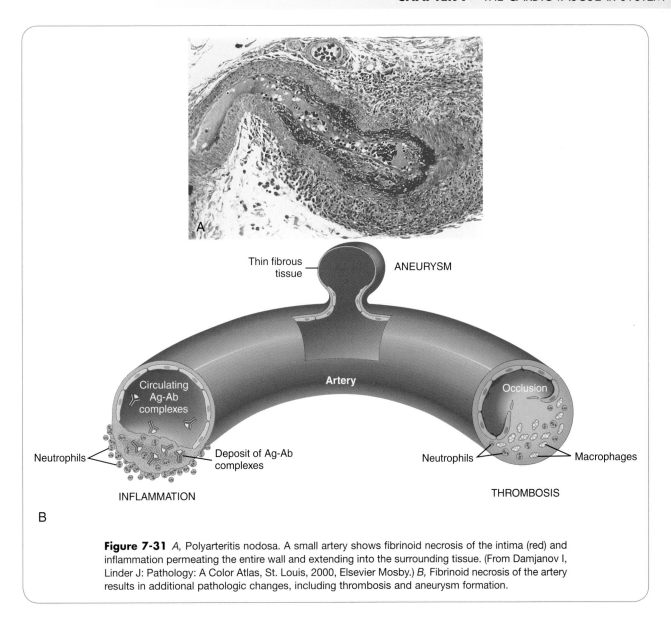

Figure 7-31 *A,* Polyarteritis nodosa. A small artery shows fibrinoid necrosis of the intima (red) and inflammation permeating the entire wall and extending into the surrounding tissue. (From Damjanov I, Linder J: Pathology: A Color Atlas, St. Louis, 2000, Elsevier Mosby.) *B,* Fibrinoid necrosis of the artery results in additional pathologic changes, including thrombosis and aneurysm formation.

diseases such as systemic lupus erythematosus and systemic sclerosis, and thus it is believed to be immunologically mediated. Vessels contract at random but especially prominently in cold weather. Contraction of arteries causes ischemia of the distant parts of the body—typically the tips of the fingers and toes—which may be painful. Upon reheating, the spasm of the arteries subsides and blood returns to the extremities. The affected blood vessels do not show any pathologic changes.

DISEASES OF THE VEINS

In considering the importance of diseases affecting the veins, it is worthwhile to reiterate the following basic facts:

- Veins have thinner and structurally different walls than arteries and do not have the capacity to contract to adjust to the blood flow or to regulate it like the arteries. Moreover,

the veins do not respond to adrenergic stimuli the same way as arteries and arterioles do. Thus veins are not directly affected by the diseases that damage arteries, such as atherosclerosis and hypertension.

- Blood flow in the veins occurs at a lower pressure than in the arteries. However, veins can more easily accommodate an increased amount of blood in their lumina. Thus backpressure from the failing heart may easily increase the pooling of blood in the veins.
- Backpressure causes retrograde flow and stagnation of blood in the veins. Veins have valves that oppose backflow of blood, but these venous valves easily become incompetent when the veins dilate.
- Once the veins have become dilated, they tend to remain so. Tortuous, dilated veins are called *varicosities* or varicose veins (the Latin *varix* meaning "dilated vein").
- The slow flow of blood in the veins predisposes an individual to clotting. Clotting is even more likely in persons

with dilated varicose veins and those in whom the back-pressure from the failing heart causes stagnation of the blood. This most often occurs in the leg veins.

Varicose veins develop most often in the lower extremities (Figure 7-32). Varicose veins are a multifactorial disease with a genetic and environmental component. They are most likely to occur in individuals from families known to have a hypothetical "connective tissue weakness." People in professions that require long hours of standing, such as hairdressing or sales, develop such changes more often than those whose jobs do not require long periods of standing. Many women develop varicose veins during pregnancy, in part as a result of the increased blood pressure in the pelvic veins compressed by the pregnant uterus; the subsequent stagnation of blood in the leg veins may prevent the outflow of venous blood and predispose individuals to varicosities.

The blood flow in the varicose veins is turbulent and slow. This favors clotting, and thrombi often form. Thrombotic occlusion of the veins may lead to an inflammation of the vessel wall *(thrombophlebitis)*. Many thrombi are organized by granulation tissue, and the lumen of the vein may become recanalized. However, some thrombi may become loosened and may be embolized to the lungs.

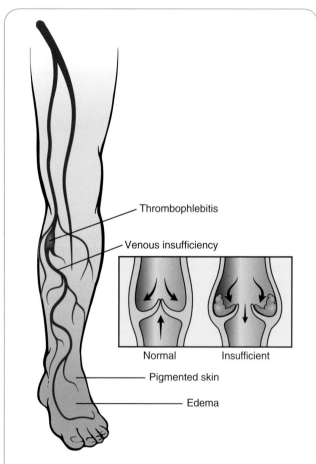

Figure 7-32 Varicose veins of the calf. The inset shows venous valvular insufficiency, which accounts for the reflux of blood and the serpiginous dilation of the veins.

Varicose veins do not drain the blood adequately from the leg, causing pooling of the blood in the lower parts of the leg. Blood leaks from the distended small capillaries and veins into the tissue. The brownish discoloration of the skin in such cases is attributable to the accumulation of blood pigment in the subcutaneous connective tissue. The skin is dry and scaly and shows small, pinpoint hemorrhages from ruptured capillaries. This is called *stasis dermatitis*. As a result of ischemia, the skin may necrotize and a stasis ulcer may form. This is also called *trophic ulcer* (in Greek, *trophein* means "feeding") because it evolves in inadequately nourished (ischemic) skin. Stasis ulcers do not heal easily, and if all treatment fails, the affected limb must be amputated.

LYMPHATIC DISEASES

As mentioned previously, the lymphatics are minute channels permeating almost all soft tissue and many internal organs. Consequently, they are involved in all inflammatory and circulatory disorders and many neoplastic disorders, affecting various tissues and organs. Diseases limited to the lymphatics are rare in clinical practice.

Lymphangitis refers to an acute inflammation confined mostly to the lymphatics of an extremity. Typically such infections are caused by pyogenic bacteria that enter a skin defect and penetrate to the local lymphatics. The subcutaneous lymphatics can be viewed as extending from the site of entry to the local lymph nodes (typically from a finger along the forearm to the cubitus or even the axilla). Enlargement of local lymph nodes is common. Lymphangitis can be readily cured by aggressive antibiotic therapy.

REVIEW QUESTIONS

1. Compare the anatomy and function of the right and left sides of the heart.

2. Compare myocardium with endocardium and pericardium.

3. Compare systole and diastole.

4. Compare arteries and veins.

5. What is the function of lymphatics?

6. How common are cardiovascular diseases?

7. What is the most common cause of heart failure?

8. How common are congenital heart diseases?

9. What is the most common cause of congenital heart disease?

10. List three well-documented causes of congenital heart disease.

11. Compatre the blood flow in the early stages of ventricular septal defect with that in the cyanotic stage.

12. Relate the pathology of tetralogy of Fallot to the clinical findings in this condition.

13. What is atherosclerosis, and how does it present clinically?

14. What are atheromas, and how are they formed?

15. Explain the role of lipids and thrombi in the pathogenesis of atherosclerosis.

16. What are the main risk factors for atherosclerosis?

17. Compare familial (primary) and secondary hyperlipidemia.

18. What is the evidence that cigarette smoking is a risk factor for atherosclerosis?

19. What are the complications of atherosclerosis?

20. Describe various forms of aneurysms.

21. What clinical symptoms could be caused by atherosclerosis of renal or intestinal arteries?

22. Explain how atherosclerosis can cause intermittent claudication or gangrene of the extremities.

23. What are the principal determinants of the clinical presentation of coronary heart disease?

24. What is the location of myocardial infarctions caused by an occlusion of the left or right coronary artery?

25. Compare the consequences of sudden occlusion of a coronary artery with those of gradual occlusion.

26. List the most important complications of myocardial infarction.

27. Compare the pathogenesis of postinfarction rupture of the myocardium and ventricular aneurysm.

28. What are the pathologic findings in congestive heart failure?

29. Explain the pathogenesis of angina pectoris.

30. How is myocardial infarct diagnosed?

31. What are the causes of primary and secondary hypertension?

32. Explain the pathogenesis of hypertension.

33. What are the main pathologic changes caused by hypertension?

34. How is rheumatic fever related to streptococcal throat infection?

35. Describe the cardiac pathology caused by rheumatic fever.

36. What are Jones' criteria for diagnosing rheumatic fever?

37. Explain the pathogenesis of infectious endocarditis.

38. List the most common complications of infectious endocarditis and relate them to typical clinical symptoms caused by these lesions.

39. Describe the pathology and list the common causes of myocarditis.

40. Describe the pathology and list the common causes of pericarditis.

41. Describe the pathology and list the common causes of cardiomyopathy.

42. Which iatrogenic heart lesions are considered to be related to treatment?

43. What is the main cause of arteritis?

44. What are the main clinicopathologic forms of arteritis?

45. What are the main diseases affecting veins?

46. What is the cause of lymphangitis, and how does this disease present clinically?

8

The Respiratory System

Chapter Outline

NORMAL ANATOMY AND PHYSIOLOGY
OVERVIEW OF MAJOR DISEASES
  Infectious Diseases
    Upper Respiratory Infections
    Middle Respiratory Syndromes
    Pneumonia
    Pulmonary Tuberculosis
    Fungal Diseases
    Lung Abscess
  Chronic Obstructive Pulmonary Disease
    Chronic Bronchitis
    Bronchiectasis
    Emphysema
  Immune Diseases
    Allergic Rhinitis
    Asthma
    Sarcoidosis
    Hypersensitivity Pneumonitis

Pneumoconioses
  Coal-Workers' Lung Disease
  Silicosis
  Asbestosis
Ventilatory Disturbances, Acute Respiratory
Distress Syndrome, and Atelectasis
  Disturbances of Ventilation
  Acute Respiratory Distress Syndrome
  Atelectasis
Neoplasms of the Respiratory Tract
  Carcinoma of the Larynx
  Lung Carcinoma
  Metastatic Cancer
Pleural Diseases
  Pneumothorax
  Pleural Effusions
  Pleural Tumors

Key Terms and Concepts

Acute respiratory distress syndrome (ARDS)
Allergic rhinitis
Asbestosis
Asthma
Atelectasis
Bronchiectasis
Bronchiolitis
Bronchitis
Bronchopneumonia
Chronic obstructive pulmonary disease (COPD)
Coal-workers' lung disease (CWLD)

Croup
Drowning
Emphysema
Histoplasmosis
Hydrothorax
Hypersensitivity pneumonitis
Interstitial pneumonia
Lobar pneumonia
Lung abscess
Lung cancer
Mesothelioma
Metastases
Pleuritis

Pneumoconioses
Pneumonia
Pneumothorax
Sarcoidosis
Silicosis
Suffocation
Tuberculosis
Upper respiratory tract infection (URI)
Ventilatory failure

Learning Objectives

After reading this chapter, the student should be able to:

1. Describe the normal respiratory system and its main functions.
2. List common causes and symptoms of upper respiratory infection.
3. Discuss the pathogenesis, etiology, and symptoms of epiglottitis and laryngitis.
4. Compare acute tracheobronchitis and bronchopneumonia.
5. List the common causes and discuss the pathogenesis of pneumonia.
6. Compare bacterial and viral pneumonia.
7. Describe the pathogenesis and typical lesions of pulmonary tuberculosis.
8. Define chronic bronchitis and describe typical lesions and complications of this disease.
9. Define emphysema, its pathologic changes, and its clinical symptoms.
10. Discuss the pathogenesis, pathologic changes, and symptoms of bronchial asthma.
11. Discuss sarcoidosis and chronic immune-mediated lung diseases.
12. Define pneumoconiosis and list three common causes of this pulmonary disease.
13. Discuss the pathogenesis of acute respiratory distress syndrome.
14. Discuss the possible causes and the public health significance of respiratory tract cancer.
15. Describe the typical location, gross appearance, and histologic findings associated with various forms of lung cancer.
16. Discuss the pathogenesis of pleuritis (pleurisy) and the differential diagnosis of pleural effusions.

The respiratory system can be divided into three parts. The upper and middle respiratory system have traditionally been the domain of *otorhinolaryngologists,* or ear-nose-throat (ENT) specialists. The lower respiratory tract is considered the domain of thoracic surgeons and respiratory disease specialists, also known as *pulmonologists.*

NORMAL ANATOMY AND PHYSIOLOGY

The upper respiratory tract comprises the *nose,* including the nasal cavity and the nares; the paranasal sinuses; the pharynx; and the larynx (Figure 8-1). The primary function of these structures is to provide entry for inhaled air, thus enabling respiration. The mucus covering the nasal mucosa serves as a trap for bacteria and foreign particles. Air passing through the upper respiratory tract is warmed and moistened and partially filtered of particles by hair and mucus in the nasal cavity.

The air may be inhaled not only through the nose but also through the mouth. From either entry site, it then reaches the *pharynx,* a structure included in the respiratory and digestive systems. From the pharynx, the air passes through the *larynx,* a highly specialized structure in the neck that also contains vocal cords enabling it to serve as a speech organ. The larynx is contiguous with the trachea, a long tube located in the midline of the thorax. The *trachea* bifurcates, giving rise to the right and left main bronchi, which enter the lung parenchyma and branch into numerous smaller bronchi. The *bronchi* extend into bronchioli, which terminate blindly in respiratory bronchioli, alveolar ducts, and *alveoli.* The alveoli and the corresponding terminal bronchiole form a functional unit called an *acinus.* Approximately five to seven acini are arranged into a pulmonary lobule, each of which is surrounded by a connective tissue septum. Pulmonary lobules are arranged into large units called pulmonary lobes. The right lung has three main lobes, whereas the left lung has two lobes, which can be readily identified in routine chest radiographs.

The outer surface of the lungs is covered by a membrane called the *pleura.* The pleura covering the outer surface of the lungs—visceral pleura—is continuous with the parietal pleura that covers the inside of the thoracic cage. These two layers of pleura enclose the pleural cavity. Pleural surfaces are moist, because the pleural cavity contains a few droplets of fluid that allow the pleural surfaces to slide over one another.

Histologically, various parts of the respiratory system are lined by distinct forms of epithelia. The nasal cavity and the paranasal sinuses are lined by cuboidal epithelium composed of ciliated and mucus-producing cells. The function of these cells is to keep the air passages moist and to filter the air by retaining large particles and bacteria. The mucus contains bactericidal substances and provides protection against infection. The movement of the cilia helps remove mucus from the air passages. This usually results in a nasal discharge, which is a common feature of upper respiratory infections (URIs).

The pharynx and larynx are lined by squamous epithelium that is identical to the epithelium of the mouth. This epithelium is sturdy and provides protection against mechanical injury. This is most important in the pharynx, which serves as a passage for air and for the food and drinks ingested through the mouth. The mucosa of the pharynx is rich in lymphoid tissue, which is part of the immune system and serves as the source of antibodies and cellular immune defense system.

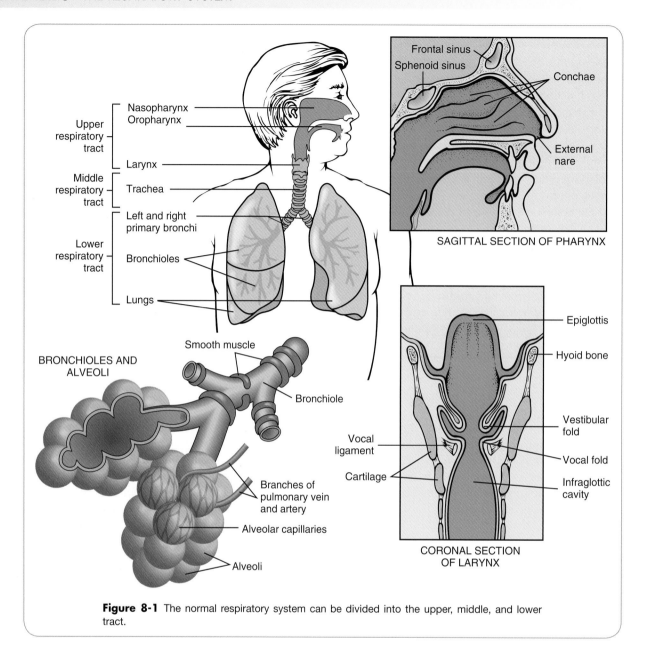

Upper respiratory tract
- Nasopharynx
- Oropharynx
- Larynx

Middle respiratory tract
- Trachea

Lower respiratory tract
- Left and right primary bronchi
- Bronchioles
- Lungs

Frontal sinus
Sphenoid sinus
Conchae
External nare

SAGITTAL SECTION OF PHARYNX

BRONCHIOLES AND ALVEOLI
Smooth muscle
Bronchiole
Branches of pulmonary vein and artery
Alveolar capillaries
Alveoli

Epiglottis
Hyoid bone
Vestibular fold
Vocal ligament
Vocal fold
Cartilage
Infraglottic cavity

CORONAL SECTION OF LARYNX

Figure 8-1 The normal respiratory system can be divided into the upper, middle, and lower tract.

Lymphoid tissue undergoes hyperplasia during infection, which contributes to swelling of the throat.

The larynx is lined by squamous epithelium, which is essential for voicing. It is enclosed in a cartilaginous box that provides support and protection. Similar cartilaginous rings provide mechanical support to the trachea, keeping it patent for the passage of air. Below the larynx, the trachea and the bronchi are lined again with cuboidal epithelium (Figure 8-2). This epithelium contains four cell types: ciliated cells, mucus-producing cells, neuroendocrine cells, and basal cells. The basal cells or reserve cells are the progenitors of all other more specialized cell forms and are thus considered developmentally pluripotent. Under pathologic conditions (e.g., with chronic cigarette smoke irritation), basal cells may proliferate and can give rise to squamous cells (squamous metaplasia). Most *lung cancers* originate from the bronchial epithelium. Histologically, these tumors

may be composed of cell types normally found in the bronchial epithelium or cells formed by metaplasia. This explains why there are several histologic types of lung cancer.

The mucosa of the branches of the bronchial tree all the way to the respiratory bronchioli are lined by the same cells as the main bronchi. All these anatomic structures also have a connective tissue–rich submucosa that contains contractile smooth muscle cells, bronchial glands, and also mucosal lymphoid tissue. The outer third of the bronchial wall, like the wall of the trachea, contains cartilage. As the caliber of bronchi diminishes on their branching, their wall becomes thinner, and finally, as the bronchi transform into bronchioli, the cartilage disappears from their wall.

The transition of bronchi into alveoli is abrupt and involves changes in the structure of the epithelium and the supporting stroma. The alveoli are lined by *pneumocytes*.

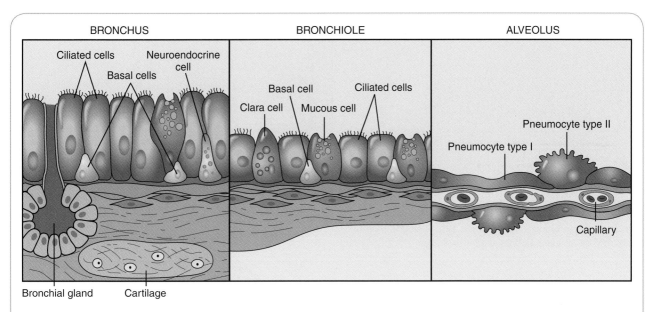

Figure 8-2 Histology of bronchi and alveoli. Bronchi are lined by cylindrical epithelium that contains ciliated, mucus-secreting, and neuroendocrine cells, all of which originate from basal cells. The wall of the bronchi also contains smooth muscle cells and cartilage. Bronchioli do not contain cartilage. The alveoli are lined by flattened type I pneumocytes and surfactant-secreting type II pneumocytes. The alveolar walls contain centrally located capillaries that are separated from the alveolar lining cells by a thin space.

Type I pneumocytes, which account for 90% of the alveolar surface, are very thin cells designed to allow the passage of air from the alveoli into the blood. *Type II pneumocytes,* which are cuboidal cells, specialize in the production of pulmonary surfactant. Pulmonary surfactant is a mixture of lipids, proteins, and carbohydrates. It coats the alveoli with a very thin film that, because of its surface tension, keeps the alveoli open and prevents them from collapsing. The alveolar septa also contain thin capillaries sandwiched between two type I pneumocytes. There is almost no connective tissue between the capillaries and the pneumocytes, an essential factor in the normal passage of air across this respiratory surface. Connective tissue is found only around the acini, in the form of septa. Because the alveoli are so thin, they can be easily ruptured and destroyed, as often occurs in chronic lung disease.

The external surface of the lungs is covered with mesothelium and underlying connective tissue, similar to that forming the interlobular septa. The mesothelium is an epithelial layer that lines both the visceral and parietal pleura.

The lungs have a dual blood supply. The pulmonary artery brings venous blood from the right ventricle into the lungs to be oxygenated in the alveolar septa. The oxygenated blood leaves the lungs through the pulmonary veins, which drain into the left atrium. This functional pulmonary circulation provides no nutrients to the lung parenchyma. Oxygen and nutrients are brought into the lungs through the bronchial arteries, which originate in the thoracic aorta. The branches of the pulmonary and bronchial arteries are interconnected by anastomoses, but these are of limited functional significance under normal circumstances.

The primary function of the lungs is respiration, which includes the transfer of oxygen across the alveolar respiratory membrane into the blood and the release of carbon dioxide and other gases generated inside the body into the ambient air (Figure 8-3). The preconditions for normal respiration are as follows:

- The airways must be patent.
- The lungs must be able to expand rhythmically during each respiratory movement.
- The alveolar respiratory membrane must be intact.
- The action of the control centers of respiration in the central nervous system (CNS), as well as of the thoracic muscles and the diaphragm, must be properly coordinated.

Any interference with these normal physiologic conditions results in impeded respiration, which is called *dyspnea.*

In addition to respiration, the respiratory system has other functions as well. The larynx produces the voice. Laryngeal pathology may result in *aphonia,* or the inability to produce voice (derived from the Greek *a,* meaning "without," and *phonos,* meaning "voice"). The mucosa of the respiratory system provides protection against infections. This is a function of the *mucosa-associated lymphoid tissue* (MALT). MALT forms tonsils in the nasopharynx and pharynx and lymphoid follicles in the wall of the bronchi. Alveolar macrophages are yet another important component of the respiratory defense system. These phagocytic cells are expectorated from the lungs and can also be seen in the sputum. Pulmonary capillaries serve as the peripheral circulatory pool for leukocytes, and these cells can be mobilized from the lungs to the site of infection within a very short time.

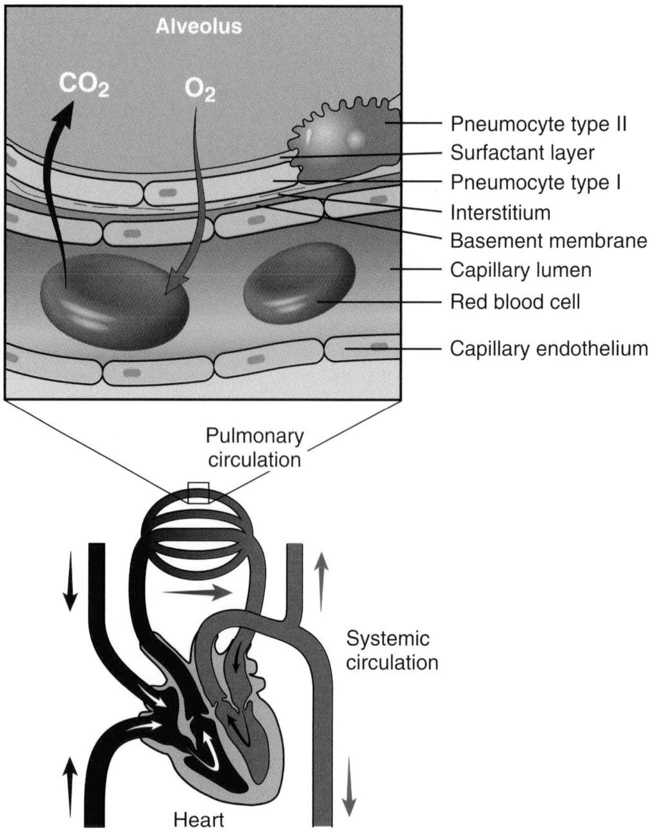

Figure 8-3 The primary function of the lung is gas exchange, which takes place in the alveoli. Oxygen enters the blood and is bound to red blood cells; this releases CO_2, which is then released into the alveolar air destined for expiration.

The major metabolic function of the lungs is the maintenance of acid–base balance. Failure of this function may result in respiratory acidosis or alkalosis. The lungs also provide compensatory mechanisms for the metabolic acidosis or alkalosis caused by pathologic changes in the kidneys or gastrointestinal tract or by systemic metabolic disorders, such as lactic acidosis secondary to diabetes mellitus.

OVERVIEW OF MAJOR DISEASES

The respiratory tract may be affected by numerous diseases, the most important of which are the following:

- Infectious diseases
- Immune diseases
- Environmentally induced diseases
- Circulatory diseases
- Tumors

Several facts important to an understanding of respiratory pathology are presented here, before a discussion of specific pathologic entities.

1. *The respiratory system is open-ended and in direct contact with the environment.* As a result, URIs are extremely common and occur from infancy to old age. URIs may become so widespread that they are considered to be airborne epidemics and even worldwide pandemics, as is often the case with influenza. Downward extension of infection into the bronchi or lungs leads to bronchitis or pneumonia. *Pneumonia* is still one of the most common causes of death in the elderly and in people with cancer or various forms of immunodeficiency, including acquired immunodeficiency syndrome (AIDS). About 2 million people in the United States develop pneumonia every year, and more than 50,000 die of this disease.

2. *The respiratory system is exposed to many allergens inhaled in air.* Immunologic diseases of the respiratory tract are very common. The most prevalent of these diseases is allergic rhinitis, or hay fever. Bronchial asthma is also common, especially among children and young adults. Many chronic lung diseases have an immune component. The immune mechanisms help eradicate infections but also may contribute to their perpetuation or progression.

3. *Inhaled air contains pollutants, airborne particles, and gases, which may cause diseases.* Many environmentally induced lung diseases are considered to be occupation related or related to air pollution. For example, *coal-workers' lung disease* is caused by particles inhaled in mines. Considerable progress has been made to reduce air pollution and the dangers of occupational diseases. Nevertheless, cigarette smoking, an avoidable yet major cause of pulmonary diseases, still accounts for most

chronic bronchitis, emphysema, and lung cancer. Pulmonary morbidity could be significantly reduced by eliminating cigarette smoking and further improving the quality of air in the human habitat.

4. *The heart and the lungs form a functional unit.* Cardiorespiratory dysfunction is prevalent especially in elderly people and in many people with chronic disease. Just as lung pathology has a profound effect on the heart, cardiac pathology almost invariably produces changes in the lungs, and many cardiac patients ultimately die with symptoms of *respiratory failure.*

The blood flow through the lungs depends on the propulsive forces of the right and left ventricle. Failure of the left ventricle results in the buildup of blood pressure within the left atrium, which is transmitted backward into the pulmonary veins and then through the entire pulmonary vascular system into the right ventricle. This clinical condition, in which the right ventricle is working against increased pulmonary resistance, is called *chronic cor pulmonale.* Chronic cor pulmonale can also develop as a result of vascular changes that develop secondary to chronic pulmonary disease. Other pulmonary vascular diseases such as pulmonary emboli may have the same results.

Massive pulmonary thromboembolism, such as saddle emboli, may block the outflow tract of the right ventricle and cause *acute cor pulmonale.* Inability of the overburdened right ventricle to overcome the block in the pulmonary artery may cause death within minutes of the occlusion.

5. *Inhaled air contains many potential carcinogens.* Malignant tumors of the respiratory system are common. The most important of these tumors is *lung carcinoma* **(lung cancer),** which usually originates from the epithelium of intrapulmonary bronchi.

All the currently available evidence indicates that lung cancer is largely related to cigarette smoking. However, not all smokers develop cancer and not all lung cancers are caused by cigarettes. The role of individual susceptibility factors, genetic changes, oncogenes, and other airborne carcinogens is being studied intensively. Mesotheliomas, malignant tumors of the pleura, are related to another important environmental pollutant, *asbestos.*

INFECTIOUS DISEASES

Infectious diseases of the respiratory tract are traditionally divided into two groups based on their location: diseases of the nose and URIs, and diseases of the lower respiratory tract (e.g., pneumonia). Pediatricians also recognize the so-called *middle respiratory syndrome* (MRS), which includes childhood diseases involving the anatomic structures between the larynx on one side and the bronchioles on the other.

Respiratory tract infections account for 75% of all human infections diagnosed clinically, at least after minor skin infections and irritations have been eliminated from consideration.

Most infections are limited to the upper respiratory tract; less than 5% involve the lungs. Lung infections are most prevalent in hospitalized patients, the elderly, drug addicts, alcoholics, and persons with AIDS. Even if one excludes those with AIDS, most of whom die of lung infection, pneumonia is listed as the cause of death of 20,000 to 30,000 persons per year in the United States.

UPPER RESPIRATORY INFECTIONS

Clinically, **upper respiratory infections (URIs)** are most often recognized as common cold. They are characterized by acute inflammation involving the nose, paranasal sinuses, throat, or larynx or all these structures together. These infections have a tendency to extend into the trachea and bronchi, and in a small number of patients they may be complicated by pneumonia. In children the infection often extends into the middle ear, causing otitis media (Figure 8-4).

Etiology and Pathogenesis

Most URIs are caused by viruses. Because it is impractical to isolate viruses in every case, the presumptive diagnosis of a viral etiology is rarely confirmed. Nevertheless, like all other acute viral diseases, URIs are short lived, heal spontaneously, and do not benefit from treatment with antibiotics. Epidemiologic studies show that the common cold is most often caused by rhinoviruses, certain echoviruses, and coxsackieviruses. Up to 50% of all these infections are caused by one of the more than 100 strains of rhinovirus. Influenza and parainfluenza viruses also may cause common cold. All these pathogens are airborne and tend to cause seasonal epidemics. Epidemics of influenza virus infection typically occur during the winter, whereas rhinovirus infections are usually the causes of spring and fall miniepidemics. Influenza epidemics can be controlled to some extent by preventive vaccination, which is especially recommended to high-risk populations, such as the elderly. There is no vaccine for rhinovirus, echoviruses, or coxsackieviruses.

URIs are popularly thought to be facilitated by exposure to cold, damp weather, or draft, but there is no scientific evidence to support this premise. On the other hand, it has been documented that physical exhaustion, old age, and general poor health predispose individuals to viral infections by lowering the body's defense mechanisms. The worldwide epidemic caused by the influenza virus H1N1 that occurred in 2009–2010 affected more younger persons under the age of 18 years than older persons because the older population was partially protected against the new virus strain by previous exposure to closely related strains of influenza viruses. Thus it seems that each new viral epidemic must be combated by new tactics. Because the antigenic structure of influenza viruses is constantly changing (called "antigenic drift"), every year the World Health Organization recommends which strains of the virus should be included in the vaccine.

Viral URIs are self-limited diseases that heal spontaneously without any specific treatment. Symptomatic relief can be obtained by antihistaminics and decongestants. Nevertheless,

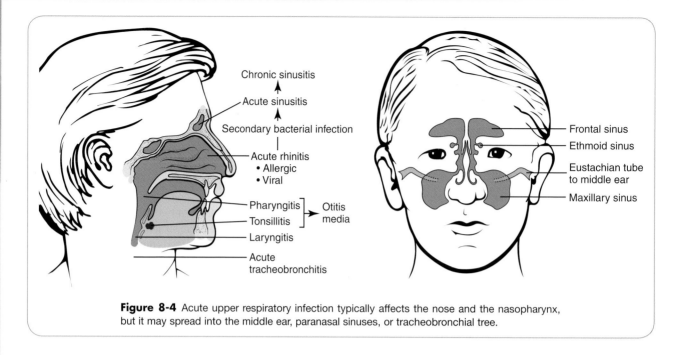

Figure 8-4 Acute upper respiratory infection typically affects the nose and the nasopharynx, but it may spread into the middle ear, paranasal sinuses, or tracheobronchial tree.

viral URIs may predispose individuals to bacterial superinfections, the best known of which is streptococcal nasopharyngitis. Bacteria may spread into the adjacent anatomic structures and cause bacterial sinusitis, otitis media, or mucopurulent bronchitis.

Pathology

The pathologic findings in URI are usually nonspecific. The mucosa of the nose and upper respiratory tract are congested, edematous, and infiltrated with inflammatory cells. In viral infections, the cell infiltrates consist of lymphocytes, macrophages, and plasma cells. Severe infections may cause ulceration of the mucosal epithelial lining, which allows the entry of bacteria. Bacterial infections elicit a reaction of polymorphonuclear neutrophils (PMNs), and many present with a fibrinopurulent exudate. This exudate may form whitish-yellow membranes on the mucosa of the throat, or purulent "plugs" in the crypts and mucosal lacunae of the tonsils.

Clinical Features

URI typically presents with nasal congestion, inflammation, and *rhinorrhea* ("runny nose"). Throat pain or discomfort, especially on swallowing; sneezing; and a hacking cough are common symptoms. General malaise, fever, headaches, and muscle pain with prostration are typical systemic manifestations of influenza infection. The disease lasts 2 to 3 days but then symptoms rapidly subside, even though fever may persist a day or two longer. The appearance of a purulent nasal discharge, sinus or ear pain, and deep throat expectoration are usually signs of bacterial superinfection. In contrast to viral infections, bacterial superinfections do not resolve without antibiotics.

? Did You Know?

The term *flu* is often incorrectly used for URI, but it should be reserved for influenza infections with systemic symptoms. Furthermore, viral URI must be distinguished from bacterial infections and especially throat infection with group A beta-hemolytic streptococci. "Strep throat" should be documented by rapid strep test and, if need be, confirmed by bacteriologic cultures of material obtained by throat swabs. It requires a 7- to 10-day treatment course with antibiotics. If not eradicated, some streptococcal infections may be complicated by rheumatic fever or acute glomerulonephritis.

MIDDLE RESPIRATORY SYNDROMES

The term *middle respiratory syndrome* is used to denote infections of the larynx, trachea, and the major extrapulmonary bronchi. These diseases are most prevalent among children and include isolated *laryngitis* presenting as croup, acute epiglottitis, and viral tracheobronchitis. Most often they result from extension of a URI into the lower parts of the respiratory system, and they are commonly associated with pneumonia. Clinically it is often difficult to determine whether the infection is limited to the trachea and major bronchi or if it has spread into the smaller pulmonary airways as well, but such a spread can be discovered with x-ray studies.

CROUP

Croup is an acute, possibly life-threatening infection that involves the larynx (Figure 8-5). This acute laryngotracheobronchitis is most common in children younger than 3 years.

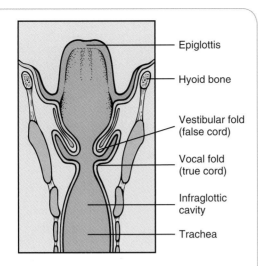

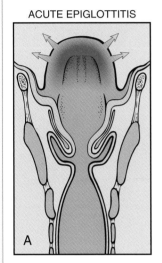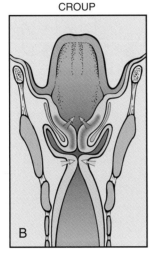

ACUTE EPIGLOTTITIS   CROUP

Figure 8-5 Acute inflammation of the larynx. *A,* Inflammation localized to the epiglottis (so-called acute epiglottitis). *B,* Inflammation of the entire larynx causing diffuse laryngeal swelling and laryngospasm (croup).

Clinically it is marked by spasm of the vocal cords, which results in inspiratory stridor described as a "barking" or "brass cough." Croup is typically caused by parainfluenza virus but may be attributable to other viral infections as well. There is no specific treatment for such viral infections. Nevertheless the child must receive intensive care; in some cases the larynx must even be intubated to prevent suffocation.

EPIGLOTTITIS

Epiglottitis that is caused by *Haemophilus influenzae* previously had a peak incidence in school-aged children and adolescents. Widespread immunization against *H. influenzae* has reduced the incidence of this disease. Clinically it is characterized by a sudden loss of voice and hoarseness and throat pain on swallowing (see Figure 8-5). Edema and redness of the epiglottis and the surrounding inflamed pharyngeal mucosa cause narrowing of the air passage. Antibiotic treatment and supportive therapy with humidified oxygen mask are usually adequate.

BRONCHIOLITIS

Bronchiolitis is a term used for the acute childhood disease involving the bronchi and bronchioles but not extending into the alveolar spaces of the lungs. Pediatricians usually lump bronchiolitis together with other middle respiratory syndromes.

Bronchiolitis is a viral infection, and in more than 80% of cases it is caused by the *respiratory syncytial virus.* Other viruses, such as parainfluenza and rhinovirus, can cause the same symptoms. The virus invades the epithelial cells of the bronchi and bronchioli, causing cell death and desquamation. It also incites an inflammatory infiltrate, which consists of lymphocytes, plasma cells, and macrophages. The edema of the small airways and the desquamation of dead cells causes obstruction of the bronchi and bronchioli.

The disease affects infants and small children and occurs in epidemics from fall until spring. Approximately 1% of all urban infants and even more of those in nurseries develop signs of bronchiolitis in the course of their first year of life. The clinical picture is dominated by wheezing respiration, low-grade fever, and shortness of breath. Unless pneumonia secondary to bacterial superinfection supervenes, spontaneous recovery occurs within 7 to 10 days.

PNEUMONIA

Pneumonia is an inflammation of the lung that occurs in two major forms: *alveolar pneumonia,* which is marked by intra-alveolar inflammation, and *interstitial pneumonia,* which primarily involves the alveolar septa (Figure 8-6).

Alveolar pneumonia may be focal or diffuse (Figure 8-7). Focal pneumonia may be limited to the alveoli, or it may involve both alveoli and bronchi. Focal intra-alveolar inflammation is typical of *hypostatic pneumonia.* It represents bacterial infection superimposed on the pulmonary edema of chronic heart failure, and it is most prevalent in debilitated elderly patients who are confined to bed. Pneumonia that is limited to the segmental bronchi and surrounding lung parenchyma is called **bronchopneumonia.** Widespread or diffuse alveolar pneumonia is called **lobar pneumonia.** Lobar pneumonia is often the end result of confluent bronchopneumonia in which the infection spreads from one lobule to another until the entire lung is involved.

Interstitial pneumonia is usually diffuse and often bilateral. In contrast to alveolar pneumonia, which is usually caused by bacteria, interstitial pneumonias are related to infections with *Mycoplasma pneumoniae* or viruses.

According to their duration, pneumonias can be classified as acute or chronic. Most bacterial and viral pneumonias are

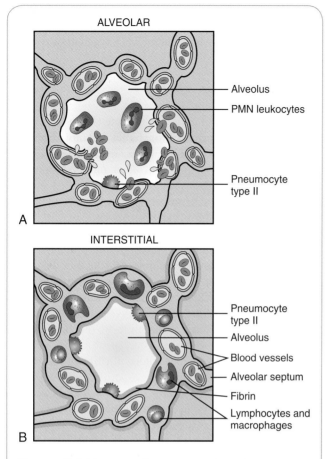

Figure 8-6 Diagrammatic representation of pneumonia. *A,* Alveolar bacterial pneumonia. *B,* Interstitial viral pneumonia. PMN, polymorphonuclear neutrophil.

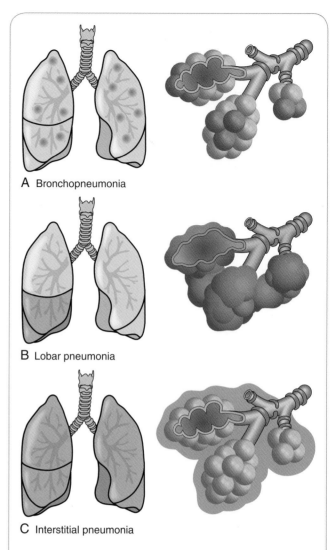

Figure 8-7 Clinically and pathologically the lung infection may be *(A)* localized (lobular pneumonia or bronchopneumonia) or *(B)* diffuse (lobar pneumonia). *C,* Interstitial viral pneumonia is often bilateral and diffuse.

acute. Untreated or incompletely cured, acute pneumonia may become chronic. Recurrent pneumonias, as may occur in children affected by cystic fibrosis, are also classified as chronic. Chronic pneumonia is typical of *tuberculosis* and certain fungal infections.

Etiology

Pneumonia may be caused by bacteria; by viruses; or, less commonly, by fungi, protozoa, or parasites (Table 8-1). Bacteria are the most important pathogens and account for 75% of the cases of clinically diagnosed pneumonia.

Pneumonias may be classified etiologically as being caused by the following:

- Upper respiratory flora
- Enteric saprophytes
- Extraneous pathogens that are not normally associated with the human body

UPPER RESPIRATORY FLORA

The normal flora of the upper respiratory tract is a mixture of bacteria. These bacteria, many of which are potential pathogens, normally exist in equilibrium within the human body and cause no disease. Nevertheless, if aspirated into the lower

respiratory tract, they will cause pneumonia. The most important among these bacteria are *Streptococcus pneumoniae, Haemophilus influenzae,* and *Staphylococcus aureus.*

ENTERIC SAPROPHYTES

Anaerobic bacteria, such as *Escherichia coli* or *Pseudomonas aeruginosa,* are part of normal enteric flora. Pulmonary infection may occur if enteric bacteria contaminate the airways or reach the lungs by blood circulation.

EXTRANEOUS PATHOGENS

Bacteria such as *Legionella pneumophila,* the cause of Legionnaire's disease, or *Mycobacterium tuberculosis,* the cause of pulmonary tuberculosis, are inhaled in an aerosol form from the environment. Various fungi are also present in the environment. Some viruses that are not normally present in the nasopharyngeal flora or on other body surfaces may

TABLE 8-1 Common Causes of Pneumonia

Causative Agents	Percentage of All Diagnosed Cases
Bacteria	
Streptococcus pneumoniae	50
Haemophilus influenzae	10
Staphylococcus aureus	5
Mycobacterium tuberculosis	5
Viruses	10
Influenza virus	—
Fungi*	
Aspergillus fumigatus	—
Candida albicans	—
Pneumocystis jiroveci	—
Bacteria-like organisms	
Mycoplasma pneumoniae	10

*Opportunistic infection; rare except in immunosuppressed, debilitated, or terminally ill patients.

cause pneumonia if inhaled in droplets exhaled by infected persons. Acute viral pneumonias are acquired by close contact with an infected person. Some viruses, such as *herpesvirus* or *cytomegalovirus* (CMV), may have entered the body many years ago and are present in a latent form to be reactivated in immunosuppressed persons, in whom they may cause pneumonia.

? Did You Know?

Legionnaire's disease was recognized scientifically as a new disease some 30 years ago. The pathogen, not known until then, was isolated from the lungs of patients who died in a miniepidemic that affected participants of an American Legion convention held in Philadelphia in 1976. Named *Legionella pneumophila* in honor of the dead legionnaires, this bacillus was found to reside in stagnant waters, such as the tanks used to store water for air conditioning. In the original epidemic in Philadelphia, the bacilli apparently spread through the hotel's air-conditioning system.

Pathogenesis

The pathogens responsible for pneumonia can reach the lung parenchyma through several routes, including the following:
- *Inhalation of pathogens in air droplets.* This is the typical means by which viral infections are spread.
- *Aspiration of infected secretions from the upper respiratory tract.* This is typical for streptococcal and staphylococcal infections.

- *Aspiration of infected particles in gastric contents, food, or drinks.* Such aspiration pneumonia is often caused by anaerobic bacteria and is common in people who are unconscious, those who have vomited, and those who have lost control of their body functions (e.g., alcoholics and drug addicts).
- *Hematogenous spread.* Bacteria may be transported to the lungs by the blood. Pneumonia is common in bacteremia (sepsis) and may develop secondary to urinary or alimentary tract infections. Contaminated foreign material introduced by intravenous self-injection is a common cause of pneumonia in drug addicts.

Pathology

Alveolar pneumonia presents in several forms. *Bronchopneumonia* typically begins with bacterial invasion of the bronchial or bronchiolar mucosa. This is usually followed by exudation of PMNs into the lumen of the airways (Figure 8-8). The inflammation spreads from the bronchi into the adjacent alveoli. In *hypostatic pneumonia* the infection is preceded by pulmonary edema. In either case the inflammation may be limited to a small number of single lobules *(lobular pneumonia),* or it may be spread through large portions of the pulmonary parenchyma *(lobar pneumonia).*

As the intra-alveolar exudate accumulates, it replaces the air and the lung parenchyma becomes consolidated. On gross examination at autopsy, affected lungs resemble the liver; therefore this process is called *hepatization.* Because consolidated lung parenchyma is denser than normal lung, pneumonia can be recognized on x-ray studies as "infiltrates" or "consolidation of parenchyma." With appropriate treatment, the pulmonary infection can be brought under control and the pneumonia cured. The exudate is resorbed or coughed out with complete restitution of the normal alveolar spaces.

Interstitial pneumonias, which are usually diffuse and often bilateral, differ from alveolar pneumonias in that the inflammation primarily affects the alveolar septa and does not

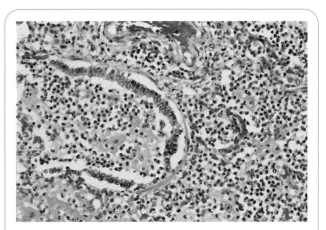

Figure 8-8 Histologic appearance of bronchopneumonia. The bronchus and the surrounding alveoli contain polymorphonuclear leukocytes.

result in exudation of PMNs into the alveolar lumen. In contrast to alveolar pneumonia, which is usually caused by bacteria, interstitial pneumonias are caused by viruses or *M. pneumoniae* that attach to the surface of respiratory epithelial cells. These pathogens cause cell necrosis and induce an infiltrate predominantly restricted to the alveolar septa. This accounts for the so-called reticular pattern, with no major consolidations typically seen on radiographic examination. Fortunately, most interstitial pneumonias cause only minor alveolar damage and resolve without consequences. However, some viral pneumonias may progress to a chronic stage that is characterized by interstitial fibrosis and a honeycomb appearance of lungs. Because viral pneumonias often have an "atypical" course and may pass undiagnosed, it is possible that some cases of "pulmonary fibrosis of unknown origin" are late complications of viral pneumonia.

Complications

Complications of bacterial pneumonia may occur in rapidly progressing cases caused by virulent pathogens, in debilitated patients, or in cases in which treatment is delayed or ineffective (Figure 8-9). The most important complications of pneumonia are pleuritis, abscess formation, and chronic lung disease.

- **Pleuritis.** Extension of inflammation to the pleural surface commonly leads to pleural effusion. Sometimes, especially with purulent bacteria, pus fills the entire pleural cavity *(pyothorax);* more often it is encapsulated by fibrous tissue into pockets called *empyema.* Suppurative pleuritis heals slowly and usually results in pleural fibrosis encasing the entire lung. Pleural fibrosis obliterates the pleural cavity. Because the lungs cannot expand during inspiration, restrictive lung disease results.
- *Abscess.* Abscesses are usually associated with highly virulent bacteria, such as *Staphylococcus,* which cause destruction of the lung parenchyma and suppuration.
- *Chronic lung disease* is an important complication of pneumonia that is unresponsive to treatment. Pus inside the bronchi causes destruction of their walls and bronchial dilation *(bronchiectasis).* Destruction of the lung parenchyma and concomitant fibrosis transform the lung into a honeycomb-like structure *("honeycomb lungs").*

Complications of viral pneumonias are rare because most of these infections heal spontaneously. Some viral pneumonias may not resolve, and in such cases, chronic pulmonary interstitial fibrosis will develop. Bacterial superinfection occurs in some cases and is an important cause of morbidity in elderly people and debilitated persons.

Clinical Features

Pneumonia is a serious infection that requires prompt and aggressive treatment. It may occur in any age group but most often affects children younger than 5 years or elderly persons older than 70 years.

The first prerequisite for diagnosing pneumonia is to suspect that it has developed. Clinicians divide pneumonias into two groups: (1) *primary* or *community-acquired pneumonias,*

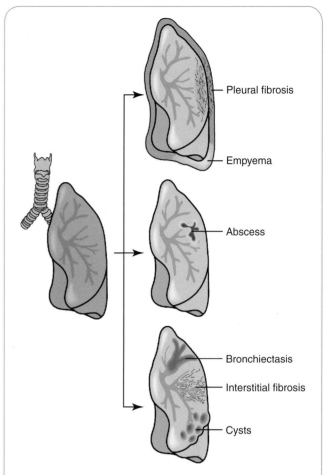

Figure 8-9 Pneumonia may extend to the pleura and cause pleuritis, which may heal in the form of pleural fibrosis. Persistence of pus in the pleural cavity is called *empyema.* Suppurative pneumonia results in abscess formation. Bronchiectasis is a consequence of chronic lung infection. Interstitial fibrosis with cysts accounts for the honeycomb appearance of lungs in chronic lung disease.

which affect previously healthy people; and (2) *secondary pneumonias,* which are hospital-acquired *(nosocomial)* infections or which arise in persons with preexisting illnesses. Elderly people and debilitated or sick people are at greater risk for developing pneumonia than are healthy persons. Other risk factors are smoking, alcoholism, and immunosuppression caused by diseases or treatment. Pneumonia is a common feature of AIDS.

The symptoms of pneumonia may be classified as follows:
- *Systemic signs of infection.* These include high fever, chills, and prostration.
- *Local signs of irritation.* These are related to bronchial inflammation and the secretion of mucus and include coughing and expectoration. Pleural inflammation causes chest pain.
- *Airway obstruction.* Impaired gas exchange in the damaged alveoli results in shortness of breath *(dyspnea)* and rapid breathing *(tachypnea).*

- *Inflammation and tissue destruction.* Inflammatory exudate causes tissue destruction and bleeding. Consequences include mucopurulent, blood-tinged "rusty sputum," or even frank hemoptysis.

 Did You Know?

The instrument hanging around the neck of many doctors and nurses is called a *stethoscope* (from the Greek *stethos,* meaning "chest"). The original stethoscope, which looked like a funnel, was invented in the nineteenth century by the French physician Laënnec, who used it as an aid for hearing pulmonary and cardiac sounds. The rubber tubes of the modern stethoscope were added in the twentieth century. Auscultation of the chest with a stethoscope is still an essential part of the physical examination. Using nothing more than this sophisticated "hearing aid," an astute clinician can diagnose many pulmonary and cardiac diseases.

On physical examination, affected patients usually appear in great distress and short of breath. Relentless coughing is a common symptom. Auscultation usually reveals rales, bronchi, and other signs of pulmonary consolidation. A presumptive diagnosis of pneumonia, made on the basis of clinical findings, must be confirmed by additional studies, such as the following:

- *Chest radiography.* Radiologic findings are essential for localizing the pulmonary infiltrates and for assessing the extent of pulmonary consolidation.
- *Bacteriologic studies of the sputum.* Sometimes the pathogens can be identified in smears of sputum examined under the microscope, but in most cases bacteriologic cultures of sputum are more reliable and yield more conclusive proof of infection. Bacteriologic data also provide the best guidance for treatment. The need to treat patients with pneumonia urgently prevents doctors from establishing their cause, and thus the cause of more than 70% of pneumonias remains unknown before onset of treatment.
- *Peripheral blood studies.* Bacterial pneumonias are accompanied by leukocytosis. Viral pneumonia does not cause leukocytosis but may be associated with an elevated number of lymphocytes in blood. Hypoxia and respiratory acidosis may be detected by blood gas analysis (oxygen and carbon dioxide content) and pH measurement of the blood.

The treatment of pneumonia is based on eradication of the bacterial infection with antibiotics and support of vital functions until the lung function has recovered.

SPECIAL FORMS OF PNEUMONIA

Infection with *S. pneumoniae* accounts for more than 50% of all bacterial pneumonias. Other forms of pneumonia that have unique features are also recognized. For example, *Staphylococcus aureus* tends to produce multiple abscesses. *Pseudomonas pneumoniae* is the most common gram-negative bacterium causing hospital-acquired pneumonia. It is characterized by vascular lesions that typically cause infarcts and necrosis of the lung parenchyma. *P. aeruginosa* is also the most common cause of lung infection in cystic fibrosis.

In immunosuppressed persons, and especially those who have AIDS, it is often caused by a fungus, *Pneumocystis jiroveci* (previously called *Pneumocystis carinii*). In patients suspected of pneumocystic infection, the alveolar contents must be aspirated by bronchoalveolar lavage and the alveolar contents sent to the pathology laboratory for microscopic examination. Such material is then stained with silver impregnation to demonstrate *P. jiroveci.*

Atypical Pneumonia

Pneumonias that do not present with classical symptoms are called *atypical.* This clinical term is used for a variety of conditions and usually implies that a bacterial pathogen cannot be identified. The best examples of atypical pneumonia are diffuse lung diseases caused by viruses or *M. pneumoniae.*

Clinical symptoms of atypical pneumonia are milder than those in classical pneumonia. The fever is less pronounced, and usually there are no chills. The cough is mild and does not produce mucopurulent or blood-stained sputum, but the patient may experience dyspnea. The x-ray findings may be minimal, and no distinct condensations are seen. Bacteria cannot be cultured from the sputum. There are usually no signs of septicemia. Purulent pleuritis and abscess formation are not among the complications of atypical pneumonia. There is also no leukocytosis. The diagnosis is made serologically by testing patient's blood for immunoglobulin M (IgM) antibodies to possible pathogens.

PULMONARY TUBERCULOSIS

Tuberculosis is a chronic bacterial infectious disease caused by *M. tuberculosis.* It was widespread in industrialized societies of the nineteenth century, but its incidence in the United States and Europe has decreased steadily since the 1950s, when the first tuberculosis drugs were introduced. Nevertheless, tuberculosis infection still affects approximately 13,000 Americans every year, most of whom have lung infection. Because primary pulmonary tuberculosis is clinically unrecognized in most instances, the true incidence of tuberculosis is probably much higher. The emergence of strains of *Mycobacterium* that are resistant to drugs has, during the last few years, refocused the attention of the public on this problem.

Etiology and Pathogenesis

Pulmonary tuberculosis is caused by *M. tuberculosis,* a rod-shaped bacterium with a waxy capsule. Because of this capsule, *M. tuberculosis* can effectively be stained only with a special Ziehl-Neelsen technique, which renders it red even after an acid wash. Therefore it is called *acid-fast bacillus.*

M. tuberculosis does not attract PMNs, and the infection is not marked by acute purulent lesions. Instead, the encapsulated bacteria elicit formation of granulomas. These granulomas are composed of lymphocytes and macrophages. Stimulated macrophages transform into epithelioid cells and often

171

fuse to form multinucleated Langerhans' giant cells. The necrotic central portion of the granulomas resembles cottage cheese on gross examination and is therefore called *caseous necrosis.*

Primary infection in a person who has not previously been exposed to *M. tuberculosis* results in a localized lung inflammation. This lesion, known as *Ghon's complex,* consists of granulomas in the lung parenchyma and the enlarged regional lymph nodes (Figure 8-10). In 95% of cases, the Ghon complex heals spontaneously, usually by undergoing calcification, which can be recognized by x-ray studies. Nevertheless, calcified primary complex may contain *M. tuberculosis,* which can be reactivated, producing secondary tuberculosis. Progressive primary tuberculosis is a rare event that occurs mostly in children and immunosuppressed persons.

Secondary tuberculosis can develop as a result of reactivation of the dormant primary infection or a reinfection. Most cases represent reactivation of a previous infection. The bacteria typically spread to the apex of the lungs, causing a granulomatous lobular pneumonia. Confluent granulomas tend to produce cavities *(cavernous tuberculosis).* Pulmonary cavities are common sources of hemoptysis, which may be fatal.

Tissue destruction facilitates additional intrapulmonary and extrapulmonary spread of infection. Dissemination of bacilli occurs through the lymphatics, the pulmonary blood vessels, or the airspaces (Figure 8-11). Typical complications resulting from dissemination of tuberculosis include the following:

- *Miliary tuberculosis.* Widespread seeding of bacteria in the lungs or in other organs results in the formation of small granulomas that resemble millet seeds (the Latin *milium* means "millet seed").

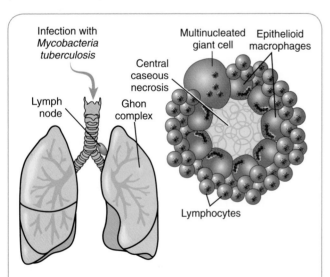

Figure 8-10 Ghon's complex, typical of pulmonary tuberculosis, consists of a parenchymal focus and hilar lymph node lesions. The detailed section of the diagram shows the typical features of tuberculous granuloma: central caseous necrosis surrounded by epithelioid cells, multinucleated giant cells, and lymphocytes.

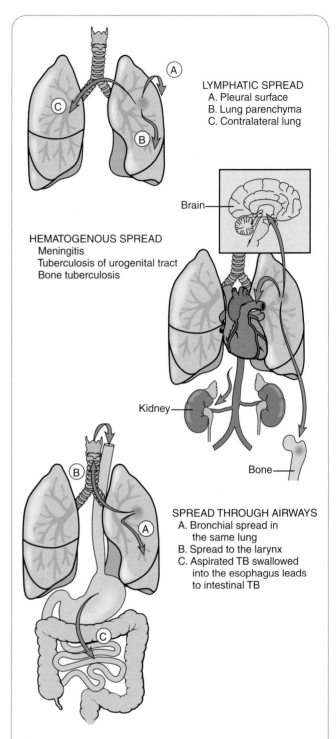

Figure 8-11 Spread of tuberculosis (TB). Reactivated bacilli can spread through the lymphatics, blood vessels, or bronchi. Hematogenous spread usually accounts for tuberculosis in distal sites, such as the urogenital tract or the brain. Expectorated bacilli may be swallowed and cause intestinal tuberculosis.

- *Tuberculous pneumonia.* Fulminant spread of bacteria through the airspaces produces a massive lobular or lobar pneumonia. It may involve the same lung as the primary infection or the contralateral lung.
- *Pleuritis.* Extension of infection to the pleura is accompanied by pleural effusion and the formation of granulomas on visceral and parietal pleura. Thick adhesions regularly form in protracted disease, resulting in obliterative pleural fibrosis.
- *Extrapulmonary tuberculosis.* Expectorated bacilli may infect the larynx and, if swallowed, may cause gastrointestinal tuberculosis, usually in the small intestine. Hematogenous spread may cause tuberculosis of essentially any organ in the body. Extrapulmonary tuberculosis is rarely seen today in Western countries.

Clinical Features

Tuberculosis may present with a variety of symptoms, most of which are nonspecific, and the diagnosis is made only if a high degree of suspicion is maintained. *Primary tuberculosis* is associated with mild pulmonary disease and low-grade fever. It remains clinically unrecognized in more than 95% of the cases. The symptoms of *secondary tuberculosis* include a nonproductive (dry) cough, low-grade fever, loss of appetite, malaise, night sweats, and weight loss. Hemoptysis from destructive cavitary lesions usually occurs later. Dyspnea may indicate the spread of infection through the parenchyma of the lungs, pulmonary destructive lesions, and pleural effusions.

Chest x-ray studies are essential for the diagnosis, which is definitively established by identifying acid-fast bacilli in sputum stained with the Ziehl-Neelsen technique or in bacteriologic cultures. The *tuberculin test,* performed by injecting 0.1 mL of diluted bacterial extract (called *tuberculin*) into the skin, is typically positive. However, this test is not absolute proof of tuberculosis. Positive and negative tuberculin test data must be interpreted in the context of other clinical and laboratory findings. For example, persons who have developed immunity because of a previous resolved infection or those who have been immunized with attenuated *M. tuberculosis* (called *bacille Calmette-Guérin* [BCG]) also react positively to injected tuberculin. Anergic patients (i.e., those whose immune system has been weakened and cannot mount an adequate immune reaction, as in people with terminal AIDS or terminal cancer) have a negative response to tuberculin.

Pulmonary tuberculosis is a treatable disease unless it is caused by drug-resistant strains of *M. tuberculosis.* Tuberculosis in immunosuppressed persons, such as those with AIDS, does not respond to treatment.

FUNGAL DISEASES

Among the causes of primary, community-acquired pulmonary infections, two fungal diseases deserve mention: *histoplasmosis* and coccidioidomycosis. **Histoplasmosis** is widespread in the Midwestern United States, and *coccidioidomycosis* is endemic in the Southwest deserts. Both diseases are acquired by inhaling dried fungi and their spores. Clinically these infections

resemble tuberculosis. The infection may be asymptomatic, as is usually the case, or it may present as solitary pulmonary lesions or even in the form of miliary nodules. Fungal infections induce the formation of granulomas, which heal by calcification.

Hospital-acquired fungal infections are common among patients who are terminally ill and those with cancer or AIDS. The most common pathogens are *P. jiroveci, Candida albicans,* and *Aspergillus fumigatus.*

LUNG ABSCESS

Lung abscess is a localized, destructive, suppurative lesion. It is most often caused by *S. aureus* and less often by other bacteria, such as *Klebsiella pneumoniae* and *P. aeruginosa.*

Lung abscesses develop under the following conditions:

- As a typical complication of necrotizing staphylococcal pneumonia
- After aspiration of infected material from the alimentary or upper respiratory tract
- Distal to bronchial obstruction by tumors
- As a result of septic lung emboli

Abscesses may be solitary or multiple. Like abscesses in other sites, lung abscesses are also cavitary lesions filled with pus. In early stages the central pus is surrounded by granulation tissue, whereas in late stages it is surrounded by a capsule composed of hyalinized collagen. In contrast to abscesses of other internal organs, which usually remain encapsulated, pulmonary abscesses tend to connect with the airways. The expanding abscesses erode the bronchial wall and extrude their purulent content into the airways. Putrid malodorous expectoration is thus typical of lung abscesses.

CHRONIC OBSTRUCTIVE PULMONARY DISEASE

The term **chronic obstructive pulmonary disease (COPD)** is a catchall clinical term used for lung diseases characterized by chronic airway obstruction. For the sake of simplicity, we shall consider COPD as a spectrum of diseases extending from chronic bronchitis on one end to emphysema on the other. Although chronic bronchitis and emphysema may occur in "pure" forms, in most cases these two diseases coexist. Patients can be classified into two groups: those who have predominantly chronic bronchitis and those who have predominantly emphysema.

CHRONIC BRONCHITIS

Chronic **bronchitis** is defined clinically as excessive production of tracheobronchial mucus causing cough and expectoration for at least 3 months during 2 consecutive years. Smoking is the cause of chronic bronchitis in more than 90% of the cases. The extent of disease correlates with the number of cigarettes smoked, and cessation of smoking is associated with improvement of clinical symptoms. Other contributory factors include air pollution, occupational exposure to toxic fumes, and various respiratory infections, especially if recurrent. It has been shown that a single bout of viral pneumonia, especially in childhood, may predispose that individual to COPD in later life.

The pathology of chronic bronchitis is relatively nonspecific. The walls of the bronchi and bronchioli are thickened, and their lumen contains thick mucus. Histologically the mucosa is infiltrated with lymphocytes, macrophages, and plasma cells. The surface epithelium is usually preserved, but it may show focal ulcerations or metaplasia of columnar into squamous epithelium. The most prominent changes involve the submucosa, which shows marked mucous gland hyperplasia, chronic inflammation, and fibrosis.

BRONCHIECTASIS

Bronchiectasis, a permanent dilation of the bronchi, is the most common complication of chronic bronchitis. It is often associated with bronchiolectasis, a dilation of the bronchioli. Such dilation occurs as a result of persistent inflammation inside the airways. Enzymes released from bacteria and leukocytes; mechanical pressure from the inside, exerted by the bronchial contents; and traction of the fibrous scars from the outside all contribute to the formation of bronchiectases.

The larger bronchi usually show *saccular* or *cystic dilation,* whereas the smaller bronchi and bronchioli show *cylindrical dilation* (Figure 8-12). The dilated bronchi and bronchioli are filled with mucopurulent material. This material stagnates and

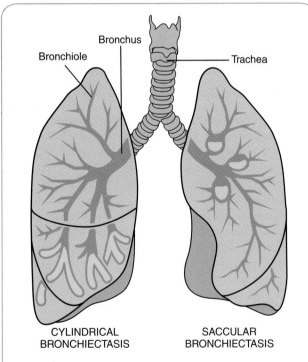

CYLINDRICAL BRONCHIECTASIS   SACCULAR BRONCHIECTASIS

Figure 8-12 Bronchiectasis. The dilation may be saccular or cylindrical. The lumina of the dilated bronchi contain pus and mucus.

cannot be cleared by coughing. Infection spreads into the adjacent alveoli, and recurrent pneumonias are common. Hematogenous spread of the infection into other organs and the systemic consequences of protracted suppuration cause low-grade fever, generalized malaise, and fatigue. These patients often develop clubbing of the fingers. Secondary amyloidosis characterized by a deposition of insoluble amyloid fibers in tissues is a well-known complication and may lead to renal or hepatic failure.

EMPHYSEMA

Emphysema is defined, in pathologic terms, as enlargement of the airspaces distal to the terminal bronchioles with destruction of the alveolar walls. Emphysema is a disease affecting chronic cigarette smokers, and like chronic bronchitis, it is pathogenetically related to the chemicals contained in smoke. Emphysema is rare in nonsmokers, and most of these patients have a genetic deficiency of alpha$_1$-antitrypsin (α_1-AT).

Pathogenesis

The exact mechanism of tobacco-induced emphysema is not known. It has been hypothesized that the irritants in the smoke provoke an influx of inflammatory cells into the alveoli. Proteolytic enzymes released from the leukocytes presumably destroy the alveolar walls. Oxygen radicals generated by the burning cigarette kill alveolar cells and leukocytes, which release even more degradative enzymes. Increased activity of leukocyte-derived elastase in these lungs probably accounts for the loss of elastic fibers from the alveolar walls. Furthermore, it has been hypothesized that the oxygen radicals inactivate the endogenous antiproteolytic enzymes. Uninhibited by natural inhibitors, the leukocytic proteases act on normal tissues and destroy alveoli.

This hypothesis, which implicates proteolytic enzymes, is supported by observations of congenital α_1-AT *deficiency.* α_1-AT is a serum protein produced by the liver. It circulates in serum and permeates tissues, where its primary function is to neutralize proteases. α_1-AT protects tissues from the adverse effects of proteases released from leukocytes. α_1-AT deficiency results in emphysema, indicating that α_1-AT has a crucial role in counteracting the potentially damaging effects of the leukocytes exudate in the pulmonary alveoli. α_1-AT deficiency is uncommon, and it accounts for less than 1% of all patients with emphysema. Nevertheless, it is an important "experiment of nature." Extrapolating from observations of this "experiment," one could assume that the inhibition of endogenous antiproteases by smoke could result in uncontrollable destruction of the alveolar walls by elastase and other proteases released from leukocytes.

Pathology

Pathologic findings in emphysema are classified according to the pattern of alveolar wall destruction. The most important forms are *centrilobular* (centriacinar) and *panacinar* emphysema (Figure 8-13).

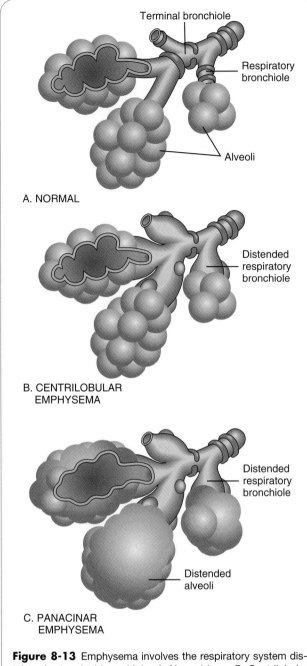

Figure 8-13 Emphysema involves the respiratory system distal to the terminal bronchiole. *A,* Normal lung. *B,* Centrilobular emphysema. *C,* Panacinar emphysema.

Centrilobular emphysema is marked by widening of the airspace in the center of a lobule and involves predominantly the respiratory bronchioles. This is the most common form of emphysema. It is typically found in cigarette smokers. The remaining respiratory bronchioles are characteristically infiltrated with anthracotic macrophages and chronic inflammatory cells. *Panacinar emphysema* involves all the airspaces distal to the terminal bronchioles. This form of emphysema typically occurs in α_1-AT deficiency but may also be caused by smoking.

Clinical Features

Clinical symptoms of COPD vary depending on the extent and duration of the disease. Patients are customarily divided into two prototypic groups: those with predominant bronchitis ("blue bloaters") and those with predominant emphysema ("pink puffers") (Figure 8-14). Table 8-2 compares the clinical features of these two conditions.

Chronic bronchitis results in prolonged bouts of coughing, expectoration of tenacious or purulent mucus, and dyspnea. Hypoxia may be so pronounced during the coughing episodes that it causes cyanosis (blue bloating). The pulmonary vasculature is affected by the peribronchial fibrosis, and this results in pulmonary hypertension and chronic cor pulmonale. Right ventricular failure is marked by peripheral venous stagnation, which contributes to cyanosis. Chest x-ray studies show increased bronchiovascular markings and an enlarged heart.

Patients with predominant emphysema have no bronchial obstructions and no irritation that would force them to cough and expectorate. Because of the reduced respiratory surface, they have compensatory tachypnea. The chest is overexpanded ("barrel-chest"), and they often must hunch forward while holding onto a table or a window frame to engage the auxiliary respiratory muscles. These patients hyperventilate and thus manage to oxygenate the blood adequately so as not to develop cyanosis or anoxia. Chest radiographs show clear lung fields and "overinflation" with a small heart.

The treatment of COPD is symptomatic and based on supportive measures. The advanced pulmonary lesions are irreversible. Even if patients stop smoking, the symptoms often persist.

IMMUNE DISEASES

Among the numerous immune disorders affecting the respiratory tract, the most important are allergic rhinitis (hay fever), bronchial asthma, *sarcoidosis,* and *hypersensitivity pneumonitis.*

ALLERGIC RHINITIS

Hay fever, or **allergic rhinitis,** is a very common disease affecting millions of people. It represents a typical IgE- and mast cell–mediated type I hypersensitivity reaction of the nasal mucosa to exogenous allergens. Among these allergens, the most common are pollens—hence the popular name *hay fever.* However, the list of potential allergens is much longer than that and includes such mundane, ubiquitous particles as animal dandruff and various industrial chemicals.

Allergic rhinitis is an acute vasomotor response mediated by histamine and related vasoactive substances released locally in the nose from mast cells coated with IgE. The attack of sneezing may be short lived or prolonged but usually stops when the histamine has been depleted. Sneezing can be stopped with antihistaminic drugs and nasal sprays.

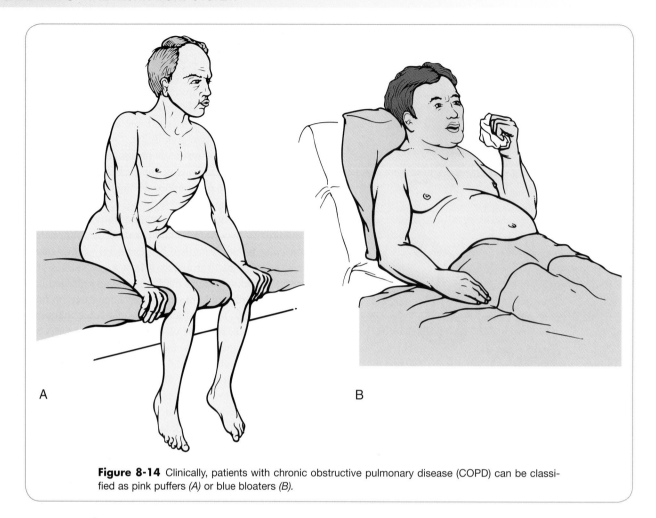

Figure 8-14 Clinically, patients with chronic obstructive pulmonary disease (COPD) can be classified as pink puffers *(A)* or blue bloaters *(B)*.

ASTHMA

Asthma is a disease characterized by increased responsiveness of the bronchial tree to a variety of stimuli. Typical "asthmatic attacks" are marked by wheezing during expiration, cough, and dyspnea. Asthma is a common disease, affecting approximately 10% of children and 5% of adults in the United States. In more than 50% of cases, the disease begins in childhood, affecting males two times more often than females. In another 30% of cases, signs of asthma develop by the age of 40 years, whereas the remaining 20% have so-called old-age asthma.

 Did You Know?

Asthma is the most common chronic childhood disease. It is the most common reason for admission of children to the emergency rooms in the United States and accounts for up to 20% of all acute admissions to pediatric hospital wards.

Etiology and Pathogenesis

Asthma is a heterogeneous, multifactorial disease. In many instances the disease has more than one cause and is mediated by more than one pathogenetic mechanism. For the sake of

TABLE 8-2 Chronic Obstructive Lung Disease		
	Predominantly Bronchitis ("Blue Bloaters")	Predominantly Emphysema ("Pink Puffers")
Chest	Normal	Barrel chest
Dyspnea	+	+ +
Cough	+ +	+
Sputum	+ + Mucopurulent	+/− Mucoid
Cyanosis	+ +	−
Pulmonary hypertension	+ +	−
Peripheral edema	+ +	−
Radiographic findings	Densities	Overinflation

simplicity, two major forms of disease are recognized: extrinsic and intrinsic asthma.

Extrinsic asthma is mediated by exposure to exogenous allergens and represents a type I hypersensitivity reaction. Extrinsic asthma typically affects children and is often associated with other allergies, such as atopic dermatitis or hay fever.

Intrinsic asthma is precipitated by nonimmune mechanisms, most of which are nonspecific and would not produce symptoms were it not for the hyper-reactivity of the bronchial tissues. These include the following:

- Physical factors, such as heat or cold
- Exercise
- Psychological stress
- Chemical irritants and air pollution
- Bronchial infection
- Aspirin

The reasons for increased reactivity of the bronchi to various stimuli remain unknown. Current evidence indicates that it is most likely caused by persistent inflammation of the bronchial mucosa. The inflammatory cells, such as lymphocytes, macrophages, eosinophils, basophils, and plasma cells, produce a variety of mediators that act on the blood vessels, increasing their permeability. These substances also act on smooth muscle cells, stimulating their contraction (Figure 8-15).

The mediators of inflammation in asthma can be divided into two groups: those involved in a rapid, immediate response and those that have a delayed but prolonged effect. In the first group, the best known are vasoactive substances, such as histamine, bradykinin, prostaglandins, and other derivatives of arachidonic acid. Leukotrienes, which are also derived from arachidonic acid, and platelet-activating factor (PAF) produce delayed and protracted smooth muscle cell contraction. In addition, the inflammatory cells in the mucosa generate chemotactic factors that continuously recruit more inflammatory cells into the bronchial mucosa. Mucous cells stimulated by a variety of mediators secrete and discharge mucus into the bronchial lumen, where the mucus forms viscous plugs. Some of the mediators stimulate nerves that trigger smooth muscle cell contraction and secretion of mucus. Neural dysfunction may play an important role in altering the responsiveness of the bronchial mucosal cells and smooth muscles to cholinergic and beta-adrenergic stimuli.

Pathology

The pathologic changes in the lungs are similar in all forms of asthma, regardless of the etiology of the disease. Histologically the bronchi show chronic inflammation and overabundance of mucus in the lumen. The mucosal infiltrates consist of nonspecific chronic inflammatory cells, but they often also contain prominent eosinophils (Figure 8-16). The bronchial walls also show bronchial gland hyperplasia, which correlates with overproduction of mucus. Smooth muscle cells are increased in number and appear to be enlarged, reflecting frequent bronchial spasms.

Autopsy examination of patients who die in status asthmaticus shows overinflation of the alveoli and mucous

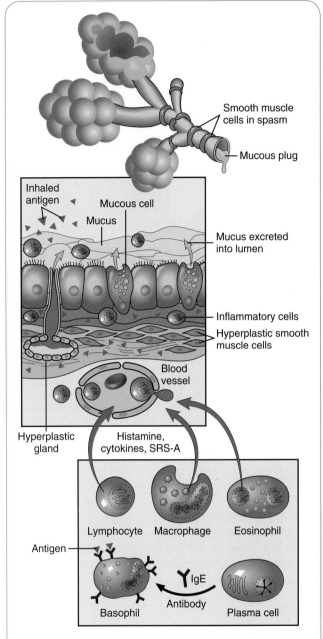

Figure 8-15 Pathogenesis of asthma. Allergens can trigger the release of mediators from mast cells, which act on the blood vessels and smooth muscle cells. The mediators released from chronic inflammatory cells in the wall of the bronchus also stimulate mucous secretion and contraction of the smooth muscle cells. IgE, immunoglobulin E; SRS-A, slow-reacting substance of anaphylaxis.

plugging of the bronchi. The lungs of asthmatic patients who die of other causes usually do not show grossly visible changes at autopsy.

Clinical Features

Extrinsic asthma typically begins before the age of 10 years and lasts for several years. Many children improve spontaneously, but in about 50% of those affected in childhood, recurrent

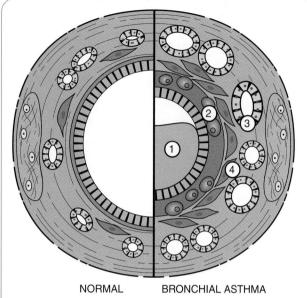

NORMAL   BRONCHIAL ASTHMA

1. Mucus in lumen
2. Inflammation and basement membrane thickening
3. Enlarged mucous glands
4. Smooth muscle hyperplasia

Figure 8-16 Histopathology of asthma. The lumen of the bronchus contains mucus. The wall is thickened and inflamed and contains hyperplastic smooth muscle cells and bronchial glands.

attacks persist throughout their life span. The disease is characterized by attacks of wheezing, dyspnea, and cough. These attacks are often precipitated by exposure to specific allergens. Most of these young patients often have a family history of asthma and other allergic diseases, such as atopic dermatitis ("eczema"). Skin testing may be useful for identifying the allergen, and an inhalation test may be used to provoke the attack and thus confirm the diagnosis. The serum of these patients contains elevated concentrations of IgE and often shows eosinophilia.

Intrinsic asthma begins in adulthood, usually before the age of 40 years. The asthmatic attacks, which are similar to those in extrinsic asthma, do not appear to be precipitated by exposure to identifiable allergens. Most attacks occur at random, but they may also be related to exposure to cold, environmental pollutants, and toxic gases. Aspirin is a well-known precipitating factor of asthmatic attacks in some people. Emotional stress and exercise can cause asthmatic attacks in others. Respiratory infections—especially chronic sinusitis—are the cause of asthmatic attacks in still others.

The treatment of asthma is symptomatic and is generally directed at preventing or reducing bronchospasm and bronchial inflammation. Drugs that prevent the degranulation of mast cells are especially beneficial. Bronchodilation with sympathomimetics is an efficient way of stopping the attacks. The prognosis is generally good, and most patients have a normal life span. Death secondary to status asthmaticus occurs only rarely.

SARCOIDOSIS

Sarcoidosis is a multisystemic granulomatous disease of unknown etiology, presumably mediated by cell-mediated immunity. It has an incidence of approximately 50 per 100,000 and affects blacks 10 times more often than people of other races. It is twice as common in black women than in men.

The cause and pathogenesis of sarcoidosis are not known. For unknown reasons, the disease has a predilection for the lungs and mediastinal lymph nodes. The lungs are infiltrated with T lymphocytes; CD4-positive T-helper cells outnumber the CD8-positive T-suppressor cells by a ratio of 10:1. The number of CD4-positive cells in the circulation is reduced, indicating that these cells have been attracted to the lungs and lymph nodes, where they contribute to the formation of granulomas. It was proposed that granulomas represent a response to putative antigens inhaled into the lungs, but the nature of these antigens has not been elucidated.

Clinical Features

Granulomas of sarcoidosis may involve any organ in the body (Figure 8-17). The lungs, the lymph nodes of the thorax and the neck, and the liver are most often involved. Granulomas of the lacrimal and salivary glands are found in one third of patients.

Pathology

The clinical symptoms of sarcoidosis vary. Approximately 50% of patients are asymptomatic and are diagnosed during routine examination. Most symptomatic patients have a low-grade fever and feel tired and anorexic. Symptoms pertaining to lung involvement are among the most common complaints and include dyspnea, cough, or wheezing respiration. In such patients, x-ray studies show pulmonary nodules and hilar lymph node enlargement. Peripheral lymphadenopathy, hepatosplenomegaly, and skin nodules are occasionally found. Enlargement of the salivary and lacrimal glands is a useful diagnostic finding, but unfortunately it is seen only in a minority of patients.

The definitive diagnosis of sarcoidosis is made on the basis of biopsy of the lymph nodes, bronchi, liver, or skin. Typical sarcoid granulomas are composed of epithelioid and giant cells surrounded, at the periphery, by a narrow rim of lymphocytes. In contrast to infectious granulomas, such as those caused by *M. tuberculosis* or fungi, granulomas of sarcoidosis do not show central necrosis (*noncaseating granulomas*).

The laboratory data are not pathognomonic but can nevertheless support the diagnosis. For example, 60% of patients have elevated serum levels of angiotensin-converting enzyme (ACE), which is released from macrophages in granulomas. Approximately 10% of patients develop hypercalcemia related to elevated serum levels of vitamin D_3. Unfortunately, these findings are not diagnostic, because similar biochemical changes can occur in other granulomatous diseases as well.

No specific therapy exists for sarcoidosis. More than 70% of patients recover spontaneously within a year or two. In

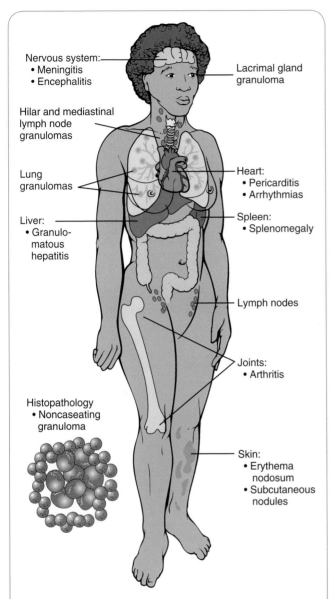

Nervous system:
• Meningitis
• Encephalitis

Lacrimal gland granuloma

Hilar and mediastinal lymph node granulomas

Lung granulomas

Heart:
• Pericarditis
• Arrhythmias

Liver:
• Granulo-matous hepatitis

Spleen:
• Splenomegaly

Lymph nodes

Joints:
• Arthritis

Histopathology
• Noncaseating granuloma

Skin:
• Erythema nodosum
• Subcutaneous nodules

Figure 8-17 Sarcoidosis. The most common sites of granulomas are the lungs and the thoracic lymph nodes. Other extrathoracic sites are less commonly involved. The inset shows a granuloma composed predominantly of epithelioid cells, macrophages, and lymphocytes. In contrast to tuberculosis, there is no central necrosis.

TABLE 8-3 Examples of Hypersensitivity Pneumonitis

Disease	Source of Antigen
Farmer's lung	Moldy hay or grain silage
Bagassosis	Sugar cane
Maple bark disease	Maple bark
Mushroom worker's lung	Mushrooms
Humidifier lung	Contaminated fluid
Pigeon-breeder's lung	Pigeon droppings
Furrier's lung	Animal pelts

also known to induce hypersensitivity pneumonitis. A short list of such diseases caused in various settings is given in Table 8-3.

Hypersensitivity pneumonitis may occur in an *acute* and a *chronic* form. *Acute pneumonitis* is mediated by antibodies that react with the inhaled antigen in the alveoli. The formation of antigen-antibody complexes activates complement, which in turn provides chemotactic signals and stimulates an influx of leukocytes. An acute pneumonitis evolves over a period of several hours after the exposure (Figure 8-18). *Chronic hypersensitivity pneumonitis* is mediated by T lymphocytes and is characterized by a typical cell-mediated reaction. Granulomas, found in most patients with chronic disease, are primarily located in the alveolar septa, causing their thickening or focal destruction. Damaged tissue cannot be repaired but is replaced by granulation tissue and fibrosis. Loss of parenchyma, scarring, and cystic dilation of the remaining airspaces is recognized on gross inspection of honeycomb lungs. Such end-stage lung disease of immune origin cannot be distinguished from other chronic lung diseases known under various names, such as fibrosing alveolitis, usual interstitial pneumonitis, idiopathic interstitial pneumonitis, and others. It is possible that some of these diseases are the consequences of an initial immune injury, but in most instances an immune pathogenesis cannot be proved.

Clinical Features

Acute hypersensitivity pneumonitis presents with dyspnea of sudden onset. Removal of the antigen usually improves the clinical picture. For example, a farmer who has hypersensitivity to silo grain contaminants should be told to avoid close exposure to the silo. Chronic hypersensitivity pneumonitis has a more ominous prognosis. In most of these chronic cases, the lung biopsy shows signs suggestive of hypersensitivity, but the inciting antigen cannot be identified. Destructive lung lesions cause chronic dyspnea, hyperventilation, and ultimately *respiratory failure*. Such end-stage lung disease can be treated only by lung transplantation.

20% of patients the disease persists, whereas in the remaining 10% it will progress and often have a lethal outcome.

HYPERSENSITIVITY PNEUMONITIS

Hypersensitivity pneumonitis, or *extrinsic allergic alveolitis,* is an immune disorder caused by repeated inhalation of foreign antigens. Most of these allergens are derived from molds and fungi growing on organic material, such as hay or tree bark, or in contaminated fluid or air-conditioning equipment. Bird droppings, animal fur dust, and wood dust are

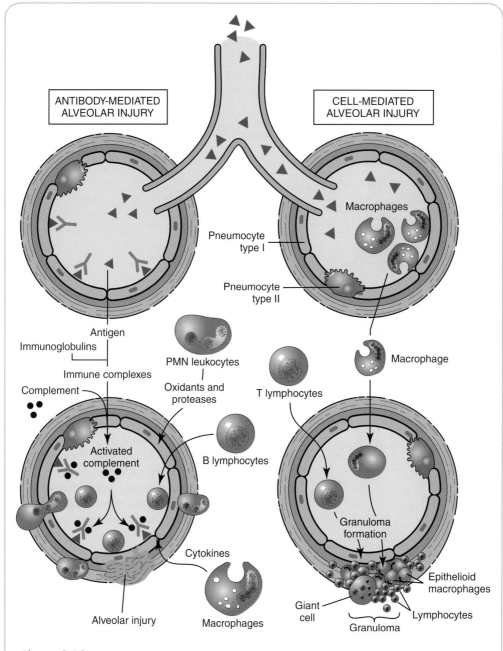

ANTIBODY-MEDIATED ALVEOLAR INJURY

CELL-MEDIATED ALVEOLAR INJURY

Macrophages

Pneumocyte type I

Pneumocyte type II

Antigen
Immunoglobulins

Immune complexes

Complement

Activated complement

Alveolar injury

PMN leukocytes

Oxidants and proteases

B lymphocytes

Cytokines

Macrophages

T lymphocytes

Macrophage

Granuloma formation

Giant cell

Granuloma

Epithelioid macrophages

Lymphocytes

Figure 8-18 Pathogenesis of hypersensitivity pneumonitis. The disease may be antibody or cell mediated. PMN, polymorphonuclear neutrophil.

PNEUMOCONIOSES

Pneumoconioses are lung diseases caused by inhalation of mineral dusts, fumes, and various organic or inorganic particulate matter. Most of these diseases are classified as occupational and are a consequence of long-term exposure in the workplace. Mineral dust pneumoconioses (most notably, coal-workers' lung disease), silicosis, and asbestosis are the most important diseases in this group. Other air pollutants are listed in Table 8-4.

The lung injury caused by mineral particles is complex, and although the exact mechanisms are unknown, it has been shown that the extent of injury depends on the following:
- Duration of exposure
- Concentration of particles
- The size of the particles, their shape, and their solubility
- The biochemical composition of the inhaled dust

Inert material, like coal particles, is less reactive; therefore coal-miners' pneumoconiosis develops only after very long exposure to high levels of polluted air. Silica particles are more reactive and apparently produce more prominent tissue

TABLE 8-4 Examples of Air Pollutants

Pollutant	Source(s)	Consequences
Gases		
Carbon monoxide (CO)	Car exhaust Gas stove	Anoxia (death)
Sulfur dioxide (SO$_2$)	Coal smoke Tobacco	Mucosal irritation
Polychlorinated biphenyls (PCBs)	Air spray Refrigerators	Undefined
Formaldehyde	Laboratory fumes House insulation	Mucosal irritation
Particles		
Carbon	Coal smoke Smog Mining	Anthracosis
Quartz (silica)	Stone cutting	Silicosis
Asbestos	Insulation Shipbuilding	Asbestosis

injury. Asbestos particles are insoluble and tend to remain lodged inside the lungs permanently.

The size of the particles is very important. Large dust particles—that is, those measuring more than 10 μm—are retained in the nasal mucus and do not reach the lower respiratory tract. However, particles smaller than 5 μm can enter the alveoli, where they are taken up by macrophages. Such particles, depending on their chemical composition, may produce lung injury.

The response of inflammatory cells to the inhaled particles is also important. Macrophages stimulated by the ingested particles release various cytokines, such as interleukin-1 (IL-1) or tumor necrosis factor (TNF), which promote inflammation and also stimulate the proliferation of fibroblasts and the formation of collagen. Destruction of tissue, the ensuing repair, and fibrosis contribute to a restructuring of the lung parenchyma, and these changes are typically associated with a loss of respiratory surfaces.

The clinical symptoms of pneumoconiosis are variable. Usually the symptoms are nonspecific and resemble those caused by other restrictive lung diseases. Progressive dyspnea ultimately leads to respiratory failure.

COAL-WORKERS' LUNG DISEASE

Coal miners working in reasonably well-ventilated mines are relatively safe or have only minor problems. At autopsy the lungs of these miners show only black discoloration, known as *anthracosis* (derived from the Greek *anthrakos,* meaning "black"), pathologic tissue changes caused by the accumulation of carbon particles in the pulmonary interstitial spaces, around the bronchi, and underneath the pleura. Clinically, anthracosis

is not associated with significant pulmonary dysfunction. Furthermore, similar blackening of the lungs can be seen in smokers and in many city dwellers.

Coal miners working in suboptimal conditions or without protective gear may develop more severe lung disease known as **coal-workers' lung disease (CWLD).** Colloquially it is also known as *black lung disease* because at autopsy the lungs of these patients appear black, fibrotic, and structurally abnormal. The black color is related to the accumulation of carbon particles, but it is suspected that other minerals, such as silica, are also present and contribute to the pathogenesis of lung destruction.

Pathogenesis

Amorphous carbon particles are innocuous; indeed, most of them never reach the lungs but instead are retained in the nasal or bronchial mucus. Those that do reach the alveoli are taken up by alveolar macrophages and, in most cases, are expectorated. If the burden of coal particles in the dust is overwhelming or if the dust contains other particles besides carbon, the macrophages cannot eliminate it through the bronchi. Dust particles accumulate in the interstitial spaces of the lung, incite fibrosis, and contribute to the destruction of normal parenchyma.

Not everybody working in the coal mines develops lung disease. It is possible that the lesions occur only after a critical threshold of exposure has been surpassed. Furthermore, some persons might be more susceptible than others. This view is supported by observations that some coal miners tend to develop rheumatoid lung disease *(Caplan's syndrome),* which is rare in the general population. Finally, it appears that persons who develop CWLD have a predisposition to pulmonary tuberculosis, which was previously prevalent among coal miners.

Pathology

CWLD is caused by prolonged inhalation of dust that is rich in carbon particles and other earth minerals. These particles are deposited in the centrolobular zones of the lung and may be associated with fibrosis or centroacinar emphysema. Fibrosis may become progressive, replacing broad fields of lung parenchyma (Figure 8-19).

Clinical Features

The symptoms of CWLD vary in clinical severity from mild to severe. There is no effective treatment, and the disease usually has a slow but unrelenting course. The only good news about this disease is that it apparently does not predispose the individual to cancer. Improved conditions in the coal mines and the protective masks that are currently used have reduced the incidence of this lung disease.

SILICOSIS

Silicosis is a lung disease caused by inhalation of small (1- to 3-μm) silica crystals, which are inhaled in dust generated during stone cutting, mining, and sand blasting. The disease typically develops only in persons exposed to silica dust for 10 to 20 years.

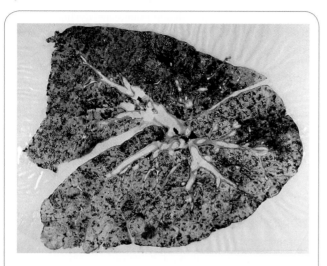

Figure 8-19 Coal-workers' lung disease. The lungs appear black because of the massive deposits of carbon particles. (From Damjanov I and Linder J: Pathology: A Color Atlas, St. Louis, 2000, Mosby.)

Silicosis is currently considered the most common lung disease caused by mineral particles from the environment.

Pathology

Silicosis is characterized by fibronodular lesions in the lung parenchyma. Silica particles are initially taken up by macrophages, which are damaged in this process and often killed. Dead macrophages release silica crystals and various biologically active substances that stimulate fibroblasts to produce collagen. This results in the formation of collagenous nodules, which are most prominent along the lymphatics draining toward the hilar lymph nodes. Because silicosis occurs only rarely in an isolated form (it usually presents as *anthracosilicosis*), these nodules are often black. Confluent silicotic nodules destroy lung parenchyma and cause massive pulmonary fibrosis, which is indistinguishable from other forms of fibrotic lung disease. Tuberculosis is a common complication, probably because silica-laden macrophages cannot effectively combat mycobacterial infections.

Clinical Features

The clinical symptoms of silicosis are generally mild unless a progressive bilateral fibrosis or tuberculosis supervenes. Once the lesions develop, they are irreversible and do not regress on treatment. Silicosis may be an incapacitating disease, but it is worth noting that it does not predispose individuals to cancer.

ASBESTOSIS

Four lung lesions have been linked to asbestos exposure:
- Pulmonary fibrosis
- Pleural fibrosis and pleural plaques
- Lung cancer
- *Mesothelioma*

Asbestos is a generic name for several fibrous silicates that form natural minerals, such as chrysotile, amosite, or crocidolite. Asbestos fibers have been used in manufacturing and industry for many years. However, only recently—several years after World War II—were the health hazards of asbestos exposure recognized. During the war and thereafter, some 10 million American workers, such as those involved in shipbuilding, the construction industry, and the manufacture of car brakes and house insulation, were exposed to asbestos in the workplace. Only a small percentage of these workers developed lung diseases, but nevertheless the actual numbers are staggering. Estimates are that approximately 10,000 deaths per year are still directly or indirectly attributable to asbestos exposure during the 1940s and 1950s.

Asbestos fibers vary in size, shape, and biochemical composition. Large and long asbestos particles are innocuous because they do not reach the lungs. Such fibers are retained in nasal and bronchial mucus. Most asbestos fibers presently used in industry, such as chrysotile, are classified as serpentines, which are curly and elongated and produce no harm. On the other hand, amphibole asbestos, the brittle, short, straight fibers of crocidolite and amosite, are potentially more dangerous. These amphiboles are not used today.

Pathogenesis

The pathogenesis of asbestos lung disease is not known. It is known that short (straight) fibers enter the alveoli and are taken up by macrophages (Figure 8-20). In contrast to silica, which is toxic to macrophages, asbestos does not kill these cells. Instead, asbestos activates the macrophages and stimulates them to release various fibrogenic cytokines and growth factors. This ultimately results in extensive pulmonary fibrosis. Fibrosis of the pleura leads to the formation of typical fibrous plaques. Asbestos is carcinogenic; it stimulates the formation of mesotheliomas of the pleura and lung cancer.

> **? Did You Know?**
>
> Asbestos is not a recent invention. Historical documents show that it was used in classical Greece and Rome. In Greek it means "inextinguishable." It was used to keep the eternal flames of the vestal virgins burning day and night. The ancients also knew that it might have adverse effects. The Greek geographer Strabo and the Roman naturalist Pliny the Elder both mentioned asbestos-related lung disease in slaves who used asbestos for weaving cloth.

Pathology

Lungs affected by asbestos show fibrosis and pleural plaques and may contain foci of lung cancer or *mesothelioma*. Fibrous tissue contains beaded bodies with knobbed ends called *asbestos bodies*. These bodies are coated with hemosiderin pigment and thus appear brown, so they are also called *ferruginous bodies*. Ferruginous bodies can be found in lungs not affected by asbestosis, but in asbestosis, such bodies are extremely abundant. It has been estimated that for every iron-coated asbestos body, there are at least 10 that are

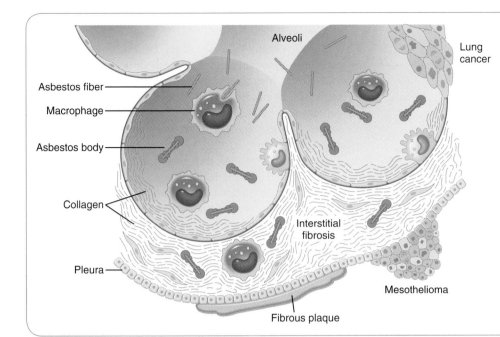

Alveoli

Lung cancer

Asbestos fiber

Macrophage

Asbestos body

Collagen

Interstitial fibrosis

Pleura

Mesothelioma

Fibrous plaque

Figure 8-20 Asbestosis. Asbestos bodies in the terminal respiratory spaces elicit interstitial fibrosis of the lung and also contribute to the formation of pleural plaques. Asbestosis plays a role in the pathogenesis of lung cancer and mesotheliomas of the pleura.

not coated and therefore cannot be seen by light microscopy. These can best be demonstrated by chemical analysis after microincineration (i.e., burning of the lung tissue sample), with subsequent analysis of the ashes. The asbestos fibers are fire resistant and will remain in the ashes.

Clinical Features

Asbestosis presents as restrictive lung disease and dyspnea. The dyspnea persists for years, but respiratory failure occurs only rarely. Solitary or small pleural plaques are usually asymptomatic. Diffuse pleural fibrosis may cause restrictive lung disease.

Lung cancer is an important complication of exposure to asbestos. Malignant tumors develop in fibrotic lungs five to six times more often than in the control population. However, when asbestos exposure is combined with cigarette smoking, the risk of lung cancer is more than 50 times higher. Mesotheliomas are yet another complication of asbestos exposure and are discussed in the section on lung tumors. These pleural tumors occur almost exclusively in persons exposed to asbestos.

VENTILATORY DISTURBANCES, ACUTE RESPIRATORY DISTRESS SYNDROME, AND ATELECTASIS

Respiratory functions of the lung depend critically on the normal inhalation of air, passage of oxygen across the alveolar membrane, and normal blood flow through the lungs. Pathologic changes involving the alveolar walls—that is, the interface between the air and the blood—have been described in the previous sections on pneumonia and interstitial pulmonary fibrosis. Pulmonary emboli and other circulatory disturbances

have previously been presented in Chapter 6. Here, only processes that affect ventilation are described. Two complex multifactorial lesions—*acute respiratory distress syndrome* (ARDS) and *atelectasis*—are also included in this discussion.

DISTURBANCES OF VENTILATION

Normal ventilation depends on the unimpeded influx of air into the lungs through the upper and middle respiratory tracts. This is effectively achieved through the action of respiratory muscles. It depends on the ability of the thorax to expand and retract with each respiratory movement. Finally, the expansion of the lungs depends on the pressure gradients: the positive pressure inside the airspaces that inflates the alveoli and the negative pressure within the pleural cavity that keeps the lungs from collapsing.

Respiratory difficulties present typically as shortness of breath *(dyspnea)*. Various causes of dyspnea are listed in Table 8-5.

Obstruction of the upper respiratory tract can occur under a variety of conditions. **Suffocation** can be caused by occlusion of the larynx with food. For example, a big bite of steak may enter the respiratory system; indeed, steaks kill approximately 30 Americans this way every month! Homicide by suffocation is a common finding in the daily practice of forensic pathology. Small children may suffocate accidentally by pulling plastic bags over their heads. *Small foreign bodies,* such as cherry pits or candy, when aspirated into the larynx and trachea, may completely block the air passage and cause death, especially in children.

Drowning is another example of obstruction of the respiratory tract. It is the third leading cause of accidental death in the United States, and current estimates indicate that more than 5000 people drown every year. The number of near-drowning

TABLE 8-5 Causes of Dyspnea

Causes	Examples
Large airway obstruction	Laryngospasm, foreign body
Small airway obstruction	Bronchiolitis, asthma
Intra-alveolar obstruction	Pneumonia, edema
Alveolar septal lesions	
Destruction	Emphysema
Increase in thickness	Interstitial fibrosis
Collapse	Atelectasis
Central nervous causes	Apoplexy of respiratory centers

victims is approximately 10 times that number, which indicates that 9 of every 10 persons thought to have drowned can be saved. Children and adolescents, mostly males, are the most common victims.

During an autopsy examination of a drowned person, one may encounter two sets of changes: a more common form, known as *wet drowning* (90% of cases), and a less common form, known as *dry drowning.* In wet drowning, the aspirated water enters the respiratory tract, filling the airways and thus preventing the entry of air. Anoxia results, and if the person is not resuscitated, death occurs within minutes. Dry drowning occurs as a result of reflex laryngospasm and closure of the glottis, which prevents fluid and air from entering the lower respiratory tract. These patients are more easily resuscitated, and many can be saved. It is believed that most persons who experience near-drowning survive because of such laryngospasm.

Aspiration of sea water, which is hypertonic in respect to the blood, causes more pronounced pulmonary edema than does aspiration of fresh water. Whereas hypertonic sea water promotes the entry of water from the circulation into the alveoli, hypotonic fresh water is absorbed into the circulation. In patients who survive near-drowning, these distinctions are of limited clinical significance, because most clinical symptoms stem from hypoxia.

Ischemic brain injury is the most common cause of death. If the patient survives, pulmonary acidosis is the most common short-term consequence of anoxia. Long-term consequences depend on the duration of oxygen deprivation. Neurologic symptoms that develop as a result of brain ischemia and focal necrosis of neurons predominate. The extent of brain injury will ultimately determine the extent to which the patient will recover.

VENTILATORY FAILURE

Ventilatory failure *secondary to alveolar hypoventilation* occurs in several conditions that may affect the following:
- Neural control of respiration
- Respiratory muscles
- Chest wall
- Airways

Neural control of respiration resides in the respiratory centers in the brainstem. It depends critically on peripheral input from chemoreceptors and the content of carbon dioxide in the blood. Brainstem lesions, such as apoplexy, may depress spontaneous breathing. Retention of CO_2 (i.e., prolonged hypercapnia and the resulting acidosis) has the same effect.

The respiratory muscles—that is, the diaphragm and the intercostal and other thoracic chest wall muscles—are striated muscles that are innervated by cranial or spinal nerves. These muscles may become dysfunctional under several conditions. Lesions affecting the nerves, the neuromuscular junction, or the muscles can impair ventilation. *Poliomyelitis,* a disease that affects the spinal cord, was previously known as the most dreaded cause of respiratory paralysis. Similar paralysis can occur after spinal cord trauma. *Tetanus* toxin causes muscle spasm. With tetanus, death is often secondary to respiratory failure because the muscles cannot move. *Myasthenia gravis* affects the neuromuscular junctions and also depresses breathing. *Muscular dystrophy,* especially in its most severe form (known as *Duchenne-type dystrophy*), is also marked by respiratory muscle failure.

Chest wall lesions that restrict the expansion of the chest wall during inspiration can also cause alveolar hypoxia. Respiratory movement is impaired in persons who have deformities of the chest cage *(kyphoscoliosis)* or pleural fibrosis and pleural tumors that encase the lungs. Extreme obesity can also depress respiration.

 Did You Know?

Impeded respiration secondary to extreme obesity is called *pickwickian syndrome,* named so after the obese boy, Joe, described by Charles Dickens in *The Pickwick Papers.* Joe was so obese that he could not move. He was constantly somnolent, presumably from hypoxia and hypercapnia, related to his shallow and depressed breathing.

Airway pathology causing alveolar hypoxia has been described previously and is mentioned here only as a reminder and for the sake of completeness. The best examples are laryngospasm (croup), the bronchial mucous plugs associated with cystic fibrosis, and the alveolar lesions typical of interstitial pulmonary fibrosis, which may be caused by a variety of factors.

ACUTE RESPIRATORY DISTRESS SYNDROME

Acute respiratory distress syndrome (ARDS) is a clinical term used to describe changes that occur in the lungs under a variety of conditions, all of which cause acute respiratory failure. The most important causes of ARDS are listed in Box 8-1.

The consequences of initial injury are increased permeability of the alveolar blood vessels, loss of alveolar lining cells, and accumulation of fluid in the alveolar spaces. All these events impair oxygenation of blood, resulting in anoxia. The disrupted pulmonary blood circulation strains the heart, and patients die of severe cardiopulmonary failure.

Injury of the *alveolar lining cells* is the initiating event in viral pneumonia or after inhalation of toxic fumes. Leukocytes forming an intra-alveolar exudate in bacterial pneumonia also can damage alveolar cells. *Endothelial cell* injury is the initiating event in patients who are septic. Cytotoxic drugs or anoxia caused by cardiogenic shock can also damage endothelial cells. In many instances, ARDS is attributable to injury of both the alveolar lining cells and the endothelial cells. Inhalation of hot air, for example, may cause pulmonary burns, which can destroy the entire alveolar wall (i.e., both the endothelial cells and the capillaries).

Etiology and Pathogenesis

ARDS may develop through several pathways, usually beginning either as an injury of endothelial cells in pulmonary capillaries or an injury of alveolar lining cells (Figure 8-21). The terminal airways (i.e., the alveolar walls) are invariably affected in either case, and their function is severely impaired.

Pathology

Regardless of the etiology of ARDS, the lungs show the typical features of diffuse alveolar damage (DAD). On gross examination at autopsy, the lungs are heavy and filled with

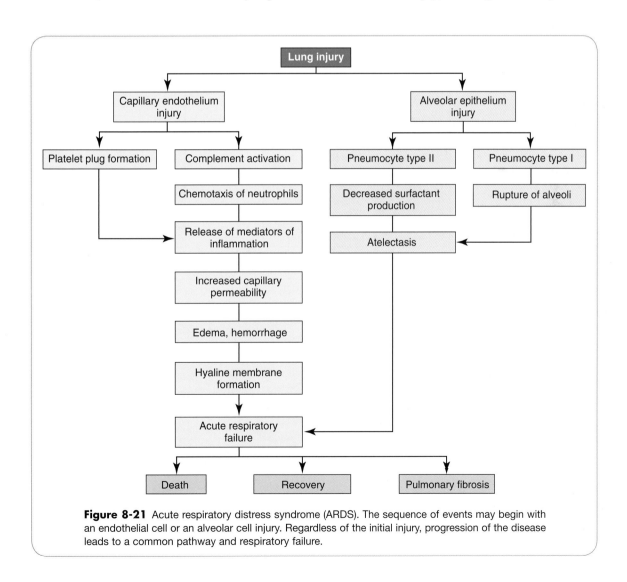

Figure 8-21 Acute respiratory distress syndrome (ARDS). The sequence of events may begin with an endothelial cell or an alveolar cell injury. Regardless of the initial injury, progression of the disease leads to a common pathway and respiratory failure.

edema fluid and are therefore airless. Histologically the alveolar spaces are dilated and filled with proteinaceous edema fluid. The plasma extravasates into the alveoli clots, forming fibrin-rich hyaline membranes (Figure 8-22). The alveolar capillaries are engorged with blood, which escapes focally into the alveoli. In disseminated intravascular coagulation (DIC), which is caused by shock, intra-alveolar hemorrhages are often associated with microthrombi in small pulmonary vessels.

Clinical Features

The symptoms of ARDS reflect the acute onset of respiratory failure. Initial symptoms usually occur within 24 hours of the inciting event. The patient is in severe distress, short of breath, and gasping for air. Laboratory findings confirm hypoxemia and hypercapnia. Chest x-ray studies show diffuse consolidation of the lungs, which appear to be airless. Most patients must receive ventilator (respirator) therapy, and even in those who survive the initial lung injury, there is still a very high mortality. These patients are prone to infections and often die of pneumonia. Those who recover completely

tend to have chronic respiratory problems related to the fibrosis of damaged alveolar septa. One third of patients die within days, one third die of pneumonia and heart failure within weeks of ARDS onset, and one third recover. Of those who recover, approximately 40% have permanent residual respiratory problems.

ATELECTASIS

Atelectasis (derived from the Greek *ateles,* meaning "incomplete," and *ectasis,* meaning "expansion") is a term used to denote incomplete expansion or, more often, collapse of alveoli. Minor focal atelectases are very common and accompany many pulmonary diseases. Massive atelectasis of the entire lungs is less common but is associated with more significant symptoms.

The most important causes of atelectasis, as shown in Figure 8-23, are as follows:
- Deficiency of surfactant
- Compression of the lungs from outside
- Resorption of air distal to bronchial obstruction

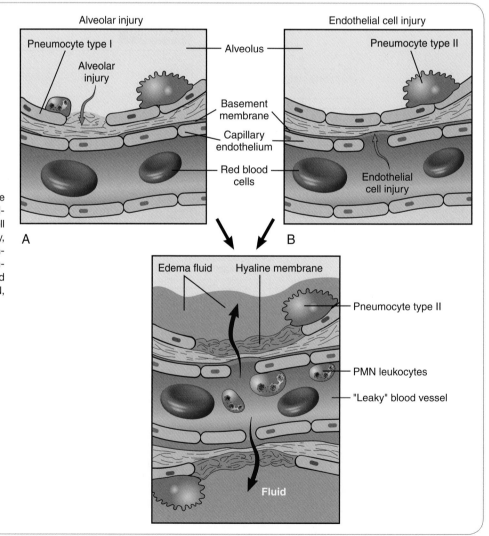

Figure 8-22 Pathogenesis of acute respiratory distress syndrome. *A,* Alveolar cell injury. *B,* Endothelial cell injury. Regardless of the initial injury, the established lesions appear identical and comprise hyaline membranes, ruptured alveolar walls, and intra-alveolar edema fluid. PMN, polymorphonuclear neutrophil.

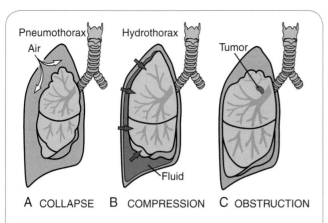

Figure 8-23 Mechanism of atelectasis. *A*, Collapse of the lung in pneumothorax. *B*, Compression of the lung by pleural fluid. *C*, Resorption of the air from alveoli distal to an obstructed bronchus. Obstructive atelectasis is usually focal. Atelectasis of premature infants, which is caused by a deficiency of pulmonary surfactant, is not shown.

Atelectasis secondary to a deficiency of surfactant occurs in premature neonates who are born before their lungs have achieved functional maturity. Alveolar type II pneumocytes of immature lungs do not produce the surfactant. Because the alveoli cannot remain open, the lungs collapse. Because the infant cannot breathe, a respiratory distress syndrome develops that is associated with high mortality.

Compression atelectasis is usually caused by fluid in the pleural cavity. It may represent transudate formed as a result of heart failure or an exudate caused by inflammation *(pleuritis)*. Tumors of the pleura, especially those that are associated with pleural effusion, also can compress the lungs. The fluid compressing the lungs prevents their expansion. Entry of air into the pleural cavity (pneumothorax) also causes massive pulmonary atelectasis.

Resorption atelectasis typically develops within a single pulmonary anatomic unit that is distal to an obstructed bronchus. The obstruction may be caused by a mucous plug, by a tumor, or by foreign material that is aspirated into the bronchial tree. The air from alveoli distal to the obstructed bronchus is resorbed, and the alveolar walls collapse.

Atelectasis is usually reversible. After the causative defect has been corrected, the alveoli expand and resume their normal function.

NEOPLASMS OF THE RESPIRATORY TRACT

The most important neoplasms of the respiratory tract are lung cancer and carcinoma of the larynx. In comparison with these two neoplasms, all the others are of lesser significance and will not be discussed in detail here.

CARCINOMA OF THE LARYNX

Carcinoma of the larynx accounts for less than 2% of all human cancers. The most important facts about carcinomas of the larynx are as follows:

- They have been pathogenetically linked to smoking and chronic alcohol intake. This accounts in part for the high prevalence of laryngeal cancer in males, who are affected seven times more frequently than females.
- Laryngeal cancer is rare in people younger than 40 years, and its incidence increases with advancing age.
- Carcinoma may originate from any part of the larynx. Tumors originating above the glottis are called *supraglottic*, whereas those arising below this demarcation line are termed *infraglottic*.
- Laryngeal tumors present as nodules or ulcerations of the mucosa (Figure 8-24). If not resected, these tumors invade locally and tend to metastasize to local neck lymph nodes. Distant metastases are a late event.

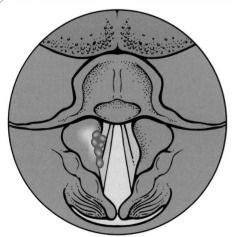

Mirror view of carcinoma of the larynx. The vocal cord is infiltrated with the tumor.

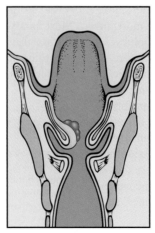

Coronal section

Figure 8-24 Carcinoma of the larynx. The tumor resembles an ulcerated nodule.

- Histologic examination reveals that essentially all laryngeal cancers are squamous cell carcinoma.

Patients with carcinoma of the larynx present relatively early in the course of the disease with symptoms such as hoarseness, loss of voice, or stridorous respiration. Because the tumors are discovered early and are mostly localized at the time of diagnosis, the overall prognosis is very good. The 5-year survival rate of patients who have been treated surgically or by radiation therapy is 75%.

LUNG CARCINOMA

Lung carcinoma is the leading cause of cancer death in the United States and most other Western industrialized countries. Until a few years ago, affected males outnumbered females by a large margin. However, changing work habits and increased smoking among women in the post–World War II era have contributed to an increased incidence of lung cancer among women. The campaign against smoking has only slightly reduced the incidence of lung cancer in the United States but very little elsewhere. In this context, it is worth remembering the following:

- Lung cancer is the most common malignant disease of internal organs and the leading cause of cancer death in the United States. It has been estimated that during 2008, approximately 170,000 people died of lung cancer.
- Lung cancer is in most cases caused by *cigarette smoking*. Although there is no definitive proof to support this statement, the epidemiologic evidence linking lung cancer to smoking is very persuasive. Approximately 90% of patients with lung cancer are smokers!
- Lung cancer is rare before the age of 40 years, but thereafter its incidence rises in direct proportion with age.
- Lung cancer still has a very poor prognosis. The overall 5-year survival rate is 10% to 15%, and in most instances, the disease is incurable.

Etiology and Pathogenesis

The events leading to the formation of lung carcinoma are not fully understood. Various chemicals in tobacco smoke probably act as the primary carcinogens. The tobacco smoke contains many potentially harmful substances, the most important of which are chemically classified as polycyclic hydrocarbons. Like the polycyclic hydrocarbons derived from tar, those in cigarette smoke are also mutagenic to bacteria *in vitro* in the Ames test. In tissue culture, these chemicals can initiate and promote malignant transformation of normal mammalian cells. It is assumed that the exposure to carcinogens in smoke initiates malignant transformation of bronchial cells and promotes their progression into invasive cancer. This probably involves the direct action of carcinogens on cellular DNA, the activation of oncogenes, or mutation and inhibition of tumor suppressor genes, such as *TP53*.

Inhaled *procarcinogens* (incomplete carcinogens) are transformed into carcinogens through the action of cytoplasmic enzymes in bronchial cells exposed to smoke. Inducibility of these enzymes, which are potentially important for carcinogenesis, is genetically determined. It is high in some persons and low in others. These genetic differences could account for the fact that not all smokers develop lung cancer and for the increased predisposition to lung cancer noted in some families.

The chemicals inhaled in tobacco smoke contain several proven carcinogens and also various irritants that could act as promoters of incipient neoplasia. Histologic studies of respiratory epithelia in smokers indicate that in most cases bronchial cancer is associated with a variety of preneoplastic lesions that are most likely caused by the combined action of carcinogens and irritants.

It has been proposed that the sequence of events begins with metaplasia of the bronchial epithelium. This reactive, benign lesion is characterized by a transformation of normal, pseudostratified, cylindrical epithelium into squamous epithelium (Figure 8-25). Metaplasia is initially a reversible lesion. If smoking is discontinued, the lesion will disappear and the normal structure of bronchial epithelium will be restored. If the carcinogenic stimuli persist, metaplasia will progress into carcinoma *in situ,* and this will give rise to invasive carcinoma, most of which will be of the squamous type. Initial squamous metaplasia explains the paradoxical appearance of a *squamous cell carcinoma* in an epithelium not normally composed of squamous cells.

If the transformed stem cells progress and become more anaplastic, the tumor will be histologically classified as an *undifferentiated large-cell carcinoma.* In some bronchial carcinomas the malignant transformation will primarily involve the neuroendocrine cells, which are normally present in the bronchial mucosa. These tumors of neuroendocrine cells may be low-grade malignancies called *carcinoids* or *neuroendocrine carcinomas.* Highly malignant neuroendocrine carcinomas are called *small-cell carcinomas* (also known as *oat-cell carcinomas*). Finally, some bronchial tumors will be composed of cylindrical cells, resembling the normal cells in the bronchus. These cells tend to form irregular glands and are classified as *adenocarcinomas.*

Macroscopic Pathology

Most tumors that surgeons or pathologists encounter in clinical practice are grossly visible masses that can be classified according to their location as *hilar* (central) or *peripheral* (subpleural).

 Did You Know?

Despite overwhelming scientific evidence linking lung carcinoma to smoking, many people continue to smoke cigarettes and the tobacco industry is making higher profits than ever. It was only in 1998 that the tobacco industry finally agreed to pay for some of the health care costs caused by smoking.

Hilar tumors are attached to the bronchi, extending into the adjacent parenchyma or protruding into the lumen

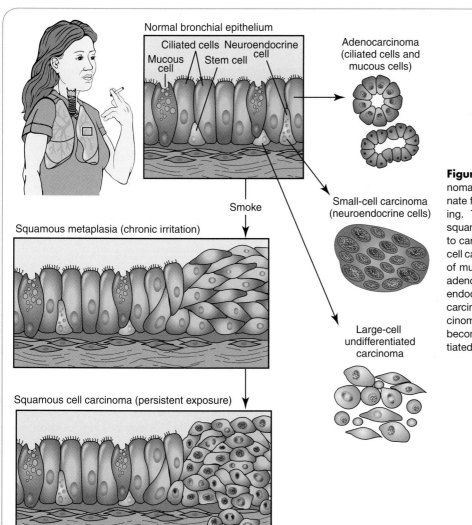

Normal bronchial epithelium

Ciliated cells Neuroendocrine cell

Mucous cell Stem cell

Adenocarcinoma (ciliated cells and mucous cells)

Smoke

Squamous metaplasia (chronic irritation)

Small-cell carcinoma (neuroendocrine cells)

Large-cell undifferentiated carcinoma

Squamous cell carcinoma (persistent exposure)

Figure 8-25 Histogenesis of lung carcinoma of the bronchus. Most tumors originate from bronchi and are caused by smoking. The columnar epithelium undergoes squamous metaplasia, which can progress to carcinoma *in situ* and invasive squamous cell carcinoma. Malignant tumors composed of mucous or ciliated cells are classified as adenocarcinomas, whereas those of neuroendocrine cells are classified as small-cell carcinomas. Large-cell undifferentiated carcinomas originate from stem cells that have become anaplastic and have never differentiated into any other cell type.

(Figure 8-26, *A*). In clinical practice, these tumors are seen on x-ray studies as nodules. Those that protrude into the bronchi and those that cause ulceration of the overlying bronchial mucosa can be recognized by bronchoscopy.

Peripheral neoplasms can form subpleural nodules or present as a consolidation of pulmonary parenchyma (Figure 8-26, *B*). Nodular cancers may originate from small bronchi or bronchiolar cells or type II pneumocytes trapped in the fibrous tissue *(scar carcinomas)*. Some tumors arising from cells in the terminal bronchioli tend to grow inside the alveoli, do not invade the stroma, and are called *bronchioloalveolar carcinomas*. Consolidation caused by these tumors may be mistaken for pneumonia.

Lung cancer is a highly malignant tumor, and it tends to metastasize early. Locally these tumors extend into the mediastinum and often spread into the pleural cavity. At the time of diagnosis, more than 70% of patients already have metastases that are apparent, and many more probably have microscopic metastases that are clinically inapparent. Approximately one half of those with tumors extending beyond the lung parenchyma have metastases to the local lymph nodes.

Distant metastases are most often found in the liver and brain (Figure 8-27). Lung cancer also has a tendency to metastasize to bones, kidneys, and, for some peculiar reason, the adrenals.

Microscopic Pathology

Lung tumors can be classified microscopically into several groups:

- Adenocarcinoma (40%)
- Squamous cell carcinoma (30%)
- Large-cell undifferentiated carcinoma (10%)
- Small-cell carcinoma (15%)
- Carcinoids (5%)

Each of these tumor types has unique histologic features, although there is some overlap between some of them. Squamous cell, small-cell, and large-cell carcinomas tend to be central, whereas adenocarcinomas predominate in the peripheral parts of the lung. For practical purposes, it is customary to separate small-cell carcinomas from all others, which are grouped under the name of *non–small-cell lung carcinoma (NSCLC)*. NSCLC are treated surgically, supplemented by

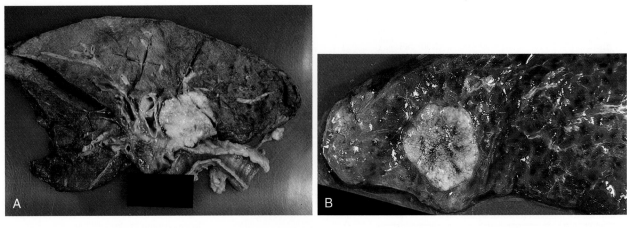

Figure 8-26 Lung cancer. *A,* Centrally located lung carcinoma. *B,* Peripheral carcinoma.

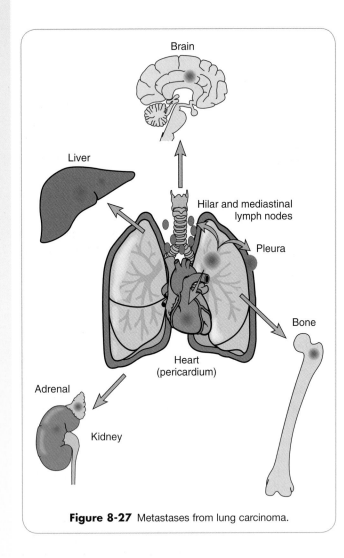

Figure 8-27 Metastases from lung carcinoma.

Carcinoid is a neuroendocrine tumor of low-grade malignancy. These tumors have a tendency to invade locally and to grow slowly, and they do not metastasize to distant places. Local resection is the treatment of choice. Cure can be achieved in 87% of cases. Tumors classified as atypical carcinoids have a less favorable prognosis, but still patients with these tumors have a 5-year survival rate of 60%. Obviously this is much better than the 5% survival rate of those with large-cell or small-cell carcinomas.

Clinical Features

Symptoms of lung cancer can be classified as being related to the following:

- Bronchial irritation or obstruction
- Local extension into the mediastinum or pleural cavity
- Distant metastases
- Systemic effects of neoplasia

Approximately 10% to 15% of patients with lung cancer have no obvious symptoms, and the tumor is discovered incidentally during routine chest x-ray examination. Among the patients who are symptomatic, approximately one third will report to the physician with symptoms pertaining to local effects of tumor in the chest, one third will present with symptoms pertaining to distant metastases, and one third will present with nonspecific systemic complaints and no localizing symptoms.

Bronchial irritation most often causes coughing; less commonly, it causes respiratory wheezing, dyspnea, and other respiratory symptoms. Hemoptysis is reported in 30% of all patients.

Local extension of the tumor into the pulmonary parenchyma tends to obstruct bronchi, cause atelectasis, and predispose the individual to lung infection. Extension to the pleural surface is typically associated with pleural effusion and progressive dyspnea secondary to lung compression. Ingrowth of tumor into the mediastinal nerves causes pain or paralysis of muscles of the diaphragm or vocal cords. Tumor may also extend into the esophagus and cause dysphagia.

radiation therapy and adjuvant chemotherapy. Small-cell carcinomas are treated primarily by chemotherapy and are not removed surgically. Overall, those with small-cell carcinomas have a more rapid downhill course than patients with NSCLCs.

Distant metastases produce symptoms that are specific to the organ(s) involved. Liver metastases cause hepatomegaly. Brain metastases result in neurologic symptoms and are associated with high mortality. Bone metastases result in fractures. Adrenal metastases may produce destruction of the glands and cause Addison's disease (i.e., adrenocortical insufficiency).

The *systemic symptoms* of lung cancer do not differ significantly from symptoms produced by other tumors and include weight loss and cachexia, anorexia, and general malaise.

Lung tumors also produce various *paraneoplastic syndromes.* The most common among these are syndromes caused by oversecretion of the following:

- Parathyroid-like polypeptide, which results in hypercalcemia
- Adrenocorticotropic hormone (ACTH), which results in overstimulation of the adrenals (Cushing's syndrome)
- Antidiuretic hormone, which results in excessive retention of water in the kidneys and dilutional hyponatremia

Lung cancer is essentially incurable. Treatment includes surgery, radiation therapy, and chemotherapy. The overall 5-year survival is around 10% to 15%. The only patients who can be effectively cured are those whose tumors are clinically inapparent and were discovered by chance on cytologic examination or bronchoscopy and those with most typical carcinoid tumors.

METASTATIC CANCER

Although lung cancer represents the most common malignant disease in humans today, primary lung carcinomas are less common than lung **metastases** from other sites. Because a large amount of blood circulates through the lungs, any tumor cell floating in the blood could be filtered out while passing through the pulmonary capillaries. Furthermore, the thoracic duct, the main lymphatic vessel, is confluent with the superior vena cava; thus tumor cells transported in the lymph will also lodge in the lungs.

Pulmonary metastases may present as the following:
- Solitary lesions
- Multiple lesions
- Diffuse lesions replacing large parts of the lung or diffusely covering the pleural surface

Solitary metastases may be resected. If the patient has no other evidence of tumor, such treatment may be beneficial and prolong life. Metastases, recognized by x-ray studies as round nodules ("cannonball lesions"), are incurable (Figure 8-28).

PLEURAL DISEASES

The pleura forms the outer covering of the lung (visceral pleura) and the inner covering of the chest cage (parietal pleura). The space between the two layers of pleura is called the *pleural cavity.* It is a virtual space because the two layers

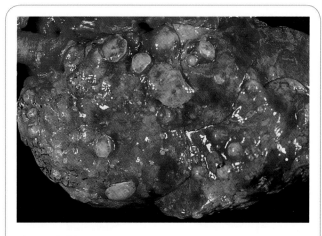

Figure 8-28 Carcinoma metastatic to the lungs. The lung parenchyma contains several round nodules. (From Damjanov I, Linder J: Pathology: A Color Atlas, St. Louis, 2000, Mosby.)

of the pleura are tightly apposed to one another and are separated only by a thin film of fluid that keeps the surfaces moist, allowing movement of the lungs during respiration. The negative pressure within the pleural cavity keeps the lungs expanded. If the traction of this negative pressure is lost, the internal elastic forces of the lung tissue will prevail and the lung will collapse toward the hilum.

PNEUMOTHORAX

Entry of air into the pleural cavity is called **pneumothorax** (Figure 8-29). This typically occurs after stab wounds of the chest wall or rupture of emphysematous lung tissue. Pneumothorax causes pulmonary atelectasis and dyspnea. It is a reversible lesion that may heal spontaneously or be cured surgically.

PLEURAL EFFUSIONS

Accumulation of fluid in the pleural cavity is called **hydrothorax** or *pleural effusion.* The fluid can be an *exudate,* caused by inflammation, or a *transudate (hydrothorax).* Exudate is a hallmark of *pleuritis* also known as pleurisy. Bacterial pneumonias typically produce a fibrinous or purulent pleuritis, whereas viral pneumonias produce serous pleuritis. Tuberculosis and other granulomatous diseases tend to produce serous or fibrinous pleuritis and do not cause exudation of PMNs. Transudate accumulates in the pleural cavity secondary to heart failure or in generalized edema.

Serous pleuritis or hydrothorax tends to resolve without any consequences. Fibrinous or fibrinopurulent pleuritis, especially if associated with inflammation of the pleura or tissue destruction, stimulates the ingrowth of granulation tissue into the pleural cavity. This leads to obliteration of the cavity and the formation of fibrous adhesions between the visceral and parietal pleura, called *fibrothorax.* Partial fibrotic obliteration

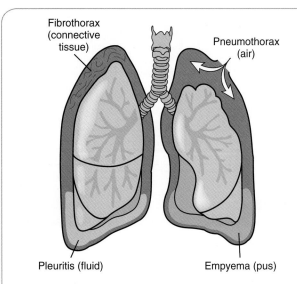

Fibrothorax
(connective
tissue)

Pneumothorax
(air)

Pleuritis (fluid)

Empyema (pus)

Figure 8-29 Pleural diseases. Pleuritis is usually associated with pleural effusion. Fibrothorax is an encasement of the lungs with fibrous tissue that obliterates the pleural cavity. Pneumothorax denotes the entry of air into the pleural cavity. Empyema involves pockets of pus enclosed in fibrous adhesions.

of the pleural cavity filled with pus results in empyema. Empyema resembles an abscess in which the pus may remain for extended periods unless surgically removed.

PLEURAL TUMORS

Tumors of the pleura may be primary or secondary. *Primary tumors* are rare. The only benign pleural tumor worth mentioning is *solitary fibrous tumor.* Malignant pleural tumors are called *mesotheliomas.*

Mesothelioma is a rare malignant tumor of the pleura (Figure 8-30). Almost invariably, mesothelioma is related to exposure to asbestos in the workplace. These tumors are

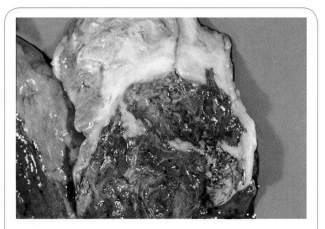

Figure 8-30 Mesothelioma. The tumor is on the pleural surface encasing the lung.

invasive locally but do not metastasize outside the thorax until late in the course of the disease. The pleural tumors encase the lung, preventing its expansion during inspiration. Mesothelioma is an incurable neoplasm with an abysmal prognosis.

Secondary tumors are either pulmonary primaries extending to the pleura or metastases from distant sites. Ovarian and breast cancers often metastasize to the pleura. These tumors are usually associated with pleural effusions, which contain floating tumor cells. The diagnosis can be made by submitting a sample of pleural fluid for cytologic examination. All malignant pleural tumors have a poor prognosis.

REVIEW QUESTIONS

1. What kind of epithelia line the respiratory tract?

2. What are the main functions of the respiratory system?

3. Describe the respiratory defense system.

4. What are the main respiratory diseases?

5. Compare the infections of the upper respiratory system with those of the so-called middle respiratory system.

6. What could cause a "runny nose"?

7. What is croup?

8. Compare epiglottitis and bronchiolitis.

9. Compare alveolar and interstitial pneumonia.

10. List the most common causes of pneumonia and give specific characteristics about each of these forms of lung infection.

11. Compare lobar pneumonia and bronchopneumonia with interstitial pneumonia.

12. Explain complications of bacterial pneumonia.

13. Compare community-acquired pneumonia and hospital-acquired pneumonia.

14. What are the clinical signs of pneumonia, and how is this disease diagnosed?

15. Explain the concept of atypical pneumonia and give specific examples of this clinicopathologic entity.

16. Compare primary and secondary tuberculosis.

17. Which fungi cause pneumonia and under what circumstances?

18. Which pathogens cause pulmonary abscesses?

19. Compare chronic obstructive pulmonary disease caused by chronic bronchitis and COPD caused by emphysema.

20. What is bronchiectasis, and how does it develop?

21. Compare centrilobular and panacinar emphysema.

22. List the most important immune diseases of the respiratory tract.

23. Explain the pathogenesis of asthma.

24. Compare extrinsic and intrinsic asthma.

25. What is sarcoidosis, and how does it affect the body?

26. List several important antigens that cause hypersensitivity pneumonitis.

27. Compare acute and chronic hypersensitivity pneumonitis.

28. What is pneumoconiosis?

29. How does inhalation of mineral particles damage the lungs?

30. Explain the effect of air pollutants on the lungs.

31. Explain the pathogenesis of coal-workers' lung disease.

32. What is silicosis, and how does it present pathologically?

33. Which lung diseases are related to exposure to asbestos?

34. Explain the pathogenesis of dyspnea caused by various mechanisms.

35. Compare the pathologic findings in wet drowning and dry drowning.

36. List four main pathogenetic mechanisms of ventilatory failure and explain how they affect respiration.

37. List common causes of acute respiratory distress syndrome.

38. Describe the pathology of acute respiratory distress syndrome and explain its pathogenesis.

39. What are the possible outcomes of acute respiratory distress syndrome?

40. What is atelectasis, and what are its possible causes?

41. What are the most important neoplasms of the respiratory tract?

42. Correlate the pathology of carcinomas of the larynx with clinical findings and prognosis of the disease.

43. How common is lung cancer?

44. How is tobacco smoking related to lung carcinoma?

45. Explain the histogenesis of various histologic types of lung carcinoma.

46. Compare hilar (central) and peripheral lung carcinoma.

47. Where do lung carcinomas metastasize?

48. What are the clinical signs of lung cancer?

49. What are the common paraneoplastic syndromes caused by lung carcinoma?

50. Compare pneumothorax and hydrothorax.

51. Explain the pathogenesis of pleuritis.

52. What is mesothelioma?

9

The Hematopoietic and Lymphoid Systems

Chapter Outline

NORMAL ANATOMY AND PHYSIOLOGY
  Peripheral Blood
OVERVIEW OF MAJOR DISEASES
  Anemia
    Aplastic Anemia
    Iron Deficiency Anemia
    Megaloblastic Anemia
    Hemolytic Anemias
    Immune Hemolytic Anemia
  Polycythemia

Leukocytic Disorders
  Leukopenia
  Leukocytosis
Malignant Diseases of White Blood Cells
  Leukemias
  Lymphoma
  Multiple Myeloma
Bleeding Disorders
  Normal Hemostasis
  Major Bleeding Disorders

Key Terms and Concepts

Anemia
Aplastic anemia
Bleeding disorders
Burkitt's lymphoma
Coagulation factors
Diffuse large B-cell lymphoma
Disseminated intravascular coagulation (DIC)
Erythrocytes
Erythropoietin
Extranodal lymphoma
Flow cytometry
Hemoglobin

Hemolytic anemia
Hemophilia
Hemostasis
Hereditary spherocytosis
Hodgkin's lymphoma
Idiopathic thrombocytopenic purpura
Immunohistochemistry
Iron deficiency anemia
Leukemia
Leukocytes
Leukocytosis
Leukopenia
Lymphadenopathy
Lymphoma

Lymphopenia
Megaloblastic anemia
Monoclonal gammopathy
Multiple myeloma
Myeloproliferative disorders
Pancytopenia
Platelets
Plasmacytoma
Polycythemia
Sickle cell anemia
Splenomegaly
Thalassemia
Thrombocytopenia

Analysis of blood represents one of the most important laboratory tests. It is routinely performed on most, if not all, hospitalized patients and many of those seen in ambulatory health care facilities. The blood reflects the pathologic changes in many internal organs and is thus a valuable source of information about body functions and health in general. General medical practitioners, highly specialized physicians, nurses, and many allied health professionals deal with hematologic data daily and are trained to interpret such findings.

The discipline concerned with the study of blood is called *hematology* (derived from the Greek words for "blood," *haima,* and "science," *logos*). The clinicians treating disorders of blood cells and coagulation factors are called hematologists and hematopathologists.

Expert hematologists are called in as consultants on complicated cases and for those patients who do not respond to standard therapy. Hematologists also treat patients with neoplastic diseases of blood-forming tissues, such as leukemia; primary deficiencies of bone marrow, such as aplastic anemia; and **bleeding disorders,** such as **hemophilia.** Hematopathologists supervise blood banks and prepare blood and blood components for transfusions, although in major medical centers there are also specialists in transfusion medicine.

NORMAL ANATOMY AND PHYSIOLOGY

Blood is a specialized tissue that consists of fluid, known as *plasma,* and cells, including white blood cells **(leukocytes),** red blood cells **(erythrocytes),** and **platelets** (thrombocytes). Plasma is the protein-rich fluid component of the blood, which contains not only albumin and globulins but also all the clotting factors. Removal of coagulation proteins transforms plasma into serum. White blood cells are further divided into granulocytes, monocytes, and lymphocytes. Granulocytes are divided on the basis of their cytoplasmic granules into neutrophils, eosinophils, and basophils. Monocytes and lymphocytes are also known as *agranulocytic leukocytes* because they do not contain cytoplasmic granules.

Hematopoiesis (from the Greek *haima,* meaning "blood," and *poiesis,* meaning "formation") begins in fetal life from stem cells located in the yolk sac (Figure 9-1). From the yolk sac, the hematopoietic stem cells migrate to the liver and then to the bone marrow and, to some extent, to the spleen, lymph nodes, and thymus. *Extramedullary hematopoiesis* in the liver and the spleen subsides after birth, and the bone marrow remains the primary blood-forming organ. As the organism matures, the red bone marrow of the long bones is replaced by fat. Only the flat bones (e.g., sternum or pelvic bones), ribs, vertebrae, and the end portions of long bone produce blood during adulthood. The thymus and lymph nodes remain sites of lymphocytopoiesis in infancy and adolescence, but the thymus usually involutes after puberty. Lymph nodes form lymphocytes, but in adults these organs do not produce red blood cells or granulocytic leukocytes. However, if the hematopoietic bone marrow is destroyed, extramedullary hematopoiesis may resume in the spleen, liver, and lymph nodes.

The mature blood cells are descendants of developmentally pluripotent hematopoietic stem cells. The term *pluripotent* means that these cells can differentiate and develop into more than one mature cell type. The mother stem cell differentiates into several developmentally committed stem cells, which are the precursors of distinct cell

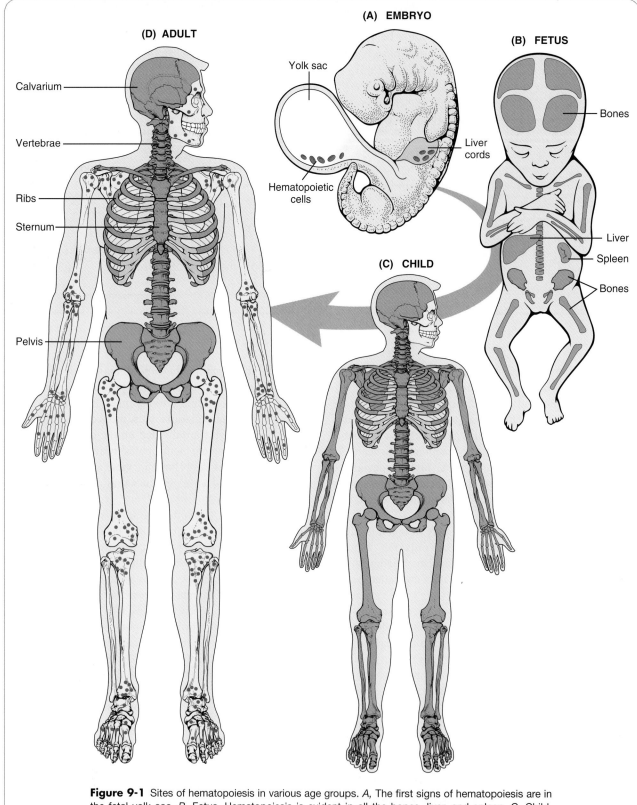

Figure 9-1 Sites of hematopoiesis in various age groups. *A,* The first signs of hematopoiesis are in the fetal yolk sac. *B,* Fetus. Hematopoiesis is evident in all the bones, liver, and spleen. *C,* Child. Hematopoiesis is evident mostly in the short and long bones. *D,* Adult. Whereas essentially all bones of the skeleton contain some hematopoietic bone marrow, bone marrow biopsy is performed only on the iliac crest of the pelvis and the sternum. The calvaria, vertebrae, and ribs and the end of long bones also contain some hematopoietic cells, but it is not practical to biopsy these bones.

lineages, the ultimate product of which are the mature blood cells. Two major cell lineages are formed: lymphoid and myeloid (Figure 9-2). The lymphoid stem cell gives rise to B cells, which finally mature into immuno-globulin-secreting plasma cells, and T cells, most of which assume their function in mediating cell-mediated immune reactions after they have passed through the thymus (T—thymus!). The myeloid stem cell, also known as the *trilineage-myeloid stem cell,* gives rise to three subsets of stem cells, which are the precursors of mature erythrocytes, megakaryocytes, and nonlymphoid white blood cells such as neutrophils, monocytes, eosinophils, and basophils.

The stem cells of various cell lineages are small, undif-ferentiated cells that are indistinguishable from one another; however, they differ with regard to their development poten-tial. This developmental potential can be realized only in the presence of specific growth factors, called *colony-stimulating factors* (CSFs). Most CSFs are produced in the bone marrow, which forms the ideal microenvironment for the growth and development of hematopoietic stem cells. Many other growth factors, such as interleukins produced by macrophages and T lymphocytes, also stimulate blood cell formation. Only the growth factor for the erythroid cell lineages—**erythropoietin**—is produced outside the bone marrow (in the kidney).

PERIPHERAL BLOOD

In living persons the blood is found in the vessels and the heart. It amounts to 7.5% of total body weight, which means that an average person has 5.5 to 6 L of blood. Taller men have more blood than shorter men, and females typically have less blood than males.

The blood cells circulate through blood vessels suspended freely in the plasma. Blood cells can be separated from the plasma by allowing the formed elements to form a sediment over a period of several hours at the bottom of a tube coated with anticoagulant. This can be achieved much faster by centrifuging the blood at high speed for 2 to 3 minutes. The volume of packed red blood cells, expressed as a percentage of the total peripheral blood, is called the *hematocrit.* In healthy adults, formed blood cell elements constitute 40% to 45% of the total blood volume, whereas the plasma accounts for 55% to 60%. Normal peripheral blood parameters are listed in Box 9-1.

BOX 9-1 Composition of Peripheral Blood

Plasma (55%)
Water (92%)
Proteins (7%)
- Albumin
- Immunoglobulins
- Enzymes
- Transport proteins
Salts
Lipids
- Cholesterol
Carbohydrates
- Glucose
Gases
- Oxygen
- Carbon dioxide

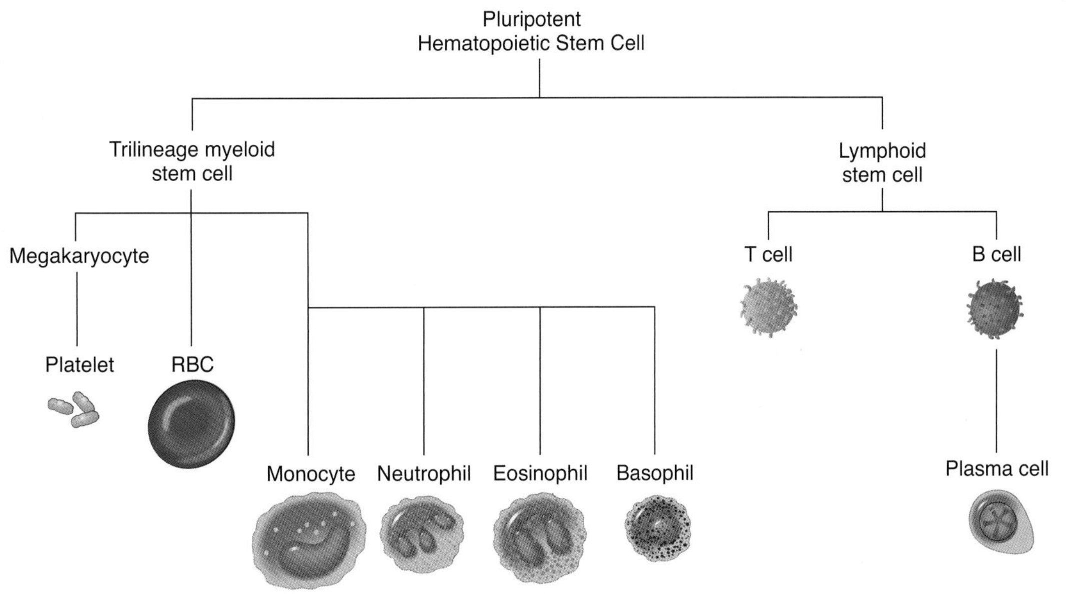

Cells (45%)
Red blood cells (erythrocytes):
  4.5 million/µL
White blood cells (leukocytes):
  5,000–10,000/µL
Granulocytes
Neutrophils (60%–70%)
Eosinophils (1%–3%)
Basophils (1%)
Monocytes (4%–8%)
Lymphocytes (20%–40%)
Platelets (thrombocytes):
  150,000–400,000/µL

Figure 9-2 Hematopoiesis. All cell lineages originate from a developmentally pluripotent stem cell. This common precursor gives rise to developmentally restricted stem cells: erythromyeloid stem cells and lymphoid stem cells. The descendants of these intermediate stem cells are mature T and B lymphocytes, erythrocytes, neutrophils, monocytes, eosinophils, basophils, and megakaryocytes (platelets).

Did You Know?

Isolation of the genes for erythropoietin and other hematopoietic growth factors made it possible for researchers to produce those recombinant growth factors in large quantities. Anemic patients who do not have endogenous erythropoietin because their kidneys have been destroyed by disease can be treated successfully with recombinant erythropoietin.

Blood that is withdrawn into a tube coated with anticoagulants can be separated by centrifugation into a fluid phase *(plasma)* and a cell-rich phase (Figure 9-3). Most of this second phase consists of red blood cells, except for the top layer, called the *buffy coat,* which contains leukocytes and platelets.

Blood cells can be separated from the fluid by allowing the blood to coagulate. The coagulation proteins are consumed in this process, which leads to transformation of plasma into serum. *Serum* is defined as defibrinated plasma. It contains all the proteins except fibrinogen, prothrombin, and other coagulation factors. Some blood tests can be performed only on plasma, whereas others can be performed on serum. The blood submitted in heparinized ("green top") tubes, tubes coated with ethylenediaminetetraacetic acid (EDTA) ("lavender top"), or tubes containing sodium citrate ("blue top") will not clot; with centrifugation, plasma will be obtained. By contrast, blood collected in "red top" tubes, which do not contain anticoagulants, will coagulate and on centrifugation will yield serum. Serum also can be obtained from serum separator tubes ("gold top"). Plasma is typically used for the study of clotting disturbances. Most other biochemical tests are performed on serum. In general, clinical laboratories specify the requirements for each test, and one must check the hospital manual before drawing blood for a specific test.

OVERVIEW OF MAJOR DISEASES

Hematologic diseases occur as a result of abnormal formation, increased destruction, or abnormal structure and function of blood cells. Principal hematologic diseases include the following:

- Anemia
- Leukemia
- Lymphoma
- Bleeding disorders

Several facts important to an understanding of the hematopoietic system are presented here, before a discussion of specific pathologic entities:

1. *Erythrocytes are ideally suited for their primary function: transport of oxygen from the lungs into the peripheral tissues.* Erythrocytes are red (in Greek, *erythros* means "red"), biconcave disks that are thinnest in the center (Figure 9-4) and thickest at the periphery. The red color is derived from **hemoglobin,** an iron-containing pigment that constitutes 90% of the dry weight of each normal, mature erythrocyte. In peripheral blood smears, the thinner central portion, spanning half the cell diameter, appears paler than the peripheral part. The erythrocytes are round but can easily be deformed while passing through small capillaries and other small vessels. Erythrocytes do not have nuclei or organelles that would interfere with their transport function. Because of their biconcave shape, they have a large surface that allows easy diffusion of gases.

2. *Hemoglobin is a complex molecule that consists of four heme groups and four globins.* Heme is composed of four pyrrole rings held together with a centrally placed iron in ferrous form (Fe^{2+}). The heme portion of hemoglobin is the oxygen-binding part of the molecule. Heme cannot be synthesized without iron. *Iron deficiency anemia* is thus marked by low hemoglobin (Hb) values.

   The globin part of hemoglobin consists of four polypeptide chains designated by the Greek letters *alpha, beta, gamma,* and *delta.* Alpha chains are present in all hemoglobins. Two alpha and two beta chains form HbA, two alpha and two delta chains form HbA_2, and two alpha and two gamma chains form HbF (see Figure 9-4).

   Each globin chain is synthesized under the control of a specific gene. Mutations of these genes cause hemoglobinopathies marked by abnormal hemoglobins; for example, **sickle cell anemia** is characterized by an abnormal B chain, and the hemoglobin is known as *hemoglobin S* (HbS).

3. *Hemoglobin synthesis requires iron, vitamin B_{12}, vitamin B_6, and folic acid.* Deficiency of these nutrients also results in **anemia.** Anemia may develop because the nutrient is

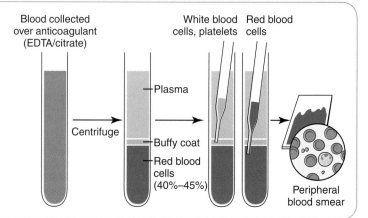

Figure 9-3 Blood drawn into a tube that contains an anticoagulant can be separated by centrifugation into plasma and formed cell elements (red blood cells and a buffy coat that contains mostly white blood cells and platelets). EDTA, ethylenediaminetetraacetic acid.

Blood collected over anticoagulant (EDTA/citrate)

White blood cells, platelets   Red blood cells

Centrifuge

Plasma

Buffy coat

Red blood cells (40%–45%)

Peripheral blood smear

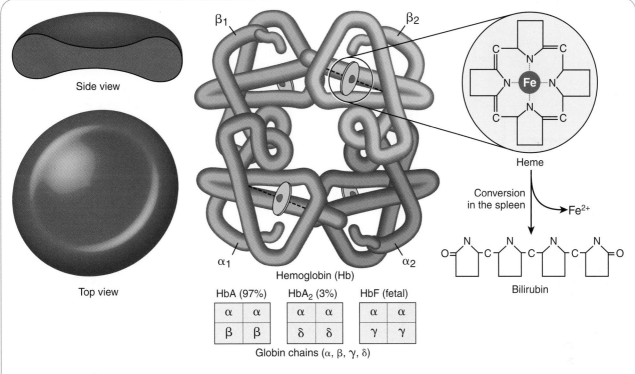

Figure 9-4 Schematic drawing of an erythrocyte and hemoglobin. The cell is biconcave and lacks a nucleus. Hemoglobin is the main component of red blood cells. Note that the molecule consists of globin and heme. The globin consists of four polypeptide chains (alpha, beta, gamma, and delta). Heme is made up of four pyrrole rings held together by iron in ferrous form (Fe^{2+}). On degradation of hemoglobin, iron and globin are reutilized immediately. Pyrrole rings give rise to bilirubin.

not available in food, because it cannot be absorbed, or because the loss exceeds the intake.

4. *Red blood cells live in the circulation for 120 days* (Figure 9-5). The aging cells are sequestered in the spleen, which removes the old and defective red blood cells from circulation and serves as their primary "graveyard." The phagocytic cells of the spleen digest the main components of the red blood cells and release them into the circulation for reutilization and excretion from the body. Essentially, all protein components and iron are reutilized. Heme is converted to bilirubin, which is excreted in bile into the intestine. The intestinal bilirubin is reabsorbed and partially reutilized or metabolized. The remainder is excreted in the form of urobilinogen and stercobilinogen in urine and feces.

5. *Objective measurements of red blood cell parameters are done with instruments that estimate the mean size of red blood cells and their hemoglobin content.* Analysis of blood has become highly automated and is performed with sophisticated instruments. The following measurements are clinically important:

   ■ *Mean corpuscular volume* (MCV) denotes the mean volume of each red blood cell. Normal values are in the range of 83 to 99 fL. MCV is calculated by dividing the hematocrit value by the red blood cell count. Low values (<80 fL) indicate microcytic anemia, whereas high values (>100 fL) indicate macrocytic anemia.

   ■ *Mean corpuscular hemoglobin* (MCH) content denotes the content of hemoglobin per each red blood cell. It is obtained by dividing hemoglobin concentration by red blood cell count. Normal values are in the range of 28 to 32 pg/cell. Low values indicate hypochromic anemia.

   ■ *Mean corpuscular hemoglobin concentration* (MCHC) denotes the concentration of hemoglobin in red blood cells. It is obtained by dividing the hemoglobin concentration by the hematocrit value. Normal values are in the range of 32 to 36 g/dL. Low values indicate hypochromic anemia.

6. *White blood cells participate in the body's defense against infections. Neutrophils are the most numerous white blood cells in the blood, accounting for 60% to 70% of all nucleated cells.* The main function of neutrophils is to defend the body against bacterial infections. Neutrophils are most qualified for this job, because they have remarkable mobility (i.e., they can *migrate* rapidly to the site of infection by ameboid movement); they respond quickly to *chemotactic* stimuli released from the site of inflammation; they are capable of *phagocytosis*

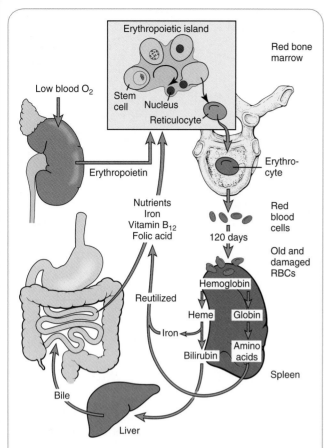

Figure 9-5 The events in the life of erythrocytes. Nucleated red blood cell (RBC) precursors, stimulated by erythropoietin, form erythrocytes in the bone marrow. Normal synthesis of hemoglobin occurs only in the presence of nutrients, iron, vitamin B_{12}, and folic acid. Mature RBCs are released into circulation. The old or defective RBCs are degraded in the spleen. Iron and globin are reutilized immediately. Bilirubin is released in bile into the intestine.

produces new neutrophils at a very fast pace. Because the life span of neutrophils is about 300 times shorter than the life span of erythrocytes, the bone marrow contains three times more white blood cell precursors than erythroid precursors. Technically, this is reported as the myeloid (white cell precursors) to erythroid ratio, or *M:E ratio*, which in normal bone marrow is 3:1.

8. *Monocytes and lymphocytes are long-lived blood cells.* Monocytes account for 4% to 8% of white blood cells. These cells are precursors of tissue macrophages. Lymphocytes form 40% of the white blood cells. Peripheral lymphocytes are predominantly T cells, but there are also B cells, natural killer (NK) cells, and stem cells.

9. *Platelets or thrombocytes are essential clotting factors.* Platelets are cytoplasmic fragments derived from megakaryocytes. *Megakaryocytes* are very large cells found only in the bone marrow. Abundant cytoplasm of megakaryocytes forms buds, which are released into the circulation as platelets. Platelets do not have nuclei; however, they survive 8 to 10 days in the circulation.

10. *Malignant transformation of hematopoietic cells may result in solid tumors or leukemia.* Lymphomas, resulting from malignant transformation of lymphoid cells, occur most often in lymph nodes. Stem cells of leukemias are most often located in the bone marrow. These malignant cells may remain localized to their site of origin, extend into the adjacent tissues, or enter the circulation. Because of the white color of blood that contains large numbers of malignant leukocytes, the malignancy of circulating white blood cells is called *leukemia*.

ANEMIA

Anemia is a reduction of hemoglobin in red blood cells below normal levels. In practice, this means less than 13 g/dL in males and 11.5 g/dL in females. This may be associated with the following:

- Appearance of abnormal hemoglobins
- Reduced number of red blood cells
- Structural abnormalities of red blood cells

Because of the reduction of hemoglobin in the circulating blood, the tissues do not receive enough oxygen and symptoms of *hypoxia* develop. These symptoms vary, because no organs are equally susceptible to oxygen deprivation. In principle, all organs show signs of slower metabolism and a reduced capacity to respond to increased demand for action. For example, hypoxia of the brain causes somnolence, and cardiorespiratory hypoxia causes shortness of breath and easy fatigability. Paleness of the skin and mucosae is a common feature of anemia, but it has almost no functional consequences.

Classification

There are two ways to classify anemias: (1) etiologically, by determining what has caused it; and (2) *morphologically* and biochemically, by assessing the size and shape of erythrocytes

(i.e., uptake of bacteria); and finally, they can kill the bacteria with the bactericidal substances contained within their cytoplasmic granules. Eosinophils form 1% to 3%, and basophils less than 1%, of all white blood cells in the blood. These cells have an important role in allergic reactions. Typically, eosinophils and basophils counteract each other's effects, but sometimes they may act synergistically, helping each other. Eosinophils are also the major inflammatory cells in parasitic infections. Basophil granules contain histamine, heparin, and serotonin. The release of these substances causes blood vessels to dilate and increases their permeability. Basophils also have receptors for immunoglobulin E (IgE), which stimulates them to react to foreign allergens, as in hay fever.

7. *Neutrophils are short-lived cells that survive no more than 4 days in the peripheral circulation.* Therefore these cells must be replaced constantly, and the bone marrow

and analyzing hemoglobin and other major constituent proteins of red blood cells.

Etiology and Pathogenesis

Anemia may be a consequence of the following:
- Decreased hematopoiesis
- Abnormal hematopoiesis
- Increased loss or destruction of red blood cells

Each of these categories includes several distinct diseases, the most important of which are listed in Box 9-2.

DECREASED HEMATOPOIESIS

Decreased hematopoiesis may be a consequence of bone marrow failure or a deficiency of essential nutrients. *Bone marrow failure* is also called *aplastic anemia.* The stem cells disappear from the bone marrow with consequent **pancytopenia** (lack of all blood cells) in the peripheral blood. Bone marrow stem cells may be damaged or replaced by infiltrates of metastatic tumor cells. This is called *myelophthisic anemia.* Similar bone marrow destruction occurs in various forms of leukemia, in which the leukemic cells infiltrate the bone marrow, replacing all normal cell components.

Deficiencies of nutrients also cause anemia. *Deficiency of iron* is the most common form of deficiency anemia. Deficiency of vitamin B$_{12}$ and folic acid—two vitamins essential for the synthesis of DNA and the maturation of hematopoietic stem cells—causes megaloblastic anemia. Protein deficiency results in decreased formation of all hematopoietic cells. Anemia and even pancytopenia are typical features of malnutrition and starvation. Intestinal malnutrition syndromes impair absorption of iron as well, thus contributing to iron deficiency anemia.

ABNORMAL HEMATOPOIESIS

Abnormal hematopoiesis is usually a consequence of genetic abnormalities. These can be inherited as Mendelian traits that affect families, but they may also occur as point mutations in individuals without a previous family history of such a disease. The best known among these is probably sickle cell anemia, caused by a gene mutation that substitutes a valine for the glutamic acid at position 6 of the beta chain of hemoglobin.

Erythrocytes that contain abnormal hemoglobins (or are abnormally shaped) cannot function properly, and affected patients suffer from chronic hypoxia. Furthermore, the abnormal hemoglobin reduces the life span of erythrocytes, which are destroyed at an increased rate in the spleen and within the blood vessels.

INCREASED LOSS AND DESTRUCTION OF RED BLOOD CELLS

Various conditions may cause increased loss or destruction of red blood cells, including bleeding, intrasplenic sequestration, immune hemolysis, and infections.

Acute blood loss (e.g., bleeding) results in anemia that is only temporary. To compensate for the loss of blood and maintain a constant volume of circulating blood, the body mobilizes fluid from the interstitial spaces into the circulation. This restores the volume of blood but dilutes it, changing the ratio of blood cells to fluid. This temporary dilutional anemia is usually corrected spontaneously within a few weeks by replenishment of the blood cells from the bone marrow. However, if the bleeding persists, as in patients with a bleeding peptic ulcer, chronic anemia will develop.

Normally, old red blood cells are removed from the circulation during their passage through the spleen. The removal of red blood cells may be accelerated in some pathologically altered and enlarged spleens. The best example of this is a condition called *hypersplenism.* This disease of unknown etiology is marked by **splenomegaly** (an enlargement of the spleen) and increased destruction of red blood cells and suppression of hematopoiesis in the bone marrow.

An important form of red blood cell destruction occurs in various autoimmune disorders and **hemolytic anemias.** Common to these disorders is an antibody-mediated injury of red blood cell membranes, which leads to their rupture *(hemolysis)* and the release of hemoglobin.

Malaria is the most common infectious cause of hemolytic anemia. It is caused by an infection with the parasite Plasmodium, which invades the red blood cells and causes their lysis. Millions of people are infected with malaria worldwide, but in the United States the disease is not common.

BOX 9-2   Etiologic Classification of Anemias

Decreased Hematopoiesis
Aplastic anemia (bone marrow failure)
Myelofibrosis
Myelophthisic anemia secondary to bone marrow replacement
 with tumor cells
  Leukemia
  Multiple myeloma
  Metastatic carcinoma
Deficiency disorders
  Iron deficiency
  Vitamin B$_{12}$ deficiency
  Folic acid deficiency
  Protein deficiency

Abnormal Hematopoiesis
Genetic hemoglobinopathies
  Sickle cell anemia
  Thalassemia
Structural protein defects
  Spherocytosis

Increased Loss or Destruction of Red Blood Cells
Bleeding
  Prolonged menstrual bleeding
  Peptic ulcer
Immune hemolytic anemia
Hypersplenism
Infection
  Malaria

Morphology of Anemia

Morphologic and biochemical classifications of anemias are based on the study of peripheral blood smears, measurement of hemoglobin content, and chemical analysis of the hemoglobins. These studies use various techniques, such as electrophoresis, immunochemistry, and, most recently, DNA analysis (by molecular biology techniques).

The blood smears provide a quick and simple approach to evaluating red blood cells' size, shape, and hemoglobin content. Normal red blood cells have a uniform biconcave shape that presents as a central pale area and a red peripheral ring (Figure 9-6). Such erythrocytes are called *normocytic, normochromic* (in Greek, *chromos* means "color"; in this case, it refers to the normal red color). Small red blood cells are called *microcytic,* whereas the large ones are called *macrocytic.* The variation in size of erythrocytes is called *anisocytosis,* whereas the variation in shape is termed *poikilocytosis.*

On the basis of crucial parameters (i.e., red blood cell count, hemoglobin content, and hematocrit), anemias can be classified into several types, the most important of which are as follows:

- *Normocytic, normochromic anemia.* The red blood cells appear to be normal. Typically this type of anemia occurs after a massive blood loss ("dilutional anemia"). Chronic infections and metabolic diseases also cause this type of anemia.
- *Microcytic, hypochromic anemia.* The red blood cells are small and pale. Most often, this anemia is caused by iron deficiency. It is also seen in **thalassemia,** a hereditary defect affecting the synthesis of hemoglobin.
- *Macrocytic, normochromic anemia.* The red blood cells are normal in color but are large. Typically this is caused by a deficiency of vitamin B_{12} and/or folic acid, but it can also occur in chronic liver disease.
- *Anemias characterized by abnormal red blood shapes.* These anemias are descriptively called by the predominant

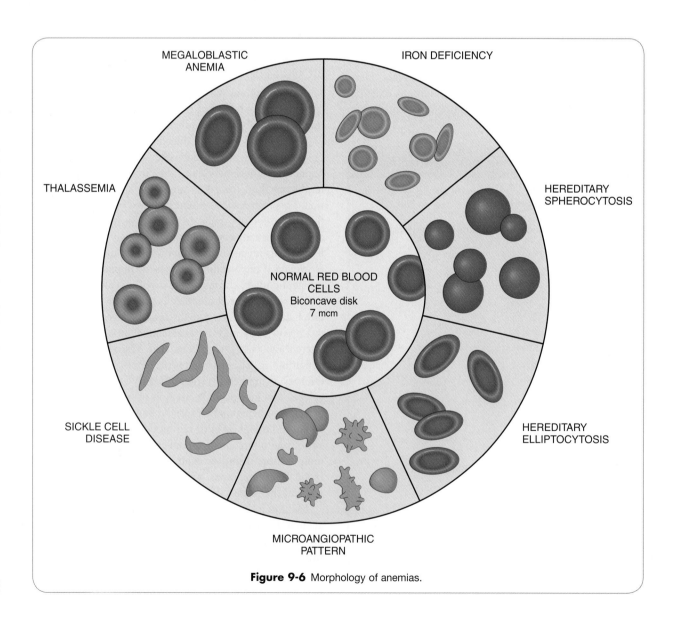

Figure 9-6 Morphology of anemias.

cell shape seen in peripheral smears and include entities such as elliptocytosis and spherocytosis. The prototype of this form of anemia is sickle cell anemia, a disease characterized by the appearance of sickle-shaped erythrocytes.

Morphologic classification of anemias is usually supplemented these days by biochemical data. For example, some microcytic anemias are caused by an iron deficiency, whereas others are a symptom of a genetic disorder of globin, the gene defect that causes thalassemia. To establish the cause of a microcytic hypochromic anemia, one would first have to exclude iron deficiency by measuring the blood iron and estimating the iron stores in the body. Thalassemia, the other cause of microcytic hypochromic anemia, can be diagnosed by demonstrating the abnormal hemoglobin levels typical of this disease. Furthermore, because there are several globin genes, encoding the alpha, beta, or delta chain of this molecule, the diagnosis may be even more specific by demonstrating the gene defect using techniques of molecular biology.

In most cases the morphologic-biochemical classification of anemia will point to the cause of the anemia, which then can be assigned to one of the categories within the etiologic-pathogenetic classification system. Once the cause of an anemia is identified, one should try to eliminate the adverse influences or provide substitutional therapy to correct the deficiency. Good response to treatment is the best confirmation of the diagnosis!

APLASTIC ANEMIA

Aplastic anemia is a rare but important disease in which the anemia is usually accompanied by leukopenia and thrombocytopenia. In other words, aplastic anemia is a pancytopenia, or generalized bone marrow failure.

Etiology and Pathogenesis

Two forms of aplastic anemia exist: idiopathic and secondary. *Idiopathic* cases—those without an identifiable cause—predominate. Secondary aplastic anemia is related to bone marrow suppression that is caused by cytotoxic drugs, radiation therapy, or viral infection. Many of these secondary aplastic anemias are reversible, and elimination of the causative agent often allows the bone marrow to recover. The prognosis for recovery in patients with idiopathic aplastic anemia is less favorable.

Pathology

Bone marrow is typically depleted of hematopoietic cells and consists only of fibroblasts, fat cells, and scattered lymphocytes. Anemia, leukopenia, and thrombocytopenia are found in the peripheral blood.

Clinical Features

Uncontrollable infections secondary to leukopenia and a bleeding tendency resulting from thrombocytopenia are usually the first symptoms. Other, general symptoms of anemia, such as chronic fatigue, sleepiness, and weakness, ensue after 4 to 5 weeks. Most patients die of overwhelming infection.

Bone marrow transplantation is the only known treatment for patients with idiopathic aplastic anemia, in whom hematopoiesis does not recover spontaneously. Transplanted new stem cells repopulate the bone marrow and reestablish normal hematopoiesis. Approximately 60% of patients so treated will improve and resume a normal life.

IRON DEFICIENCY ANEMIA

Iron deficiency anemia is the most common form of anemia. In most cases it is associated with a depletion of body iron stores caused by chronic blood loss. Without iron, which is the essential component of heme molecule, hemoglobin synthesis is impeded. Moreover, newly formed red blood cells are small and contain less hemoglobin than normal.

Etiology

Iron deficiency can be caused by the following:

- Increased loss of iron (e.g., chronic bleeding)
- Inadequate iron intake or absorption (e.g., faulty diet or gastrointestinal disease)
- Increased iron requirements (e.g., childhood growth and pregnancy)

Pathogenesis

To understand how iron deficiency develops and how it can be corrected, one should first review the metabolism of iron in the body, as well as a few important facts about iron in general (Figure 9-7).

Iron is an essential nutrient. Many food ingredients, such as meat, liver, beans, and most vegetables and fruits, contain iron. Because iron is added to many packaged and processed foods, the typical American daily diet contains about 15 mg of iron, which is far above the daily requirements for iron.

Iron is absorbed in the intestine through two independent pathways. Iron that is part of heme or respiratory enzymes in animal cells is taken up as part of these molecules by the intestinal cells. The iron is then dissociated from the pyrrole rings within the intestinal cell cytoplasm. Free iron is absorbed through a receptor mechanism. This mechanism is less efficient, and only 1% to 2% of free iron is absorbed from the intestines.

From the intestines, the iron is transported to other sites bound to a transport protein called *transferrin.* Iron delivered to the bone marrow is incorporated into the hemoglobin. Circulating red blood cells contain approximately 60% to 80% of the total body iron. The rest of the iron is bound to *ferritin,* a storage protein, which aggregates to form granules of brown pigment, known as *hemosiderin.* Hemosiderin is especially prominent in the stroma of the bone marrow, where it can be demonstrated by a special histochemical stain called the Prussian blue reaction.

Iron is lost primarily through cell loss. Aging red blood cells are destroyed in the spleen, but most of the iron released from them is reutilized. Intestinal epithelial cells and skin cells, which also contain iron in the form of ferritin or

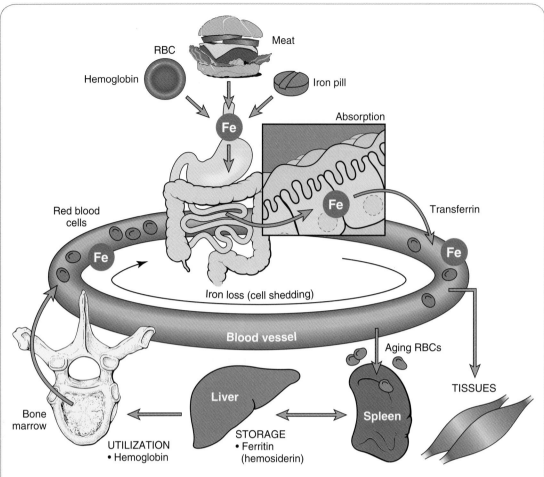

Figure 9-7 Iron metabolism. Uptake of heme iron or ferrous iron occurs in the intestine. From the intestine, iron is transported on transferrin to the liver or the bone marrow. Transferrin binds to red blood cell (RBC) precursors in the bone marrow and delivers iron for incorporation into hemoglobin. RBCs in the circulation contain 60% to 80% of body iron. Old RBCs are destroyed in the spleen. The iron is bound to transferrin for recirculation. Approximately 20% to 30% of iron is stored in the form of hemosiderin in the spleen, liver, and bone marrow. The remaining iron is in the respiratory enzymes of somatic cells. Iron is lost by desquamation of skin and intestinal cells.

respiratory enzymes, are shed in large quantities through desquamation. In addition, women lose iron during menstrual bleeding.

Pathology

Iron deficiency causes hypochromic microcytic anemia. The total iron stores in the body are reduced. The bone marrow shows normal hematopoiesis but contains a reduced number of hemosiderin-laden macrophages.

Clinical Features

Iron deficiency anemia is more prevalent among women than among men. It has been estimated that 20% of women in the United States have iron deficiency. Menstruating women lose 50 to 70 mL of blood every month, and if the iron lost in this blood is not replenished, iron deficiency develops. Pregnant women may develop iron deficiency if their increased requirements are not satisfied by iron supplements. In adult males, iron deficiency anemia is often

caused by occult bleeding. Typically the origin of the bleeding is a peptic ulcer in the stomach and duodenum or a carcinoma in the large intestine. Other causes of iron deficiency, such as diseases of the small intestine that prevent absorption, are rare.

Anemia caused by iron deficiency responds well to iron intake. In many cases anemia is only a symptom of another, more serious disease marked by chronic bleeding or intestinal malabsorption. Such diseases should be treated appropriately, and once the bleeding stops, anemia will disappear. Children and pregnant women, who have increased needs, should receive dietary iron supplements.

MEGALOBLASTIC ANEMIA

Megaloblastic anemia is caused by a deficiency of vitamin B_{12} or folic acid, two essential cofactors for DNA synthesis and blood cell production. Both these deficiencies adversely affect hematopoiesis and delay the normal maturation of blood cells. Red blood cell precursors—normoblasts—do not mature but are instead transformed into megaloblasts. In these cells the nucleus does not mature normally and remains large. Because hematopoiesis is ineffective, many of these megaloblasts are destroyed before they reach maturity. The slowdown of erythropoiesis and the loss of megaloblastic cells combine to cause anemia.

Etiology and Pathogenesis

Vitamin B$_{12}$, also known as *cobalamin,* is an essential nutrient found in meats, eggs, and dairy products. Because a normal diet usually contains enough vitamin B$_{12}$, a nutritional deficiency almost never occurs unless absorption is impaired.

The absorption of vitamin B$_{12}$ occurs in several steps (Figure 9-8). Dietary vitamin B$_{12}$ is released from the food in the stomach, where it binds to the intrinsic factor produced by the gastric parietal cells. The soluble intrinsic factor–B$_{12}$ complex remains in the lumen and is passed into the small intestines. It is absorbed in the terminal ileum, from which it is transferred by blood to the bone marrow. Excess B$_{12}$ is stored in the liver. If any of these phases in the uptake of vitamin B$_{12}$ is disturbed, a deficiency can develop.

The most common form of vitamin B$_{12}$ deficiency—*pernicious anemia*—develops as a result of a lack of the gastric intrinsic factor. Although the pathogenesis of pernicious anemia is not completely understood, it is known that these patients have atrophic gastritis. Because of a reduced number of gastric parietal cells, they do not produce sufficient amounts of intrinsic factor. Antibodies to the parietal cells of the stomach can be demonstrated in the serum of most of these patients. Many patients also have antibodies to the intrinsic factor. Presumably these antibodies destroy the parietal cells or inactivate the intrinsic factor, thereby preventing it from binding to vitamin B$_{12}$. Antibodies may also inhibit intestinal absorption of the intrinsic factor–B$_{12}$ complex.

Other forms of vitamin B$_{12}$ malabsorption are less common. Resection of the stomach for cancer or peptic ulcer may cause B$_{12}$ deficiency. Conditions that interfere with protein absorption in the small intestine in general, such as celiac disease, will also interfere with B$_{12}$ absorption. Crohn's disease affects the terminal ileum and is typically associated with vitamin B$_{12}$ malabsorption. Finally, some parasites, such as the flatworm *Diphyllobothrium latum,* thrive on vitamin B$_{12}$. Because these parasites reside in the small intestine, they may compete with the body for this vitamin in the food and cause anemia.

Folic acid deficiency develops because of inadequate intake in the diet or because of malabsorption caused by diseases of the duodenum and proximal jejunum, where it is absorbed under normal circumstances. During pregnancy and lactation and in infancy, there is an increased need for folates; if these needs are not met by increased intake, deficiency ensues. Certain drugs used in cancer treatment, known as *folic acid antagonists* (e.g., methotrexate), may interfere with utilization of folic acid.

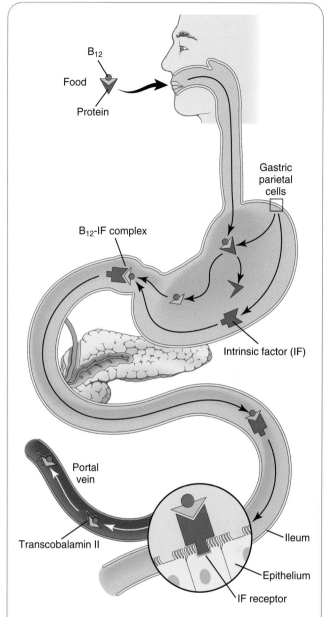

Figure 9-8 Megaloblastic anemia. Anemia develops as a result of vitamin B$_{12}$ or folate deficiency. The absorption of vitamin B$_{12}$, which must undergo several modifications and bind to the intrinsic factor, occurs in the terminal ileum. Folate is absorbed in the duodenum and jejunum. Several factors may interfere with folate and vitamin B$_{12}$ absorption and utilization.

Pathology

The pathologic findings are diagnostic. The bone marrow is hypercellular and contains numerous megaloblasts. The peripheral blood count shows a decreased number of erythrocytes, which are larger than normal (macrocytic anemia). Defective nuclear maturation of leukocytes results in hypersegmentation of neutrophils, which contain five to six nuclear segments instead of the normal three to four segments.

The pathologic changes causing vitamin deficiency are usually identifiable and include either atrophic gastritis or small intestinal or liver disease. Pernicious anemia caused by B_{12} deficiency is often associated with spinal cord disease. The spinal cord lesions typically involve demyelination of the posterior and lateral columns.

Clinical Features

Symptoms of anemia, such as fatigue, shortness of breath, and weakness, may be prominent. Destruction of posterior and lateral columns in the spinal cord results in a loss of the senses of vibration and proprioception, as well as loss of the deep tendon reflexes. Because of these losses, affected patients cannot walk without looking at their legs.

Folic acid deficiency is readily treated with oral intake of folic acid. However, vitamin B_{12} must be injected intravenously because it cannot be absorbed if administered orally. Anemia responds well to treatment, but the neurologic symptoms may persist.

Did You Know?

Pernicious anemia was a fatal disease until scientists discovered that it could be treated by eating raw liver. Later it was found that liver contains vitamin B_{12}, which was isolated from the liver and then synthesized *de novo* in the laboratory. Today patients suffering from pernicious anemia do not have to eat raw liver because the synthetic vitamin can be injected intravenously.

HEMOLYTIC ANEMIAS

Hemolytic anemias occur as a result of increased red blood cell destruction (hemolysis). Hemolysis results from two main abnormalities: intracorpuscular and extracorpuscular red blood cell defects. Intracorpuscular defects include structural abnormalities of the red blood cells, as in sickle cell anemia, thalassemia, and hereditary spherocytosis. Extracorpuscular defects include antibodies, infectious agents, and mechanical factors. Extracorpuscular causes of hemolysis have been identified in a variety of conditions, such as autoimmune hemolytic anemia, hemolytic disease of the newborn, transfusion reactions, malaria, hemolytic anemia caused by cardiac valve prosthesis, and disseminated intravascular coagulation.

Common to all these conditions are the following:
- Anemia (i.e., low erythrocyte count)
- Compensatory erythroid hyperplasia of the bone marrow
- Hyperbilirubinemia and jaundice

The low erythrocyte count is attributable to the destruction of red blood cells. The erythroid hyperplasia is an attempt of the bone marrow to compensate for the red blood cell loss. Bilirubin released from red blood cells causes hyperbilirubinemia. Jaundice appears when the levels of bilirubin in serum exceed 2 to 3 mg/dL.

SICKLE CELL ANEMIA

Sickle cell anemia is caused by a genetic defect in the synthesis of the beta chain of hemoglobin. This defect has been traced to a mutation in the sixth position counting from the N term in a portion of the molecule. Substitution of glutamic acid by valine at this site results in synthesis of an abnormal beta chain. The abnormal beta chain can still combine with alpha chains, but instead of normal HbA, an abnormal hemoglobin (HbS) is formed. In homozygous persons who have two mutated genes for the beta globin, both beta chains are replaced by the product of the mutated gene. Persons who have less than 40% of HbS are asymptomatic, those with 40% to 80% HbS have mild to moderate disease, and those who have more than 80% of HbS show all the typical symptoms of the disease. Thus, although the sickle cell trait is inherited as an autosomal recessive gene, symptoms occur only in homozygotes, which obviously represent a minority of the population with HbS.

Sickle cell anemia is most prevalent among blacks: 8% of African Americans and 30% of black Africans have the disease. In the United States, approximately 50,000 persons have sickle cell anemia, which means that approximately 1% of all African Americans have symptoms of this disease. The disease also affects some inhabitants of the Mediterranean countries and their descendants in America. However, the prevalence of the mutated gene in these populations is relatively low.

Did You Know?

Sickle cell anemia was the first human disease linked to a single amino acid substitution. Linus Pauling received the Nobel Prize for this epochal discovery, which changed the way we view genetic diseases.

Pathogenesis

HbS undergoes polymerization at low oxygen tension, which causes the red blood cell deformities known as *sickling*. The aggregates of sickle cells occlude the small blood vessels, causing ischemia in the affected tissue. At the same time, these abnormal blood cells are hemolyzed at an accelerated rate, and the patients develop signs of chronic anemia and jaundice. The bone marrow undergoes compensatory erythroid hyperplasia.

The pathologic findings and the clinical symptoms in patients with sickle cell anemia can be deduced from what is known about the primary defect in this disease. Symptoms usually are first noted in children 1 to 2 years of age, which is the age at which fetal hemoglobin (HbF) is normally replaced by HbA. Affected patients present with signs of chronic anemia, and the course of the disease is marked by typical periodic exacerbations that are clinically classified as *sickling crisis* or *hemolytic crisis* (Figure 9-9). These may occur spontaneously but are usually induced or aggravated

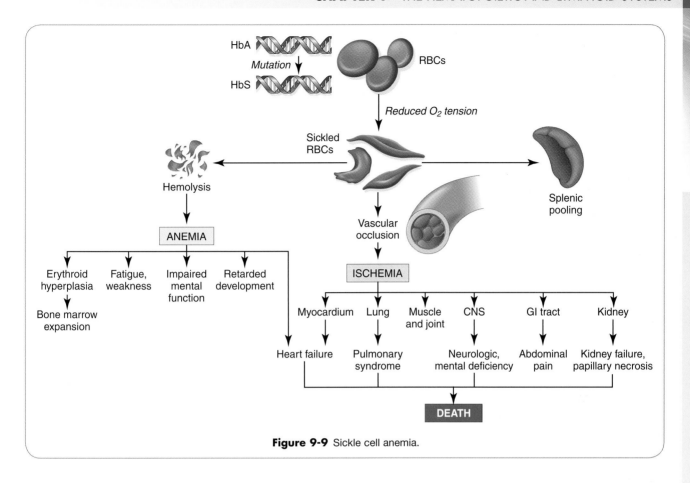

Figure 9-9 Sickle cell anemia.

by fever, respiratory diseases, or some other cause of anoxia. Sickling is accelerated under low oxygen tension, so all situations characterized by reduced oxygen tension can induce a sickling crisis. Thus these patients should avoid mountain climbing, strenuous exercise, and activities that make them breathless. Pregnancy also may cause sickling.

Pathology

Most of the pathologic findings are related to repeated attacks of sickling crisis, which causes multiple infarcts in various organs (Figure 9-10). Such infarcts in the brain cause neurologic defects; infarcts in the bones, spleen, and extremities cause sharp pain. Retinal infarcts are common and cause visual problems. As a consequence of repeated infarcts, the spleen becomes fibrotic and shrinks. This process, called *autosplenectomy,* renders the spleen nonfunctional.

Hemolysis results in hyperbilirubinemia and jaundice. Increased excretion of bilirubin in bile leads to the formation of bile stones. Foci of ischemic necrosis, which heal by fibrous scarring, can be detected in all organs.

Clinical Features

Repeated sickling attacks severely damage the vital organs. The most important consequences include the following:

- Retarded intellectual development and neurologic deficits
- Cardiopulmonary insufficiency
- Recurrent infections

Retarded intellectual development is a consequence of brain ischemia and multiple infarcts. Most often these infarcts are microscopic; however, larger infarcts causing symptoms of *stroke* can also occur.

The attempt of the heart to compensate for inadequate oxygen transport results in cardiac hypertrophy and ultimately *heart failure.* The occlusion of peripheral small blood vessels with sickle cells and thrombi aggravates the circulatory situation even more by increasing the peripheral resistance. Pulmonary edema is common as a result of heart failure, and it tends to predispose the individual to pneumonia.

Other infections are both common and recurrent. These typically include osteomyelitis in the foci of aseptic bone necrosis and pyelonephritis evolving for renal cortical infarcts of papillary necrosis. Ischemic skin ulcers also may become infected. Infections are facilitated by the loss of the phagocytic cells in the spleen destroyed by autosplenectomy. Accumulation of hemosiderin from hemolyzed RBCs in Kupffer cells and other macrophages further reduces the body's defense mechanisms. Moreover, the infections themselves can predispose the patient to even more sickling. The vicious cycle cannot readily be interrupted, and even with the best medical care, sickle cell anemia has a high mortality. Most patients die in early adulthood. No definitive therapy is yet available. The pain and suffering associated with this disease can be reduced only by avoiding conditions that cause sickling and by combating infections.

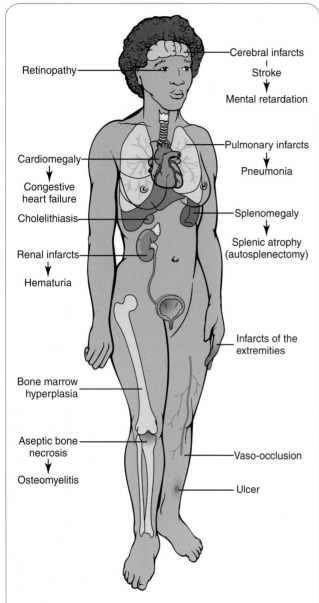

Figure 9-10 Clinicopathologic findings in sickle cell anemia. The findings are a consequence of infarctions, anemia, hemolysis, and recurrent infections.

The diagnosis of sickle cell is made clinically and confirmed with laboratory tests. Severe disease can be recognized by examining peripheral smears, which contain abnormally shaped erythrocytes. The sickling of red blood cells can be induced in a test tube by exposing the blood to low oxygen tension, which is typically done by adding an oxygen-binding chemical, such as metabisulfite. HbS can be demonstrated by electrophoresis because it migrates differently than normal HbA. The complementary DNA (cDNA) probes for the beta chain can be applied to DNA extracted from patients' nucleated cells or the amniotic cells obtained by amniocentesis prenatally. These Southern blots can detect the gene in homozygotes and heterozygotes and are most useful for genetic counseling.

THALASSEMIA

Thalassemia is a genetic defect in the synthesis of HbA that reduces the rate of globin chain synthesis. In contrast to sickle cell anemia, no abnormal hemoglobin is produced—that is, the defect is quantitative rather than qualitative (Figure 9-11).

HbA has four chains: two alpha and two beta chains. There are two genes for the beta chains (one on each chromosome) and four genes for the alpha chain. Each of these genes can be affected. *Thalassemia beta* refers to a reduced synthesis of the beta chain, whereas *thalassemia alpha* indicates reduced synthesis of the alpha chain of globin. The hemoglobin molecule cannot be assembled without alpha or beta chains, and a hypochromic anemia develops. In heterozygotes, in whom only one of the four chains is missing, only mild anemia ensues; in this population the disease is called *thalassemia minor* or *thalassemia trait*. Homozygotes develop thalassemia major, a severe, usually lethal form of anemia. Because there are only two genes for the beta chain, compared with four genes for the alpha chain of globin, mutations or deletions of the beta genes produce anemia of greater severity than do mutations of the alpha genes, which can partially be compensated for by the two remaining normal genes.

The deletion of a beta chain gene can be partially compensated for by the gamma chain. The gamma chain may combine with the alpha chain, resulting in the formation of HbF. However, if all four genes for the alpha chain are deleted, the disease is so severe that it causes intrauterine death of the fetus. As may be remembered, the alpha chain is present in all four hemoglobins (α, β, γ, δ), and without it no species of hemoglobin can by synthesized. Such a condition is incompatible with life, and death occurs *in utero* or shortly after birth.

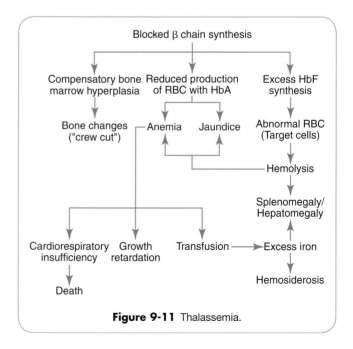

Figure 9-11 Thalassemia.

Thalassemia beta is more common than thalassemia alpha, and thalassemia minor is more common than thalassemia major. All forms of this disease are most prevalent in Mediterranean peoples; therefore it is sometimes called *Mediterranean anemia.* People of North Africa and Southeast Asia can also be affected; in the United States it is mostly reported in descendants of immigrants from these countries.

Clinical Features

Thalassemia minor presents with mild and nonspecific symptoms. Often the disease is diagnosed only after hematologic examination reveals microcytic hypochromic anemia. In such cases it is important to distinguish thalassemia from the more common forms of microcytic hypochromic anemia, such as iron deficiency anemia. The latter responds readily to iron supplementation, whereas thalassemia will not. Treatment with iron may even cause signs of iron overload, because the defective globin synthesis hinders its utilization. The mild or subclinical forms of thalassemia require no treatment.

Thalassemia major is a severe and serious disease that has a high mortality in children. Erythrocytes are not produced in sufficient numbers, and those carrying the abnormal hemoglobin are prone to hemolysis. Red blood cell counts are low, and unless transfusions are given, most patients die during childhood. Hemolysis is accompanied by splenomegaly, hemosiderosis, and hepatomegaly (which result from increased amounts of hemosiderin in the phagocytic cells and hepatocytes). The bone marrow undergoes compensatory hyperplasia and widening. The newly formed bone spicules on the calvarium project perpendicular to the broad basis of the bone, resembling "crew-cut" hair on radiographic study. Hemolysis results in hyperbilirubinemia and jaundice.

Chronic anemia retards the growth of children. Ischemia of the brain impairs their normal intellectual development. Cardiorespiratory insufficiency develops early. These children are always short of breath and tired. Finally, when the heart reserve and its ability to compensate have been exhausted, heart failure occurs.

There is no treatment for thalassemia. Molecular biology probes make it possible to diagnose these diseases *in utero,* but currently, genetic counseling is the only way to reduce the incidence of this disease among at-risk populations.

HEREDITARY SPHEROCYTOSIS

Hereditary spherocytosis is a heterogenous group of genetic defects involving one of several genes encoding the structural proteins that form the cytoskeleton of red blood cells. The mutations most often involve the genes encoding ankyrin, band 3, and spectrin, or band 4.2 (Figure 9-12). These mutations cause destabilization of the red blood cell membrane and a loss of its pliability, ultimately resulting in a lysis of red blood cells during their passage through the spleen.

Hereditary spherocytosis is the most common hereditary disease of red blood cells in whites. Usually inherited as an autosomal dominant disease, it affects 1 in 5000 whites in the United States. As a result of the structural defect of the cell membrane, the erythrocytes "round up" to form spheres rather than normal biconcave disks. Spherocytes can be recognized in peripheral blood smears. Such erythrocytes appear dark red and either do not have a central pale zone or have a very small one. The smears also show marked anisocytosis. The fragility of spherocytes may be demonstrated by suspending them in hypotonic solutions and measuring the rate of their hemolysis. In hypotonic solutions, normal red blood cells swell because of the influx of water across their cell membranes. Because spherocytes are already round, they cannot swell much more;

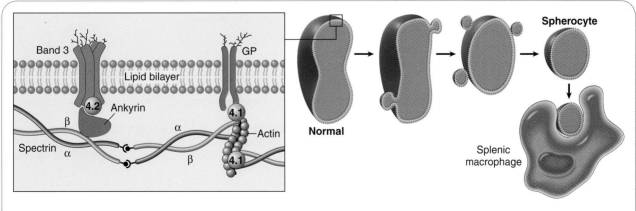

Figure 9-12 Spherocytosis. The disease results from mutations of genes encoding the proteins forming the membrane skeleton. (From Kumar V, Abbas AK, Fausto N, Aster JC: Robbins and Cotran Pathologic Basis of Disease, 8th ed, Philadelphia, 2010, Saunders.)

thus the abnormal cell membranes rupture faster than the membranes of normal erythrocytes do. These rounded erythrocytes are less deformable. Because of the rigidity of their membranes, they do not deform readily and do not adapt to the requirement of microcirculation. During their passage through the spleen, many spherocytes are retained in the sinusoids, where they undergo hemolysis.

The clinical course of spherocytosis, like other hemolytic anemias, is marked by hemolytic or aplastic crises. Symptoms of anemia are, in such instances, accompanied by splenomegaly and jaundice. Splenectomy is currently the preferred treatment for this disease, although clearly it does not correct the basic cellular defect.

IMMUNE HEMOLYTIC ANEMIA

Immune hemolytic anemias are mediated by antibodies that destroy red blood cells. These antibodies may be directed to an autoantigen, which is normally expressed on a patient's own red blood cells, or an *alloantigen,* which is foreign to the host producing the antibodies. Neoantigens are newly formed antigens that are produced by fusion of a normal tissue component with a nonimmunogenic foreign substance that acts as a hapten. Attached to the body's own proteins, haptens may transform such proteins into immunogens.

Mismatched blood transfusion is an example of an immune reaction to a foreign antigen. Red blood cells carry on their surface major blood group antigens of the ABO type (Figure 9-13). Persons of the A blood group express the A antigen on the surface of their erythrocytes and at the same time have natural antibodies to blood group B antigens. Individuals with blood group B have B antigens on their erythrocytes and antibodies to blood group A in their serum. Mismatched transfusion of B blood into an A person will result in almost instantaneous hemolysis of the donor's B erythrocytes. The natural anti-B antibodies will bind to the red blood cells, forming an antigen-antibody complex. These complexes activate complement in the serum and cause hemolysis of red blood cells. Massive hemolysis may result in shock and even death.

Autoimmune hemolytic anemias develop as a consequence of an immune reaction to red blood cell autoantigens or neoantigens formed between the body's own proteins and hapten (Figure 9-14). Red blood cells express numerous blood antigens, but these are not recognized as foreign by the body's immune system and therefore are innocuous. For unknown reasons, some people react to their own red blood cells' antigens, and this causes autoimmune hemolytic anemia. This is a typical antibody-mediated immune reaction in which the immunoglobulins bind to the cell surface and form an immune complex with the red blood cell antigen. Antigen-antibody complexes activate complement, which lyses the cells. In most cases the reasons for the production of these autoreactive antibodies are not evident. However, because those affected usually have other autoimmune disorders or lymphoma, complex disturbances of the entire immune system may be involved.

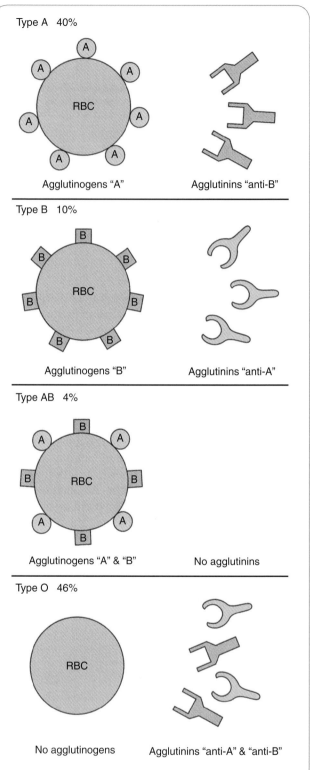

Figure 9-13 Blood group antigens A and B expression results in four blood groups: A, B, AB, and O. (From Applegate EJ: The Anatomy and Physiology Learning System, 4th ed, St. Louis, 2011, Saunders.)

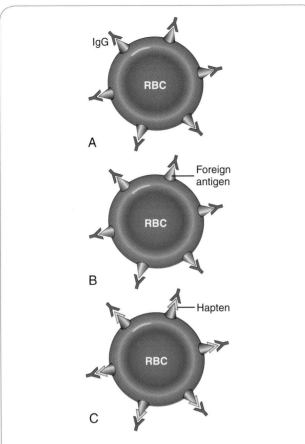

Figure 9-14 Hemolytic anemias. *A,* Autoantigens present on red blood cells (RBCs) are normally not recognized as foreign by the body. In some persons the body produces antibodies to its own antigens on RBCs. This occurs in some autoimmune disorders for no obvious reasons. *B,* Alloantigens are foreign antigens. For example, blood group B RBCs are recognized as foreign by group A persons. *C,* Neoantigens are formed from the body's own proteins linked to a nonimmunogenic hapten. IgG, immunoglobulin G.

Some hemolytic anemias are related to drugs or environmental chemicals. Ingestion of a drug that is not immunogenic has no effect on red blood cells. However, some of these chemicals may attach to the surface of red blood cells and act as a hapten, forming neoantigens that will induce production of antibodies. Drugs rarely cause hemolytic anemia. Nevertheless, it is important to consider this possibility because drug-induced hemolysis can be prevented by discontinuing use of the drug in question.

POLYCYTHEMIA

Polycythemia, also called *erythrocytosis,* denotes an increased number of red blood cells. Typically, affected patients have more than 5.5 million red blood cells per microliter, more than 15.5 g of hemoglobin, and a hematocrit that exceeds 55% of the total blood volume.

Polycythemia occurs in two forms: primary and secondary (Figure 9-15). *Primary polycythemia* or *polycythemia vera* is a clonal proliferation of hematopoietic stem cells resulting in an uncontrolled production of red blood cells and an increased total red blood cell mass. The disease belongs to the spectrum of **myeloproliferative disorders** and is considered neoplastic. The proliferative stem cells show clonal genetic abnormalities and proliferate independently of erythropoietin. In contrast, *secondary polycythemia* denotes an increased red blood cell volume as a result of erythroid bone marrow hyperplasia caused by erythropoietin. Increased concentration of erythropoietin can be demonstrated in blood. Secondary polycythemia is usually caused by prolonged hypoxia. Living at high altitudes, anoxia secondary to chronic lung disease, and congenital heart disease are all causes of secondary polycythemia. Renal carcinoma also can cause secondary polycythemia.

Clinical Features

The symptoms of polycythemia vera are related to the hyperviscosity of blood that contains too many red blood cells. Such blood flows sluggishly and tends to clot more readily than does normal blood. Hypertension is usually present. Patients appear dark red or flushed in the face and have headaches, visual problems, and neurologic symptoms. Pathologic examination usually reveals disseminated thrombi and foci of bleeding, and splenomegaly is prominent. The bone marrow is hypercellular. The superfluous red blood cells can be removed by phlebotomy (blood-letting from the veins) in both primary and secondary polycythemia. In polycythemia vera, this confers only temporary relief, and, as in other leukemias, the disease must ultimately be treated with cytotoxic drugs.

The distinction between primary and secondary polycythemia is made on the basis of clinical findings and laboratory data. In primary polycythemia, the bone marrow cells are

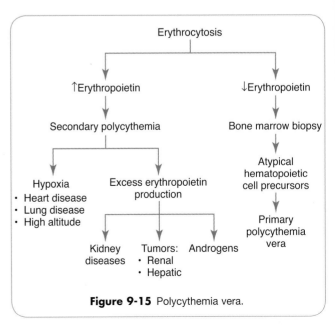

Figure 9-15 Polycythemia vera.

neoplastic and appear atypical. In some cases the proliferation of neoplastic erythroid cells is associated with neoplastic white blood cells that are all part of a myelodysplastic syndrome. In contrast to the neoplastic red blood cell precursors of primary polycythemia, which proliferate on their own without external stimuli, secondary polycythemia depends on erythropoietin stimulation. Serum erythropoietin levels are invariably elevated in such patients.

LEUKOCYTIC DISORDERS

Disorders of leukocytes include benign reactive disorders characterized by too few or too many leukocytes and malignant diseases, such as leukemias and lymphomas.

LEUKOPENIA

Leukopenia is a reduction in the white blood cell count to below normal levels (in Greek, *penia* means "lack of"). In contrast to the common occurrence of anemias, leukopenia is rare. Several forms of leukopenia are known. The most important of these is *neutropenia,* also known as *agranulocytosis,* which is marked by low numbers of neutrophils in the peripheral blood, and **lymphopenia,** which is characterized by a reduction in the numbers of lymphocytes. *Selective lymphopenia* is the term used to denote a condition in which a subset of lymphocytes is reduced in number, as in the helper T-cell deficiency that occurs in acquired immunodeficiency syndrome (AIDS).

Leukopenia may be induced by many means. In general, any substance that is toxic to the bone marrow cells can provoke leukopenia. The most important among these are various drugs (e.g., the cytotoxic drugs used in cancer therapy) and environmental and industrial chemicals. Radiation therapy and many chronic diseases also damage the bone marrow and cause leukopenia. Deficiency of leukocyte precursors is often combined with a loss of erythroid precursors (aplastic anemia). As mentioned earlier, aplastic anemia is a disease affecting the bone marrow stem cells, which are common precursors of both white and red blood cells.

The symptoms of leukopenia relate to the primary function of white blood cells: the body's defense against infections. Neutropenia is typically marked by overwhelming bacterial infections. Lymphopenia deprives the body of its defense against bacterial, viral, fungal, and parasitic pathogens. Short-term leukopenia is treated with antibiotics to prevent massive infections. Long-term leukopenia and the leukopenia of aplastic anemia are often fatal.

LEUKOCYTOSIS

Leukocytosis is an increased number of white blood cells in the peripheral blood, typically exceeding 10,000/μL. The number of all white blood cells can increase proportionally, or some subsets of white blood cells may be increased more than others. *Granulocytosis* (or neutrophilia) is an increased number of

granulocytes that typically occurs in response to acute bacterial infection. Eosinophilic leukocytosis (or eosinophilia) usually accompanies allergies, such as hay fever, asthma, and some skin diseases or parasitic infections. In many cases eosinophilia is associated with a normal white blood cell count and an increase only in the number of eosinophils (from 2% or 3% to 5% and more). Lymphocytosis is common in viral infections and in chronic infections, such as tuberculosis. It is also a feature of some autoimmune disorders, such as SLE.

Leukocytosis is usually a benign, reactive condition that requires no treatment. Persistent leukocytosis requires thorough investigation because it may represent the first manifestation of a hematologic malignant disease (lymphoma or leukemia).

Reactive leukocytosis is often associated with splenomegaly. In patients with bacterial infection, such an enlarged spleen is called *septic spleen.* Lymphocytosis is often accompanied by a lymph node enlargement, termed **lymphadenopathy.** Histologically, such lymph nodes show enlargement of the germinal follicles, widening of the perifollicular (paracortical) cell zone, sinusoidal histiocytosis, or changes in all these lymph node compartments.

Lymph node enlargement in the neck is especially common in children with upper respiratory diseases. Lymph node enlargement is also common in infectious mononucleosis, a disease caused by the Epstein-Barr virus (EBV) (the so-called kissing disease). Generalized lymphadenopathy occurs in the early stages of AIDS. As the disease progresses, the lymphoid tissue is depleted and the lymphadenopathy disappears.

Lymph node enlargement is typically one of the most common presenting symptoms of lymphoma. Any persistent lymphadenopathy, especially if unaccompanied by signs of infection, should be evaluated carefully; if persistent for a long time, a lymph node biopsy should be performed. Only lymph node biopsy can definitively confirm the diagnosis and identify reasons for the lymph node enlargement.

MALIGNANT DISEASES OF WHITE BLOOD CELLS

Malignant diseases of the white blood cells present as *leukemias* and *lymphomas.* Malignant diseases of plasma cells, which are closely related to lymphocytes, are known as **plasmacytoma** or multiple myeloma.

Classification

Malignant diseases involving white blood cell precursors in the bone marrow, when associated with an increased number of malignant white blood cells in the peripheral blood, are called *leukemias* (in Greek, *leukos* means "white"; hence, "white blood"). Lymphoid cell malignant diseases predominantly involve the lymph nodes and thus are called *lymphomas.* Leukemias can be grouped into two major classes: myeloid and lymphoid lymphocytic.

Clinically both myelocytic and lymphocytic leukemia can be classified as acute or chronic. Acute leukemias have a relatively sudden onset and, before the modern era of chemotherapy, were often fatal within 3 to 6 months. Chronic leukemias have a more insidious onset, and many patients are actually asymptomatic, although laboratory findings indicate that they have the disease.

Lymphomas occur in several forms, which can correspond to acute and chronic lymphocytic leukemia. A special form of lymphoma is called *Hodgkin's lymphoma*. Multiple myeloma is a malignant disease of plasma cells. Although related to lymphoma and leukemia, it represents a clinically and pathologically distinct entity.

Etiology and Pathogenesis

The causes of most lymphomas and leukemias, like the causes of most other malignant tumors, are unknown. However, there is considerable evidence that at least some of these malignant diseases are caused by viruses, and some are related to the activation of endogenous oncogenes.

Among the viruses, the greatest attention has been devoted to those that infect B or T lymphocytes. Two of these have received special scrutiny: human T-cell leukemia/lymphoma virus 1 (HTLV-1) and EBV.

HTLV-1 is a T-lymphotropic retrovirus from the same family as human immunodeficiency virus (HIV), the virus of AIDS. This virus was originally isolated from a rare form of lymphoma discovered in Japan, but it was found later in other parts of the world as well. HTLV-1 isolated from patients can infect normal lymphocytes and transform them into malignant lymphoma cells, thus proving that the virus is truly cancerogenic.

EBV has a predilection for infecting B lymphocytes. This virus has been implicated as the possible cause of Burkitt's lymphoma, but the final proof for its pathogenetic role in this disease is still lacking. EBV is a widespread pathogen that in most persons produces only a mild flulike disease that often passes unnoticed. In others it causes infectious mononucleosis. Lymphoma develops in a small number of infected persons, most of whom are children or are from sub-Saharan Africa, suggesting that the neoplastic potential of EBV can be realized only under certain conditions.

Endogenous oncogenes probably play an important role in the pathogenesis of leukemias and lymphomas, as evidenced by the data published daily by various laboratories. Nevertheless, it would be premature to blame endogenous oncogenes for all the malignant diseases of the hematopoietic system. Activation of cellular oncogenes has been related to several chromosomal breaks and translocations noted in hematopoietic malignant diseases. The translocation of fragments of chromosome 8 and 14 seen in Burkitt's lymphoma is a good example of such changes. The *Philadelphia chromosome,* a shortened chromosome 22, is a well-known marker for chronic myelogenous leukemia. The long arm of chromosome 22 is transposed to chromosome 9 and replaced with a fragment of chromosome 9. This leads to juxtaposition of *ABL* oncogene (normally present in chromosome 9) and *BCR* oncogene (normally present in chromosome 22). The product of the hybrid *BCR-ABL* gene has tyrosine kinase activity and is considered to promote uncontrollable proliferation of leukemia cells. Similar cutogenetic and molecular changes have been identified in most leukemias and lymphomas and are widely used for precise laboratory diagnosis of these diseases in clinical medicine.

LEUKEMIAS

The term **leukemia** means "white blood." The blood becomes milky white only after the number of white cells has reached approximately 1 million/μL. This is rarely seen today because patients are usually diagnosed and treated early in the course of the disease.

Clinical Features

All leukemias have several features in common:

- The bone marrow is infiltrated with malignant cells. The involvement of the bone marrow can be best demonstrated by bone marrow biopsy.
- The peripheral blood contains an increased number of immature blood cells. Peripheral blood smears may be the first indication that the patient has leukemia.
- Leukemias are clonal diseases, and accordingly the neoplastic stem cells show chromosomal or genetic changes that are specific for each disease. These genetic changes are important for the diagnosis of various forms of leukemia and in some cases are important for choosing the right treatment and for formulating the prognosis.
- Complications common to all leukemias include anemia, recurrent infections, and uncontrollable bleeding. These can be explained by the fact that malignant cells replace the precursors of erythrocytes, white blood cells, and platelets. As a result of these disturbances and normal hematopoiesis, patients exhibit signs of anoxia, cannot effectively combat infections, and develop a bleeding tendency. Overwhelming infection is the most common cause of death in all forms of leukemia.

Leukemia may occur at any age, from birth through old age. However, certain forms of leukemia are more common in certain age groups (Figure 9-16). Most leukemias (85%) affecting children present in an acute form. By contrast, chronic leukemias are more common in adults.

Acute lymphoblastic leukemia (ALL) has its peak incidence in children younger than 5 years, but the incidence again rises in the elderly population. It accounts for only 20% of all leukemias but is the most common form of leukemia in children.

Acute myelogenous leukemia (AML) is, overall, the most common leukemia (40%). It occurs in all age groups, but it is most common in older persons.

Chronic myelogenous leukemia (CML) accounts for 15% of all leukemias. It rarely occurs before adolescence. It affects adults, and its incidence increases with advancing age.

Chronic lymphocytic leukemia (CLL) accounts for 25% of all leukemias. It is almost unknown in patients younger than 40 years, but its incidence rises progressively thereafter.

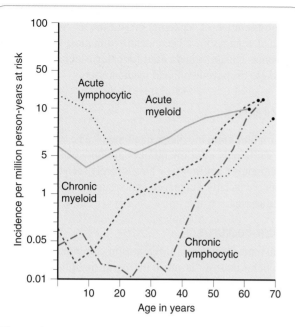

Figure 9-16 Age distribution of leukemias. Acute lymphocytic (lymphoblastic) leukemia is the most common form affecting children younger than 5 years. Acute myeloid (myelogenous) leukemia occurs in all age groups. Chronic myeloid (myelogenous) leukemia is a disease of adulthood. Chronic lymphocytic leukemia is a disease of older persons. (From Upton AC: Comparative aspects of carcinogenesis in ionizing radiation, Natl Cancer Inst Monogr 14:221, 1964.)

Specific Forms of Leukemia

Each form of leukemia has specific clinical and pathologic features.

ACUTE LYMPHOBLASTIC LEUKEMIA

ALL is characterized by massive infiltration of the bone marrow with immature lymphoid cells (blasts). Blast cells, which correspond to precursors of T and B lymphocytes, also spill over into the blood. Therefore the peripheral blood contains an increased number of malignant lymphoid cells.

 Did You Know?

Leukemia was discovered almost simultaneously in 1845 by Rudolf Virchow in Berlin and John Hughes Bennett in Edinburgh. Virchow's name for the disease (*Leukamie* in German) proved to be more popular than the somewhat convoluted term *leukocythaemia* proposed by Bennett.

The following are the most important aspects of ALL:
- Overall, ALL accounts for approximately 30% of all acute leukemias. However, it is the most common form of leukemia in children and the most common malignant disease in children younger than 5 years.

- The disease has a rapid course and is marked by recurrent infections, generalized weakness, and bleeding into the skin and major internal organs. Lymph nodes are enlarged, and there is mild splenomegaly.
- The presence of certain cytogenetic findings, deemed unfavorable, is associated with worse prognosis.
- With modern chemotherapy, remission can be induced in essentially all patients, and at least two thirds of all patients can be permanently cured. Without chemotherapy, ALL is lethal within 3 to 6 months.
- The prognosis is better for children than for adults.

ACUTE MYELOGENOUS LEUKEMIA

Acute myelogenous leukemia (AML) is a heterogenous group of neoplastic diseases characterized by clonal proliferation of myeloblasts in the bone marrow and their entry into the blood or other tissues. To establish the diagnosis of AML, one must find at least 20% myeloblasts in the bone marrow biopsy. In addition, the disease must be subclassified by analyzing the malignant myeloblasts by means of cytochemistry, karyotyping, and molecular biology.

On the basis of cell markers and cytogenetic findings, it is possible to classify AML into several categories. According to the World Health Organization (WHO), there are four forms of AML:
1. AML with recurrent genetic abnormalities
2. AML evolving from multilineage dysplasia
3. Therapy-related AML
4. AML not otherwise specified

Most AMLs do not show recurrent genetic abnormalities and belong to the last category. This group is further subdivided into eight subtypes using the modified FAB (French-American-British) classification system. These subcategories—known as M0, M1, M2, M3, M4, M5, M6, and M7—reflect the fact that the malignant cells correspond to specific white cell lineages or precursors of various hematopoietic cells. For example, M0 is minimally differentiated AML, M4 is acute myelomonocytic, M6 is acute erythroid leukemia, and M7 is acute megakaryoblastic leukemia.

The most important aspects of AML are as follows:
- AML is the most common form of acute leukemia in adults.
- AML has an acute course, and without treatment most patients die within 6 months after the onset of symptoms. Chemotherapy can induce remission in approximately 60% of patients, but unfortunately only 15% to 30% remain free of disease for 5 years.
- Following high-dose irradiation and chemotherapy, patients undergoing bone marrow transplantation during the first remission have a 70% 3-year survival. It is not known whether, over the long term, this treatment has any significant advantages over chemotherapy alone.

CHRONIC MYELOGENOUS LEUKEMIA

Chronic myelogenous leukemia (CML) is a malignant disease of pluripotent hematopoietic stem cells capable of differentiating into neutrophilic leukocytes. The bone marrow is overgrown with malignant stem cells and their descendants, which can be classified morphologically as promyelocytes, metamyelocytes, and so on. These cells are also found in the peripheral blood, which typically shows high white cell counts (Figure 9-17).

The most important aspects of CML include the following:

- CML is a disease of adulthood; 85% of all affected patients are older than 30 years.
- Clinically, CML has a slow onset marked by nonspecific symptoms that include mild anemia and signs of hypermetabolism. Patients with CML are tired, lack endurance, and are prone to infections. Splenomegaly and thrombosis secondary to accelerated clotting are common.
- Three phases of the disease are recognized. The *chronic phase* of the disease lasts 2 to 3 years. There is marked leukocytosis with an increased number of eosinophils and basophils. The bone marrow contains less than 10% blasts. The platelets are increased in circulation, and the bone marrow contains an increased number of megakaryocytes, usually in the form of so-called micromegakaryo-

cytes. In about one half of all patients, the disease may then progress into an *accelerated* phase, characterized by greater than 10% bone marrow blasts, more than 20% basophils in the peripheral blood, and increasing unresponsiveness to therapy. This phase usually ends in a *blast crisis* that resembles acute leukemia and is characterized by an increased number of blasts in the bone marrow (more than 20%). In the remaining one half of patients in the chronic phase, the onset of the blast crisis is sudden and is not preceded by an accelerated phase. The blast crisis cannot be treated adequately and usually heralds death. Classical chemotherapy yields unsatisfactory results in patients with CML, and most patients die within 3 to 5 years of the onset of the disease. Bone marrow transplantation, when combined with radiation therapy and chemotherapy, yields a 70% chance for 3-year disease-free survival. However, most promising results have been recently achieved using *tyrosine kinase inhibitors* (e.g., imatinib [Gleevec]), drugs that can induce remission in 90% of cases.

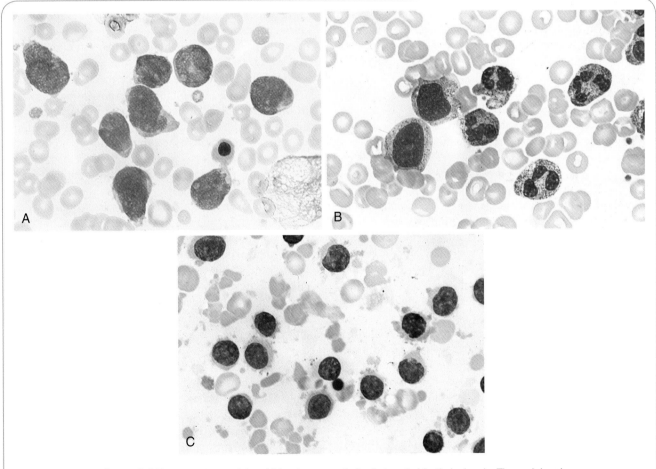

Figure 9-17 Leukemia—peripheral blood smears. *A,* Acute lymphoblastic leukemia. The peripheral blood contains numerous nonsegmented, immature, atypical white cell precursors. *B,* Chronic myelogenous leukemia shows a variety of immature precursors of neutrophils. *C,* Chronic lymphocytic leukemia. The cells resemble mature lymphocytes.

- Approximately 90% of patients with CML have the Philadelphia (Ph[1]) chromosome, with *BCR-ABL* gene rearrangement. The 10% of patients who do not have Ph[1] have a worse prognosis than those who do have this marker.

CHRONIC LYMPHOCYTIC LEUKEMIA

Chronic lymphocytic leukemia (CLL) is a malignant disease involving lymphoid cells. The most important aspects of chronic lymphocytic leukemia are as follows:

- CLL is a disease of older people. Most patients are older than 50 years.
- CLL cells are indistinguishable from normal mature lymphocytes. Normal blood contains less than 4000 lymphocytes/μL. CLL should be suspected if the number of lymphocytes exceeds 5000/μL. Bone marrow biopsy confirms the diagnosis.
- CLL has many features in common with small-cell lymphocytic lymphoma. Both are slowly progressive diseases. Many patients have only peripheral lymphocytosis or lymph node enlargement and are otherwise asymptomatic. Others may have reduced resistance to infections because the neoplastic abnormal B lymphocytes are not as efficient in combating infections as are normal lymphocytes.
- The course of the disease is prolonged, and most patients survive 7 to 9 years from the time of diagnosis. Because CLL cells do not proliferate rapidly, they are unresponsive to chemotherapy.
- After many years CLL can transform into a more aggressive form of lymphoma/leukemia. Resulting disease may be more responsive to chemotherapy, but in general it usually follows a progressive and lethal course.

LYMPHOMA

Lymphoma is a term that can be applied to an entire spectrum of malignant diseases involving lymphocytes and their precursors. There is no need to preface this term with *malignant,* because all lymphomas are malignant and no benign forms are recognized.

Lymphomas account for approximately 3% of all malignant diseases in humans. Pathologically and clinically they are a heterogenous group of diseases that can occur in any age group. As stated earlier, lymphomas are closely related to some forms of leukemia. The malignant cells often infiltrate the lymph nodes, spleen, thymus, or bone marrow, but they may also involve any other organ in the body. Lymphomas originating outside the lymph nodes in solid organs, the gastrointestinal system, or the brain, eyes, or skin are called **extranodal lymphomas.**

Lymphomas are divided into two large categories: non-Hodgkin's lymphoma (NHL) and Hodgkin's lymphoma. Both can be further subclassified on the basis of histopathologic features, clinical manifestations, and tumor cell biology.

NON-HODGKIN'S LYMPHOMAS

Several classifications of NHLs (referred to here simply as *lymphomas*) have been proposed. One of these classifications, the Revised American European Classification of Lymphoid Neoplasms (REAL), has been used as the basis for the most recent WHO classification that is currently recommended for clinical purposes.

The WHO classification of NHL divides lymphoid neoplasms according to their resemblance to normal B and T or NK cells and their precursors. Accordingly, there are two major categories of tumors: B-cell neoplasms and T-cell and NK-cell neoplasms. In each category, there are numerous subsets, corresponding to precursor B or T cells and mature B or T cells. It is important to remember the following facts:

- There are no benign lymphomas. All lymphomas are malignant, but the degree of their malignancies varies.
- Most lymphomas have a B-cell phenotype.
- Lymphomas can occur in all age groups, but in general they are more common in adults than in children.
- Lymphomas can spill over into the blood and present as leukemia.
- Lymphomas most often involve lymph nodes, bone marrow, spleen, and thymus but can also be of extranodal origin. The most common site of extranodal lymphomas is the gastrointestinal system.

The diagnosis of lymphoma requires a lymph node biopsy, which is first examined by the pathologist. Ideally the lymph node is divided into three parts: one part that is fixed immediately for histologic examination, a second part that is freshly frozen for possible molecular biology studies, and a third part that is dispersed into tissue culture media in a single-cell suspension for flow cytometry and cytogenetic methods or specialized molecular biologic techniques. In most cases, an experienced pathologist can provide the diagnosis of lymphoma on the basis of light microscopic examination alone; the other studies are performed only for "fine-tuning" the diagnosis and subclassifying the tumors. If the pathologists cannot agree on the correct diagnosis, additional immunochemical and molecular biologic studies in a reference center are required for a definitive diagnosis.

In addition to the light microscopy, pathologists use several ancillary methods of modern cell biology and molecular biology.

Light Microscopy

It should be remembered that this classification requires a lymph node biopsy and is dependent on the pathologist's ability to recognize, with the aid of a light microscope, the typical morphologic signs of lymphocytic maturation. Among these features, two are most important: (1) the size and shape of the cell nuclei; and (2) the growth pattern of neoplastic lymphoid cells, which may completely obliterate the normal lymph node architecture or impart to it a nodular (follicular) appearance (Figure 9-18).

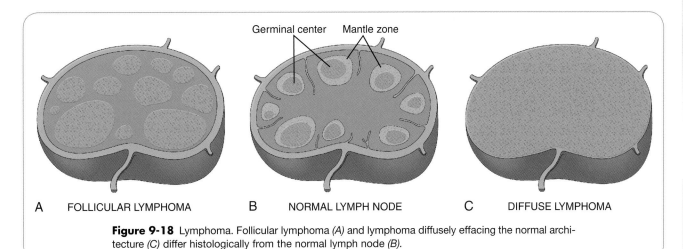

Figure 9-18 Lymphoma. Follicular lymphoma *(A)* and lymphoma diffusely effacing the normal architecture *(C)* differ histologically from the normal lymph node *(B)*.

Ancillary Techniques

Modern diagnostic workup of lymphoid neoplasms mandates that the biopsy be stained with immunohistochemical methods, a piece of tissue be prepared for flow cytometry, and if possible, a cytogenetic analysis be performed.

IMMUNOHISTOCHEMISTRY

Immunohistochemistry is a technique in which labeled antibodies are used to analyze the tissues for the presence of specific tumor cells. Using this technique, it is possible to determine whether the tumor is a B-cell lymphoma involving the typical B-cell areas of the lymph node, such as the germinal center of the follicles or the mantle zone, or whether it is a T-cell lymphoma, involving the paracortical zones normally occupied by T cells.

FLOW CYTOMETRY

Flow cytometry is a technique for sorting cells according to their surface properties. The biopsied lymph node is dispersed into a single-cell suspension and then stained with monoclonal antibodies to specific surface antigens known as clusters of differentiation. Cells treated this way can be separated into subsets that correspond to lymphocytes at various stages of maturation. Because lymphomas retain many normal cell surface markers and also acquire some additional markers, it is possible to cytochemically separate the neoplastic population from reactive lymphocytes and determine the immunophenotype of the tumor.

CYTOGENETIC ANALYSIS

Cytogenetic analysis is based on the karyotyping (chromosomal analysis) of tumor cells. The lymphoma cells are cultured and chromosomes are prepared from cells that have been arrested in metaphase. Many, if not most, lymphomas have abnormal karyotypes, which may be diagnostic of specific malignancy.

On the basis of the light microscopic findings, the immunophenotype as determined by immunohistochemistry, and the flow cytometry or cytogenetic findings, malignant lymphomas are further classified into one of the categories of the WHO classification. The schemes and algorithms that are used to this end are too complicated to be explained here, but this workup is essential for treatment of lymphoma patients. Once categorized, these patients are then entered into nationally approved treatment protocols, which include cytotoxic drug combinations, radiation therapy, and even some new treatment modalities, such as intravenous infusion of monoclonal antibodies.

Clinical Features

The symptoms of NHL vary. The most prevalent symptoms and clinical findings are as follows:

- *Lymph node enlargement,* which is typically painless and which may be solitary or diffuse (Figure 9-19). It may be

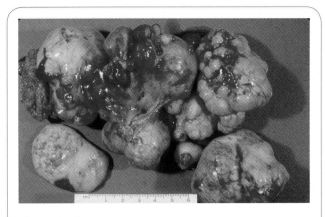

Figure 9-19 Lymphoma. Lymph node enlargement is typical.

associated with splenomegaly and lymphocytosis or lymphocytic leukemia.

- *Systemic constitutional symptoms,* including fatigue, malaise, fever, weight loss, pruritus, and sweating. These are attributable to hypermetabolism (i.e., the rapid turnover of proliferating tumor cells); anemia, leukopenia, and associated infections; and autoimmune phenomena that occur with increased frequency in persons with these disorders.
- *Extranodal tumor spread,* whereby tumor cells infiltrate and compress major organs, causing functional disturbances. The best example is lymphoma that infiltrates the brain, causing compression and destruction of parts of the brain.

A few typical examples of low-grade and high-grade lymphomas are discussed to describe the salient points.

FOLLICULAR LYMPHOMA

Follicular lymphoma is the most common form of lymphoma in the United States, accounting for approximately 45% of all cases. It occurs mostly in older people. It shows histologic and cytologic signs of differentiation; that is, the follicular structure of the lymph nodes is partially preserved and the tumor cells resemble mature lymphocytes or follicular center–activated lymphocytes (see Figure 9-18). Thus it is a slow-growing tumor, and most patients survive 7 to 9 years after the onset of the disease. Most patients present with long-standing enlargement of the lymph nodes and only mild constitutional symptoms. The slow-growing tumor cells do not react to most currently available cytotoxic drugs. In the terminal stages of this disease, the body becomes overwhelmed with the tumor mass, or a higher-grade lymphoma develops that spreads rapidly through the vital organs. Such accelerated forms of lymphoma may temporarily respond to chemotherapy, but overall these patients have a rapid downhill course.

DIFFUSE LARGE B-CELL LYMPHOMA

Diffuse large B-cell lymphomas (DLBL) occur in several forms. As a group these lymphomas represent the most common aggressive form of NHL. Histologically, DLBL show complete effacement of the normal lymph node architecture. Instead of normal lymphocyte, the tissue is infiltrated with large lymphoid cells that have irregular nuclear outlines and prominent nucleoli. The tumor cells infiltrate the perinodal tissue, and a spread into the parenchyma of major organs is common.

Complete remission can be induced by chemotherapy in 75% of patients, and approximately 50% of those that respond may be free of disease for several years. However, the complete cure rate remains low.

BURKITT'S LYMPHOMA

Burkitt's lymphoma is a highly malignant tumor composed of small B cells that divide rapidly. Cells are also prone to apoptsis, which gives the lymph node a microscopic appearance of a "starry sky." Burkitt's lymphoma may originate from the lymph nodes or the bone marrow. Neoplastic lymphoid cells may infiltrate other tissues, and extranodal masses are often more prominent than enlarged lymph nodes.

Burkitt's lymphoma is common in sub-Saharan Africa, where it is endemic among children infected with EBV. The disease presents most often as a tumor involving the mandible and facial soft tissue. Outside the endemic areas Burkitt's lymphoma is rare, affecting children and young adults. It presents often as an abdominal mass (e.g., ovarian or intestinal mass) rather than involving the orofacial structures. Burkitt's lymphoma responds well to chemotherapy, and most children and young adults can be cured.

HODGKIN'S LYMPHOMA

Hodgkin's lymphoma is a form of malignant disease that is pathologically distinct from other lymphomas. It affects all age groups. Nevertheless, the age distribution curve is bimodal, with one peak at 25 years and another at 55 years.

Pathologically there are five types of Hodgkin's lymphoma, four classical forms and a "nonclassical" form, as follows:
- nodular sclerosis (65%–70%)
- mixed cellularity (20%–25%)
- lymphocyte predominance (5%)
- lymphocyte depletion (5%)
- lymphocyte rich (uncommon "nonclassical" form)

Common to the four classical forms of Hodgkin's lymphoma are the pathognomonic Reed-Sternberg cells (Figure 9-20). Typically the Reed-Sternberg cells have a bilobed or multilobed nucleus and prominent nucleoli surrounded by a clear halo that is reminiscent of an owl's eye. The diagnosis of classical Hodgkin's lymphoma should not be made unless Reed-Sternberg cells are found. In lymphocyte-rich nonclassical Hodgkin's lymphoma there are, however, no typical Reed-Sternberg cells; instead the lymph nodes contain lymphohistiocytic cells with "popcorn nuclei."

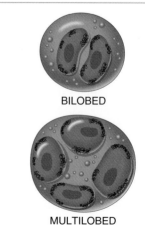

BILOBED

MULTILOBED

Figure 9-20 Diagnosis of Hodgkin's lymphoma. Reed-Sternberg cells are binucleated or multinucleated and have prominent nucleoli.

The histologic subtyping of Hodgkin's lymphoma was important before modern chemotherapy was introduced. Today the prognosis of the disease depends primarily on the extent of spread of the disease throughout the body. Histologic typing of lesions is less important, even though lymphocyte depletion has the poorest prognosis.

To facilitate prognosis determination and treatment, it is important to *stage the disease* accurately. This is done by clinically determining which parts of the body are involved. Multiple lymph nodes are sampled and biopsies of the liver, spleen, or bone marrow are performed.

Clinical Features

The clinical features of Hodgkin's lymphoma are not distinct from those in other lymphomas. Most patients exhibit lymph node enlargement, which may be associated with nonspecific symptoms. The neck nodes are most often involved. Mediastinal lymph nodes are also commonly involved, as the disease seems to spread from one group of lymph nodes to another in continuity. Overall, the central lymph nodes (i.e., those on the body) are more often involved than those on the extremities. Extranodal involvement is generally less common than in other lymphomas and occurs only in advanced disease. Leukemic spread is very rare.

Stage I disease signifies involvement of a single lymph node region (Figure 9-21). Stage II disease signifies involvement of two or more lymph node regions on the same side of the diaphragm. Stage III disease signifies involvement of lymph node regions on both sides of the diaphragm, with or without splenic lesions. Stage IV disease signifies widespread dissemination of the disease with involvement of one or more extranodal tissues and nonlymphoid organs (e.g., liver or intestine). The overall 10-year survival rate for all patients is more than 80%. In general, stage I and II tumors are associated with an excellent prognosis and a high rate of cure (greater than 90%) achieved with chemotherapy. Advanced disease has a less favorable prognosis. Nevertheless, 50% of patients with stage IV disease survive 5 years.

MULTIPLE MYELOMA

Multiple myeloma is a malignant disease of plasma cells. It is believed that the disease begins with malignant transformation of a single plasma cell. Clonal expansion of the descendants of this malignant cell leads to an overgrowth of the bone marrow by neoplastic cells, all of which share the same features. Because all neoplastic cells are descendants of a single cell that has undergone malignant transformation, the condition is called *monoclonal.* Other lymphomas are probably also monoclonal. The monoclonality of the plasma cell population in multiple myeloma is much more easily detected because plasma cells secrete immunoglobulins, which can be detected in the serum.

In the normal bone marrow, 5% of all cells are plasma cells. These cells are descendants of B lymphocytes. With

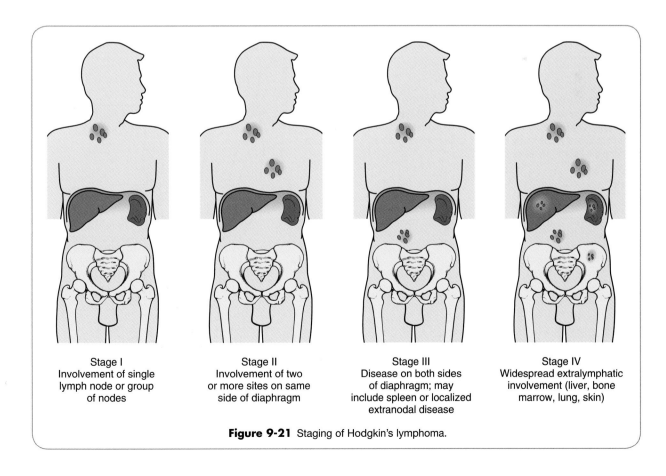

| Stage I | Stage II | Stage III | Stage IV |
| Involvement of single lymph node or group of nodes | Involvement of two or more sites on same side of diaphragm | Disease on both sides of diaphragm; may include spleen or localized extranodal disease | Widespread extralymphatic involvement (liver, bone marrow, lung, skin) |

Figure 9-21 Staging of Hodgkin's lymphoma.

antigenic stimulation, plasma cells proliferate and produce antibodies. Numerous clones of plasma cells are stimulated, with the result that numerous forms of immunoglobulins are produced. Infection causes a polyclonal activation of plasma cells, and the increased immunoglobulins appear as a broad-shaped globin "hump" in the serum electrophoresis pattern. After malignant transformation of a single plasma cell, as occurs in multiple myeloma, the bone marrow descendants of this malignant cell secrete all the same form of immunoglobulin. This can be detected as a "monoclonal spike" in serum protein electrophoresis. This spike is typical of multiple myeloma, which is therefore also called **monoclonal gammopathy**. Light chain of the immunoglobulin secreted by tumor cells appears in urine as Bence Jones protein.

Did You Know?

Dr. Bence Jones reported some 150 years ago that the urine of multiple myeloma patients contains a peculiar protein. This protein turned out to be a fragment of the immunoglobulin secreted by the neoplastic plasma cells and is still known as *Bence Jones protein*. Dr. Bence Jones is credited in medical history books for discovering the first biochemical tumor marker.

Multiple myeloma is a disease of old age, with most patients being older than 45 years. The malignant plasma cells typically proliferate in the bone marrow and, through this process, destroy the surrounding bone. Punched-out holes in the blood-forming bones, such as the calvaria and the vertebrae, can be detected by x-ray studies (Figure 9-22).

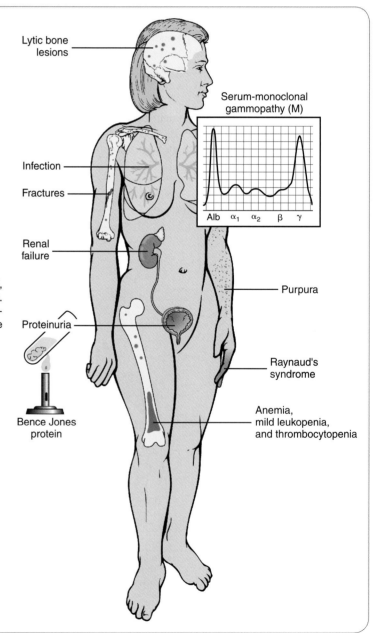

Figure 9-22 Multiple myeloma. Radiographs of the skull, ribs, and vertebrae show multiple punched-out lesions. There is anemia secondary to suppression of hematopathology. Kidney failure is the most common cause of death. The urine contains Bence Jones protein.

Calcium released from the bones contributes to hypercalcemia and the deposition of calcium in many organs, especially the kidneys. In addition, the immunoglobulin secreted by the plasma cells is also excreted in the kidney, where it damages the tubules and contributes to deterioration of renal function. Renal failure ensues. Most other symptoms and complications of multiple myeloma are related to the proliferation of malignant plasma cells in the bone marrow. These cells partially replace the normal hematopoietic marrow and also suppress the maturation of remaining hematopoietic cells. Typically there is normochronic anemia, mild leukopenia, and thrombocytopenia. Bone fractures are also common because of widespread bone destruction and weakening.

The diagnosis of multiple myeloma is based on x-ray studies, serum electrophoresis data, and ultimately bone marrow biopsy. Multiple lytic defects seen on radiographs typically contain numerous plasma cells that can be identified in bone marrow biopsy specimens. The monoclonal spike on electrophoresis supports the diagnosis of monoclonal proliferation of plasma cells.

The course of the disease is variable, but overall the prognosis is grim. Chemotherapy is ineffective. Most patients die within 3 to 4 years, primarily of kidney failure or infection.

BLEEDING DISORDERS

To move through the vessels, the blood must remain fluid. On the other hand, if the integrity of the blood is disrupted, it is in the best interest of the entire organism to prevent unnecessary bleeding. The process that prevents uncontrolled bleeding is called **hemostasis,** whereas pathologic alterations of bleeding are termed *bleeding disorders* or *hemorrhagic disorders.*

NORMAL HEMOSTASIS

Normal hemostasis depends on the closely integrated, coordinated action of the following:
- Vascular factors
- Platelet factors
- Coagulation factors

After an injury that disrupts the integrity of a vessel wall (e.g., a knife wound), the small arteries supplying blood to the area undergo vasoconstriction. This is mediated by a neural reflex and results in a slowdown of blood flow. At the same time, the blood extravasated into the surrounding tissue exerts pressure on the damaged vessels, compressing them from outside. The slowdown of blood flow promotes aggregation of platelets, which leads to the formation of a hemostatic plug. Substances released from platelets act on the circulating coagulation factors of the plasma and initiate the coagulation cascade. Additional clotting factors are released from the damaged endothelium and the surrounding tissue, all of which contribute to the formation of a definitive clot.

The formation of this definitive clot is critically dependent on the activation of the plasma coagulation factors (Figure 9-23). The salient features of these factors are listed here:
- There are 12 factors (Table 9-1). Note that there is no factor VI. All except factor IV (calcium) are proteins that are produced by the liver. They circulate in plasma as precursors or in an inactive form.
- The activation of factors occurs sequentially through an intrinsic or an extrinsic pathway. These two pathways converge, and both generate the activated factor Xa. In the common pathway of coagulation, factor Xa catalyzes the conversion of prothrombin to thrombin. Thrombin promotes the conversion of fibrinogen to fibrin. Final polymerization of fibrin results in a definitive thrombus.
- The intrinsic pathway is activated through several substances ("intrinsic" to the blood itself) that act on factor XII, also known as *Hageman's factor.* The extrinsic pathway is activated through the factor VII action of extraneous tissue-derived substances on factor VII. Prothrombin time

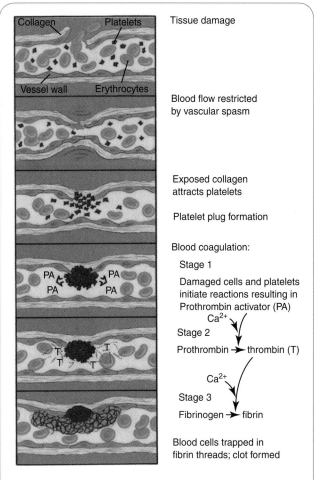

Figure 9-23 Normal hemostasis is accomplished through the interaction of platelets and plasma clotting factors and substances released from endothelial cells and perivascular tissue. (From Applegate EJ: The Anatomy and Physiology Learning System, 4th ed, St. Louis, 2011, Saunders.)

TABLE 9-1 Coagulation Factors

Factor	Name
I	Fibrinogen
II	Prothrombin
III	Tissue factor
IV	Calcium
V	Proaccelerin
VII	Proconvertin
VIII	Antihemophilic factor
IX	Plasma thromboplastin component
X	Stuart-Prower factor
XI	Plasma thromboplastin antecedent
XII	Hageman's factor
XIII	Fibrin stabilizing factor

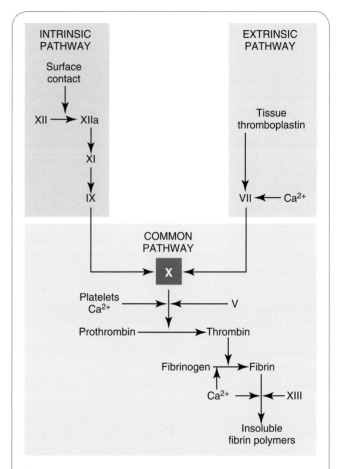

Figure 9-24 Plasma clotting factors are activated in a sequence that corresponds to the intrinsic and extrinsic pathways.

(PT) is used to measure the extrinsic and common pathway, whereas the activated partial thromboplastin time (aPTT) is used to measure the intrinsic and the common pathways of coagulation (Figure 9-24).

- The action of clotting factors is counterbalanced by the action of natural anticoagulants, the most important of which are heparin, antithrombin, and plasminogen. Heparin acts on several steps of the coagulation cascade and is therefore used to prevent clotting in patients. It is also used to prevent clotting of blood in test tubes. Antithrombin inactivates thrombin and prevents its action on fibrinogen. Plasmin can lyse fibrin and is therefore used to dissolve clots.

MAJOR BLEEDING DISORDERS

Hemorrhage, or the escape of blood from the vessels or the heart, can occur in several forms. It is considered *external* if the blood flows outside of the body (wound) or *internal* if the blood enters the tissues or body cavities. Hemorrhages from multiple sites are called *purpura.*

Bleeding disorders occur as a result of the following defects:
- Vascular
- Platelet related
- Clotting factor related

Often, all these aspects of normal hemostasis are involved.

VASCULAR DISORDERS

The most important vascular causes of bleeding are mechanical trauma, vessel wall weakness, and immune injury.

MECHANICAL TRAUMA

Mechanical trauma to the blood vessels is the most common cause of hemorrhage. It is a feature of everyday life, manifesting as small bruises and wounds or skin hematomas caused by known and unnoticed minor and major injuries.

VESSEL WALL WEAKNESS

Vessel wall weakness is an important cause of spontaneous and trauma-induced hemorrhages. It is well known that some persons tend to bruise more readily than others. Apparently, individuals do not have equally strong connective tissue; therefore some of us are more prone to bleeding and cannot withstand trauma as readily as others ("devil's pinches"). With aging, the vessels become more fragile, and minor hemorrhages are thus more common in older people ("senile purpura"). Some metabolic disorders, such as Cushing's syndrome, or congenital disorders of connective tissue are characterized by easy bleeding. Hypovitaminosis C (scurvy) is marked by multiple hemorrhages because the intercellular matrix of the blood vessels cannot be formed properly without vitamin C.

IMMUNE MECHANISMS

Immune mechanisms may damage the blood vessels and cause hemorrhage. Any vasculitis will thus present with hemorrhages, which are most noticeable in the various autoimmune disorders that involve the capillaries and small arteries and veins of the skin. The best example is provided by various allergic drug reactions, the presenting sign of which is skin purpura.

PLATELET DISORDERS

Platelet disorders can be classified as quantitative or qualitative. That is, they may be caused by either a decreased number of platelets or an abnormality in structure and function.

Normal blood contains 150,000 to 300,000 platelets/μL. A decrease to levels below 70,000/μL is considered abnormal and is called **thrombocytopenia**. A bleeding tendency develops only in severe thrombocytopenia, when the platelet count drops to less than 10,000 to 20,000/μL.

Thrombocytopenia develops as a result of decreased production or increased destruction, removal, or utilization of platelets.

Decreased production of platelets occurs in many disorders affecting the bone marrow. Under normal circumstances, the platelets are formed from the megakaryocytes. They represent anuclear fragments of megakaryocytic cytoplasm that survive in the peripheral blood for several days. Any disease or agent that affects megakaryocytes will cause thrombocytopenia. The most important among these are the following:

- Aplastic anemia, marked by a loss of all hematopoietic cells
- Leukemia, marked by the replacement of normal hematopoietic cells with tumor cells
- Drugs that damage megakaryocytes
- Infectious agents, such as rubella virus (and probably many others), which affect the megakaryocytes

These patients develop a bleeding tendency and require blood or platelet transfusions.

The primary cause of failure must be identified before any treatment. Drug-induced thrombocytopenia may respond to withdrawal of the drug. Virus-related disease may improve upon cure of the infection. In severe thrombocytopenia of aplastic anemia, the only definitive treatment promising survival is bone marrow transplantation.

Increased intravascular destruction of platelets or their increased consumption can also result in thrombocytopenia. Destruction of platelets is a feature of many autoimmune disorders. Antibodies to platelets occur in SLE, various forms of hemolytic anemias, and drug-induced hematologic disorders. Such antibodies are also the major features of **idiopathic thrombocytopenic purpura** (ITP), a disease of unknown etiology.

Immune thrombocytopenia also may develop after some blood transfusions because the platelets carry not only the major blood group antigens expressed on the red blood cells but also some platelet-specific antigens that can induce formation of antibodies.

Thrombocytopenia also develops in some children who are born to mothers immunized with paternal platelet antigens in a manner similar to the hemolytic disorder caused by maternofetal Rh incompatibility.

Increased removal of platelets typically occurs in the spleen. The platelets that have been coated or damaged by antibodies are removed at a faster rate. This occurs in hypersplenism, a syndrome characterized by splenomegaly and pooling of blood in the enlarged spleen. There is also an increased removal of platelets and of other blood cells.

Consumption of platelets occurs at an accelerated rate in various conditions that cause **disseminated intravascular coagulation (DIC).** DIC may be triggered by infection, tumors, or any form of shock (Figure 9-25). Formation of thrombi in the small blood vessels is typically associated with trapping of platelets and thrombocytopenia. Once the platelets and plasma clotting factors have been used up, the blood cannot coagulate any longer and bleeding ensues.

Disorders of platelet function may be classified as either congenital or acquired. The congenital disorders are rare and involve some of the major platelet functions. These include, for example, defective platelet aggregation *(thrombasthenia),* adhesion to solid surfaces, and the release of biologically active substances. Acquired disorders of platelet function are relatively common but are rarely severe enough to cause clinical problems. Chronic renal failure is the prototype of a metabolic disease associated with abnormal platelet function, probably related to the accumulation of metabolites that are not excreted through the kidney. *Aspirin* prevents platelet aggregation and release of thromboplastin. However, aspirin intake is rarely associated with clinical bleeding problems.

CLOTTING FACTOR DEFICIENCIES

Deficiencies of clotting factors can be congenital or acquired. Congenital clotting factor defects are relatively common. Each of the proteins that participate in the coagulation cascade is

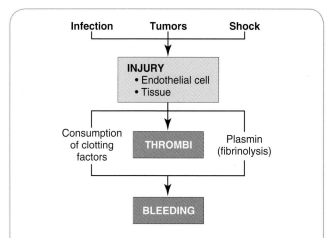

Figure 9-25 Disseminated intravascular coagulation (DIC). Various diseases causing endothelial cell or tissue injury trigger the formation of thrombi in small blood vessels, or bleeding.

encoded by a distinct gene. Mutation or deletion of these genes results in a bleeding disorder. Although there are many such disorders, only *hemophilia* is discussed here, because it is the most important clinical disorder of this type. Acquired clotting factor deficiencies are more common and also deserve to be noted.

Hemophilia is a sex-linked congenital clotting factor deficiency that occurs in two forms: (1) hemophilia A, or the deficiency of factor VIII; and (2) hemophilia B, or the deficiency of factor IX.

Both these genes are located on the X chromosome. The gene is recessive, so it cannot be expressed in women who have two X chromosomes. Women who carry the gene (asymptomatic carriers) can transmit the hemophilia gene to their daughters as well as to their sons. The daughters will be asymptomatic carriers. The sons whose Y chromosome does not carry the normal allele that could overshadow the recessive hemophilia gene will have the bleeding disease. The sons of hemophiliacs acquire from their fathers the normal Y. They are asymptomatic and do not carry the gene, whereas the daughters of hemophiliac males are always asymptomatic carriers. Hemophilia A affects 1 in 5000 males. Hemophilia B is 10 times less common than hemophilia A and is generally less severe.

The deficiency of factor VIII or factor IX results in uncontrollable bleeding after trauma. Affected males tend to bruise and often develop subcutaneous hematomas or hemarthrosis. Bleeding during surgery cannot be stopped in such individuals, and even minor surgery, such as tooth extraction, can cause profuse blood loss. Joint deformities are common late consequences of repeated hemarthrosis.

The diagnosis of hemophilia may be suggested by the family history. However, it should be noted that at least 20% of cases represent newly acquired mutations and are not associated with a previous family history of hemophilia. Thus the bleeding disorder must be diagnosed by applying several tests. Typically, the most significant abnormality is a prolonged aPTT, an abnormality of the intrinsic pathway. Bleeding time and prothrombin time are normal. Specific tests measuring the functions of factor VIII and IX must be performed to distinguish hemophilia A from hemophilia B. Genetic testing by molecular biology techniques may be used to further characterize the nature of the defect and the extent of the mutation or deletion. The gene for factor VIII is an especially large one, so different parts of the gene can be affected. Depending on the extent of the genetic defect, the disease may present as a mild, moderate, or severe bleeding disorder. The clinical syndrome develops only if blood levels of factor VIII have been reduced below 1% of normal.

 Did You Know?

The Babylonian Talmud, the holy Jewish scripture, contains the first reference to hemophilia, although not under that name. The scripture quotes Rabbi Judah, a well-known scholar who allowed a boy not to have ritual circumcision because three of his brothers had bled to death from this procedure. The cause of this familial bleeding disorder remained obscure for more than two millennia thereafter.

Patients with hemophilia need frequent transfusions of fresh blood, which places them at high risk for acquiring various bloodborne infections. Previously many hemophiliacs were infected with hepatitis virus B or C or HIV, but improved screening of blood donors has almost completely eliminated these complications.

Acquired clotting factor defects occur in many clinical situations. In general these are attributable to inadequate production of clotting factors, excessive consumption, or the action of anticoagulants.

Decreased production of clotting factors is typically found in patients with chronic liver disease. Essentially all proteins of the coagulation cascade are synthesized in liver cells, the exception being von Willebrand factor, which is produced by the endothelial cells. Therefore chronic liver disease results in a deficiency of these factors. Because fibrinogen represents the most abundant of these factors, this condition is often referred to as *hypofibrinogenemia*.

The synthesis of several clotting factors requires vitamin K. Without vitamin K, the liver cannot synthesize factors II, VII, IX, and X. Vitamin K is a fat-soluble vitamin produced by the bacteria in the intestines. Neonatal hemorrhagic tendency occurs in children in whom the maternally acquired stores of vitamin K have been depleted before their intestines are colonized with bacteria. In adults, hypovitaminosis K occurs if the bacteria that produce vitamin K in the intestines have been eliminated by antibiotics, or if the absorption of fat, which is essential for the uptake of vitamin K, is impaired by biliary or pancreatic disease. Finally, vitamin K utilization in the liver can be inhibited medically. The best known of these anticoagulants is warfarin (Coumadin), a drug used to prevent thrombosis in persons at risk for infarcts or thromboemboli.

Did You Know?

Vitamins carry the names of letters, and it seems that they have been labeled alphabetically, at least for vitamins A to E. Vitamin K seems to be out of sequence. How come? Although it is important for coagulation, it could not be given the letter *C* because that letter was already given to ascorbic acid. The Nobel Prize–winning discoverers, Henrik Dam of Denmark and Edward Doisy of the United States, settled for the letter K, because in Danish, "blood clotting" is spelled *koagulation.*

Increased consumption of clotting factors leads to excessive bleeding. Consumption of coagulation factors occurs during the formation of thrombi of any type and is most prominent in DIC. This syndrome is typically triggered by thromboplastins released from injured endothelial cells or from tissue or some substances that are foreign and are not supposed to be in contact with the circulating blood. Any form of shock could induce DIC, primarily because the perfusion of the peripheral circulatory system has been compromised. The ischemic endothelial cells themselves promote thrombosis, or they allow the leakage of thrombogenic stimuli from the adjacent tissues into the blood. Infections also damage blood vessels and tissues. On the other hand, many bacteria can themselves initiate formation of clots. Massive tissue injury caused by trauma is yet another source of tissue thromboplastins. Amniotic fluid embolism (i.e., entry of amniotic fluid into the maternal circulation) also can cause DIC. Tumors are often associated with DIC because they release cells or necrotic material into the circulation, thus initiating clotting.

Regardless of the initiating event, DIC is always a consumptive coagulopathy. In the first stages of the disease, the small blood vessels are occluded with numerous thrombi composed of platelets, fibrin, and other coagulation factors. As a result of this increased consumption, the blood is depleted of platelets and clotting factors. Plasminogen activators released from ischemic tissue activate plasmin, which acts as a fibrinolytic agent, dissolving the microthrombi. As the blood rushes through the newly reopened blood vessels whose endothelial cells were damaged by ischemia, bleeding occurs. This bleeding cannot be stopped because the circulating blood does not have any more **coagulation factors**. These factors must be replenished by transfusions, but often this is to no avail and the patient dies of exsanguination. Laboratory tests show low values of all coagulation factors and platelets. Fibrin split products are found in the urine of these patients.

Anticoagulants are important causes of acquired clotting factor deficiencies. Some of these anticoagulants are produced by the body, whereas others are injected for therapeutic purposes. Many exogenous anticoagulants, such as heparin or warfarin, are widely used in clinical practice. It is important to monitor the effects of these anticoagulants because overdoses can cause uncontrollable bleeding and major mishaps, such as brain bleeding.

REVIEW QUESTIONS

1. Describe the sites of hematopoiesis in various age groups.
2. How is hematopoiesis regulated?
3. Describe the pathways of differentiation of pluripotent hematopoietic stem cells.
4. Compare serum and plasma and explain which one you would collect for various blood tests.
5. Explain the molecular structure of hemoglobin.
6. Describe the major events in the life of erythrocytes.
7. Explain the significance of various erythrocytic parameters, such as MCV, MCH, and MCHC, and describe how they are measured.
8. What are the normal values for a white blood cell count?
9. Compare neutrophils and lymphocytes.
10. What is the function of platelets?
11. What is anemia?
12. Provide an etiologic and a morphologic classification of anemias.
13. Which anemias are caused by decreased hematopoiesis?
14. Which anemias are caused by abnormal hematopoiesis?
15. Which anemias are caused by increased loss or destruction of red blood cells?
16. List typical examples of normocytic, microcytic, and macrocytic anemia.
17. List typical examples of anemias that present with abnormal red blood cell shapes.
18. Explain the pathogenesis and pathology of aplastic anemia.
19. List the causes of iron deficiency anemia.
20. What are the critical events in the metabolism of iron in the human body?
21. Explain the pathogenesis of megaloblastic anemia.
22. Compare anemia caused by vitamin B_{12} with anemia caused by folic acid deficiency.
23. Compare hemolytic anemia caused by intracorpuscular defects with anemia caused by extracorpuscular factors.
24. Explain the pathogenesis of sickle cell anemia.
25. Correlate the pathologic findings in sickle cell anemia with the clinical symptoms of this disease.
26. Explain the pathogenesis of thalassemia.
27. Compare thalassemia minor and thalassemia major.
28. Why are red blood cells spherical (round) in hereditary spherocytosis?
29. Explain the pathogenesis of immune hemolytic anemia.
30. Compare primary and secondary polycythemia.
31. What is leukopenia, and what are its causes?
32. What is leukocytosis, and what are its causes?
33. What are the possible causes of lymph node enlargement?
34. What is the difference between lymphoma and leukemia?
35. What causes lymphomas and leukemias?
36. What are the common features of all leukemias, and what distinguishes acute from chronic leukemia and lymphocytic from myelogenous leukemia?
37. List the most important features of acute lymphoblastic leukemia and correlate the pathologic findings with the clinical features of this disease.
38. List the most important features of acute myelogenous leukemia.
39. List the most important features of chronic myelogenous leukemia.
40. List the most important features of chronic lymphocytic leukemia.
41. How are non-Hodgkin's lymphomas classified?
42. List the most common symptoms and clinical findings of non-Hodgkin's lymphomas.

43. Compare follicular lymphoma with diffuse large-cell lymphoma and Burkitt's lymphoma.

44. What is Hodgkin's lymphoma?

45. How is Hodgkin's lymphoma classified histologically?

46. How is Hodgkin's lymphoma staged?

47. What is multiple myeloma?

48. How is multiple myeloma diagnosed?

49. How do vascular platelet and coagulation factors interact to ensure normal hemostasis?

50. Compare the mechanism of the activation of the intrinsic and extrinsic pathway of coagulation.

51. What are the three major groups of bleeding disorders?

52. Which bleeding disorders are caused by vascular diseases?

53. What is thrombocytopenia, and what is its clinical significance?

54. What are the main causes of thrombocytopenia?

55. What is thrombasthenia?

56. What is hemophilia, and how is it diagnosed?

57. Why is hypofibrinogenemia a sign of a chronic liver disease?

58. Why is disseminated intravascular coagulation accompanied by a bleeding tendency?

The Gastrointestinal System

10

Chapter Outline

NORMAL ANATOMY AND PHYSIOLOGY
OVERVIEW OF MAJOR DISEASES
  Diseases of the Oral Cavity
    Developmental Abnormalities
    Inflammation
    Oral Cancer
  Salivary Gland Diseases
    Sialadenitis
    Neoplasms
  Diseases of the Esophagus
    Developmental Abnormalities
    Hiatal Hernia
    Motility Disorders of the Esophagus
    Esophagitis
    Circulatory Disturbances
    Carcinoma of the Esophagus

Diseases of the Stomach and Duodenum
  Developmental Abnormalities
  Gastritis
  Peptic Ulcer
  Gastric Neoplasms
Diseases of the Small and Large Intestine
  Developmental Abnormalities
  Diverticulosis
  Intestinal Vascular Diseases
  Inflammatory Bowel Disease
  Gastrointestinal Infections
  Intestinal Obstruction
  Malabsorption Syndromes
  Intestinal Neoplasms

Key Terms and Concepts

Achalasia
Angiodysplasia of the intestines
Appendicitis
Barrett's esophagus
Carcinoembryonic antigen (CEA)
Carcinoids
Carcinoma of the esphagus
Carcinoma of the stomach
Celiac sprue
Cleft lip
Colorectal cancer
Crohn's disease
Dental caries
Diarrhea
Diverticulosis
Dysphagia
Esophageal atresia

Esophagitis
Familial adenomatous
  polyposis coli
Gastritis
Hematemesis
Hematochezia
Hemorrhoids
Hernias
Hiatal hernia
Hirschsprung's disease
Ileus
Inflammatory bowel disease (IBD)
Intestinal strictures
Intussusception
Ischemic bowel disease
Malabsorption

MALToma
Meckel's diverticulum
Melena
Norovirus
Oral cancer
Peptic ulcer
Periodontal disease
Peritonitis
Polyps (intestinal)
Pseudomembranous colitis
Rotavirus
Sialadenitis
Stomatitis
Ulcerative colitis
Volvulus
Whipple's disease

Learning Objectives

After reading this chapter, the student should be able to:

1. Describe the normal gastrointestinal tract and its functions.
2. List the most common alimentary diseases in infants, young adults, and the elderly.
3. Discuss dental decay and periodontal disease in terms of etiology, pathology, and clinical presentations.
4. Explain the etiology and clinical presentations of inflammatory diseases of the mouth.
5. Explain the risk factors for oral cancer.
6. Discuss the main diseases affecting the salivary glands.
7. Discuss the inflammatory diseases of the esophagus.
8. Discuss cancer of the esophagus in terms of etiology, gross and microscopic pathology, and clinical presentation.
9. Discuss the pathogenesis of acute and chronic gastritis and peptic ulcer.
10. List three causes of hematemesis and melena and explain their pathogenesis.
11. Describe the pathology of various forms of gastric cancer.
12. Describe the pathology and complications of diverticulosis of the colon.
13. Discuss inflammatory bowel disease and compare Crohn's disease and ulcerative colitis.
14. List and discuss various causes of diarrhea.
15. Define peritonitis, ileus, and hernia and explain their pathogenesis.
16. Discuss the etiology and pathogenesis of malabsorption syndromes.
17. Describe the pathology of colon cancer and list the most important prognostic factors, comparing the lesions of the right and left colon.

NORMAL ANATOMY AND PHYSIOLOGY

The normal gastrointestinal tract, also called the *alimentary* or *digestive tract,* can be divided into two sections: the upper and lower tract. The upper part includes the mouth, pharynx, esophagus, stomach, and duodenum (Figure 10-1, *A*). The lower gastrointestinal tract includes the small and large intestine, appendix, rectum, and anus. Clearly this division is arbitrary and is based more on current medical practice than on scientific principles. Diseases of the mouth are treated by dentists and otorhinolaryngologists, who also treat the diseases of the salivary glands. Gastroenterologists are concerned with the diseases involving the remainder of the gastrointestinal tract, including the liver and the pancreas. The surgical lesions of the esophagus are in the domain of thoracic surgeons, whereas general surgeons operate on the abdominal parts of the gastrointestinal tract.

The gastrointestinal tract can be perceived as a hollow tube that has essentially the same structural organization from one end to the other (Figure 10-1, *B*). From the mouth to the anus, the gastrointestinal tract has four layers: mucosa, submucosa, muscularis, and serosa (or adventitia). In the upper gastrointestinal tract, the epithelium of the mucosa is squamous; from the stomach to the anus, it is cuboidal glandular epithelium, and then it again becomes squamous. In the supradiaphragmatic part of the upper gastrointestinal tract, the muscle layer is covered by connective tissue called *adventitia.* The outer surface of the stomach and the intestines is covered with a serosal surface called *peritoneum.* Visceral peritoneum covering the gastrointestinal organs is in continuity with the parietal peritoneum, which covers the rest of the abdominal cavity.

The gastrointestinal tract has a complex blood supply. It is important to remember that the upper and lower mesenteric arteries, which provide blood to most of the abdominal gastrointestinal organs, receive approximately one sixth of the arterial cardiac output and that blood flow can be upregulated or downregulated according to physiologic needs. The *portal system* drains most of the venous blood from the small and large intestine.

The intestines have a rich supply of lymphatics, which begin as lacteals in the mucosal wall and drain into local lymph nodes and larger lymphatic channels that enter the thoracic duct. This lymphatic system is important for the absorption of nutrients from food, and plays a critical role in the body's immune response. Under pathologic conditions, it is the main route for the spread of cancer.

The gastrointestinal tract has a complex innervation that regulates the movements of its various parts. The innervation is mostly derived from the autonomic nervous system and is both vagotonic and sympathomimetic. The autonomic ganglia are located partially outside the gastrointestinal system and partially inside the wall of these organs *(myenteric plexus).*

Developmentally the gastrointestinal tract is derived from the embryonic gut, which has three parts: foregut, midgut, and hindgut. The foregut gives rise to the pharynx, esophagus, and stomach, as well as to the respiratory tract. The midgut gives rise to the small intestine, but it also represents the primordium of the liver and pancreas. The hindgut gives rise to the colon. The mouth and the anus (i.e., the beginning and end of the gastrointestinal tract) have a complex developmental relationship with adjacent structures and develop somewhat independently of the remainder of the gastrointestinal tract.

The main functions of the gastrointestinal tract are the digestion of food and alimentation. Each section of the

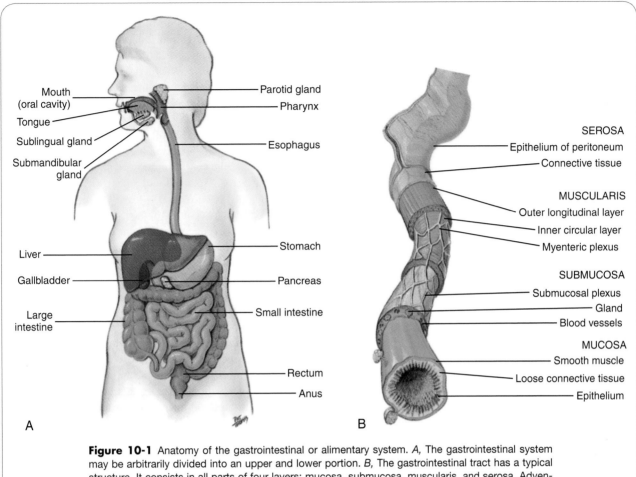

Figure 10-1 Anatomy of the gastrointestinal or alimentary system. *A,* The gastrointestinal system may be arbitrarily divided into an upper and lower portion. *B,* The gastrointestinal tract has a typical structure. It consists in all parts of four layers: mucosa, submucosa, muscularis, and serosa. Adventitia rather than serosa forms the outer layer of the upper alimentary tracts. (From Applegate EJ: The Anatomy and Physiology Learning System, 4th ed, Philadelphia, 2011, Saunders.)

gastrointestinal tract has a specialized role in preparing the food for absorption. Digestion can be divided into the following specific phases. These phases are listed by their technical, Latin-derived names, with brief explications:

- *Ingestion.* The food is taken in through the mouth.
- *Mastication.* Chewing is accomplished by the strength of facial muscles compressing the food between the maxilla and the mandible. The *teeth* have a crucial role in mincing of food, which is at the same time mixed with the digestive juices of the *salivary glands.*
- *Deglutition.* Swallowing is a function of the pharyngeal and *esophageal* muscles. In the beginning, it is voluntary, but once the food enters the esophagus, it is accomplished by *peristalsis* (i.e., contraction of the smooth muscles of the esophagus under the control of autonomic reflexes).
- *Digestion.* Chemical breakdown of nutrients begins in the mouth, where the food is mixed with saliva. The food entering the stomach is permeated with hydrochloric acid and gastric enzymes, and it is mechanically propelled into the duodenum. In the duodenum the food is mixed with bile, pancreatic juice, and intestinal enzymes. Digestive enzymes ensure appropriate lysis of proteins, carbohydrates, and

lipids, each of which is absorbed under specific circumstances and in different parts of the intestines.
- *Absorption.* The taking in of chemically digested food components into the cells of the intestinal mucosa occurs mostly in the small intestine. However, other organs are also involved in the absorption of nutrients. For example, alcohol is absorbed in the stomach, and the colon absorbs water and electrolytes.
- *Excretion.* Elimination of undigested food, various secretions, and the waste excretory products of metabolism occurs through the anus in the form of feces. This is called *defecation.*

The processing of food occurs in a highly regulated manner that is under neural and neuroendocrine control. Various neural reflexes regulate salivation, production of gastric juices, and release of bile, as well as the motility of the esophagus, stomach, and intestines. The most important digestive juices and polypeptide hormones secreted by the digestive system are listed in Table 10-1. For example, cholecystokinin that is released from the duodenum, which is distended by food, stimulates the contraction of the gallbladder, release of bile into the intestine, and secretion of bicarbonate in the pancreas.

TABLE 10-1 Main Exocrine and Endocrine Products of the Gastrointestinal Tract

Organ	Secretory Product	Function
Salivary gland	Amylase	Digestion of starch
Stomach	Pepsin	Digestion of proteins
	Hydrochloric acid	
	Gastrin	Stimulates secretion of hydrochloric acid
	Intrinsic factor	Mediates absorption of vitamin B_{12}
Small intestine	Enterokinase	Activates pancreatic enzymes
	Cholecystokinin	Stimulates gallbladder contraction and pancreatic secretion of bicarbonates
	Secretin	Stimulates secretion of pancreatic trypsin and chymotrypsin

Gastrin, a polypeptide hormone released from the pyloric glandular cells, stimulates the production of hydrochloric acid in the stomach. These polypeptide hormones are secreted by neuroendocrine cells that are distributed throughout the entire gastrointestinal tract. These cells are loosely integrated into a complex, diffuse network called the *gastrointestinal neuroendocrine system.* Endocrine control of digestion is coordinated neurally and involves several cranial and spinal nerves and the autonomic nervous system.

OVERVIEW OF MAJOR DISEASES

Gastrointestinal diseases are very common. Approximately 20 million Americans consult their physicians yearly about some problems caused by these diseases. In addition to those diseases that require medical treatment, minor discomforts, such as excessive burping *(eructation),* flatulence (passing of gases), or bad breath *(halitosis),* are common.

The most important diseases of the upper and lower gastrointestinal tract are as follows:

- Dental caries and gum disease
- Infectious gastroenteritis
- Circulatory disorders and hemorrhagic lesions
- Multifactorial disorders, such as peptic ulcer and inflammatory bowel disease
- Obstructive disorders, such as hernias and ilea
- Functional disorders that result in malabsorption, such as celiac sprue
- Neoplasms

Several facts important to an understanding of gastrointestinal disease are presented here, before a discussion of specific pathologic entities:

1. The function of the normal gastrointestinal tract depends on the normal development of anatomic structures and the functional differentiation of their components. The development of the gastrointestinal tract occurs at two levels: structural (anatomic) and functional (physiologic). Structural development of various anatomic segments of the gastrointestinal tract is largely completed during the first 3 months of fetal development. It can be disturbed by many external influences that cause complex malformation, and it is often associated with developmental anomalies of other organs. For example, cleft lip ("harelip") may be associated with abnormalities of the palate (cleft palate) and nose. Likewise, **esophageal atresia** (obliterated lumen) is often associated with abnormalities of the trachea (esophagotracheal fistula).

   Functional inadequacy of the gastrointestinal cells is usually related to a congenital enzyme deficiency. For example, in congenital abetalipoproteinemia, an enzymatic defect in the small intestinal cells prevents the absorption of fats from food, causing steatorrhea.

   Abnormal development of the intestinal ganglia, which is a structural defect, may have profound functional consequences. The best example of this is congenital megacolon or **Hirschsprung's disease,** in which the intramural ganglia of the rectum do not develop. This leads to spasmodic constriction of the aganglionic segment of the large intestine and the dilation of the intestine above the obstruction.

2. The gastrointestinal tract is open ended and thus is readily accessible to bacteria and other pathogens and allergens. In contrast to many other organ systems that are sterile, the gastrointestinal tract is largely colonized by bacteria. The bacterial flora is site specific; that is, it is different in the mouth than in the stomach or the rectum. The flora also changes with age, depending on the site, the environment, and the function of the alimentary tract. For example, neonates have a different intestinal flora than do older children and adults. Normally the host maintains a balance with the saprophytes, but disease may alter that balance. For example, broad-spectrum antibiotics change the colonic flora and facilitate the overgrowth of toxigenic bacteria, such as *Clostridium difficile,* which leads to pseudomembranous colitis. *Candida albicans* infection of the mouth or esophagus is common in debilitated cancer patients.

   Many bacteria, protozoa, and parasites that are not normal components of the intestinal flora reach the intestines via the food that is ingested. Cholera, a severe watery **diarrhea** caused by ingested *Vibrio cholerae,* is a good example of such infection.

   The immune system of the body, especially the mucosa-associated lymphoid tract (MALT), may react against foreign pathogens and saprophytes. Immune reactions also occur against various components of food (food allergy). Allergens present in the food produce functional or structural changes in the gastrointestinal tract. These are most prominent in children and account for most food allergy in neonates and small children.

3. The intestinal mucosa is an interface and a barrier between the external and the internal milieu that requires energy to be maintained actively. The mucosa of the gastrointestinal

tract resembles skin in that it protects the body from adverse external influences. Thus it is essential that the mucosal barrier by kept intact. The intestinal tract can be breached mechanically, by infection, or even chemically. Small defects of the oral mucosa, especially around the teeth, are common sites of bacterial invasion. One infection may lead to another. For example, oral mucosal ulceration caused by herpesvirus may become infected with bacteria. The esophageal mucosal barrier can be breached also by the hydrochloric acid in the gastric juice regurgitated from the stomach. The breakdown of the mucosal defense mechanisms is an important cause of peptic ulcers in the stomach and duodenum.

4. The gastrointestinal tract is a tube that can dilate or become obstructed. Obstruction of the gastrointestinal tube may be anatomic or functional. In achalasia of the esophagus, a spasm of the lower esophageal sphincter (LES) prevents the passage of food and causes dilation of the lumen proximal to the obstruction. A similar obstruction may be caused by "esophageal webs" and "rings" that protrude into the lumen and are composed of connective tissue and smooth muscles. Congenital spasm of the pylorus is a cause of vomiting in neonates and infants, but this condition can be surgically corrected if it does not correct itself. Tumors are probably the most important cause of gastrointestinal obstruction.

The lumen of the gastrointestinal tube may also dilate. Megacolon has already been mentioned. Megaesophagus, as in achalasia, represents similar dilation proximal to a structural or functional obstruction. An irregular focal outpouching of the intestinal or esophageal wall is called a diverticulum.

5. Gastrointestinal diseases may disturb one or more of the basic functions of the gastrointestinal tract. Loss of teeth affects chewing. Diseases of the salivary glands reduce the moistening of food during mastication and cause "dry mouth," or xerostomia (from the Greek *xeros,* meaning "dry," and *stoma,* meaning "mouth"). Stiffening of the esophagus affected by the connective tissue disease scleroderma will cause **dysphagia** (abnormal or strained swallowing). Abnormal secretion of hydrochloric acid can result in achlorhydria (lack of hydrochloric acid) or hyperacidity of the gastric content. The term *dyspepsia* is generally used for defective digestion. It has many causes, such as the lack of pepsin that occurs secondary to gastric mucosal atrophy or the lack of trypsin associated with chronic pancreatitis.

Malabsorption (i.e., abnormal absorption of intestinal contents) may involve carbohydrates, peptides, lipids, or all the basic food ingredients. Malabsorption of fat is associated with a deficiency of the fat-soluble vitamins: A, D, E, and K. The absorption of essential minerals can also be disturbed.

6. The movement of the intestines depends on the autonomic contraction of smooth muscles, which is under neural and hormonal control. Smooth muscle contraction that mediates the swallowing and propulsion of food through the gastrointestinal tract is highly regulated by cranial, spinal, and autonomic nerves. Disturbances of motility result from smooth muscle disease or loss of neural cells in the intestine (e.g., after irradiation). Carcinoid tumors secrete polypeptide hormones, which could also cause motility problems as a result of neuroendocrine dysregulation. Symptoms include dysphagia (abnormal swallowing), constipation (lack of defecation), diarrhea (frequent passing of stools), and colic (intestinal spasm).

7. Abundant blood flow through the gastrointestinal tract and the superficial location of the blood vessels in the mucosa make it prone to hemorrhage or ischemia. The gastrointestinal tract receives a large amount of blood through large-caliber arteries that originate directly from the aorta. These arteries are prone to atherosclerosis; therefore, with advancing age, the blood supply to the intestine diminishes. This is one of the reasons why elderly adults often have problems with digestion and constipation. They often develop ulcerations and ischemic atrophy of the mucosa.

The abundant blood supply irrigates the mucosa of the gastrointestinal tract diffusely, which facilitates absorption of nutrients. This mucosal vascularity makes the stomach and intestines vulnerable to bleeding secondary to mechanical trauma. Furthermore, the mucosal injury of peptic ulcer or other ulcerative diseases is also associated with bleeding, which stems from the sheared mucosal capillaries and even the larger submucosal vessels.

Gastrointestinal hemorrhage may be clinically apparent or occult. Occult hemorrhage may cause iron deficiency anemia secondary to chronic blood loss. Upper gastrointestinal bleeding that leads to a mixing of blood with hydrochloric acid in the stomach will result in melena (from the Greek *melas,* meaning "black"). Massive bleeding from the stomach, duodenum, or esophagus may cause vomiting of blood, called **hematemesis.** Bleeding from the rectum is called **hematochezia.**

8. The gastrointestinal tract is an important source of enzymes, hormones, and biologically active polypeptides. Each portion of the gastrointestinal tract produces unique biologically active substances. For example, the intestines secrete immunoglobulin A (IgA), which has an important role in mucosal immunity. The stomach secretes the intrinsic factor, which is essential for the absorption of vitamin B_{12}. The small intestines synthesize chylomicrons and release them into the blood circulation, which is essential for the transport of absorbed food lipids to the liver. Loss of these anatomic parts (i.e., from resection of the stomach or intestine) affects the well-being of the entire body.

Some intestinal secretory products may be used as markers of disease. For example, the fetal intestinal cells secrete a complex glycoprotein called **carcinoembryonic antigen (CEA),** which is not produced by the normal intestine. CEA is produced by adenocarcinomas of the intestine, and it can be measured in the serum of adult patients. CEA is thus a valuable tumor marker.

TABLE 10-2	Incidence and Mortality from Malignant Tumors of the Gastrointestinal System, Liver, and Pancreas in the United States	
Organ	**Incidence**	**Mortality**
Large intestine	150,000	55,000
Pancreas	33,000	32,000
Oral cavity and pharynx	31,000	7,500
Stomach	22,000	11,000
Liver and biliary system	18,000	16,000
Esophagus	16,000	14,500

NOTE: Data are based on 200 reports for 2008. The figures have been rounded up and thus represent approximations.

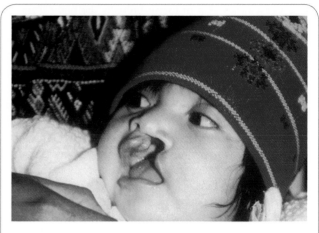

Figure 10-2 Cleft lip. The upper lip is separated into two parts by a cleft.

9. The gastrointestinal tract is exposed to environmental carcinogens in food. Carcinomas of the gastrointestinal tract are among the most common human malignant diseases (Table 10-2). It is believed that carcinogens in food play an important pathogenetic role and are directly responsible for most of these malignant diseases. Differences in diet account for many of the differences in the incidence of various cancers in various parts of the world. For example, **colorectal cancer** is the most important gastrointestinal cancer in the United States. The incidence of gastric carcinoma, which was very common a century ago in the United States, has decreased here, but it is still high in Japan.

DISEASES OF THE ORAL CAVITY

The most important diseases of the oral cavity are *dental caries, periodontal disease,* and cancer. Developmental defects can also affect the oral cavity, as can other inflammatory diseases.

DEVELOPMENTAL ABNORMALITIES

Cleft lip is a congenital abnormality that occurs with increased frequency in some families; it is considered to be inherited as a polygenic trait. It results from a lack of fusion of the fetal nasal and maxillary processes that form the upper lip (Figure 10-2). It may be associated with cleft palate, in which a fissure forms between the mouth and the nasal cavity. Cleft lip is more common in males than in females.

Teeth abnormalities are common. These may involve delayed or irregular dentition and abnormally shaped or abnormally positioned teeth, such as impacted wisdom teeth.

INFLAMMATION

Bacterial infection leads to tooth decay known as *dental caries.* Bacterial infections also affect the gums and tissue surrounding the tooth, thus causing **periodontal disease.** Inflammation of the oral mucosa is called *stomatitis.*

DENTAL CARIES

Dental caries (from the Latin *caries,* meaning "dry rot") is one of the most common diseases of humans. It is most prevalent in children and adolescents, but it occurs in older persons as well. Caries has been considered a disease of modern civilization, but archeologists have demonstrated caries in ancient Egyptian mummies and the frozen remains of Neanderthal men as well. Lifestyle and diet probably influence the development of caries, because the disease is less prevalent among Eskimos and some jungle dwellers of South America. Widespread fluoridation of water has decreased the occurrence of caries in the United States.

Dental caries is a multifactorial disease mediated by oral saprophytic bacteria. The predisposition to caries varies from one person to another, and it may have a genetic basis. Resistance to caries can be bolstered by fluoridation of the drinking water. It is thought that fluoride promotes formation of enamel that has increased resistance to bacteria. Saliva that contains various antimicrobial substances, such as lysozyme and lactoferrin, provides additional protection. Xerostomia is associated with an increased incidence of caries. Dental hygiene, involving regular brushing and flossing of teeth, also reduces caries. This reduction is achieved by removing the bacteria and by preventing the formation of bacterial *plaque.* Sugar-containing food should be avoided, because the bacterial action on teeth is facilitated by lactic acid formed locally from carbohydrates in food.

Caries begins after the bacteria that are forming plaque on the surface of the tooth have eroded the enamel (Figure 10-3).

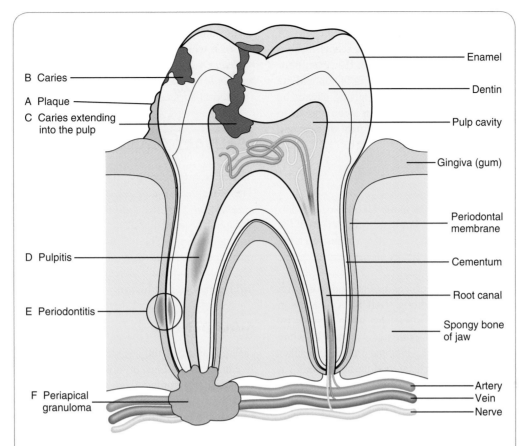

B Caries

A Plaque

C Caries extending into the pulp

D Pulpitis

E Periodontitis

F Periapical granuloma

Enamel

Dentin

Pulp cavity

Gingiva (gum)

Periodontal membrane

Cementum

Root canal

Spongy bone of jaw

Artery
Vein
Nerve

Figure 10-3 Dental and periodontal diseases. Caries begins as a bacterial plaque *(A)*, which leads to a defect in the enamel *(B)*. Deeper defects allow the entry of bacteria into the pulp cavity *(C)*. Pulpitis is a bacterial infection that may extend into the root canal *(D)*. Periodontal disease is caused by bacteria that colonize the gingival pockets *(E)*. Extension of infection into the periapical bone leads to the formation of periapical granuloma *(F)*.

The defect extends into the dentin, which becomes decalcified and disintegrates, allowing the bacteria to penetrate deep into the tooth and invade the pulp chamber. Because the inside of the tooth contains nerves and blood vessels, pulpitis and inflammation of the root canal are accompanied by pain.

Superficial caries and pulpitis may be treated and the affected tooth salvaged. However, if the infection extends into the root canal, it evokes an inflammatory response in the periodontal tissue known as *periapical granuloma*. Massive suppuration is accompanied by formation of a *periapical abscess,* and this may extend into the jaws, provoking bone infection *(osteomyelitis)*. These complications of caries usually require extraction of the tooth and often jaw surgery with antibiotic coverage. Less extensive disease may heal spontaneously; in such cases the periapical granuloma or abscess is transformed into a *pseudocyst* (i.e., a cavity lined by granulation tissue and filled with fluid). The ingrowth of the gum epithelium may transform the granuloma cavity into a cyst lined by squamous epithelium *(radicular cyst)*.

PERIODONTAL DISEASE

Periodontal inflammation *(periodontitis)* is a common disease, accounting for more tooth loss than caries and all other dental diseases combined. It is related to the colonization of periodontal pockets with bacteria. This leads to the formation of plaque, which calcifies and transforms into *tartar.* Bacteria, plaque, and tartar together cause inflammation of the overlying gingiva, which loosens the tooth ligaments and allows bacterial invasion of the tooth socket and the root canal. This impedes the blood supply to the pulp and devitalizes the tooth. The gums are initially swollen and tender, but as the infection progresses, loosening of teeth occurs. Loss of teeth and massive inflammation of the gums predominate in chronic cases. Profuse infection may cause oozing of pus from the gums *(pyorrhea)*.

Although the mouth flora contains more than 300 bacterial species, periodontitis is caused in most instances by only three species. These pathogens carry almost unpronounceable names, which are listed here just in case you want to show off your erudition *(Aggregatibacter actinomycetemcomitans,*

Porphyromonas gingivalis, and *Prevotella intermedia).* It is not known why these microbes colonize the mouth cavity of some individuals and spare others, but there seems to be a familial predisposition to periodontal disease. However, poor oral hygiene is the most common predisposing factor, and the importance of regular teeth and mouth cleansing cannot be overemphasized. Preventive dental care has been shown to significantly reduce the incidence of periodontal disease and prevent tooth loss.

STOMATITIS

Stomatitis is an inflammation of the mouth. It often occurs during the course of systemic disease, but it may also represent the only sign of infection. It is caused by various viruses, bacteria, and fungi. Herpesvirus infection typically causes vesicles on the lips that may extend into the mouth. *C. albicans stomatitis* (thrush) is common in debilitated cancer patients and those with acquired immunodeficiency syndrome (AIDS). Colonization with *C. albicans* can also occur in patients using steroids by metered dose inhaler for bronchial asthma. It is marked by white surface layers covering the mucosa. *Aphthous stomatitis* (canker sores) are painful, recurrent, superficial, oral ulcers of unknown etiology that cause considerable distress but heal spontaneously.

ORAL CANCER

Oral cancer is common and may involve the lips, tongue, soft palate, or just about any other structure in the mouth (Figure 10-4). It is a well-known complication of smoking, especially pipe smoking, and of chewing tobacco. Chronic alcoholism is also a risk factor. Males predominate among patients with lip carcinoma (10:1) and those with carcinoma of the oral cavity (2:1). The average age at diagnosis is 55 to 60 years.

Carcinoma of the lips and oral cavity presents in the form of mucosal abnormalities, such as the following:

- *Leukoplakia,* a white, slightly elevated plaque that covers the mucosal surface

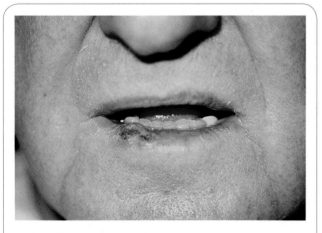

Figure 10-4 Carcinoma of the lip. On gross examination the tumor appears to be ulcerated.

- *Erythroplakia,* a red plaque that appears distinct from the surrounding mucosa
- *Ulcer,* which appears as a shallow defect
- *Crater,* which appears as a defect with raised margins
- *Nodule or plaque,* an induration that protrudes from the mucosal surface

SALIVARY GLAND DISEASES

Saliva is produced by major and minor salivary glands. There are three major salivary glands: the *parotid,* the *submandibular,* and the *sublingual*—each of which is paired and readily identifiable by palpation or gross examination during surgery. The small salivary glands are scattered throughout the oral cavity, mostly on the floor of the mouth. The most important diseases of the salivary glands are inflammations and tumors.

SIALADENITIS

Inflammation of the salivary glands is called **sialadenitis.** It can be infectious or immunologically mediated. Infections usually spread from the mouth. *Staphylococcus aureus* and *Streptococcus viridans* are the most common causes of suppurative sialadenitis. *Mumps* is the most common viral infection. Enlargement of the salivary glands in children is a typical feature of mumps. Mumps is less common in adults.

Infections cause pain and enlargement of the salivary glands, the latter usually being asymmetric. Functionally the disease may present with *sialorrhea* (i.e., overproduction of saliva) or *xerostomia* (dry mouth). Acute sialadenitis typically heals on its own and has few residual effects. Chronic sialadenitis of infectious origin is rare and usually represents a complication of salivary duct obstruction. This may be caused by periductal fibrosis or ductal stones, a condition known as *sialolithiasis* (from the Greek *sialos,* meaning "saliva," and *lithos,* meaning "stone").

Immunologically mediated sialadenitis is a typical feature of Sjögren's syndrome. This autoimmune disease presents with systemic symptoms but invariably involves the salivary or the lacrimal glands. *Xerostomia* and *xerophthalmia* (dry eyes) are thus typical symptoms. Enlargement of the glands is attributable to infiltrates of lymphocytes and plasma cells, which slowly replace the normal acinar cells and ultimately cause glandular insufficiency. In the later stages of the disease, the glands become fibrotic and shrink in size. An increased incidence of lymphoma has been reported in patients with salivary glands affected by Sjögren's syndrome.

NEOPLASMS

Tumors of the salivary glands are not common. Their peak incidence is in patients who are 40 to 60 years of age. These tumors may originate from either the major or the minor salivary glands. The parotid gland, which is the largest of all, is involved most often. Two additional facts worth remembering are as follows:

- Tumors of the major salivary glands are more often benign than malignant. Only 25% of these tumors are malignant, whereas 50% of the tumors in the minor salivary glands are malignant. However, even the benign tumors are often difficult to remove without mutilating surgery or transection of nerves. If incompletely removed, they tend to recur. Follow-up is thus important for all patients with salivary gland tumors.

- *Pleomorphic adenoma* is the most common histologic tumor type, accounting for 70% of all tumors in the major salivary glands and 50% of tumors in the minor salivary glands. It is benign and composed of epithelial and myoepithelial cells and areas resembling cartilage (hence the name pleomorphic adenoma). In a small number of cases, pleomorphic adenoma may evolve into carcinoma.

Salivary gland tumors present as slow-growing masses, compressing the normal facial structures and often causing pain. Surgery is the treatment of choice. Although recurrences are common, the overall prognosis is excellent.

DISEASES OF THE ESOPHAGUS

The most important diseases of the esophagus are *esophagitis,* circulatory disturbances, and neoplasms. Typical symptoms of esophageal disease include the following:

- *Dysphagia,* or difficulty in swallowing. This includes an inability to initiate swallowing and the sensation that the swallowed food cannot pass. Some patients have true obstruction to the passage of food.
- Esophageal pain. This may present as a colic (a spasmodic substernal pain) that occurs spontaneously, presumably as a result of muscular spasm, or it may present as retrosternal burning ("heartburn").
- Aspiration and regurgitation of food and liquids. Food or liquid may reenter the oral cavity from the esophagus and reach the lower respiratory tract.

DEVELOPMENTAL ABNORMALITIES

The most important developmental anomaly involving the esophagus is congenital *atresia* (lack of lumen), an abnormality that presents shortly after birth and is often associated with abnormal connections between the esophagus and trachea *(esophagotracheal fistula)* (Figure 10-5). Because food cannot pass into the stomach, affected babies vomit ingested milk. If the defect is not repaired, these babies die of hunger or aspiration pneumonia.

HIATAL HERNIA

Several conditions predispose individuals to gastroesophageal reflux. The most common cause of reflux esophagitis is **hiatal hernia.** It occurs in several forms (e.g., sliding hiatal

hernia or paraesophageal hernia), all of which lead to displacement of the cardiac portion of the stomach from the abdominal cavity into the thoracic cavity through the diaphragmatic hiatus. Hiatal hernia alters the function of the LES and facilitates reflux of gastric juice into the esophagus. The tone of the LES also may be reduced by smoking and caffeine. Heartburn is common in pregnancy, which causes physiologic relaxation of the LES.

MOTILITY DISORDERS OF THE ESOPHAGUS

A large number of functional motility problems affect the esophagus. These disorders have no visible pathologic substrate but can be diagnosed by measuring the pressure inside the esophagus (by manometry) or by barium swallow examination with x-ray studies. The best known of these disorders is the *nutcracker esophagus,* named so because of its typical wavy appearance on radiographs. Scleroderma, a connective tissue disease characterized by replacement of the smooth muscle of the esophagus with fibrous tissue, also causes motility problems.

Achalasia (from the Greek term meaning "lack of relaxation") is the antithesis of LES insufficiency. Achalasia is marked by a spasm of the LES, a dilation of the esophagus proximal to the site of the spasm, and an inability to swallow food *(dysphagia).* In most instances, achalasia is idiopathic.

ESOPHAGITIS

Esophagitis, or inflammation of the esophagus, may be caused by the following:

- Infection
- Reflux of gastric juice ("peptic esophagitis")
- Exogenous irritants, chemicals, and drugs

Infectious esophagitis is typically caused by viruses or fungi, and it occurs usually in immunosuppressed or debilitated persons. Normal squamous epithelium is resistant to pathogens, and the rapid passage of food through the esophagus does not favor contact between the pathogens and the mucosa, so infections usually do not take place. However, if the general health or the immune response of the patient has been compromised, infections may occur. Such infections are caused by viruses, such as herpesvirus or cytomegalovirus, or fungi, such as *C. albicans.* These infections produce superficial lesions (shallow ulcers). Bacterial infections are uncommon in the intact esophagus but may become superimposed on viral or fungal ulcerations.

Peptic esophagitis is caused by a reflux of gastric juice into the esophagus. Normally the LES prevents the reflux of gastric juices into the esophagus. However, if the function of the sphincter is compromised, reflux may occur and ulcerations of the esophagus mediated by pepsin and hydrochloric acid may develop.

Peptic esophagitis is histologically characterized by nonspecific inflammation and ulceration of the squamous epithelium. The defects are often repaired by metaplastic epithelium

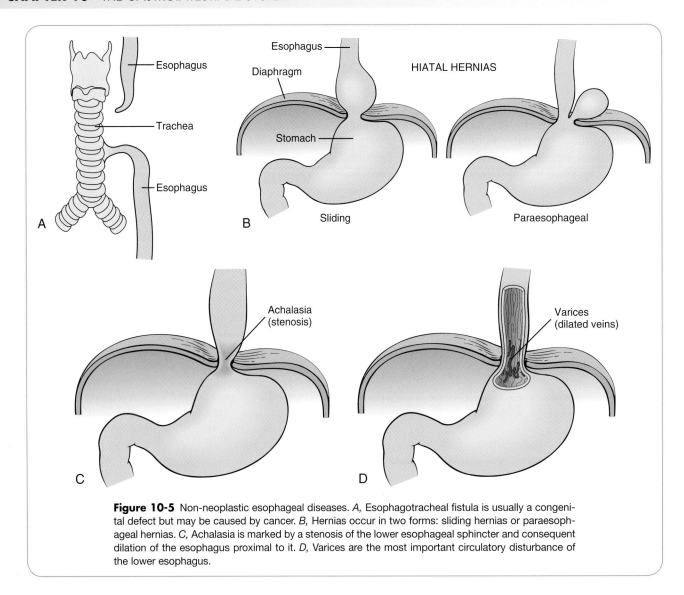

Figure 10-5 Non-neoplastic esophageal diseases. *A,* Esophagotracheal fistula is usually a congenital defect but may be caused by cancer. *B,* Hernias occur in two forms: sliding hernias or paraesophageal hernias. *C,* Achalasia is marked by a stenosis of the lower esophageal sphincter and consequent dilation of the esophagus proximal to it. *D,* Varices are the most important circulatory disturbance of the lower esophagus.

that appears glandular and resembles the columnar epithelium of the stomach or intestine. Foci of esophageal mucosa, composed of metaplastic glandular epithelium, are called **Barrett's esophagus.** This mucosa is more sensitive to injury than normal squamous epithelium and may give rise to peptic ulcers, which are indistinguishable from similar ulcers in the stomach. Furthermore, Barrett's esophagus is a risk factor for cancer, which develops in a significant number of patients.

Chemical esophagitis, caused by accidental swallowing of inorganic acids or lyes, is typically encountered in children. Suicide attempts are another cause of such changes. Esophagitis may also be caused mechanically by permanently placed nasogastric tubes that are used for feeding terminally ill patients.

CIRCULATORY DISTURBANCES

Circulatory disturbances of the esophagus are important because they may cause hematemesis. Esophageal varices, typically caused by cirrhosis of the liver and other diseases marked by portal hypertension, are among the most common causes of upper gastrointestinal bleeding and are associated with high mortality. Laceration of the small blood vessels at the gastrointestinal junction is typical of the *Mallory-Weiss syndrome,* a clinical syndrome marked by hematemesis. Mallory-Weiss syndrome is caused by tears in the mucosa that occur during strenuous vomiting. Understandably, it is most often encountered in alcoholics.

CARCINOMA OF THE ESOPHAGUS

Carcinoma of the esophagus is the most important neoplasm of the esophagus. Benign tumors of the esophagus, such as leiomyoma or neurofibroma, are rare and thus do not warrant detailed consideration.

Although less common than other major gastrointestinal cancers, it is still an important malignant lesion because of its extremely unfavorable prognosis. In certain parts of the world, such as China, Iran, and South Africa, the incidence of esophageal cancer is 10 to 15 times higher than that in the

United States. In those countries it is one of the most common cancers.

The etiology and pathogenesis of esophageal cancer are poorly understood. The best clues about the origin of esophageal cancer are derived from epidemiologic studies. Interesting epidemiologic data include the following:

- Geographic differences. The high incidence of esophageal cancer in China, Iran, and South Africa points to a possible carcinogen in the soil or food. In China even the domestic fowl have a high incidence of esophageal cancer, a fact that further points to some potential environmental carcinogens in the soil.
- Racial differences. For unknown reasons, esophageal cancer is three times more common in blacks than in whites in the United States.
- Gender differences. The male to female ratio is 4:1 in the United States. In China and South Africa, males and females are affected equally.
- Correlation with tobacco and alcohol abuse. In the United States a large number of patients with esophageal cancer have a documented history of chronic alcoholism and tobacco use.

Pathology

Most carcinomas originate from the lower portion of the esophagus. Tumors tend to grow into the lumen as endophytic masses or to infiltrate the wall as a result of exophytic growth. The part of the esophagus that is infiltrated with tumor is usually indurated and ulcerated (Figure 10-6), which accounts for the associated pain on swallowing, dysphagia, and bleeding.

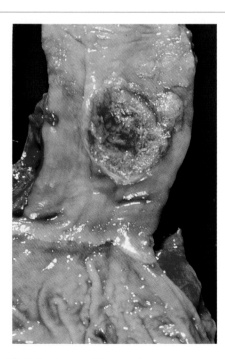

Figure 10-6 Carcinoma of the esophagus appears as an indurated mucosal defect.

Esophageal tumors are locally invasive. By the time of diagnosis, most tumors have already spread through the adventitia into the lymph nodes and the surrounding mediastinal organs. Distant metastases are a late event. Histologically, almost all upper and middle esophageal cancers are squamous cell carcinomas. In the lower third, adenocarcinomas originating in Barrett's esophagus predominate, but even here approximately 40% of cancers are squamous cell carcinomas.

Clinical Features

The clinical symptoms of esophageal cancer include dysphagia, pain, and, occasionally, bleeding or malodorous breath. Patients have pain upon swallowing, and as the obstruction becomes more severe, they are unable to ingest any solid food at all. The diagnosis is established by barium swallow x-ray examination or esophagoscopy accompanied by biopsy. The prognosis is dismal. Less than 25% of patients survive 5 years.

DISEASES OF THE STOMACH AND DUODENUM

The most important diseases of the stomach are *gastritis*, peptic ulcer, and carcinoma. The symptoms of gastric diseases include the following:

- Pain. This is typically related to ulceration of the mucosa, the caustic action of hydrochloric acid, and the enzymatic action of pepsin in the gastric juice.
- Vomiting. Obstruction of the exit portion of the stomach (pylorus) or irritation and disturbed motor function of the gastric musculature result in vomiting. Vomiting is based on a reflex, and although it is an important and common finding in gastric diseases, it may occur in other diseases of the upper gastrointestinal tract and in many systemic and central nervous system disorders; it may even be initiated voluntarily.
- Bleeding. Gastric ulceration may lead to *hematemesis* or **melena.**
- Dyspepsia. Abnormal function of the stomach may result in digestive problems, such as the inability to digest food. This may be associated with nausea, loss of appetite, or aversion to food.
- Systemic consequences. For example, chronic bleeding ulcers may cause iron deficiency anemia. Lack of intrinsic factor, a gastric protein essential for the absorption of vitamin B_{12}, results in pernicious anemia.

DEVELOPMENTAL ABNORMALITIES

Developmental abnormalities of the stomach and duodenum are rare. The most important is congenital stenosis of the pylorus. Symptoms appear early in the neonatal period. Boys are affected four times more often than girls are. Stenosis prevents emptying of the stomach and results in projectile vomiting. Surgical correction by incision of the contracted gastric muscle usually relieves the symptoms and permanently cures the disease.

GASTRITIS

Gastritis may be classified as acute or chronic. *Acute gastritis (erosive gastritis)* is a self-limiting disease of short duration that usually heals spontaneously. In contrast, *chronic gastritis,* which is also known as *nonerosive gastritis,* lasts longer.

Acute gastritis is characterized by shallow mucosal defects limited to the upper layers of the epithelium. These defects are called *erosions* if they are superficial or *ulcers* if they are somewhat deeper and extend through the entire thickness of the mucosa.

Mucosal erosions and ulceration of the stomach develop under a variety of circumstances, the most important of which are circulatory disturbances and exposure to exogenous irritants. Circulatory disturbances, such as shock, typically change the blood flow through the gastric mucosa, rendering the superficial parts of the mucosa ischemic and thus making the mucosa susceptible to the adverse effects of gastric juices. This may result in multiple superficial bleeding erosions (acute erosive gastritis), or deeper ulcerations. *Curling's ulcers,* which extend through the entire mucosa and cause profound bleeding, are related to extensive burns of external body surfaces. *Cushing's ulcers* (named after the famous neurosurgeon who described them in patients with brain tumors) are large stress ulcers. These ulcers heal if the circulatory disturbances that have caused them are corrected. On the other hand, they may persist in terminally ill patients and are often found at autopsy.

Exogenous irritants that cause gastritis include several drugs, alcohol, and chemicals ingested by accident or suicidally. The most important among these is aspirin, which often causes superficial erosions in the stomach.

Chronic gastritis is a term used to describe several pathologic processes with differing pathogenesis. Most often it presents as atrophic gastritis, with or without intestinal metaplasia, but it may occur also in a hyperplastic form. In both forms there are signs of chronic mucosal inflammation.

The cause of chronic gastritis is unknown. The disease is more common in older persons. In some cases, as in pernicious anemia, chronic atrophic gastritis is probably mediated by an immunologic mechanism. In others it may be related to infection with Helicobacter pylori. The disease is much more common in some countries, such as Japan, China, and East European countries, than in the United States.

Chronic gastritis produces mild digestive symptoms related to gastric atrophy and reduced secretion of pepsin and hydrochloric acid. The symptoms are usually nonspecific and are labeled as *dyspepsia* ("indigestion"). Immune-mediated gastric atrophy results in reduced production of the intrinsic factor and impaired absorption of vitamin B_{12}. Vitamin B_{12} deficiency results in pernicious anemia and a variety of neurologic symptoms. Immune-mediated gastric atrophy and concomitant gastric metaplasia also predispose affected individuals to gastric cancer.

PEPTIC ULCER

Peptic ulcer is a chronic multifactorial disease characterized by mucosal ulceration that extends through the entire gastric epithelial layer and into the muscularis. It can occur in any part of the gastrointestinal tract exposed to peptic juice. Most often it is located in the duodenum or the stomach; less often it involves the esophagus and small intestine. Peptic ulcer is a very common disease, affecting approximately 4 million people in the United States at any one time. It accounts for 10% of all the money spent for the treatment of gastrointestinal diseases. Approximately 1% to 2% of all Americans have a peptic ulcer during their life span.

Etiology and Pathogenesis

The etiology and pathogenesis of peptic ulcer are poorly understood, although there is general agreement that several factors play a crucial role. These include the following:

- Gastric juice. Peptic ulcer develops only in parts of the gastrointestinal tract that are exposed to pepsin and hydrochloric acid. The dictum "no acid, no ulcer" still holds true. Inhibition of gastric secretion with histamine-2 (H_2) blockers, such as cimetidine, promotes ulcer healing.
- Mucosal barrier. The normal gastric and duodenal mucosa are resistant to the chemical and enzymatic action of gastric juice. Reduced resistance and frank breakdown of the mucosal barrier occur under a variety of conditions, such as shock and even prolonged psychological stress. Smoking and alcohol also have adverse effects. Drugs, such as aspirin or nonsteroidal anti-inflammatory drugs (NSAIDs), cause mucosal erosions and shallow ulcers.
- *H. pylori* infection. *H. pylori* is found in the stomach or duodenum of most patients with peptic ulcer. Eradication of the bacterial infection with antibiotics can cure ulcers in most instances.

In patients who are genetically predisposed (50% of duodenal patients have a family history), the disease can evolve under a variety of circumstances. For example, hyperacidity of the gastric juice, coupled with rapid emptying of the stomach, may overburden the duodenum. Because the acid cannot be neutralized, it destroys the mucosa, causing duodenal ulcer. Atrophy of the gastric mucosa in antral gastritis also predisposes the patient to ulceration. A stressful lifestyle, smoking, and chronic intake of aspirin and other NSAIDs promote ulcer formation. Corticosteroids are ulcerogenic if taken as medication, and they are probably also important when internally oversecreted. Gastrin, a polypeptide hormone that stimulates the secretion of hydrochloric acid, is a well-known cause of ulcers in some patients. Psychological stress and vagal stimulation of gastric secretions and motility can also have an adverse effect. Thus it is best to consider peptic ulcer as an imbalance between the adverse influences that could damage the mucosal barrier and the protective forces that preserve its integrity.

Pathology

All peptic ulcers have the same typical appearance, regardless of their location. They appear as sharply punched-out, round defects of the mucosa extending into the deep layers of the stomach or duodenum. The bottom of the ulcer consists of glandular amorphous material formed from tissue destruction by hydrochloric acid and occasionally from larger blood vessels that have an eroded wall and appear gaping (Figure 10-7). The caustic action of the hydrochloric acid keeps the bottom of the ulcer "clean" and devoid of necrotic tissue. The margins of the ulcer seem to be sharp, in contrast to ulcerated carcinomas of the stomach, which have irregular margins and a necrotic shaggy surface.

Histologically the ulcers vary in appearance, which usually reflects the duration of the disease. Acute ulcers and those of short duration are shallower and show little healing. On the other hand, chronic ulcers extend deeper into the muscle layer where they evoke tissue response. In a cross-sectioned ulcer, one can actually recognize several layers, including, from top to bottom: (1) surface composed of necrotic tissue, (2) a zone of acute and chronic inflammation, (3) vascular granulation tissue, and (4) fibrous scar tissue (see Figure 10-7, *B*).

Peptic ulcers can be cured with appropriate medication, especially in the early stages of the disease. In some cases, the disease is resistant to treatment. The most important complications of such chronic ulcers are as follows:

- *Hemorrhage.* Hemorrhage is common in all peptic ulcers. However, it is usually mild, causing melena rather than hematemesis. Large ulcers may erode arteries in the wall of the stomach and duodenum, causing massive and occasionally even lethal hemorrhage. Such arterial bleedings represent an emergency and require gastroscopic or even open surgical intervention.
- *Penetration.* Peptic ulcers of the duodenum can erode the entire wall and penetrate into the pancreas. This is typically associated with intractable pain and reactive, smoldering pancreatitis.
- *Perforation.* Duodenal ulcers may extend through the intestinal wall and form a hole. Intestinal contents pass through this hole into the peritoneal cavity and cause *peritonitis.* This is also a surgical emergency. Such perforations can be sutured, but the peritonitis may be much more difficult to treat with antibiotics.
- *Cicatrization.* Healing of duodenal ulcers is occasionally associated with extensive scarring, which may cause *intestinal stenosis* (narrowing) or obstruction.

Clinical Features

Most peptic ulcers are located in the distal portion of the stomach and the proximal duodenum. Duodenal ulcers are four times more common than gastric ulcers. Gastric ulcers affect persons older than age 50, whereas duodenal ulcers can occur any time during adult life and affect younger persons as well. The disease typically presents with pain 1 to 3 hours after a meal or during the night. The patient can typically point to the site of the maximum pain, which is usually in the midline of the epigastrium. The pain can be alleviated with alkaline agents or food but often recurs at regular intervals. Other symptoms are nonspecific and include nausea, vomiting, and loss of appetite or weight. Melena and associated iron deficiency anemia are common in chronic disease. Hematemesis and peritonitis are complications that could lead to death and therefore require vigorous treatment.

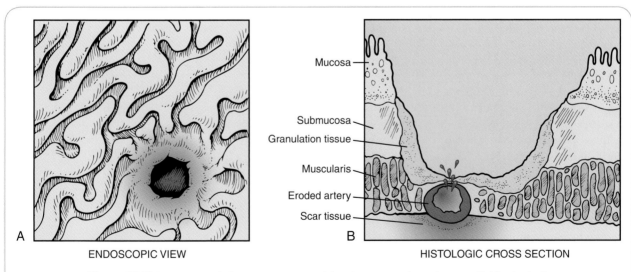

ENDOSCOPIC VIEW HISTOLOGIC CROSS SECTION

Figure 10-7 Peptic ulcer. *A,* Gross appearance of the ulcer as seen by endoscopy. *B,* Histologically the bottom of the ulcer replacing the mucosa consists mostly of granulation tissue and admixed necrotic cell debris and inflammatory cells. Peptic ulcer may bleed from eroded mucosal blood vessels. The tissue underlying the ulcer shows fibrosis and scarring.

The treatment of peptic ulcer is based on eradication of *H. pylori* infection and suppression of gastric acid secretion with H_2 antagonists, such as cimetidine. Peptic ulcers have a tendency to recur, but overall the prognosis for cure is excellent and major complications requiring surgery are rare.

GASTRIC NEOPLASMS

Benign epithelial tumors, known as *hyperplastic* and *adenomatous polyps,* are mostly asymptomatic. These tumors are usually discovered during gastroscopy performed for some other, unrelated reason. Although gastric polyps are rare, their significance is twofold:

- These benign tumors may progress to carcinoma and are actually 10 times more common in patients with pernicious anemia (another condition that predisposes to cancer) than in the population at large.
- Gastric polyps may be associated with cancer in adjacent mucosa. The discovery of a polyp warrants a detailed search for carcinoma.

CARCINOMA OF THE STOMACH

Carcinoma of the stomach is the most important neoplasm of the stomach, and it accounts for 90% of all malignant tumors in this organ. Other malignant neoplasms, such as lymphoma, gastrointestinal stromal tumors (GISTs), and smooth cell tumors *(leiomyosarcoma),* represent the remaining 10% of these tumors.

The incidence of gastric cancer has decreased significantly in the United States over the past 70 years. In the United States the incidence is now 10 per 1 million, which is approximately 8 times lower than the incidence in Japan or Chile. The fact that U.S. immigrants from these high-prevalence areas have a lower incidence of gastric cancer than their relatives or predecessors in the country of their origin suggests a possible role for environmental carcinogens. Most likely the exogenous carcinogens are in the food. However, none of these has yet been identified.

Etiology and Pathogenesis

Most studies of possible environmental carcinogens have concentrated on *nitrosamines,* which are known to produce cancer in animals. It has been proposed that the current American diet contains less nitrosamines than before. Previously, when most food was not refrigerated, bacterial overgrowth could indeed have generated excessive nitrosamines in such food. Smoked fish, consumed in some of the countries with a high incidence of gastric cancer, contains more nitrosamines than most cooked fish eaten in the United States. Furthermore, the current methods of food processing in the United States eliminate many potentially dangerous bacteria. Bacteria can convert nitrates to nitrites that in turn are the source of carcinogenic nitrosamines. Prevention of bacterial growth and proper food processing may be instrumental in gastric cancer prevention.

Environmental carcinogens probably act in concert with several endogenous factors that are poorly understood. Atrophic gastritis, pernicious anemia, and gastric adenomatous polyps carry an increased risk, but the pathogenic chain of events linking these conditions to cancer has not been elucidated.

Pathology

Most carcinomas are found in the distal stomach (i.e., pylorus and antrum). Cardia is involved in 25% of cases. Early gastric carcinoma begins as a mucosal lesion that may be raised, indented, or ulcerated. Once an invasive carcinoma develops, four growth patterns can be recognized (Figure 10-8):

- Superficial
- Polypoid
- Ulcerating
- Diffusely infiltrating

Superficial cancers resemble those in the early preinvasive stages and are typically flat. Polypoid tumors protrude into the lumen of the stomach. Ulcerating tumors resemble peptic ulcers but are usually more irregular in shape and larger. They may resemble craters that have indurated margins around a central ulceration. Diffusely infiltrating tumors permeate the gastric wall and transform it into a leather-bottle–like, stiff organ. This type of cancer is also called *linitis plastica.*

Microscopically, all gastric carcinomas are *adenocarcinomas.* Some tumors are composed of well-formed glandular structures (so-called intestinal type of adenocarcinoma), whereas others are poorly differentiated and highly invasive (diffuse type). Diffuse-type adenocarcinoma is usually composed of "signet-ring" cells, so called because the mucin

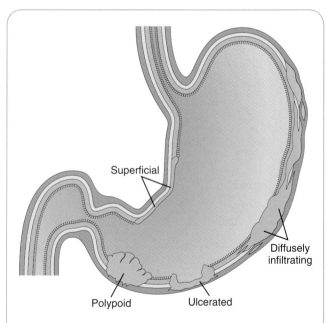

Figure 10-8 Gastric cancer. Tumors may present as superficial, polypoid, ulcerated, or diffuse carcinoma.

filling the cytoplasm displaces the nucleus to the periphery and gives the cell the appearance of a signet ring.

Gastric carcinomas metastasize to regional lymph nodes and to the liver. Through the thoracic duct, gastric carcinoma often reaches the supraclavicular lymph nodes on the left, which are called *Virchow's nodes,* in honor of the German pathologist who recognized these metastases as a characteristic sign of gastric carcinoma. Carcinoma of the stomach can also spread to other abdominal organs and to the lungs. Bilateral involvement of the ovaries, occasionally recognized by gynecologists as *Krukenberg's tumor,* is a rare but characteristic presenting sign of gastric carcinoma that has metastasized to the ovaries.

Clinical Features

Carcinoma of the stomach presents with nonspecific symptoms. Because patients do not usually seek medical assistance early, by the time of diagnosis most tumors are in advanced stages and thus are inoperable. Symptoms include nonspecific signs of tumor growth, such as weight loss, anemia, and weakness. Local tumor growth provokes gastric irritation, vomiting, loss of appetite, and dysphagia. Ulceration leads to bleeding. Sometimes the tumors are diagnosed on the basis of distant metastases, such as to the supraclavicular lymph nodes or ovaries.

Gastric carcinoma carries a very poor prognosis, except for patients diagnosed with early or preinvasive carcinoma. The 5-year survival rate is less than 20%. Active screening for gastric cancer, involving systematic gastroscopies combined with gastric brushing and cytologic examination, is widely used in Japan with most encouraging results. Early detection of gastric cancer by these techniques and an early gastrectomy seem to be the only way to combat this cancer.

GASTROINTESTINAL LYMPHOMA

Lymphomas may involve the gastrointestinal tract in the course of dissemination of disease that usually begins in the lymph nodes or the bone marrow. In contrast to these secondary gastrointestinal lymphomas, some tumors begin in the stomach or the intestines and are therefore called *primary gastrointestinal lymphomas.* These tumors originate in the mucosa-associated lymphoid tissue (MALT) and typically present as localized masses, which can be resected surgically. Most **MALTomas** of the stomach are related to *H. pylori* infection, which obviously plays a pathogenetic role in the development of these tumors. It is also worth remembering that the stomach is the most common site of gastrointestinal lymphomas. Gastrointestinal lymphomas are found in the stomach in 60% of cases; in 25% of cases, in the small intestine; and in 10%, the large intestine.

DISEASES OF THE SMALL AND LARGE INTESTINE

The most important diseases of the intestines are infections, idiopathic inflammations, vascular disturbances, obstructions of the lumen or changes in the wall of the intestine

(e.g., diverticulosis), various forms of malabsorption, and tumors.

DEVELOPMENTAL ABNORMALITIES

In view of the length of the intestines, it is remarkable that developmental abnormalities do not occur more often; of those that do occur, only a few are clinically significant.

Atresia of the intestine—that is, complete obstruction of the lumen—can occur in any part of the intestine. It can be surgically resected, with end-to-end anastomosis of uninvolved intestinal segments. *Atresia of the anus* prevents defecation but also can be corrected surgically.

Hirschsprung's disease is an abnormality in the innervation of the rectum and the sigmoid colon. Because the intramural ganglion cells do not develop, the segment of the intestine lacking innervation remains in a permanent spasm (Figure 10-9). This spasm prevents the passage of feces that accumulate proximal to the obstructed segment, causing dilation of the large intestine *(megacolon).* The aganglionic segment must be resected with an end-to-end anastomosis of the proximal and distal normal intestine. Such operations usually relieve all symptoms.

Congenital diverticula are outpouchings of the intestine. The best known of these is **Meckel's diverticulum,** which represents an incompletely obliterated embryonic connection between the intestine and the umbilicus *(omphalomesenteric duct).* Like other diverticula, it may become filled with food and rupture, or it may become infected. Symptoms of Meckel's diverticulitis resemble those of acute appendicitis, except that the pain has its epicenter in the left lower quadrant (i.e., on the opposite side of appendicitis).

DIVERTICULOSIS

Diverticulosis is a disease characterized by the formation of diverticula (i.e., outpouchings of the intestinal wall). These diverticula may be solitary or multiple, congenital or acquired. Diverticula occur in all parts of the gastrointestinal tract, but from a clinical point of view the most important are those involving the sigmoid colon.

Diverticula of the sigmoid colon are protrusions of the mucosa and submucosa through a hole in the weakened wall of the large intestine (Figure 10-10). This usually occurs at the point where the arteries penetrate through the muscle wall from the subserosal space along the teniae coli. Diverticula typically occur in older persons, especially those with chronic constipation. The weakening of the intestinal wall at the point of arterial entry through the muscle layer, combined with increased intraluminal pressure generated by straining during defecation, contributes to evagination of the mucosa between the muscle fibers. Such outpouchings, which typically measure less than 1 cm in diameter, are easily obstructed with fecal material. Obstruction may cause bleeding or inflammation *(diverticulitis).*

Perforation of diverticula may lead to the formation of pericolonic abscesses, fistulas, or pericolonic fibrosis, all of

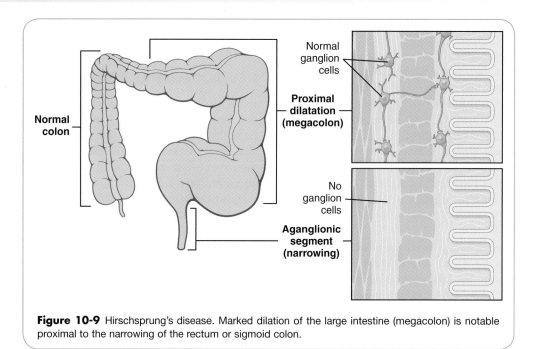

Figure 10-9 Hirschsprung's disease. Marked dilation of the large intestine (megacolon) is notable proximal to the narrowing of the rectum or sigmoid colon.

which are common complications of extensive diverticulitis. Massive pericolonic inflammation may encase the affected sigmoid colon and cause symptoms indistinguishable from those of carcinoma. Intestines that are severely deformed by diverticulitis may require surgical resection, which is often the only way to relieve intestinal obstruction.

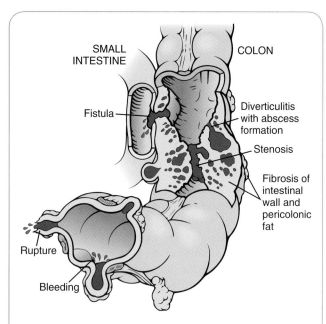

Figure 10-10 Diverticulosis of the colon. Complications include bleeding, abscess formation, perforation and rupture, fistula formation with adjacent structures (e.g., small intestine), and fibrosis extending into the pericolonic fat.

INTESTINAL VASCULAR DISEASES

Of the many vascular disorders of the intestine, only three prototypical diseases are discussed here: exemplifying venous, arteriovenous, and arterial lesions. These include the following conditions:

- Hemorrhoids
- Angiodysplasia of the intestines
- Ischemic bowel disease

HEMORRHOIDS

Hemorrhoids, or *piles,* are varicosities of the anal and perianal region that affect approximately 5% of all adults, and that means that millions of people require medical treatment for this disease. Lesions of the lower hemorrhoidal plexus (i.e., below the anorectal line) are called *external,* whereas those above the line are termed *internal* hemorrhoids. The pathogenesis of hemorrhoids is complex. A congenital, hereditary predisposition may be based on the looseness of connective tissue. For example, hemorrhoids are more common in persons whose parent also had hemorrhoids. An association between hemorrhoids and varicose veins of the lower extremities and inguinal hernias has also been noted. The increased pressure in the hemorrhoidal plexus plays an important role. This may be related to constipation and is often seen in pregnant women. Cirrhosis of the liver and other causes of portal hypertension also cause hemorrhoids because the veins of the hemorrhoidal plexus represent the site of anastomosis between the portal and the systemic circulation.

On gross examination, hemorrhoids appear as dilated veins or nodules filled with blood and thrombi. The mucosa overlying the thrombosed hemorrhoids may ulcerate, and bleeding is common. Protruding hemorrhoids may become incarcerated and infarcted. Surgical resection (closed or open hemorrhoidectomy) is a widely used treatment although there are newer techniques that seem more efficient, such as rubber band ligation or infrared coagulation of hemorrhoids, which also give very good results.

ANGIODYSPLASIA OF THE INTESTINES

Angiodysplasia of the intestines is a localized vascular lesion of the colon that may cause unexplained bleeding in elderly persons. It consists of dilated, thin-walled blood vessels that serve as an anastomosis between the arterial and venous circulation in the mucosa and submucosa of the colon. The reasons for the formation of dilated vascular channels are not known, and it is also not known why they occur preferentially in the cecum and the ascending colon. Recurrent bleeding from foci of angiodysplasia may be difficult to control, and resection of the involved intestine may be the only way to correct this condition.

ISCHEMIC BOWEL DISEASE

Ischemic bowel disease includes several disorders that compromise blood flow through segments of the intestine. Such ischemic changes may involve the entire thickness of the intestine and result in transmural infarction, or they may be limited to the mucosa.

 Did You Know?

Diverticula of the large intestine are common in elderly persons in Western Europe and in the United States but are less common in underdeveloped countries. This could possibly result from the higher prevalence of constipation in people who eat low-residue diets, as is often the case in the United States. Scientists have shown that the passage of intestinal contents is much faster in natives of Africa, who eat a lot of roughage, than in Americans, who eat sugar and rich and fatty foods. It has been suggested that increased roughage could protect against the development of colonic diverticula and also against colonic cancer. Many authorities believe that a bowl of bran every morning could "do the trick." Why not try it yourself?

Clinically these disorders are classified as chronic or acute. Chronic ischemia secondary to atherosclerosis of intestinal arteries is very common but often remains undiagnosed because it usually produces only nonspecific, mild symptoms. Acute obstruction is less common but is usually of sudden onset and associated with high mortality.

Pathologically, ischemic bowel disease can be classified as *occlusive* or *nonocclusive.* Occlusive disease is caused by thrombi or emboli, whereas nonocclusive disease is caused by atherosclerotic narrowing of arteries.

Thrombosis of the mesenteric arteries, usually a common complication of atherosclerosis, is the most important cause of transmural infarction. It typically affects the small intestine (Figure 10-11). The thrombus is most often found in the superior mesenteric artery. Under normal circumstances, occlusion of one artery is compensated for by collateral anastomoses from other arteries. However, if these are not able to compensate for the cessation of blood flow because they are extremely narrowed by atherosclerosis, a transmural infarction of the entire small intestine can occur. The intestinal loops appear bluish red and edematous. Histologically the entire intestinal wall is necrotic and permeated with extravasated blood. This catastrophic event is accompanied by high mortality.

Mucosal ischemia is caused by hyperfusion of the intestines, attributable either to vascular narrowing or to central circulatory insufficiency. The narrowing of arteries is usually caused by atherosclerosis. Repeated episodes of hypotension secondary to heart failure can cause similar changes. These "nonocclusive" intestinal infarcts are typically multiple, limited to the mucosa and submucosa, and scattered through parts of the small or large intestine. Initially they appear as small hemorrhagic patches that subsequently ulcerate and undergo fibrosis. Ischemic colitis or enteritis is common in elderly persons, accounting in part for the intestinal problems affecting this population.

INFLAMMATORY BOWEL DISEASE

Inflammatory bowel disease (IBD) is a term used for two closely related but nevertheless distinct diseases: *Crohn's disease,* or *regional enteritis*, and *ulcerative colitis.* These diseases are characterized clinically by recurrent inflammation of the intestines and a chronic, unpredictable course. In

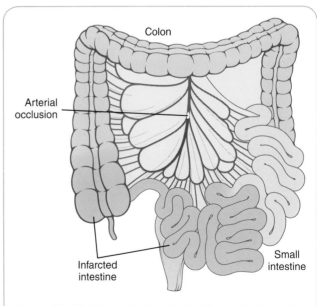

Figure 10-11 Mesenteric thrombosis with intestinal infarction.

the classical form, each of these diseases is easily distinguished from the other. However, in many cases the symptoms and findings overlap, and in 20% of cases it is not possible to tell them apart on the basis of clinical, radiologic, or pathologic findings. Ulcerative colitis is two or three times more common than Crohn's disease, with a prevalence of 70 to 150 cases per 100,000. Crohn's disease has a prevalence of 20 to 40 cases per 100,000 in Western countries.

Etiology and Pathogenesis

The etiology and pathogenesis of IBD are unknown. It has been suggested that these diseases have a strong emotional basis and that they may have a genetic basis. The pathogenetic role of immune factors and bacteria, postulated by some authorities, has not been elucidated.

It is unknown whether Crohn's disease and ulcerative colitis are distinct pathogenetic entities or only variants of a single disease that might take different forms under different conditions. Some authorities consider Crohn's disease and ulcerative colitis to be part of a spectrum, whereas others maintain that they are two distinct diseases.

In favor of a single pathogenetic entity are the following facts:

- Both diseases affect the same population; that is, they are more common among whites than blacks or Asians and are especially common among Jews of East European origin. Both diseases have a peak incidence in the third decade of life (i.e., between 20 and 30 years of age).
- Both diseases show a familial predisposition. Actually, in some families, some members have typical Crohn's disease, whereas others have ulcerative colitis.
- Both diseases have the same extraintestinal complications.
- Both diseases have an immunologic component.
- Morphologic changes in the mucosa are often indistinguishable from one another, especially in the early stages of the disease.

Keeping in mind these similarities, we shall nevertheless try to differentiate between these two diseases, limiting our description to the classical manifestations of each.

CROHN'S DISEASE

Crohn's disease is a chronic inflammation of the gastrointestinal tract that most often involves the terminal ileum and the colon. In about 50% of cases the disease affects both the terminal ileum ("terminal ileitis") and colon, in 30% of cases it is limited to the ileum, and in 20% of cases it is limited to the colon. The appendix is involved in most cases, and occasionally, Crohn's disease even may present clinically as acute appendicitis. In a small number of cases (1% to 2%), the disease involves the esophagus, stomach, or other abdominal organs such as the fallopian tubes. Approximately one third of all patients also have extraintestinal inflammatory lesions in the joints, skin, liver, or eyes.

Pathology

The earliest pathologic changes in typical Crohn's disease involve the terminal ileum and are known under the name of *aphthous ulcers* (an oxymoronic term because *aphthous* means "ulcerative" in Greek). These shallow mucosal defects typically overlie the lymphoid aggregates forming the Peyer's patches, which suggests that immune cells may be involved in their pathogenesis. The inflammation does not remain limited to the mucosa but extends through the entire wall of the intestine *(transmural inflammation)*. This is often associated with the formation of granulomas (50% of cases). Chronic inflammation is also associated with fibrosis of the muscularis and serosa. The wall of the intestine is thickened and rigid (Figure 10-12). The mucosa has a cobblestone appearance in which the fibrotic defects appear as "seams" surrounding the remaining patches of mucosa ("the cobbles"). The fibrotic intestine may be narrowed **(intestinal strictures).** The inflammation of the serosa leads to

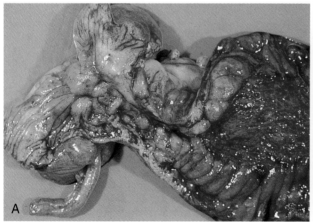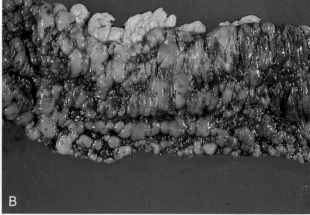

Figure 10-12 Crohn's disease. *A,* A thickened intestinal wall and a narrowed lumen are shown. *B,* The mucosa has a cobblestone-like appearance.

adhesions with adjacent intestinal loops and the formation of *fistulas*. Anal involvement is often associated with formation of *fissures*.

Clinical Features

The clinical presentation of Crohn's disease is variable. The initial symptoms are often so nonspecific that the diagnosis may be delayed by several months. The most common symptoms are diarrhea, abdominal pain, and weight loss. Bleeding is more common with rectal involvement. Fever occurs in one third of patients. In later stages of the disease, there might be constipation because of intestinal narrowing, fistulas, and adhesions. Weight loss, vitamin deficiency, and anemia secondary to malabsorption are common in the chronic stages of the disease. The most common extra-abdominal manifestations, found in one third of patients, are arthritis, skin lesions, liver disease, and eye lesions. The diagnosis is established by colonoscopy, x-ray studies, and mucosal biopsy. Crohn's disease has a chronic course. Cases that are resistant to medical therapy require surgical treatment, which includes resection of the involved intestine.

ULCERATIVE COLITIS

Ulcerative colitis is an intestinal inflammation of unknown etiology that most often involves the large intestine. The rectum is invariably affected. From initial rectal lesions, the inflammation spreads proximally, ultimately involving the entire colon. In contrast to Crohn's disease of the colon, which is typically segmental, ulcerative colitis is a diffuse disease. Furthermore, it does not extend into the ileum, although 10% of patients will show mild inflammation in the terminal ileum, called *backwash ileitis*. However, the appendix is involved in about 30% of patients.

Pathology

Ulcerative colitis is a disease principally limited to colonic mucosa. The earliest lesions seen by rectoscopy appear like flattened edematous patches involving the entire circumference of the rectum. Clinicians observing the intestine through the endoscope describe the mucosa as "sandpapered" and prone to bleeding, especially if wiped gently. This fragile mucosa appears edematous and inflamed on histologic examination. However, these changes are nonspecific and the diagnosis is not easily made. As the disease progresses, the mucosal lesions become more prominent. On rectoscopy the mucosa appears flattened and pitted, like pig skin or a football. Histologically such mucosa shows atrophy of crypts and aggregates of leukocytes in the bases of the crypts *(crypt abscesses)*. Ulcerations begin appearing in the colon proximal to the initial rectal lesions, which themselves rarely ulcerate in early stages of the disease. The ulcerated mucosa bleeds easily and is often infected. Colonic ulcerations spread through the entire colon and become confluent *(serpiginous ulcerations)*, leaving behind only small remnants of mucosa (Figure 10-13). The remnants of inflamed mucosa that have not been destroyed appear to be elevated over the base of the surrounding ulcerations and are *inflammatory polyps. Pseudopolyps* is a more appropriate term because they are not tumors but consist of residual, heavily inflamed mucosa. Some polyps represent foci of mucosal regeneration. Regeneratory foci of epithelium may undergo malignant transformation, which is the most significant late complication of ulcerative colitis.

Clinical Features

Ulcerative colitis usually begins with mild symptoms that evolve into bouts of diarrhea, rectal bleeding, and pain. In 70% of all patients the disease has a chronic course, with

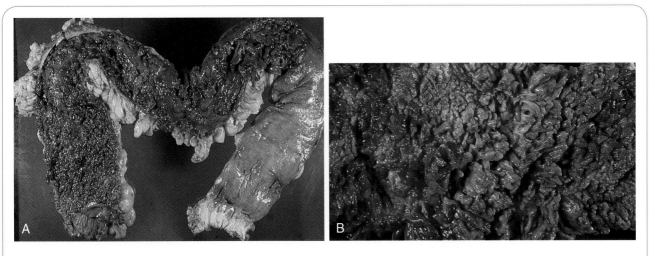

Figure 10-13 Ulcerative colitis. A: There is diffuse involvement of the intestine. B: The colon shows marked ulceration and pseudopolyposis, which account for the irregularity of the internal intestinal surface.

alternating periods of recrudescence and asymptomatic intervals. In about 10% of cases the disease has only a single episode and heals spontaneously. In about 20% of cases the disease has a fulminant course and is resistant to medical treatment. These patients often require surgical treatment, and only colectomy—resection of the entire large intestine—is lifesaving.

The diagnosis of ulcerative colitis is based on clinical, radiographic, and pathologic data. Several criteria are useful for distinguishing ulcerative colitis from Crohn's disease (Table 10-3). Ulcerative colitis predominantly affects the left side of the colon, whereas Crohn's disease tends to involve the right side of the colon and the ileum. The patterns of involvement also differ: The lesions of ulcerative colitis are diffuse, whereas Crohn's disease presents with numerous skip areas. Ulcerative colitis is limited to the mucosa, whereas Crohn's disease is transmural. Granulomas are diagnostic of Crohn's disease, but unfortunately they occur only in 50% of cases. Mucosal ulcers in ulcerative colitis are wide, leaving a few small patches of uninvolved mucosa that protrude as inflammatory polyps; by contrast, in Crohn's disease, the ulcers are linear and resemble cobblestones. The broad ulcers of ulcerative colitis tend to bleed more.

The transmural inflammation of Crohn's disease contributes to thickening of the intestinal wall and peri-intestinal fibrosis, as well as formation of adhesions and fistulas. The thinner wall of the colon in ulcerative colitis predisposes the patient to intestinal dilation and "megacolon." *Toxic megacolon,* a sudden dilation of the large intestine, is a dangerous complication of ulcerative colitis; it occurs only exceptionally in Crohn's disease. Anal lesions are found in 80% of patients with Crohn's disease but only in 20% of patients with ulcerative colitis. The extraintestinal complications of ulcerative colitis are identical to those of Crohn's disease and are therefore not useful in the differential diagnosis of these two diseases.

GASTROINTESTINAL INFECTIONS

The gastrointestinal system contains in its lumen saprophytic bacteria that live in equilibrium with the host. Diseases may develop under the following conditions:

- When the balance between the host and the intestinal flora has been lost and the ecosystem has been disturbed. The best example of this is *pseudomembranous colitis,* caused by an overgrowth of *C. difficile* in the colon of patients treated with broad-spectrum antibiotics.
- When new pathogens have been introduced into the system. This is typical of several diarrheal diseases caused by viruses, bacteria and their toxins, or protozoa.

Gastrointestinal infections are very common and vary from mild "stomach upset" to severe "food poisoning" and debilitating diarrhea. For practical purposes, it is useful to consider diarrheal disease as either small intestinal or colonic (Table 10-4). It is almost impossible to cover all the gastrointestinal infections systematically. Instead, only a few of the

TABLE 10-3 Features of Crohn's Disease and Ulcerative Colitis

	Crohn's Disease	Ulcerative Colitis
Clinical Features		
Familial predisposition	++	++
Jewish ancestry	++	++
Peak age (years)	15–25	15–25
Immune disturbances	+	+
Extraintestinal complications	+	+
Treatment efficacy	+	+
Pathology		
Diffuse (colon)	0	++
Segmental		
Colon	++	0
Ileum	++	0
Transmural inflammation	++	0
Granuloma	++ (50%)	0
Fistulas, fissures	+	0
Megacolon	–	+
Cancer	+	++

TABLE 10-4 Comparison of Diarrhea in Diseases of Small Intestine and Large Intestine

PATHOLOGIC LESIONS/INVOLVEMENT		
	Small Intestine	**Large Intestine**
Cause		
Bacteria	*Escherichia coli* *Vibrio cholerae*	*E. coli, Shigella sp.*
Viruses	Rotavirus Norwalk virus	
Parasites	*Giardia lamblia*	*Entamoeba histolytica*
Stool Characteristics		
Volume	Large	Small
Appearance	Watery	Mucoid
Blood	Rare	Common
Leukocytes	—	+/–, +, or ++
Proctoscopic Findings		
	—	+ (ulcers, hemorrhage)

more common ones, along with their underlying pathology, are discussed.

BACTERIAL DIARRHEA

Bacterial diarrhea may be caused, as illustrated in Figure 10-14, by the following:

- *Bacterial toxins.* These may be ingested preformed in food, as in food poisoning, or released by bacteria growing inside the intestine.
- *Lytic action of bacteria.* This follows colonization of the intestines by bacteria that have the capacity to invade the intestine and destroy tissue.

Preformed bacterial toxins account for typical food poisoning. This occurs after ingestion of food contaminated with

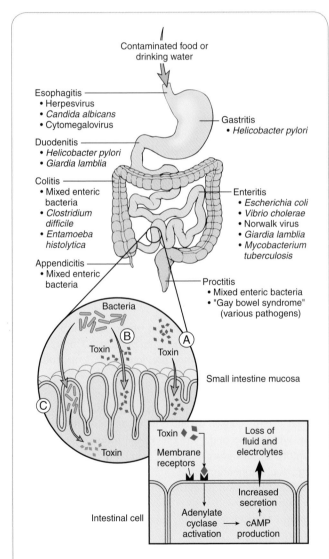

Figure 10-14 Bacterial diarrhea may be caused by an ingested toxin *(A)*, toxins formed by bacteria colonizing the intestine *(B)*, or bacteria that invade the wall of the intestine *(C)*. Cyclic adenosine monophosphate (cAMP) is essential for transduction of toxic signals that lead to watery diarrhea.

S. aureus or *Escherichia coli.* For example, food poisoning occurs following ingestion of unrefrigerated leftovers or "spoiled" fish. A rare but highly lethal food poisoning is *botulism,* caused by the ingestion of canned food contaminated with Clostridium botulinum.

Enterotoxigenic bacteria produce enterocolitis by colonizing the intestinal lumen. This is typical of so-called traveler's diarrhea, which is most often caused by enterotoxigenic strains of *E. coli* consumed in contaminated food or water. Tourists in Mexico call it *Montezuma's revenge. V. cholerae* is another enterotoxigenic bacterium that causes epidemic diarrheal disease in parts of Asia.

Invasive bacteria, such as Shigella and Salmonella, produce intestinal ulcerations that are often associated with bleeding, mucopurulent inflammation, and even intestinal perforation. Such bacteria may enter the blood or lymphatics and may cause a systemic infection ("typhoid fever").

PSEUDOMEMBRANOUS COLITIS

Pseudomembranous colitis is an acute infectious disease marked by the formation of pseudomembranes on the surface of the intestinal mucosa. It predominantly involves the colon. In more than 90% of cases it is caused by *C. difficile.* Clostridial overgrowth usually follows broad-spectrum antibiotic therapy. In a small number of cases, pseudomembranous colitis is not related to antibiotic therapy but to some other predisposing cause, such as vascular insufficiency, debilitating diseases of elderly persons, or abdominal surgery.

In typical cases, pseudomembranous colitis is a complication of antibiotic treatment. Broad-spectrum antibiotics, such as clindamycin, eradicate the normal bacterial flora and allow the intestine to be overgrown with *C. difficile.* The exotoxin produced by *C. difficile* acts on epithelial cells of the intestine, causing foci of necrosis and superficial ulcers. These ulcers are covered with a layer consisting of exudated fibrin, inflammatory cells, remnants of destroyed cells, and mucin. The pseudomembranes adhere firmly to the mucosa but can also be shed, leaving behind bleeding mucosal ulcerations.

Clinical Features

Pseudomembranous colitis presents as an acute diarrhea that may contain blood. The diagnosis may be made on the basis of a history of recent broad-spectrum antibiotic treatment. Rectoscopy is indicated only in less obvious cases. Biochemical tests for *C. difficile* toxin in bloody feces are useful in questionable cases. Eradication of *C. difficile* with antibiotics, such as vancomycin, yields good results, except in debilitated patients and those with persistent extraintestinal problems.

VIRAL GASTROENTERITIS

Viral infections of the gastrointestinal tract occur more often than one would assume from health statistics, because most of these infections are unreported. The gastrointestinal disease is usually mild, and the pathogens are rarely isolated. The most commonly documented causative agents are *rotavirus* and *norovirus,* previously known as Norwalk virus.

Rotavirus is a common cause of viral gastroenteritis in infants and children, infecting 140 million children worldwide every year and causing over 100,000 deaths of children in underdeveloped countries. During the first 6 months of their life, children are protected by maternal antibodies; thus most infections affect children from 6 months to 2 years old. Virus destroys mucosal cells of the small intestine, but the dead cells are readily replaced and the immune cells clear the infection. Clinically the disease presents with watery diarrhea. A newly available vaccine should reduce the rate of this viral infection.

Norovirus is a common cause of acute viral gastroenteritis in children and adults. Occasionally epidemics occur in nursing homes or cruise ships because the virus is extremely infectious and spread easily in closed communities. In underdeveloped countries, small epidemics are spread by contaminated water or close person-to-person contact. The disease presents with watery diarrhea, nausea, vomiting, and abdominal pain. There is no need for a biopsy because the virus produces only temporary minor nonspecific tissue damage and the infections typically heal without consequences.

PROTOZOAL ENTERITIS

Giardia lamblia is a noninvasive protozoan that infests the small intestine. The infection is typically acquired by swallowing the cysts in contaminated food or water. It presents as diarrhea or malabsorption secondary to heavy colonization of the duodenum and the proximal small bowel.

Amebiasis is an infection with *Entamoeba histolytica.* This protozoan is widespread in the tropics. Most infected persons are asymptomatic, and the clinical disease occurs only under exceptional circumstances, which are not fully understood. Tourists traveling to southern countries are at greater risk than natives. Ingested amoebas reach the cecum, where they invade the colonic mucosa and form flask-shaped ulcers extending into the submucosa. Because of histolytic properties, amoebas can penetrate into even deeper layers of the intestine, or they can invade vessels and spread to the liver, where they produce metastatic amebic abscesses. Amebiasis responds well to chemotherapy.

ACUTE APPENDICITIS

Bacterial infection of the appendix is one of the most common acute intestinal infections and the only one that requires prompt surgical intervention. It may occur at any age, but it is most common in children and adolescents.

Acute **appendicitis** is usually caused by enterogenic bacteria of the normal intestinal flora that become pathogenic after an obstruction of the lumen of the appendix. This may be caused by a hardened piece of feces, a worm, or enlarged lymph nodes or intramural lymphoid tissue of the appendix. The bacteria trapped inside the appendix

multiply and reach a critical number, at which time they become noxious, causing ulceration and invading the wall of the appendix. This usually evokes a purulent inflammation (Figure 10-15). The swollen and inflamed appendix may necrotize *(gangrenous appendicitis)* or rupture and cause *peritonitis,* which may be life threatening. This may be diffuse or localized to the right lower quadrant. The inflammation may become encapsulated, leading to an accumulation of pus around the appendix *(perityphlitic abscess).*

> ## ? Did You Know?
>
> Persons suffering from AIDS often have symptoms pertaining to the gastrointestinal tract, and all parts of the gastrointestinal tract may be involved. Such diseases may be caused by viruses, bacteria, fungi, or protozoa. Some infections, such as enteritis and intestinal malabsorption caused by *Mycobacterium avium intracellulare,* are found almost exclusively in people with AIDS.

Clinical Features

Acute appendicitis is marked by sudden fever, leukocytosis, and abdominal pain. The pain is typically strongest in the lower abdominal quadrant *(McBurney's point)* but may be referred to the umbilical area. Tenderness and rebound pain on palpation may be found in patients who have already developed serosal inflammation of the appendix, i.e., localized peritonitis. Appendectomy is the treatment of choice and should be performed immediatedly to prevent gangrene and potentially serious complications of rupture, such as purulent peritonitis.

PERITONITIS

Acute **peritonitis,** an inflammation of the peritoneal lining of the abdominal cavity, can be localized or diffuse. Chronic *tuberculous peritonitis* was common previously but is rare today.

Etiology and Pathogenesis

Peritonitis is classified as *infectious* or *sterile.* Infectious peritonitis is usually caused by bacterial invasion of the abdominal cavity, which is secondary to one of the following events:

- Rupture of the stomach (e.g., peptic ulcer) or intestines (e.g., acute appendicitis)
- Spread of infection from the fallopian tubes (e.g., gonococcal salpingitis)
- Rupture of an abscess (e.g., subphrenic abscess)
- Infection of preexisting ascites (e.g., in alcoholic cirrhosis)

Sterile peritonitis is mediated by chemical irritation. This occurs in the following:

- Acute pancreatitis, resulting from a spill of pancreatic enzymes
- Rupture of the gallbladder secondary to entry of bile into the peritoneum

- Postsurgical peritonitis caused by talc or chemicals used during operation

Pathology

In acute peritonitis the serosal surface of the intestines and the parietal peritoneum are congested and edematous. This is associated with exudation of fluid into the abdominal cavity. The fluid may be cloudy or markedly purulent and thick yellow-green. In acute pancreatitis the fluid is typically brownish yellow as a result of hemorrhage and enzymatic tissue digestion. In biliary peritonitis the fluid may be greenish from biliverdin.

Histologically, acute peritonitis is characterized by inflammatory exudates containing polymorphonuclear leukocytes and fibrin. Prolonged inflammation is marked by granulation tissue extending into the fibrinopurulent inflammatory exudate. The healing of acute inflammation results in fibrous adhesions between the intestines, which may cause intestinal obstruction.

Clinical Features

Symptoms of acute peritonitis are typical and include sharp abdominal pain, rebound tenderness, and voluntary guarding of the abdominal muscles. Intestinal peristalsis slows down until the intestines become paralyzed. Treatment of peritonitis usually requires surgical exploration to remove pus and to repair the site of rupture. All forms of peritonitis still have a high mortality.

INTESTINAL OBSTRUCTION

Intestinal obstruction, also called **ileus** (from the Greek *eilo,* meaning to "roll up"), may be of two basic types: paralytic and obstructive. Various causes of intestinal obstruction are listed in Box 10-1.

Paralytic ileus results from neuromuscular paralysis, usually related to inflammation or the disruption of innervation, or simply cessation of intestinal peristalsis as a result of exhaustion. Thus paralytic ileus is a common feature of acute peritonitis and spinal cord injury, and regularly occurs for a few hours after major abdominal surgeries.

Obstructive ileus may be caused by intraluminal material (e.g., gallstones, fecaliths, or inspissated meconium in children with cystic fibrosis) or abdominal adhesions secondary to peritonitis. Ileus may also be caused by hernia, intussusception, or volvulus (Figure 10-16).

HERNIA

A **hernia** is a protrusion of the abdominal contents through the abdominal wall. Pathogenetically, hernias relate to a weakness or a defect in the abdominal wall. The best known are the following:

- *Inguinal hernia,* which protrudes through the inguinal canal and extends into the subcutaneous tissue or into the scrotum
- *Femoral hernia,* which occurs through the femoral canal in the groin

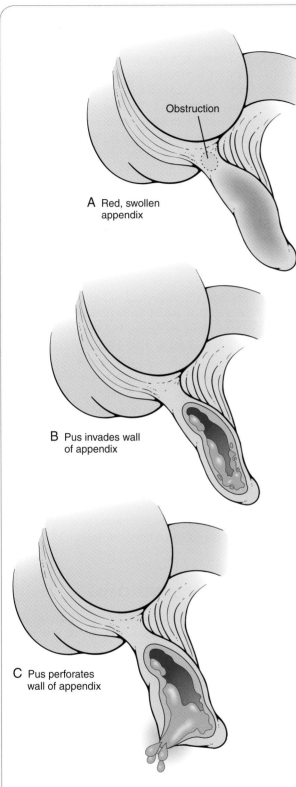

Figure 10-15 Acute appendicitis. *A,* The disease is caused by an obstruction of the appendix. *B,* The trapped bacteria invade the wall of the intestine, causing transmural inflammation. *C,* Rupture of the appendix leads to localized or diffuse peritonitis.

A Red, swollen appendix

B Pus invades wall of appendix

C Pus perforates wall of appendix

Obstruction

249

BOX 10-1 Causes of Intestinal Obstruction

Paralytic ileus
Mechanical (obstructive) ileus
   Atresia
   Stenosis
   Strictures
   Intussusception
   Volvulus
   Hernia
   Adhesions
   Neoplasms

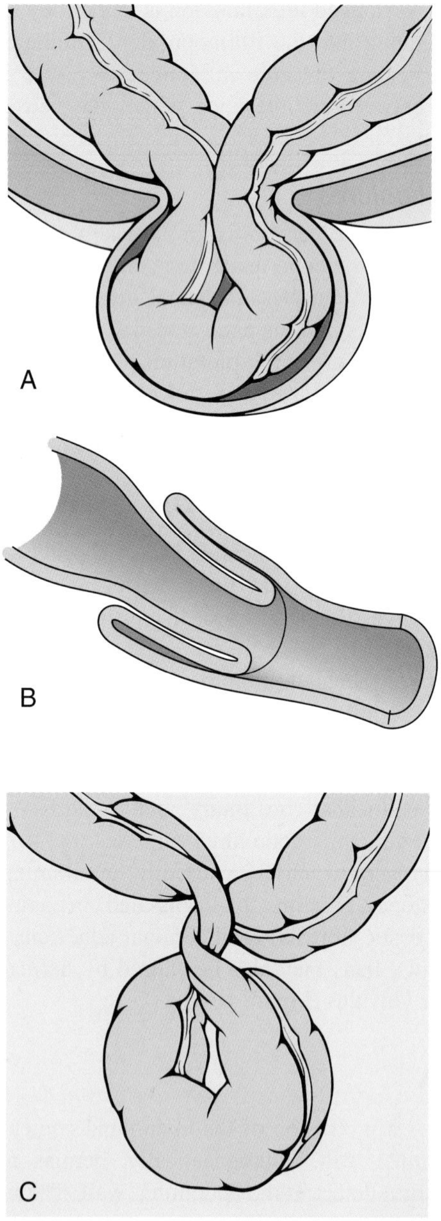

Figure 10-16 Intestinal obstructions. *A,* Hernia. *B,* Intussusception. *C,* Volvulus.

- *Periumbilical hernia,* which protrudes through the anterior abdominal wall, around the umbilicus
- *Diaphragmatic (hiatal) hernia,* which occurs through the hiatus of the diaphragm and extends into the thoracic cavity

Inguinal hernia is the most common of these. The intestinal contents are easily repositioned surgically and the abdominal wall defect is repaired. However, an untreated hernia may lead to the formation of adhesions between the hernia sac contents and the pouch in which they are located, with subsequent *incarceration.* The neck of the hernia may compromise blood flow, causing strangulation and gangrene of the intestinal loop.

INTUSSUSCEPTION

Intussusception is an invagination of one segment of the intestine into another. The blood flow to the invaginated segment may be compromised because of constriction by the outside segment, and this could lead to necrosis. In children, intussusception is usually caused by hyperactive peristalsis or enlarged lymphoid tissue in the wall of the intestine that is propulsed into the loop distal to it. In adults the leading margin of the intussuscepted intestine usually contains a tumor. Obstruction caused by intussusception can be repaired by repositioning the intestinal loops. If the inside loop is necrotic, it may need to be resected, followed by an end-to-end anastomosis of viable intestinal segments.

VOLVULUS

Volvulus is a rotation of the intestine around its mesenteric attachment site. This leads to twisting of the arteries and veins and an infarction of the rotated intestinal loop. Most often, volvulus involves the loops of the small intestine or the sigmoid colon.

MALABSORPTION SYNDROMES

Malabsorption syndromes, characterized by an inability of the intestines to absorb nutrients from food, result from abnormalities involving the following:
- Intraluminal digestion of the food
- Uptake and processing of nutrients within the intestinal cells
- Transport of the nutrients from the intestine to the liver

Malabsorption is usually caused by more than one mechanism (Figure 10-17). For the sake of simplicity, we shall classify malabsorptions on the basis of the predominant pathogenetic mechanism (Box 10-2).

The intraluminal digestion of food depends on the proper secretion of digestive juices, most notably gastric and pancreatic juice and bile. It may be disturbed in many conditions. Atrophic gastritis from resection of the stomach will reduce the gastric production of hydrochloric acid and pepsin. Chronic pancreatitis or cystic fibrosis of the pancreas reduces the output of pancreatic enzymes and bicarbonate. Lack of lipase affects the absorption of lipids, and the lack of peptidases, such

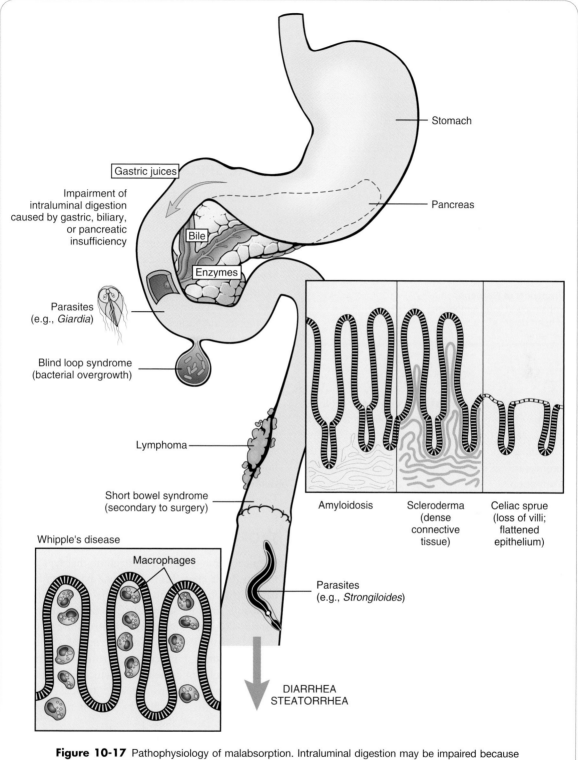

Stomach

Gastric juices

Impairment of
intraluminal digestion
caused by gastric, biliary,
or pancreatic
insufficiency

Bile

Enzymes

Pancreas

Parasites
(e.g., *Giardia*)

Blind loop syndrome
(bacterial overgrowth)

Lymphoma

Short bowel syndrome
(secondary to surgery)

Whipple's disease

Macrophages

Parasites
(e.g., *Strongiloides*)

Amyloidosis

Scleroderma
(dense
connective
tissue)

Celiac sprue
(loss of villi;
flattened
epithelium)

DIARRHEA
STEATORRHEA

Figure 10-17 Pathophysiology of malabsorption. Intraluminal digestion may be impaired because of a gastric, biliary, or pancreatic insufficiency or bacterial overgrowth and parasites. Uptake of the nutrients in the intestine may be affected by intestinal diseases, such as celiac sprue or Whipple's disease, or systemic diseases, such as scleroderma and amyloidosis. Partial resection of the intestine also causes malabsorption. Transport of nutrients from the intestine may be affected by gastrointestinal lymphoma.

BOX 10-2 Causes of Malabsorption Syndromes

Inadequate Intraluminal Digestion
Exocrine pancreatic insufficiency
   Chronic pancreatitis
   Cystic fibrosis
Reduced intestinal bile salt concentration or impaired micelle formation
   Liver disease
   Cholestasis (intrahepatic or extrahepatic)
   Abnormal bacterial proliferation in the small bowel (blind loop syndrome)
Postgastrectomy states

Primary Mucosal Absorptive Defects
Celiac sprue
Enteritis
Abetalipoproteinemia
Intestinal resection
Endocrine and metabolic disorders

Impeded Transport of Nutrients
Lymphatic obstruction (e.g., lymphoma)
Congestive heart disease
Intestinal ischemia

---

as trypsin and chymotrypsin, affects the absorption of proteins. Reduced bile flow from the liver because of obstructive jaundice also impairs absorption of lipids. In patients with Crohn's disease, or in those undergoing small bowel resection, the normal enterohepatic circulation is interrupted, also interfering with lipid absorption.

The uptake of nutrients and their further processing inside the intestinal epithelial cells is markedly affected in primary intestinal diseases. The best examples are celiac sprue and Crohn's disease. Another example is congenital abetalipoproteinemia, a deficiency of beta-lipoprotein synthesis that prevents the passage of lipids from the intestinal cells into the circulation. Such patients cannot form chylomicrons and therefore cannot prepare the absorbed intestinal lipids for transport to the liver.

The transport of nutrients from the intestine to the liver may be obstructed in the intestinal wall. This occurs, for example, in gastrointestinal lymphoma that infiltrates the intestinal wall and prevents its normal function. Congestive heart failure and intestinal ischemia could adversely affect the portal circulation, thus impeding the transport of nutrients from the intestine.

Pathology

Pathologically it is possible to divide the malabsorption syndrome into three major groups:

- Those that have characteristic pathologic findings involving the intestine, including diseases of unknown origin, such as celiac sprue or Crohn's disease; congenital metabolic defects, such as *abetalipoproteinemia*; infection with bacteria or protozoa, such as *G. lamblia* or *Cryptosporidium parvum;* and tumors, such as lymphoma.

- Those that have nonspecific pathologic findings involving the intestine, including a variety of systemic diseases, such as atherosclerosis, diabetes, scleroderma, radiation enteritis, and others.

- Those that have no pathologic findings involving the intestines; these functional disorders could be caused by intestinal bacterial overgrowth, oversecretion of hormones that alter intestinal motility (e.g., vasoactive intestinal polypeptide [VIP]), or pancreatic insufficiency.

CELIAC SPRUE

Celiac sprue, also known as *gluten-sensitive enteropathy,* is an intestinal disease characterized by hypersensitivity to gliadin in dietary grains. Gliadin, or its breakdown products, may be directly toxic to the intestine, or it may act as an allergen. Symptoms appear in early childhood, after the child is exposed to cereals. There is a familial clustering of cases that suggests a genetic predisposition, but the inheritance pattern seems to be complex. The serum of these patients contains diagnostic antibodies to tissue transglutaminase, deamidated gliadin, or endomysium. Symptoms can be induced by a diet containing grain, and they disappear on removal of grains from the diet.

Small intestinal biopsy is useful in diagnosis because it shows typical changes. These include mucosal atrophy with flattening of villi. There is also marked infiltration of the epithelium of the small intestine with T lymphocytes. After withdrawal of gliadin from the diet, the mucosa returns to normal. Follow-up of patients is important because some patients may develop a highly aggressive enteropathy-related T-cell lymphoma.

TROPICAL SPRUE

Tropical sprue is caused by bacteria that typically affect visitors to the tropics. More than one pathogen has been implicated. Morphologic changes in the intestine may be indistinguishable from those in celiac sprue but are often milder. In contrast to celiac sprue, which affects the proximal intestine more than the distal intestine, tropical sprue is more pronounced distally. Furthermore, it responds favorably to broad-spectrum antibiotic treatment, which presumably eradicates the offending pathogens. Because tropical sprue is not caused by hypersensitivity to gliadin, there is no need to restrict the intake of cereals in these patients.

WHIPPLE'S DISEASE

Whipple's disease is malabsorption caused by *Tropheryma whippelii,* a bacterium that invades the small intestinal mucosa. The disease predominantly affects middle-aged men and shows typical familial clustering. Small intestinal biopsy is diagnostic. It shows accumulation of bacteria-laden macrophages in the lamina propria mucosae. The bacteria can be seen by electron microscopy. Treatment with antibiotics cures the malabsorption.

Clinical Features of Malabsorption Syndromes

All malabsorption syndromes are characterized by a deficiency of nutrients that evolves over variable periods. The most prominent are deficiencies of protein and lipids. Protein deficiency results in anemia. This may be accentuated as a result of abnormal iron absorption, which occurs concomitantly in small intestinal diseases. Hypoalbuminemia may be severe enough to cause edema. In the most severe cases there might even be growth retardation in children and weight loss in adults. Amenorrhea, impotence, and general muscle weakness may also be present. Malabsorption of fat results in bulky, fatty stools (*steatorrhea;* from the Greek *steatos,* meaning "fatty," and *rheo,* meaning to "flow") and deficiency of fat-soluble vitamins A, D, K, and E. As a result of small stores of vitamin K, *bleeding disorders* caused by vitamin K deficiency appear the earliest. Vitamin D deficiency results in metabolic bone disorders *(osteomalacia)* and hypocalcemia, which is also caused in part by reduced intestinal uptake of calcium.

INTESTINAL NEOPLASMS

Intestinal neoplasms can be subdivided into three groups: non-neoplastic polyps, benign neoplasms, and malignant neoplasms (Box 10-3).

Neoplasms of the intestines are important causes of morbidity and mortality in the United States and the entire Western world. These tumors are less common in underdeveloped countries and the Far East. The significance of intestinal tumors can be illustrated by the following statistical data:

- Cancer of the intestines is one of the three most common malignant diseases, exceeded in incidence only by lung tumors in men and lung and breast tumors in women.
- Benign intestinal tumors outnumber malignant tumors two-fold to threefold. Because the benign tumors may progress to cancer, they must be removed as soon as detected. Early diagnosis and regular surveillance of persons at risk are the only currently available means of combating colon cancer.

BOX 10-3 Classification of Intestinal Tumors

Non-Neoplastic Polyps
Hyperplastic polyp
Inflammatory polyp
Juvenile polyp
Peutz-Jeghers polyp
Lymphoid polyp

Neoplastic Benign Polyps
Tubular adenoma
Villous adenoma
Tubulovillous adenoma

Malignant Neoplasms
Adenocarcinoma
Carcinoid
Lymphoma
Sarcoma

Three additional facts are worth remembering about intestinal neoplasia:

- In more than 95% of the cases of epithelial origin, the tumors protrude into the lumen of the intestine and can be seen by endoscopy, which is the method of choice for early detection as well as the prevention of colonic tumors.
- The intraluminal location of intestinal tumors makes them vulnerable to mechanical trauma by the intestinal contents and accounts for the frequent bleeding that is a common presenting sign of these tumors. Surveillance for blood in the stools is an effective approach to early diagnosis of intestinal cancer.
- Most tumors are located in the large intestine; indeed, the small intestine is involved in only 2% of all cases of gastrointestinal cancer.

Etiology and Pathogenesis

Any discussion of etiology and pathogenesis of intestinal tumors must take into consideration two important sets of potential carcinogenic influences: genetic factors and nutritional factors.

GENETIC FACTORS

Genetic factors play an important role in the pathogenesis of intestinal tumors. It has been estimated that at least 20% of all intestinal cancers have a genetic basis. This is most evident in families with polyposis *syndromes,* such as **familial adenomatous polyposis coli** (FAP) or *Gardner's syndrome.* In these rare autosomal dominant diseases, the colon shows multiple adenomas, which predictably evolve into adenocarcinomas. More common are the families with hereditary nonpolyposis colorectal cancer (HNPCC), which accounts for about 5% of all colorectal cancers. In these patients, colonic cancers do not evolve from preexisting polyps but rather from apparently normal mucosa. Tumors develop as a result of DNA mismatch repair deficiency, a genetic condition in which the early neoplastic genetic changes cannot be corrected. Mutatrion accumulate, resulting in cytogenetic microsatellite instability. In some families with HNPCC, colon carcinoma occurs in association with carcinoma of the ovary, uterus, and pancreas.

DIETARY FACTORS

Dietary factors are considered important in the pathogenesis of intestinal cancer, because over 80% of patients have neither familial predisposition nor an obvious genetic basis for their cancers. All aspects of dietary carcinogenesis are not fully understood, but there is enough circumstantial evidence to incriminate several key aspects of the typical Western diet as major causes. What one eats is as important as what one does not eat. A typical Western diet—rich in red meat, fat, and refined carbohydrates and low in vegetable fibers—is considered most damaging. It is not known why red meat consumption carries this high risk. Fat presumably can be degraded to potential carcinogens during food processing or during intestinal digestion. Red meat that is barbecued on a charcoal grill apparently contains more carcinogens than white meat cooked in the same manner. Fried fat is presumably degraded to potential carcinogens, which act on intestinal epithelial cells. Fat in the food also stimulates the release of bile, which is a potential source of intestinal carcinogens, presumably derived from degraded bile acids.

Oncogenes and tumor suppressor genes play an important role in pathogenesis of intestinal tumors. Most tumors develop from epithelial cells lining the crypts and villi. It has been proposed that the epithelial cells undergo malignant transformation through the action of oncogenes or because of a loss of tumor suppressor genes. The most attractive hypothesis actually combines these two pathogenetic mechanisms, suggesting that the tumors evolve through several sequential events. Accordingly, a loss of the tumor suppressor gene on chromosome 5 or hypomethylation of the tumor suppressor gene DNA in this area could deregulate the normal proliferation–maturation sequence of the epithelial cells. Normally these cells multiply in the intestinal crypts and then migrate toward the tip of the villi until they are shed at the end of their life span. Mitoses are limited to the crypts. In neoplastic mucosa, the cell divisions may be seen not only in the crypts but also in higher zones of the epithelium. At the same time, programmed cell death *(apoptosis)* does not occur. All this results in an irregular accumulation of cells that form benign adenomas. Initially the lesions are flat, but as they evolve, the tumors begin to protrude into the lumen of the intestine as villous or tubular polyps. These **polyps** (in Greek, literally meaning "with many feet" because of their attachment to the mucosa) are benign tumors. A "second hit" must occur to transform the polyp into a malignant tumor. This could involve activation of oncogenes or deletion and/or inactivation of a tumor suppressor gene. Most current evidence implicates the tumor suppressor gene *TP53* and the *KRAS* oncogene as the crucial factors in colonic neoplasia.

Molecular biologists have discovered several genetic changes that apparently occur during the transformation of polyps into carcinoma. These have been most extensively studied in patients with FAP, who develop cancer in a predictable manner. Such tumors develop as a consequence of a germ-line mutation involving the *adenomatous polyposis coli (APC)* gene mapped to the long arm of chromosome 5. The polyps appear early in life, and by the time the patient is 20 years of age, some of them already contain malignant cells. This probably occurs as a result of a second hit, which is not well defined and could involve oncogenes, tumor suppressor genes, or chemical carcinogens. It is unknown whether nonfamilial colon cancer evolves in a similar polyp-to-cancer sequence, but one can assume that there is a common pattern of development of malignant disease in both familial and nonfamilial cases.

NON-NEOPLASTIC POLYPS

This group of lesions includes hyperplastic, hamartomatous, and inflammatory polyps.

Hyperplastic Polyps

Hyperplastic polyps are the most common non-neoplastic polyps. These innocuous, benign lesions are usually discovered accidentally during endoscopy or at autopsy. More than 80% are located in the rectosigmoid area. On gross examination, they appear as dew droplet–like protrusions on the mucosa and measure less than 5 mm in diameter. They are often multiple but may be solitary as well. Histologically the polyps are composed of hyperplastic glands made up of well-differentiated absorptive and mucin-rich goblet cells surrounded by stroma. Hyperplastic polyps are considered to be "cosmetic defects" or "minor imperfections" that do not progress to true neoplasia.

Hamartoma

Juvenile polyps are hamartomas (i.e., they are developmental abnormalities in which the normal components of the tissue aggregate in an abnormal manner). As one might expect, most of them are found in children younger than 5 years. Most are solitary, with diameters of 1 to 3 cm, and are located in the rectum. These lobulated sessile lesions are composed histologically of glands lined by normal epithelium and a well-developed stroma. The glands tend to dilate cystically because of the obstructed flow of mucus—hence the name *retention polyps*. These polyps are often inflamed and ulcerated, giving rise to symptoms such as rectal irritation and bleeding. Juvenile polyps have no malignant potential.

Peutz-Jeghers polyps are also hamartomatous. These histologically distinct polyps may occur in any part of the intestine and are often multiple. These polyps are part of an autosomal dominant hereditary disease, which also includes melanotic pigmentation around the mouth, genitals, and palmar surface of the hand. The polyps are not preneoplastic. However, Peutz-Jeghers syndrome predisposes individuals to malignant disease in general; thus some patients may even develop colon cancer unrelated to preexisting polyps.

Inflammatory Polyps

Inflammatory polyps, also known as *pseudopolyps,* are encountered in IBD, especially ulcerative colitis. They represent multiple fragments of normal or regenerating mucosa surrounded by broad ulcers. On histologic examination, inflammatory polyps consist of colonic glands and granulation tissue.

NEOPLASTIC POLYPS

In contrast to non-neoplastic polyps, which are composed of normal glandular and stromal cells, neoplastic polyps are composed of neoplastic epithelium that shows no evidence of normal differentiation. Their incidence increases with age and they are often multiple. On the basis of gross and microscopic features, the neoplastic polyps are classified as tubular, villous, and tubulovillous adenomas (Figure 10-18). Although distinct from each other, these polyps are best considered as premalignant because all of them can progress to adenocarcinomas. For small tubular adenomas this risk is only 4%, but for larger villous adenomas it reaches 40%.

Tubular adenomas are the most common benign tumors, accounting for 75% of all neoplastic polyps. They are typically attached to the mucosa by a stalk (Figure 10-19). In addition to these pedunculated polyps, which have a slender

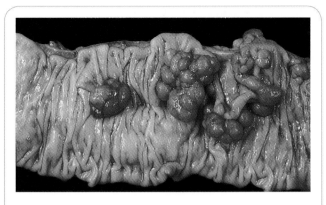

Figure 10-18 Multiple polyps of the large intestine. The polyps are round and protrude into the lumen of the intestine.

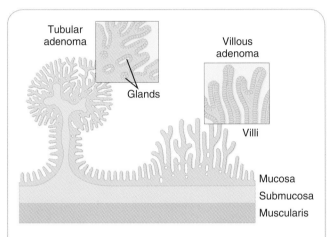

Figure 10-19 Neoplastic polyps. Tubular adenoma is pedunculated and has a stalk. Villous adenoma is sessile and has fingerlike villi projecting from its base toward the lumen of the intestine. (Modified from Kumar V, Abbas AK, Fausto N: Robbins and Cotran Pathology Basis of Disease, 7th ed, Philadelphia, Saunders, 2005, with permission.)

stalk and a lobulated "head," the smaller polyps tend to be sessile. The size of polyps and the length of the stalk vary, but most are less than 2.5 cm in diameter and have a short stalk measuring less than 5 mm in length.

Histologically, tubular adenomas are lined by cuboidal epithelium that shows signs of dysplasia, such as hyperchromasia, elongation, and stratification of nuclei. Malignant transformation can be histologically recognized by nuclear atypia; vesiculation and irregular distribution of chromatin; presence of abnormal mitotic figures; and formation of back-to-back glands. Intramucosal carcinoma developing in tubular adenomas can be recognized by its tendency to invade the lamina propria mucosae or the stalk.

Tubular adenomas can readily be resected through an endoscope. The size of the tumor is a very important risk factor for subsequent malignancy. Tubular adenomas measuring less than 1 cm have a 2% chance of being malignant, those mea-

suring 1 to 2 cm have a 10% chance, and those exceeding 4 cm have a 40% chance.

Tubulovillous adenomas are defined as predominantly tubular tumors that appear villous on at least 25% of their surface. These tumors tend to be sessile and larger than typical tubular adenomas. Histologically the tumors contain tubular and villous elements. Malignancy may be found in 25% to 40% of tubulovillous adenomas.

Villous adenomas are sessile, broad-based tumors composed of epithelial cells aligned into elongated villi. These project into the lumen of the intestine, forming fingerlike protrusions. On gross examination they have a velvety appearance. Most villous adenomas measure more than 2 cm in diameter, and many are quite large. Histologically the neoplastic villi are reminiscent of the normal villi of the small intestine. In contrast to normal small intestinal mucosa that contains several cell types, tumorous villi are lined with a single cell type that cannot be classified and does not show signs of differentiation. Invasive carcinoma is found in almost 50% of these tumors. Because of their size and broad base, these tumors usually cannot be resected through the endoscope. A segmental resection of the involved intestine is curative if performed before the malignant transformation takes place.

ADENOCARCINOMA

Adenocarcinoma accounts for 95% of malignant tumors of the intestine; the remaining 5% comprise carcinoids, sarcomas, and lymphomas. Adenocarcinomas are 50 times more common in the large intestine than the small intestine, which contains less than 2% of these tumors. For practical purposes, only colorectal adenocarcinomas are considered here.

The incidence of colorectal cancer shows great variation and thus tumors are 10 times more common in the United States and Western countries than in Asia and Africa. The peak incidence is during the ages of 50 to 70 years. Most cases occur spontaneously without any identifiable risk factors, but in 20% of cases there is a familial or genetic predisposition or tumors develop in context of hereditary cancer syndromes, as discussed earlier.

Pathology

Adenocarcinomas may develop in any part of the large intestine but are more commonly found on the left part of the intestinal loops than on the right side. Approximately 45% of cancers develop in the rectosigmoid area, 25% in the cecum and ascending colon, and the remaining 30% in other parts of the colon (Figure 10-20). Most adenocarcinomas of the intestine originate in neoplastic polyps, and many are actually found only on histologic examination of surgically removed polyps. Established invasive carcinomas can present also as mucosal plaques, ulcerations, or endophytic protruding masses. The tumors of the right colon tend to grow as fungating masses or ulcerated, shallow, craterlike lesions (Figure 10-21, *A*). In contrast, adenocarcinomas of the sigmoid and rectum tend to infiltrate the intestine circumferentially, producing so-called

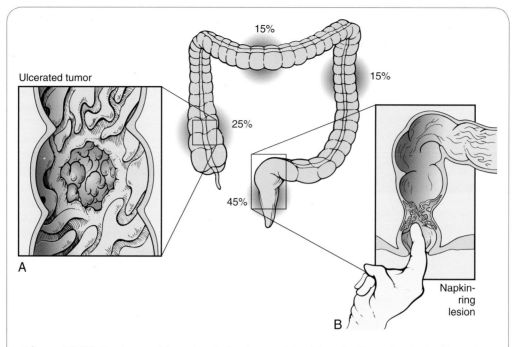

Figure 10-20 Carcinoma of the colon. *A,* Carcinoma of the right colon forms intraluminal fungating or ulcerating masses. *B,* Carcinoma of the left colon produces "napkin-ring" stenotic lesions.

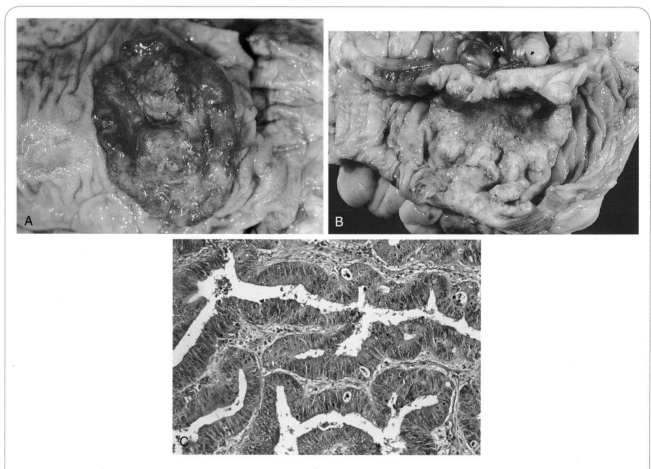

Figure 10-21 Surgically resected carcinomas of the large intestine. *A,* This carcinoma of the cecum appears like a localized craterlike ulcer limited to a portion of the intestinal surface. *B,* This carcinoma of the sigmoid colon has diffusely infiltrated the entire circumference of the intestine. *C,* Histologically these tumors are adenocarcinomas.

napkin-ring concentric narrowing (see Figure 10-21, *B*). Adenocarcinomas of the large intestine are staged according to the TNM system, which has evolved from the system devised by Dukes in the 1930s and modified by many other surgeons thereafter (e.g., the Astler-Coller modification). Patients with TNM stage 1 tumors have a 93% 5-year survival rate; those with stage 2, 70–85%; stage 3, 45–80%; and those with stage 4 tumors have less than 10% 5-year survival rate. Obviously, early detection is the only viable approach to combating colon cancer.

Clinical Features

Symptoms of intestinal cancer vary depending on the location, size, and shape of the lesion. Early cancer may produce no symptoms at all. Such lesions are typically diagnosed by endoscopy followed by biopsy or by screening of feces for occult blood. Adenocarcinoma of the right colon and cecum tend to be clinically silent, producing only nonspecific signs, such as weakness and fatigue. Chronic blood loss may cause anemia. The left-sided lesions, especially those in the rectum, tend to narrow the intestine and obstruct the passage of feces. Constipation; narrow, pencil-like feces; and blood in the feces are the characteristic findings. Hematochezia may also occur, although it is usually a sign of far-advanced lesions.

> **Did You Know?**
>
> Occult blood—that is, blood that is not visible by the naked eye—is an important early sign of colonic cancer. The test can easily be performed by smearing a small amount of feces onto a test strip that changes color on contact with blood. Early detection is the only efficient way to combat carcinoma of the intestines.

The diagnosis of intestinal cancer depends on visualizing the tumor by colonoscopy or rectoscopy, x-ray studies combined with barium enema, and computed tomography. The final diagnosis depends on histologic examination of the tissue (see Figure 10-21, *C*).

Most adenocarcinomas of the intestine release CEA into the circulation. CEA is normally produced by the embryonic intestines but is not found in the intestinal cells of the adult except in special circumstances, such as in the regenerating epithelium of ulcerative colitis. CEA produced by tumor cells enters the blood circulation and can be measured in serum. Unfortunately, CEA cannot be used for early detection or for the screening of populations at risk because it is also elevated in chronic ulcerative colitis and other nonspecific intestinal inflammations. The test is useful in the follow-up of patients whose carcinoma has been resected. A rise in serum CEA level in these patients usually heralds a recurrence of tumor.

GASTROINTESTINAL CARCINOIDS

The term **carcinoid** is used for neuroendocrine tumors of low malignancy, meaning that they are malignant but not as malignant as true carcinomas. Carcinoids can occur in all intra-abdominal parts of the gastrointestinal tract, including the stomach, small intestine, appendix, and large intestine. Approximately 40% of all carcinoids are found in the small intestine.

Pathology

Carcinoids are typically located in the submucosa, where they form small nodules elevating the overlying mucosa. Most carcinoids are small, measuring less than 2 cm, and are often found accidentally during endoscopy, in surgically resected tissue, or at autopsy. Tumors larger than 2 cm may be symptomatic and also tend to metastasize to local lymph nodes and to the liver. Carcinoids, especially those in the terminal ileum and the stomach, are often multiple.

Histologic examination reveals that carcinoids are composed of small neuroendocrine cells arranged into islets or cords and trabeculae (Figure 10-22). The neuroendocrine nature of the tumor cell is best demonstrated by immunohistochemistry or electron microscopy. With use of immunohistochemical methods, it is possible to demonstrate that these cells contain polypeptide hormones, such as secretin, gastrin, or VIP, and biogenic amines, such as serotonin. Electron microscopy reveals that the tumor cells contain neuroendocrine granules, which have a dense central core surrounded by a clear halo and a limiting membrane.

Clinical Features

Carcinoids are low-grade malignant tumors. This is evident histologically because tumor cells typically invade the normal tissue, often metastasizing to local lymph nodes. The propensity to metastasize correlates with the size of the tumor and its location. Metastases are most common with tumors larger than 2 cm in diameter, especially those localized in the right colon, small intestine, or stomach. Carcinoids of the appendix are usually small and tend to remain localized.

Clinical symptoms of carcinoid tumors include those related to local growth, which are not different from the symptoms produced by other malignant tumors, and those related to their secretory neuroendocrine activity. Secretory products of intestinal carcinoid tumors that are released into the portal circulation are detoxified during their passage through the liver. Carcinoids that have metastasized to the liver release their secretory product into the venous blood; this causes a systemic disease known as *carcinoid syndrome.* Symptoms, which are probably caused by a release of serotonin, bradykinin, and histamine, include episodes of facial blushing, bronchial wheezing, attacks of intestinal colics, and bouts of watery diarrhea. In long-lasting carcinoid syndrome, there is also endocardial fibrosis of the right ventricle and tricuspid valve. Carcinoids are slow-growing, low-grade malignant neoplasms, and the 5-year survival rate of treated patients exceeds 80%.

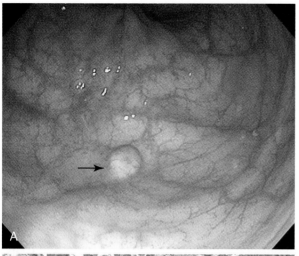

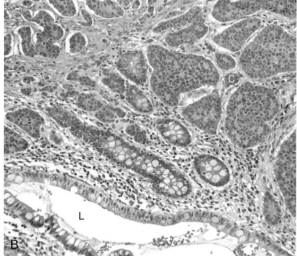

Figure 10-22 Carcinoid. *A,* Like most carcinoids, this small subucosal nodule (*arrow*) measures less than 2 cm in diameter. *B,* Microscopically the tumor is composed of solid nests of neuroendocrine cells (C) that have uniform round nuclei. L, intestinal lumen.

REVIEW QUESTIONS

1. Compare the structure and function of the upper and the lower digestive tract.

2. List the main exocrine and endocrine products of the gastrointestinal tract and their functions.

3. How do developmental anomalies affect the function of the digestive tract?

4. What is dental caries, and how can it be prevented?

5. What are the main complications of dental caries?

6. What causes periodontal disease?

7. What is stomatitis, and what are its causes?

8. What is the significance of oral leukoplakia and erythroplakia?

9. What are the risk factors for oral cancer?

10. How does oral cancer present clinically?

11. What is sialadenitis, and what are its causes?

12. How does Sjögren's disease affect the salivary glands?

13. Are salivary gland tumors mostly benign or malignant?

14. What is the most common salivary gland tumor?

15. What are the clinical signs and symptoms of esophageal disease?

16. What is dysphagia, and what are its causes?

17. What is esophagitis, and what are its causes?

18. What is a hiatal hernia, and how does it present clinically?

19. What is achalasia, and what are its causes?

20. What is the most common cause of esophageal varices?

21. What are the risk factors for esophageal cancer, and how do they account for the differences in the incidence of this disease in various parts of the world?

22. Correlate the pathologic and clinical features of esophageal carcinoma.

23. What are the main forms of gastritis?

24. What causes gastritis?

25. Explain the pathogenesis of peptic ulcer, placing special emphasis on the role of gastric juice, the mucosal barrier, and *H. pylori.*

26. Describe the gross and microscopic pathology of peptic ulcer and correlate these morphologic findings with the clinical signs and symptoms of the disease.

27. What are the main complications of peptic ulcer?

28. How common is gastric cancer in the United States in comparison with the incidence of this neoplasm in other parts of the world?

29. How does gastric carcinoma present on macroscopic (naked eye) examination?

30. Where do gastric carcinomas metastasize?

31. What are the clinical signs and symptoms of gastric carcinoma?

32. How is gastric lymphoma related to MALT?

33. Compare atresia of the small intestine with Hirschsprung's disease.

34. Describe diverticula of the large intestine and their complications.

35. Compare hemorrhoids and intestinal angiodysplasia.

36. Compare occlusive and nonocclusive ischemic bowel disease.

37. How common is inflammatory bowel disease?

38. Compare Crohn's disease and ulcerative colitis.

39. What is pseudomembranous colitis?

40. List the most important bacterial and protozoal infections of the intestines.

41. Compare diarrhea caused by small intestinal disease with diarrhea caused by large intestinal disease.

42. What are the clinical and pathologic features of acute appendicitis?

43. Compare infectious and sterile peritonitis.

44. Describe the pathogenesis and pathology of acute peritonitis.

45. List the most common causes of intestinal obstruction.

46. What are the most common types of hernia?

47. Compare intussusception and volvulus.

48. Classify malabsorption syndromes according to their pathogenesis.

49. Compare iliac sprue and tropical sprue.

50. What are the clinical features of malabsorption syndrome?

51. How common are intestinal neoplasms, and where are they most often located?

52. Classify intestinal neoplasms.

53. What are the risk factors for intestinal neoplasms?

54. What are polyps, and how are these intestinal lesions classified?

55. Compare neoplastic and non-neoplastic polyps.

56. What are the clinical features of large intestinal cancer?

57. Compare adenocarcinomas of the right and left colon.

58. What is CEA, and what is the clinical value of this tumor marker?

59. How do carcinoids differ from adenocarcinoma of the large intestine?

60. What is carcinoid syndrome?

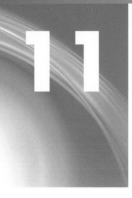

11

The Liver and Biliary System

Chapter Outline

NORMAL ANATOMY AND PHYSIOLOGY
OVERVIEW OF MAJOR DISEASES
  Jaundice
  Acute Viral Hepatitis
    Forms of Hepatitis
  Cirrhosis
  Drug- and Toxin-Induced Liver Diseases
  Alcoholic Liver Disease
  Hereditary Diseases of the Liver
    Gilbert's Disease
    Hemochromatosis
    Wilson's Disease
    Alpha$_1$-Antitrypsin Deficiency

Immune Disorders
  Autoimmune Hepatitis
  Primary Biliary Cirrhosis
  Primary Sclerosing Cholangitis
Bacterial, Protozoal, and Parasitic Infections
Gallstones
Hepatobiliary Neoplasms
  Hepatocellular Carcinoma
  Bile Duct Cancer
  Carcinoma of the Gallbladder
  Metastases to the Liver
Liver Transplantation

Key Terms and Concepts

Alcoholic hepatitis
Alpha$_1$-antitrypsin deficiency
Alpha-fetoprotein (AFP)
Anastomoses
Ascites
Autoimmune hepatitis
Bile duct carcinoma
Bleeding tendency
Carcinoma of the gallbladder
Cholecystitis

Cholelithiasis
Cirrhosis
Esophageal varices
Fatty liver
Gallstones
Gilbert's disease
Hemochromatosis
Hepatic encephalopathy
Hepatitis
Hepatocellular carcinoma

Hepatorenal syndrome
Hyperbilirubinemia
Jaundice
Liver transplantation
Portal hypertension
Primary biliary cirrhosis
Primary sclerosing cholangitis
Steatohepatitis
Wilson's disease

Learning Objectives

After reading this chapter, the student should be able to:

1. Describe the normal liver and biliary tract.
2. List the cells of the hepatobiliary tract and describe their primary functions.
3. Describe the formation of bile and explain the main disorders that can cause jaundice.
4. List and explain the principal biochemical changes typical of acute liver disease.
5. Describe the principal clinical, biochemical, and pathologic findings in chronic liver disease.
6. Describe the pathologic changes induced by hepatitis virus and compare the effects of hepatitis virus A, B, and C.
7. Define cirrhosis and describe the most important pathologic findings in this disease.
8. Describe three forms of alcohol-induced liver disease.
9. Compare predictable and nonpredictable drug-induced liver disease.
10. Describe three hereditary diseases affecting the liver.
11. Discuss the pathogenesis of immunologic liver diseases and compare primary biliary cirrhosis with primary sclerosing cholangitis.
12. List typical infectious liver diseases caused by bacteria, protozoa, and parasites.
13. Describe the morphology of gallstones and discuss their pathogenesis.
14. List the symptoms and biochemical findings caused by biliary tract diseases and relate these to pathologic changes in the gallbladder and extrahepatic biliary ducts.
15. Name three malignant liver tumors and compare their features.
16. Compare the features of gallbladder cancer and cancer of the extrahepatic bile ducts.
17. Describe the benefits and hazards of liver transplantation.

NORMAL ANATOMY AND PHYSIOLOGY

The liver is the largest parenchymal organ in the body, weighing about 1500 g. It is located in the right upper abdominal quadrant in a space limited cranially by the diaphragm, on the anterior side by the rib cage, and on the posterior side by bones and muscles of the abdominal wall. The normal liver has a smooth surface and is firm. The anterior lower edge of the liver can be palpated below the right costal margin, at the peak of deep inspiration, when the entire liver is pushed caudally by the diaphragm. Because of its anatomic relationship to the chest cage, the liver can be reached by a biopsy needle inserted through the intercostal muscles.

On the inferior side, the liver is attached to the gallbladder and the extrahepatic bile ducts, which connect it to the duodenum (Figure 11-1). The point at which the bile ducts exit from the liver is called the *hilus.* Through the hilus, the liver receives its dual blood supply—arterial oxygenated blood through the hepatic artery and venous blood rich in nutrients

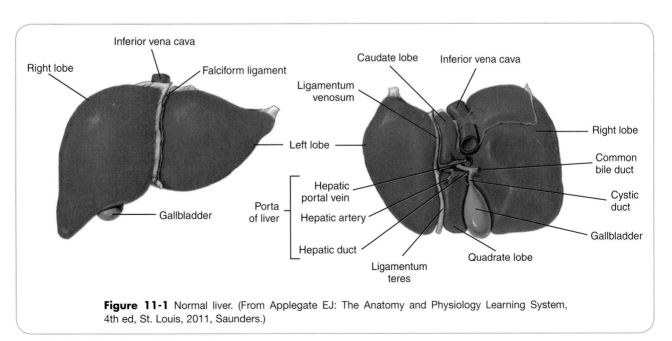

Figure 11-1 Normal liver. (From Applegate EJ: The Anatomy and Physiology Learning System, 4th ed, St. Louis, 2011, Saunders.)

absorbed from food through the portal vein. The portal circulation is separate from the systemic circulation, to which it is interconnected with narrow, nonfunctioning anastomoses. These carry little blood but are able to expand if the pressure in the portal system increases as a result of portal hypertension. The hepatic vein drains into the inferior vena cava.

The liver is primarily composed of liver cells, also known as *hepatocytes,* which constitute 90% of the total mass. The other cells are bile ductal cells and the vascular cells lining the sinusoids, veins, and arteries (Figure 11-2). Connective tissue forms the capsule of the liver *(Glisson's capsule)* and portal tracts.

The hepatocytes are arranged into functional units called *lobules* (see Figure 11-2). Blood enters the lobules from the periphery through the portal tract and flows through the sinusoids toward the central vein. The portal tract is also called the portal triad because it contains a small branch of the hepatic artery, portal vein, and bile duct. The lobular blood spaces and the sinusoids are lined by Kupffer cells and a discontinuous basement membrane. This allows easy passage of nutrients and metabolites from the blood into the liver cells and vice versa. The *Kupffer cells* are fixed phagocytes and serve as the main scavengers for foreign and internal particulate material (e.g., bacteria and blood cell fragments).

The liver has several major functions that can be classified as the following:
- Excretory
- Metabolic
- Storage
- Synthetic

Bile is the main excretory product of the liver. Bile is a complex mixture of bilirubin, bile salts, lipids, and many other minor components. It is produced by liver cells and excreted through the bile ducts into the intestine or stored in the gallbladder. On reaching the intestine, the bile is mixed with food and pancreatic and intestinal enzymes. The bile that is not used up during intestinal digestion is transformed into urobilinogen, which is reabsorbed into the portal circulation and returned to the liver (enterohepatic circulation of bile).

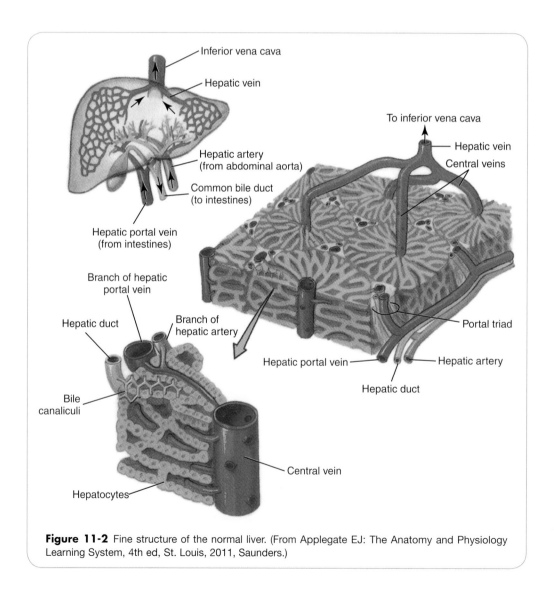

Figure 11-2 Fine structure of the normal liver. (From Applegate EJ: The Anatomy and Physiology Learning System, 4th ed, St. Louis, 2011, Saunders.)

The liver has multiple metabolic functions. It is considered the main "processing factory" for all food components, and its normal function is essential for the intermediary metabolism of carbohydrates, fats, and proteins. The liver is also the major storage site of carbohydrates and lipids.

The liver is the site of synthesis of all major plasma proteins except the immunoglobulins. Albumin, the most copious plasma protein, as well as the coagulation proteins, and all the transport proteins essential for the transfer of hormones, vitamins, and other biologically active substances are synthesized in the liver.

OVERVIEW OF MAJOR DISEASES

The most important diseases affecting the liver and the biliary tract are the following:

- *Jaundice syndromes.* These include abnormal formation, processing, or excretion of bilirubin.
- *Hepatitis.* Inflammation of the liver can be caused by viruses, as well as drugs, alcohol, and immune mechanisms.
- *Toxic/metabolic hepatic injury.* Liver cells may be injured by exogenous chemicals or endogenous metabolites.
- *Cirrhosis.* This condition may result from a variety of liver diseases. The term *cirrhosis* is used as a synonym for end-stage liver disease.
- *Diseases of the extrahepatic bile ducts and gallbladder.* The most important among these diseases are those that are caused by gallstones.
- *Tumors.* Tumors of the liver and the biliary tract can be classified as benign or malignant, primary or secondary.

Several facts important to an understanding of liver disease are presented here, before a discussion of specific pathologic entities.

1. The liver is a part of the digestive tract, to which it is connected by two important links: the portal veins and the bile ducts. The liver is involved in processing nutrients that are absorbed in the intestines. These nutrients reach the liver through the portal vein. The portal vein circulation is a low-pressure venous system that is self-contained and does not have functional communications with the systemic blood flow. However, if the blood flow through the liver is obstructed as a result of liver disease, such as cirrhosis, the increased pressure in the portal system will open up the nonfunctioning anastomoses between the portal and the systemic circulation. Through these **anastomoses,** the portal blood will bypass the liver and enter the systemic circulation. This has two important consequences: (1) The blood that has bypassed the liver contains various metabolites and toxic substances that may have deleterious effects on other organs, and (2) at the same time, such blood lacks the essential metabolites formed in the liver. For example, the blood concentration of ammonia absorbed from the intestine might be high, whereas the blood glucose level, which is not released from the liver, might be low.

   Portal hypertension widens the venous channels connecting the portal and systemic circulation. Increased pressure in these anastomoses results in the formation of varicosities (i.e., tortuous, dilated veins). These varicosities, which are prone to rupture and tend to bleed profusely, are typically located in the esophagus, in the hemorrhoidal venous plexus of the rectum, and in the umbilical venous plexus of the anterior abdominal wall (Figure 11-3).

   Portal hypertension has two other important consequences. Because the portal vein receives venous blood from the spleen, portal hypertension causes chronic passive congestion in the spleen and splenomegaly. The transudation of fluid into the abdominal cavity contributes to the formation of ascites.

   The bile ducts connect the liver to the duodenum and serve as the main route for the excretion of bile into the intestine. Obstruction of the bile ducts results in jaundice. Lack of bile in the intestines adversely affects digestion, particularly the absorption of fats and fat-soluble vitamins (A, D, E, and K). The bile ducts may also serve as the site of entry of ascending bacterial infections. Even worms, such as the common roundworm, *Ascaris lumbrocoides,* or the Chinese liver fluke, *Clonorchis sinensis,* may reach the liver through the bile ducts.

   The terminal portion of the bile duct passes through the head of the pancreas, where it becomes confluent with the main pancreatic duct, entering the wall of the intestine at the papilla of Vater. Diseases of the duodenum or the pancreas may also obstruct the extrahepatic bile ducts. Obstructive jaundice is an important symptom of carcinomas involving the head of the pancreas.

2. The liver is an encapsulated, self-contained organ that is loosely attached to adjacent structures. This is important to bear in mind, especially today when the diseased liver can easily be removed and replaced with a newly transplanted organ by an expert liver transplantation surgeon. As mentioned before, the liver moves down with each inspiration and can be palpated underneath the right costal margin. The external surface of the normal liver is smooth and covered with Glisson's capsule. Glisson's capsule contains nerves. Distention of this capsule secondary to chronic passive congestion, which is typical of congestive heart failure, causes pain that is usually dull and diffuse over the entire liver. Tumors and hepatitis also can distend Glisson's capsule and cause pain.

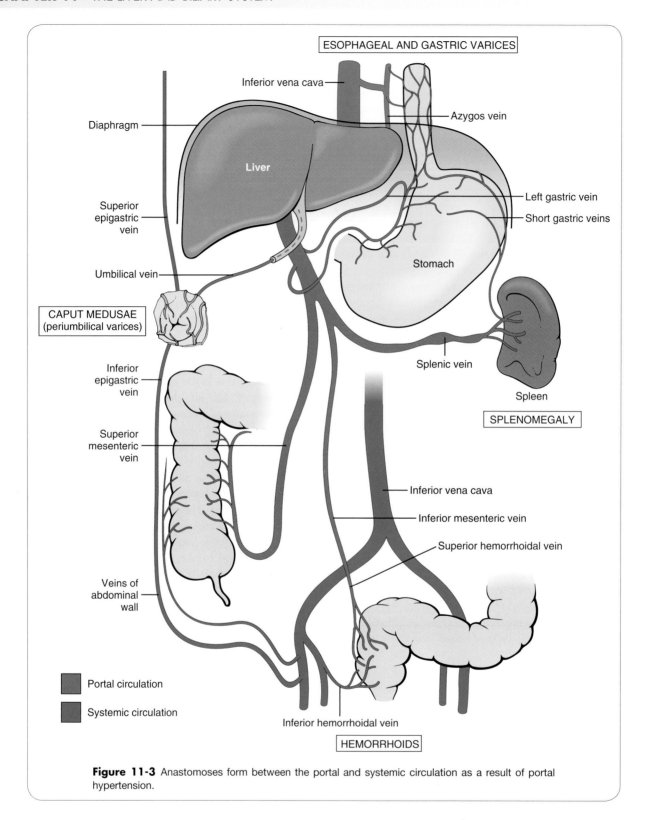

ESOPHAGEAL AND GASTRIC VARICES

Inferior vena cava

Diaphragm

Azygos vein

Liver

Left gastric vein

Superior epigastric vein

Short gastric veins

Umbilical vein

Stomach

CAPUT MEDUSAE (periumbilical varices)

Splenic vein

Inferior epigastric vein

Spleen

SPLENOMEGALY

Superior mesenteric vein

Inferior vena cava

Inferior mesenteric vein

Superior hemorrhoidal vein

Veins of abdominal wall

Portal circulation

Systemic circulation

Inferior hemorrhoidal vein

HEMORRHOIDS

Figure 11-3 Anastomoses form between the portal and systemic circulation as a result of portal hypertension.

3. The liver is essential for the uptake, processing, and excretion of bilirubin released from aged red blood cells (RBCs). Bilirubin is the degradation product of heme, the principal component of hemoglobin in RBCs. Bilirubin released from senescent RBCs is taken up by the liver and excreted in bile. Hyperbilirubinemia (i.e., a serum bilirubin level exceeding the normal concentration of 1.2 mg/dL) is one of the most common biochemical abnormalities in liver diseases. Retained bilirubin diffuses into tissues and binds to connective tissues in various organs. In the skin and mucosa this is recognized as jaundice.

4. The liver is the major source of most plasma proteins. Essentially all major plasma proteins, except the immunoglobulins, are produced by the liver. Liver diseases result in hypoproteinemia. Lack of albumin, which is the most abundant plasma protein, reduces the oncotic capacity of the plasma, resulting in edema. Decreased production of coagulation factors, such as fibrinogen, prothrombin, and factors VIII, IX, X, XI, and XII, which are all synthesized in the liver, results in a **bleeding tendency.**

5. Liver cells are rich in enzymes, which are released into the circulation on liver cell injury. Liver cell injury results in a release of aspartate aminotransferase (AST) and alanine aminotransferase (ALT) into the circulating blood. AST and ALT are ubiquitous enzymes whose levels are elevated in blood after injury of many other organs and in myocardial infarction. Because the liver represents the major source of AST and ALT, these enzyme levels are commonly used as indicators of liver function and are the common liver function tests. Alkaline phosphatase, another enzyme that is also not restricted to the liver, is used as a marker of bile duct obstruction.

6. The liver removes from circulation, metabolizes, and detoxifies or modifies many drugs, hormones, cytokines, and biologically active metabolites. The liver removes from circulation various metabolites, such as carbohydrates, lipids, and proteins, derived from the food or peripheral storage sites; immunoglobulins and various other proteins; hormones, such as androgens and estrogens; biogenic amines, such as histamine or serotonin; and many other substances. If uptake into the liver cells is blocked or cannot take place because of liver cell insufficiency, these substances persist in the blood in high concentrations and may have adverse effects on other tissues. The best example of such a condition is the accumulation of ammonia and other presumptive neurotoxins in the intestines; on absorption, these substances may act on the brain and even cause coma **(hepatic encephalopathy).**

   Chronic liver disease is associated with disturbances in the metabolism of sex hormones. Excess estrogen that has not been removed appropriately from the circulation is considered the cause of dilated arterioles surrounded by dilated capillaries, known in the skin as spider nevi. Testicular atrophy, loss of libido, and gynecomastia, which are seen in some alcoholic patients with cirrhosis, have also been attributed to hyperestrinism.

7. Certain viruses have exclusive tropism for the liver. The liver may be affected by various bacterial, viral, protozoal, fungal, and parasitic infections that reach this organ via the blood or through the bile ducts. Most of these pathogens cause disease in other organs as well. Certain viruses, such as hepatitis virus A, B, C, D, and E, show hepatotropism (i.e., they preferentially affect the liver). The reasons for this tropism are not known, but apparently the liver cells provide an ideal environment for their growth and replication.

8. Liver cells can regenerate. Liver cells are facultative mitotic (labile) cells, and lost liver cells are readily replaced by new hepatocytes derived from the remaining healthy cells. For example, a liver lobe that is injured in a car accident can be resected because it will regenerate; within a few weeks the liver will regain its normal size. Regeneration takes place in cirrhotic livers as well. However, because of concomitant fibrosis, this results in formation of nodules rather than the restoration of normal parenchyma.

9. The liver can give rise to tumors, but it is even more often involved by tumor metastases. **Hepatocellular carcinoma** is common in parts of the world in which hepatitis B (HBV) viral infection is endemic, such as the Far East or sub-Saharan Africa. Worldwide it is probably the most common human malignant disease, with more than 1 million new cases reported every year. In the United States the liver is more often affected by metastatic cancer than by primary liver cell tumors. Because the liver receives blood from two sources, and thus serves as a major blood thoroughfare, it is a common site of metastasis of tumors originating in other organs.

10. Bile can form gallstones. Gallstones are formed, under a variety of circumstances, from the normal components of bile. These stones may cause obstruction or inflammation and are the most important cause of pathologic changes in the biliary tract.

JAUNDICE

Jaundice (*icterus* in Latin) is a symptom and not a disease. It is characterized by yellow discoloration of the skin and mucosa caused by **hyperbilirubinemia**—that is, elevation of blood bilirubin levels above the upper limit of normal, which is 1.2 mg/dL. In practical terms, jaundice becomes apparent only after the concentration of bilirubin has exceeded 3 mg/dL.

Pathogenesis

As shown in Figure 11-4, jaundice may be classified as follows:
- Prehepatic
- Hepatic
- Posthepatic

Bilirubin is derived mostly from the heme portion of hemoglobin; 70% of hemoglobin is of RBC origin, whereas the remaining 30% stems from the respiratory enzymes in various tissues or the precursors of the hemoglobin in bone marrow that are not utilized (as a result of "inefficient hematopoiesis").

The senescent RBCs are taken up by the phagocytic cells of the spleen and the Kupffer cells of the liver. Within these cells the hemoglobin is degraded into heme and globin. Heme loses the iron and is transformed into yellow pigment bilirubin. Bilirubin is released into the blood, where it binds to albumin. This unconjugated bilirubin, which is not water soluble, is taken up by the liver cells and conjugated to glucuronide. Bilirubin bound to glucuronide becomes water soluble. This conjugated bilirubin is excreted in bile and into the intestine, where it participates in the digestion of dietary fats. Bilirubin that is not used up in the intestine is converted by bacteria into urobilinogen, which is reabsorbed. Most of it is

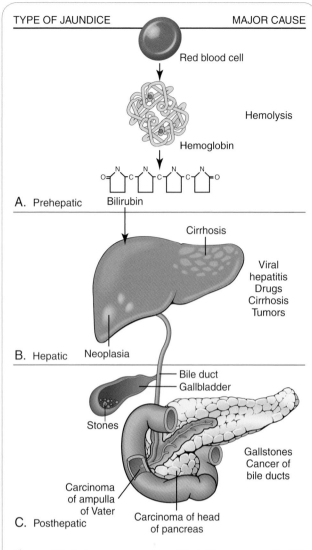

TYPE OF JAUNDICE   MAJOR CAUSE

Red blood cell

Hemolysis

Hemoglobin

A. Prehepatic   Bilirubin

Cirrhosis

Viral
hepatitis
Drugs
Cirrhosis
Tumors

B. Hepatic   Neoplasia

Bile duct
Gallbladder

Stones

Gallstones
Cancer of
bile ducts

Carcinoma
of ampulla
of Vater

C. Posthepatic   Carcinoma of head
of pancreas

Figure 11-4 Jaundice may be attributable to prehepatic *(A)*, hepatic *(B)*, or posthepatic *(C)* causes.

TABLE 11-1   Common Causes of Jaundice

Prehepatic	Hepatocellular	Posthepatic (Obstructive)
Hemolysis	Viral hepatitis	Gallstones
Hematoma	Alcoholic liver disease	Carcinoma of the pancreas or bile ducts
Gilbert's disease	Drug-induced liver disease Cirrhosis	

In *obstructive jaundice,* the bile does not reach the intestine and the feces appear clay colored or tan, rather than their normal brown. Such stools are called *acholic* and are associated with *steatorrhea.*

Mixed conjugated and unconjugated hyperbilirubinemia is a feature of various diseases marked by liver cell necrosis and destruction of liver parenchyma. It occurs in viral **hepatitis** or drug-induced hepatitis, as well as in various metabolic liver diseases, alcoholic hepatitis, and cirrhosis.

? Did You Know?

Jaundice is best recognized on the sclera. The sclera is normally white, even in blacks and Asians, but in those with jaundice it becomes yellow.

If the blood is allowed to clot in a test tube, the red blood cells (RBCs) separate from the plasma. Plasma, which consists of water and solutes, is yellow because it normally contains small amounts of bilirubin. In cases of jaundice the plasma becomes even more yellow or turns brown.

Bilirubin excreted in the urine of jaundiced persons makes the urine appear brown and bubbly. Bilirubin is a surface active substance, like detergents. Urine that contains bilirubin is similar to bubble bath and could be used for cleansing. In ancient times, bathing in animal urine was a part of certain religious rituals and beautification rites. Bilirubin-rich urine would have been more efficient.

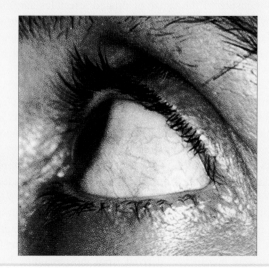

recirculated into the liver, whereas a small portion is excreted in urine.

Hyperbilirubinemia is biochemically classified as predominantly conjugated, unconjugated, or mixed (Table 11-1). *Unconjugated hyperbilirubinemia* is prehepatic and mostly caused by excessive bilirubin formation secondary to hemolysis, which is typically found in various hemolytic anemia. Worldwide, malaria is the most common cause of hemolytic jaundice. **Gilbert's disease,** a common autosomal dominant genetic defect in the hepatic conjugation of bilirubin, can also cause mild periodic unconjugated hyperbilirubinemia. *Conjugated hyperbilirubinemia* reflects disturbances in the excretion of bilirubin that has been conjugated to glucuronide in liver cells. Typically this occurs as a result of obstruction of bile flow, usually at the level of the common bile duct. Gallstones that are impacted in the extrahepatic bile ducts and tumors of the bile ducts, pancreas, or duodenum are the most common causes of obstructive jaundice.

Clinical Features

Bilirubin, both conjugated and unconjugated, binds to connective tissue and stains it yellow. This is best seen on the sclera, which is normally white. Other mucous membranes and the skin become yellow as well. Jaundice is usually accompanied by itching, but otherwise it has few serious consequences.

The unconjugated bilirubin is bound to albumin. Thus it does not cross the blood–brain barrier and does not appear in the cerebrospinal fluid or in the brain. It does not filter into the urine either. In hemolytic jaundice, urine is thus of normal color. However, conjugated bilirubin, which is water soluble, is excreted in urine. Because of its high bilirubin content, the urine of patients with viral hepatitis appears brown and foamy. Brown urine is often reported as the first sign of viral hepatitis.

As mentioned earlier, jaundice is not a disease but a symptom of several liver diseases. The underlying cause of jaundice can be identified by establishing whether the jaundice is attributable to unconjugated or conjugated hyperbilirubinemia, whether the liver disease is acute or chronic, whether there are other signs of liver cell injury, and whether there is evidence of obstruction of the bile ducts. In viral hepatitis, jaundice is usually short lived and disappears on its own. In cirrhosis the jaundice is usually mild but persistent. In primary biliary cirrhosis the jaundice may be mild or severe; severe jaundice usually predicts an unfavorable outcome. Obstructive jaundice caused by biliary stones is associated with spastic contractions (known as *biliary colics*), which abate upon surgical removal of the stone. Jaundice caused by carcinoma of the pancreas may be surgically relieved by shunting the bile flow into the intestine, but the patient has almost no chances of surviving because carcinoma of the pancreas has an abysmal prognosis.

ACUTE VIRAL HEPATITIS

Acute viral hepatitis is a clinical syndrome of variable severity caused by one of several hepatotropic viruses known as *hepatitis A, B, C, D,* and *E.* It is the most prevalent liver disease in the world. In the United States, hepatitis affects, on average, 2 persons per 1000 every year. The disease is often asymptomatic; 40% of all Americans have antibodies to hepatitis A (HAV) virus, and 5% to 10% have antibodies to HBV virus, although most of these individuals do not remember ever having had hepatitis. In addition, the estimates are that approximately 5 million Americans are infected with HCV, and most of them do not even know that they have the infection.

Acute hepatitis may also occur in the course of several systemic diseases. These "other" forms of hepatitis must be distinguished from hepatitis caused by hepatotropic viruses. The best-known examples of nonspecific hepatitis are infectious mononucleosis, caused by the Epstein-Barr virus; herpesvirus; and cytomegalovirus infection. All these viruses and many others cause hepatitis, especially in immunosuppressed patients with acquired immunodeficiency syndrome (AIDS). Childhood viral diseases (measles, rubella, varicella) may also affect the liver, although such hepatitis is usually overshadowed by other symptoms. The virus of yellow fever is an important cause of acute hepatitis in the tropics but is rare in the United States. In clinical practice the term *viral hepatitis* is reserved for the disease caused by hepatitis A, B, C, D, and E viruses.

 Did You Know?

Jaundice is a symptom characterized by yellow skin and mucosa. Yellow skin can also be a consequence of hypercarotenemia, an excess of the yellow pigment carotene found in carrots and other yellow fruits and vegetables. Overindulgence in these foodstuffs can cause yellowing of the skin, which must be distinguished from clinical jaundice. Beware of people who are overly fond of pumpkins, mangos, or paw paws!

Etiology and Pathogenesis

The main features of hepatitis viruses are listed in Table 11-2. From this table one may see that hepatitis viruses vary in size and belong to several viral families. HBV is a DNA virus, whereas all the others are RNA viruses. The duration of *viremia*, the mode of infection, the duration of incubation, and the clinical presentation are distinct for each virus. Three viruses (HBV, hepatitis C virus [HCV], and hepatitis D virus [HDV]) can also cause a chronic disease, and at least two of these (HBV and HCV) predispose the infected individual's liver cells to malignant transformation. At present, vaccines exist for HAV and HBV, and these can be used for preventive immunization of persons who are at increased risk. For example, travelers to tropical countries are immunized against HAV. In addition, health professionals are usually immunized against HBV because they are at increased risk of infection through exposure to blood or blood products.

FORMS OF HEPATITIS

HEPATITIS A

Hepatitis A virus (HAV) is a 27-nm, nonencapsulated RNA virus similar to other picornaviruses, such as poliovirus and some enteric viruses. The infection is transmitted by the fecal-oral route, and it may occur in sporadic or epidemic form. The sources of the virus are sewage, contaminated food and drinks, and shellfish. The disease is most prevalent among children in underdeveloped countries. Tourists traveling to Mexico and South America or Africa are also at risk.

Symptoms usually develop after a short incubation period of 15 to 50 days. Clinically, HAV infection is characterized by short-lived, mild, enteric fever with vomiting, loss of appetite, and jaundice. Recovery occurs within days, usually without any long-term consequences. Transition to chronic hepatitis

TABLE 11-2 Features of Known Human Hepatitis (A, B, C, D, and E) Viruses

Feature	HAV	HBV	HCV	HDV	HEV
Family	Picorna	Hepadna	Flavi	(Viroid)	Hepe
Genome	RNA	DNA	RNA	RNA	RNA
Size (nm)	27	42	30–60	35	32
Viremia	Brief	Long	Long	Like HBV	Brief
Transmission	F/O	Par/sex	Par/sex	Par/sex	F/O
Incubation (days)	15–45	40–180	15–150	30–50	14–60
Fulminant hepatitis risk (%)	0.1	1	0.1	10	1–2 (if pregnant, 20)
Chronicity	No	10%	50%	10%	No
HCC association	No	Yes	Yes	No	No
Chronic carrier state	No	Yes	Yes	Yes	No
Vaccine available	Yes	Yes	No	No	No

F/O, fecal/oral; HAV, hepatitis A virus; HBV, hepatitis B virus; HCC, hepatocellular carcinoma; HCV, hepatitis C virus; HDV, hepatitis D virus; HEV, hepatitis E virus; Par/sex, parenteral/sexual.

or cirrhosis never occurs. The fulminant form of the disease, accompanied by hepatic failure, is extremely rare. HAV infection thus has a favorable prognosis.

HEPATITIS B

Hepatitis B virus (HBV) is an encapsulated DNA virus that is species specific for humans and higher primates. Nevertheless, it is closely related to other Hepadna family viruses that cause hepatitis in woodchucks, ducks, and ground squirrels. The DNA of HBV is partially double-stranded and contains four partially overlapping genes that encode the message for the synthesis of the protein components of the virion, colloquially known as the *Dane particle*. These include hepatitis B surface antigen (HBsAg), hepatitis B *core* antigen (HBcAg), and hepatitis B *e* antigen (HBeAg). These antigens are important for serologic diagnosis and monitoring of the disease.

HBsAg is secreted and released into circulation early in the disease and can be detected in the serum 1 week after the onset of infection (Figure 11-5). HBsAg disappears from the blood during the convalescent period, which is marked by the appearance of antibody to HBsAg (anti-HBs). HBsAg persists in circulation only in patients who develop chronic hepatitis. These patients do not produce anti-HBs and apparently cannot clear the virus from the body.

HBeAg appears in the serum during acute infection but disappears faster than HBsAg, usually during the icteric stage of the disease. Persistence of HBeAg in serum is found in patients with chronic hepatitis, and its presence is a good marker of infectivity of such serum.

HBcAg and viral DNA are not released into the blood. However, antibodies to this antigen (anti-HBc) appear in all infected persons, usually a few days before the onset of jaundice. Initially, the antibodies are IgM, after which IgG antibodies appear. Patients with chronic hepatitis also have anti-HBcAg. This antibody may be the only serologic evidence of viral infection in such patients.

Clinical Features

Symptoms of HBV appear 40 to 180 days after infection. Infection follows transfusion of blood, exposure to contaminated blood or blood products, or sexual contact. The disease has three phases: preicteric, icteric, and convalescent (see Figure 11-5). In the preicteric phase there is weakness, nausea, and vomiting, which are occasionally associated with mild enlargement and tenderness of the liver. Some patients develop a measles-like skin rash. Darkening of the urine, which contains bilirubin, is a useful diagnostic finding. Jaundice, a symptom found in less than 30% of affected patients, usually appears 2 months after exposure and is associated with worsening of clinical symptoms and laboratory findings. Typically these include elevated serum levels of bilirubin, ALT, and AST. The jaundice persists for several weeks and in most patients disappears spontaneously. The more profound the jaundice, the more likely it is that the disease will enter an uneventful period of recovery. Mild jaundice may herald a protracted course of the disease and a transition to chronic hepatitis.

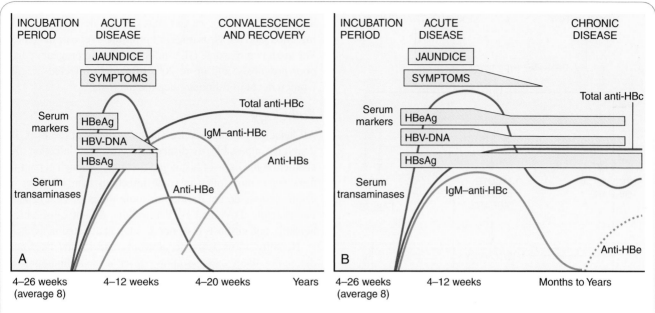

Figure 11-5 Serologic findings in acute hepatitis B viral infection. *A,* Acute infection with resolution. *B,* Acute viral hepatitis in progression to chronic hepatitis. (From Kumar V, Abbas AK, Fausto N, Aster JC: Robbins and Cotran Pathologic Basis of Disease, 8th ed, Philadelphia, 2010, Saunders.)

? **Did You Know?**

Hepatitis viruses are the most common cause of jaundice in clinical practice. Do not neglect to ask a jaundiced patient whether he or she has recently traveled abroad (hepatitis A virus [HAV]) or had a blood transfusion from or sexual intercourse with an unknown person (hepatitis B virus [HBV] and hepatitis C virus [HCV]). Information regarding drug use should also be elicited for two reasons. Jaundice could be drug induced, or it could also be the result of a viral infection transmitted by shared hypodermic needles.

The outcome of HBV infection is outlined in Figure 11-6. The disease may be symptomatic (icteric) or asymptomatic (subclinical). HBV produces clinically recognizable symptoms in one third of infected persons. The remaining two thirds have subclinical disease, which is recognized only by the subsequent appearance of antibodies to HBs and HBc. Most infected patients (90%) recover completely. Acute fulminant hepatitis develops in 1%, and chronic hepatitis in less than 10% of those with clinically evident infection. Chronic hepatitis may develop even without an acute icteric phase. *Chronic hepatitis* is subclinical in 75% of cases. These patients have no symptoms. HBsAg in the serum of affected patients and mild portal tract inflammation seen on liver biopsy are the only signs of disease. These persons show histologic signs of mild chronic persistent hepatitis and are classified as asymptomatic HBsAg carriers. Chronic active hepatitis, which develops in about 25% of patients with serologic evidence of chronic hepatitis, is a more serious form and may progress to cirrhosis. Hepatocellular carcinoma is a rare but well-known late complication of chronic HBV and cirrhosis that develops in some infected persons.

HEPATITIS D

Hepatitis D virus (HDV) is an incomplete RNA virus (viroid) that requires HBV for its own replication. Infection with these two viruses can occur simultaneously *(coinfection),* or the HDV infection may occur as a superinfection, following a preexisting HBV infection. Coinfection produces symptoms that are indistinguishable from HBV hepatitis, although the symptoms may be more prominent and there is a greater likelihood of fulminant hepatic necrosis. Superinfection of asymptomatic HBV carriers may activate the disease, and in those with active chronic hepatitis, progression to cirrhosis may be accelerated. HDV infection is best documented by demonstrating antibodies to HDV. The HDV antigen appears only briefly in the blood, so it is impractical to search for it.

HEPATITIS C

Hepatitis C virus (HCV), a flavivirus, is an RNA virus of variable size (30 to 60 nm) that encodes a single polypeptide, which on post-translational cleavage gives rise to the typical HCV proteins. Antibodies to these proteins are used to diagnose HCV infection. The infection can be confirmed by isolating the virus and measuring the number of viral particles in blood with molecular biology techniques.

HCV infections are most often acquired by blood contaminating the needles used during intravenous drug abuse.

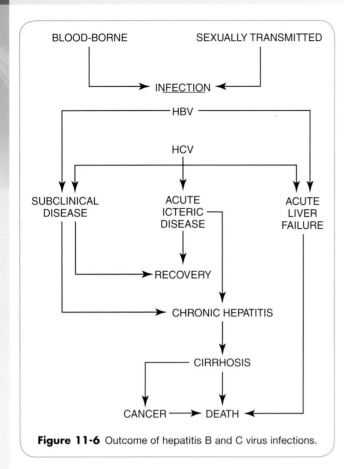

Figure 11-6 Outcome of hepatitis B and C virus infections.

Other risk factors are multiple sex partners, surgery, accidental needle stick or scalpel injuries, and multiple close contacts with HCV infected persons. Doctors, nurses, dentists, and other health professionals are at a small but definitive risk and account for 1.5% of all HCV infected persons in the United States. It is worth mentioning that approximately 30% of all HCV patients do not have any of these risk factors and do not know the source of their infection.

The clinical presentation of HCV infection is indistinguishable from that of HBV infection. Generally, however, the disease is less severe. It is often anicteric, and it is commonly associated with mild abnormalities in laboratory test results. Despite the mild course associated with the acute infection, HCV has a tendency to progress to chronic hepatitis in 50% of affected individuals. Approximately 25% of patients with chronic HCV infection will develop cirrhosis. Hepatocellular carcinoma develops in some persons as a late complication of cirrhosis.

HEPATITIS E

Hepatitis E virus (HEV) is an RNA virus transmitted by the fecal-oral route. The virus is endemic in parts of Asia, Africa, and South America, and even as close to the United States as Mexico. It tends to cause waterborne epidemics, especially during the rainy season. HEV resembles HAV in many aspects. The infection is usually asymptomatic or mild and transient. It heals without serious consequences. Chronic hepatitis and chronic carrier states do not develop after HEV infection, and the virus does not promote liver carcinogenesis. For unknown reasons, HEV infection during pregnancy has a poor prognosis, and up to 20% of acutely infected pregnant women develop fulminant hepatic necrosis.

Pathology

All hepatitis viruses produce similar changes in the liver. It is therefore impossible to distinguish one viral infection from another on the basis of histologic findings, although certain features occur more often in some infections than in others and certain lesions do not develop in some forms of viral hepatitis. For example, HAV and HEV infections do not cause chronic hepatitis, and cirrhosis does not develop in affected individuals.

Hepatitis viruses are hepatotropic and invade liver cells, damaging them and disrupting their normal functions and finally promoting cell death by apoptosis. Hepatocytes infected with HBV and HCV evoke an immune reaction that also results in apoptosis of infected cells. This process is usually associated with obvious morphologic changes, which are evident on histologic examination of liver biopsy specimens (Figure 11-7). These changes include the following:

- *Reversible hepatocellular changes.* Affected liver cells have normal nuclei and a well-preserved cell membrane but show cytoplasmic changes, such as granularity or *vacuolation* ("ballooning degeneration"). Intracellular and intercellular bile stasis may be prominent.
- *Irreversible hepatocellular changes.* Dying liver cells lose their nuclei and are transformed into round, anuclear, cytoplasmic fragments called *eosinophilic* or *apoptotic bodies.* In many instances these apoptotic cells cannot be identified because they are phagocytized by scavenger cells. In acute fulminant infection, hepatotropic viruses may induce massive liver cell necrosis.
- *Inflammatory infiltrates.* Damaged and dead liver cells are phagocytized by macrophages that invade the liver lobule, forming small foci within the disrupted strands of liver cells. Kupffer cells also proliferate, and enlarged polymorphonuclear leukocytes (PMNs) are not seen in acute viral hepatitis.
- *Regeneration of hepatocytes.* Liver cells have a high capacity for regeneration, and any loss is usually accompanied by regeneration, which occurs at random. The newly formed liver cells are relatively smaller and have more basophilic cytoplasms.

Acute hepatitis may resolve without any consequences; in a small number of patients with HBV and HCV infections, it may progress to chronic hepatitis.

Histologically, chronic hepatitis may be classified as mild, moderate, or severe. Mild inflammation is limited to the portal tracts. There is very little, if any, intralobular inflammation. In more prominent chronic hepatitis the portal tract inflammation is accompanied by spilling of inflammatory cells across the limiting plate ("interface hepatitis") and all the way into the lobule. Severe chronic hepatitis is characterized by disruption of the lobular architecture secondary to an

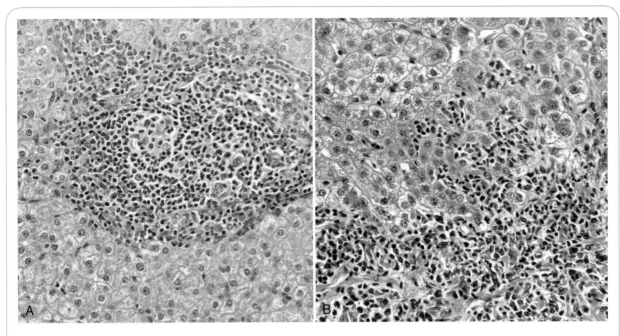

Figure 11-7 Chronic viral hepatitis C. *A*, Mild chronic hepatitis with inflammation limited to portal tracts. *B*, Severe chronic hepatitis with inflammation and fibrosis extending from portal tracts into the lobule.

aggressive inflammation and fibrosis that accompanies liver cell death. Fibrous tissue strands may form connective tissue bridges between adjacent portal tracts or portal tracts and centrolobular areas. This so-called bridging fibrosis may progress to cirrhosis.

CIRRHOSIS

Cirrhosis is a chronic liver disease characterized by a loss of normal liver structure and function. The term *cirrhosis* is a synonym for end-stage liver disease; it is irreversible and incurable except by liver transplantation. Morphologically it is characterized by fibrosis and regenerating liver cell nodules that replace the normal parenchyma.

Etiology

The most important causes of cirrhosis are listed in Box 11-1. In the United States, cirrhosis is a finding in 5% of the autopsies performed in general hospitals or in medical examiners' offices. A large number of these cases are related to abuse of alcohol. Alcoholic cirrhosis is the fourth most common cause of death in men 40 to 60 years of age. Viral hepatitis B and C are also important causes of cirrhosis. HCV is currently the most common viral cause of hepatitis in the United States. Recent studies have shown that many alcoholic patients have been infected with HCV, and in such cases it would appear that the cirrhosis has a dual etiology. Alcohol abuse and hepatitis virus infections probably account for 65% of all cases of cirrhosis in this country. Hereditary metabolic diseases, autoimmune diseases, drug use, and biliary obstruction

BOX 11-1 Causes of Cirrhosis

Alcohol
Hepatitis virus (B, C, and D)
Hereditary metabolic diseases
    Hemochromatosis
    Wilson's disease
    Alpha$_1$-antitrypsin deficiency
Autoimmune diseases
    Primary biliary cirrhosis
    Primary sclerosing cholangitis
    Autoimmune hepatitis
Drugs
Biliary obstruction
    Cystic fibrosis
    Gallstones
Cryptogenic

account for a small number of cases. In approximately 20% of cases the etiology of cirrhosis cannot be established. Such cirrhosis is thus labeled *cryptogenic.*

Pathogenesis

The exact pathogenesis of cirrhosis is unknown. However, it is generally accepted that the main pathologic processes include the following:

- Necrosis of liver cells
- Repair by fibrosis
- Regeneration

Morphologically there are two basic patterns of cirrhosis: portal cirrhosis and biliary cirrhosis. *Portal cirrhosis* is believed

271

to result from liver cell necrosis followed by an ingrowth of fibrous tissue from the portal tracts (Figure 11-8). Experimentally it is possible to produce portal cirrhosis in laboratory rats by treating them with carbon tetrachloride (CCl₄). CCl₄ produces liver cell necrosis, which is repaired by regeneration. Continuous exposure to this toxin impairs the ability of liver cells to regenerate, and parenchymal losses caused by liver cell necrosis are replaced by fibrous scars. With time the amount of fibrous tissue increases, encircling parts of the remaining liver parenchyma and thus inhibiting its ability to regenerate. This dual repair by regeneration and fibrosis alters the normal architecture of the liver. The liver becomes irregularly shaped, shrunken, firm, and nodular. Such pathogenetic mechanisms probably cause the human disease as well, although in the latter the course might be much more protracted. It takes 10 to 20 years of alcohol abuse before symptoms of cirrhosis develop. Viral

hepatitis–induced liver injury requires less time, but, on average, cirrhosis secondary to viral hepatitis becomes evident 10 to 15 years after the initial infection. Occasionally cirrhosis develops within months or a few years after massive liver necrosis caused by fulminant viral hepatitis.

Hereditary inborn errors of metabolism, such as Wilson's disease or alpha₁-antitrypsin deficiency, produce cirrhosis over a period of 10 to 20 years. However, because these diseases are congenital, the first signs of liver failure usually appear early (i.e., in the second or third decade of life).

Biliary cirrhosis results from diseases of the biliary tree. It may be primary or secondary. Primary biliary cirrhosis is an autoimmune disease affecting the bile ducts. Secondary biliary cirrhosis develops after prolonged partial or complete obstruction of bile flow. The obstruction is most often caused by biliary stones in the common bile duct. Such stones may

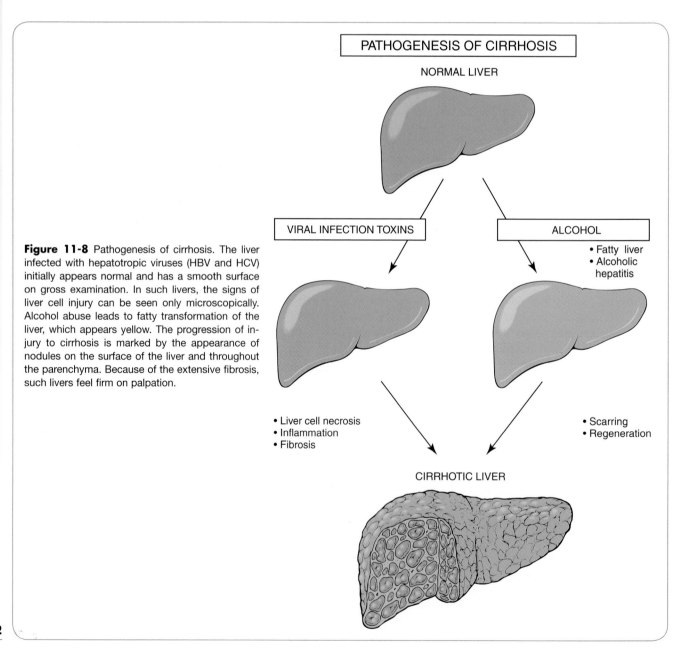

Figure 11-8 Pathogenesis of cirrhosis. The liver infected with hepatotropic viruses (HBV and HCV) initially appears normal and has a smooth surface on gross examination. In such livers, the signs of liver cell injury can be seen only microscopically. Alcohol abuse leads to fatty transformation of the liver, which appears yellow. The progression of injury to cirrhosis is marked by the appearance of nodules on the surface of the liver and throughout the parenchyma. Because of the extensive fibrosis, such livers feel firm on palpation.

mechanically occlude the duct, or they may cause chronic inflammation and fibrosis that eventually leads to obliteration of the ductal lumen. Primary sclerosing cholangitis, a disease of unknown etiology characterized by destruction of the larger bile ducts and fibrosis, also leads to secondary biliary cirrhosis. In the tropics, secondary biliary cirrhosis develops as a result of bacterial cholangitis and infections with parasites, such as Opistorchis sinensis or Schistosoma mansoni.

Pathology

Cirrhosis of the liver can be diagnosed on gross examination at autopsy; during surgical exploration of the abdomen (laparotomy); or by laparoscopy, a procedure that allows inspection of the abdominal organs through a needle-sized optical instrument called a *laparoscope*. The final diagnosis is made on the basis of histologic findings.

Cirrhosis is a progressive disease that relentlessly destroys the liver cells, replacing them with fibrous scars (Figures 11-9 and 11-10). In some forms of cirrhosis, such as those caused by chronic alcohol abuse, the liver is fatty, yellow, and usually enlarged. In most other forms of cirrhosis the liver progressively shrinks to approximately one half its normal size, weighing 600 to 800 g.

Histologic findings are diagnostic of cirrhosis, which is typically diagnosed by correlating the clinical and liver biopsy data. Histologic findings rarely provide a reliable clue about the causes of the disease. The normal liver architecture is lost. Instead, the parenchyma consists of liver cells arranged into nodules separated from each other by dense connective tissue strands. The presence of fat in liver cells and Mallory's hyaline favors the diagnosis of alcoholic cirrhosis. The presence of cytoplasmic granules in hepatocytes is a feature of α_1-AT deficiency. Iron accumulation favors the diagnosis of hemochromatosis.

Clinical Features

Symptoms and complications of cirrhosis may be seen in the liver, in the abdominal organs, and in extra-abdominal sites (Figure 11-11).

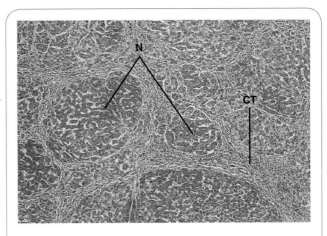

Figure 11-10 Histology of cirrhosis. The parenchyma consists of nodules (N) of liver cells surrounded by strands of connective tissue (CT).

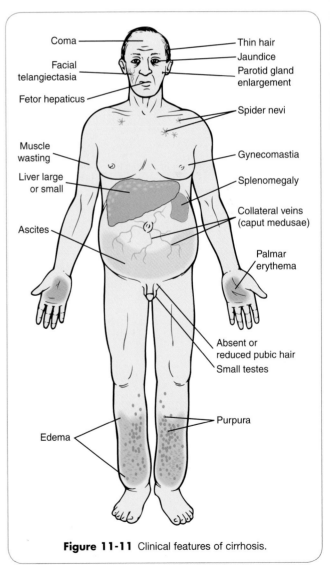

Figure 11-11 Clinical features of cirrhosis.

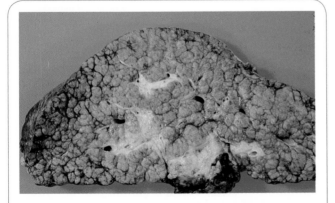

Figure 11-9 Alcoholic cirrhosis. The normal liver parenchyma has been replaced by nodules that are yellow because of their high fat content.

Fibrosis and nodularity of the liver impede blood flow and cause portal hypertension. Portal hypertension has three major anatomic consequences:

- Ascites
- Splenomegaly
- Anastomoses between the portal and systemic circulation

Ascites (from the Greek *askos,* meaning "bag") is an accumulation of fluid in the abdominal cavity. Because it can also be considered a peritoneal transudate or edema limited to the abdominal cavity, it is also called *hydroperitoneum.* Ascites develops as a result of the interaction of several mechanisms, the most important of which are portal hypertension and hypoproteinemia (Figure 11-12). Backpressure in branches of the portal

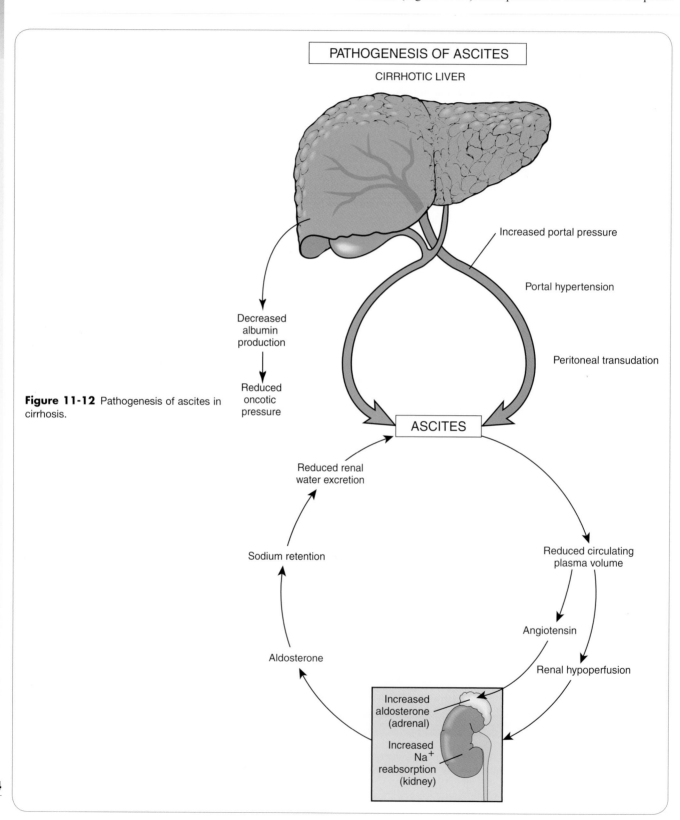

Figure 11-12 Pathogenesis of ascites in cirrhosis.

PATHOGENESIS OF ASCITES

CIRRHOTIC LIVER

Increased portal pressure

Portal hypertension

Peritoneal transudation

Decreased albumin production

Reduced oncotic pressure

ASCITES

Reduced renal water excretion

Sodium retention

Reduced circulating plasma volume

Angiotensin

Renal hypoperfusion

Aldosterone

Increased aldosterone (adrenal)

Increased Na⁺ reabsorption (kidney)

vein results in the transudation of fluid from the serosal surfaces of the intestines, liver, and peritoneal surfaces lining the abdominal cavity. Reduced oncotic pressure of the plasma secondary to hypoalbuminemia facilitates the passage of fluids from the circulation into the abdominal cavity. This results in relative hypovolemia (i.e., reduced volume of circulating blood), which triggers the release of aldosterone from the adrenal cortex. Aldosterone acts on the kidneys, causing sodium and water retention, which further compounds the problem. All this adversely affects the kidneys, which eventually stop producing urine. The patient becomes anuric and develops a hepatorenal syndrome.

Ascites is resistant to treatment, and drainage of the fluid from the abdominal cavity does not have any beneficial effects. The hepatorenal syndrome is also resistant to treatment, although the kidneys appear normal and will resume normal function if transplanted to another individual after the death of the patient. Ascites may become infected, which will lead to bacterial peritonitis.

? Did You Know?

Ascites causes bulging of the anterior abdominal wall. Portal hypertension may be associated with dilated periumbilical veins, known in the medical literature as *caput medusae* (i.e., Medusa's head). In Greek mythology, Medusa was a woman who had snakes emanating from her head instead of hair. The tortuous veins on the abdomen reminded a literary physician of Medusa's head. The term is still used, although the comparison with snakes is a bit farfetched.

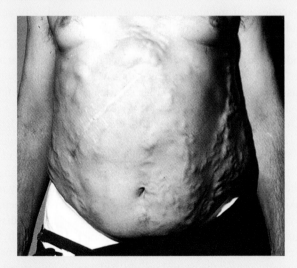

(Photograph courtesy Dr. Olav Hilmar Iversen. From Basic Text in Pathology. Universitetsforlaget, Oslo, Norway, 1974.)

Splenomegaly is very common in cirrhosis. The spleen, which normally weighs 150 g, enlarges three to six times to a weight of 500 to 1000 g. The affected patient will perceive the enlarged spleen as heavy and painful. The enlarged spleen has a tendency to sequester and destroy blood cells, which results in anemia, leukopenia, or thrombocytopenia. These hematologic consequences are aggravated by *hypersplenism*, a poorly

understood syndrome characterized by inhibition of hematopoiesis in the bone marrow.

Anastomoses between the portal and systemic circulation develop as a result of shunting of the portal blood into systemic veins in the lower esophagus, hemorrhoidal plexus, and periumbilical venous plexus. The most important of these vessels are the veins of the lower esophagus, which undergo dilation and transform into *varices* (see Figure 11-3). **Esophageal varices** (dilated veins that appear at the lower end of the esophagus) are prone to bleeding, which results in hematemesis or melena. Massive hemorrhage is one of the most common causes of death in patients with cirrhosis.

Shunting of blood from the portal to the systemic circulation is accompanied by serious metabolic consequences and corresponding clinical symptoms. The most important of these is *hepatic encephalopathy,* a syndrome marked by clouded mentation and distinct neurologic symptoms. Cerebral dysfunction is thought to be caused by ammonia and putative neurotoxins absorbed from the intestine. Because the shunts allow the enteric venous blood to bypass the liver, neurotoxic substances are not detoxified and therefore act directly on susceptible cells in the brain. The diseased brain shows edema and altered astrocytes but no other morphologic changes that would explain the pathogenesis of neurologic symptoms. Hepatic coma is associated with a high mortality rate, and the patient's life can be saved only by emergency liver transplantation.

The diagnosis of cirrhosis is made on the basis of clinical findings, but it must be confirmed by laboratory studies and liver biopsy. Associated symptoms and findings reflect the following:

- *Liver cell injury and death.* ALT and AST levels are the best markers of liver cell injury. Acute liver injury is characterized by an elevation of these liver enzymes in serum, but as the acute injury ceases, the levels of ALT and AST may revert to normal. In end-stage liver disease, often there is no ongoing liver cell death. ALT and AST concentration in blood may be only mildly elevated.
- *Loss of liver cell function.* Decreased output of albumin leads to hypoalbuminemia, which contributes to the formation of ascites and edema. Decreased synthesis of coagulation proteins results in a bleeding tendency. Defective excretion of bilirubin may result in jaundice, which is usually mild.
- *Portal hypertension.* The principal consequences of portal hypertension are ascites, splenomegaly, and anastomoses between the portal and systemic circulation (which tend to bleed). The blood from ruptured esophageal varices is a major source of ammonia. Ammonia formed from degraded blood proteins is absorbed in the intestines and thus contributes to hepatic encephalopathy.

In addition to these most important signs of cirrhosis, affected patients also have numerous other symptoms involving the cardiorespiratory, renal, endocrine, and hematopoietic systems. Ascites and secondary hyperaldosteronism and hypernatremia cause a fluid overload, with consequent cardiopulmonary failure and pulmonary edema. Hypoperfusion of the kidneys and sodium retention secondary to the action of aldosterone may precipitate renal failure (**hepatorenal syndrome**). Endocrine symptoms, such as impotence or gynecomastia in males and anovulation in females, reflect abnormal metabolism of sex hormones. Osteodystrophy is related to abnormal vitamin D metabolism and calcium homeostasis, whereas hypothyroidism may result from a deficiency of thyroid hormone–binding protein and abnormal metabolism of thyroglobulins. Anemia is very common in cirrhosis, in part as a result of a subnormal supply of metabolites from the liver and in part because of splenomegaly.

DRUG- AND TOXIN-INDUCED LIVER DISEASES

The liver is the primary site for the metabolic conversion and inactivation of drugs and various toxins. In this process, the liver cells may be injured by the chemical that is metabolized or by the toxic derivatives formed inside the liver cells. For example, carbon tetrachloride, a chemical component of brass polish and a cause of accidental poisoning in children, is metabolized into carbon trichloride, a toxic radical that may cause liver cell necrosis, as discussed in Chapter 1.

Hepatic drug reactions can be classified either as *predictable* (those that are dose related) or *unpredictable* (those that occur without obvious explanation) (Table 11-3). An example of the former can be found in the painkiller acetaminophen (Tylenol). This drug, which occasionally is ingested in suicide attempts, always produces liver necrosis if ingested in a dose exceeding 15 g. Likewise, tetracycline, an antibiotic widely used for acne, invariably produces fatty changes in liver cells, fortunately without any serious consequences. Predictable liver cell injury can be prevented by avoiding the possibly toxic substance.

Unpredictable drug reactions can take place in any setting and can induce a variety of histologic changes. In some sensitive persons the anesthetic halothane will induce an acute

TABLE 11-3 Drug-Induced Liver Disease

Pathology	Drug
Predictable (Dose-Related) Reaction	
Necrosis	Acetaminophen
Fatty changes	Tetracycline
Unpredictable Reaction	
Viral hepatitis–like changes	Halothane
Cholestasis	Chlorpromazine
Chronic hepatitis–like changes	Methyldopa
Granuloma	Phenylbutazone
Tumor	Estrogens

febrile jaundice resembling that associated with acute hepatitis. Isoniazid, used for the treatment of tuberculosis, is a well-known cause of a mild hepatitis-like disease that most often occurs in older persons. Chlorpromazine, a psychoactive drug, occasionally causes intrahepatic bile stasis and conjugated hyperbilirubinemia. Methyldopa, used for the treatment of Parkinson's disease, may induce chronic hepatitis-like changes. Phenylbutazone, an anti-inflammatory drug used for arthritis, may induce granulomas. Estrogens (and even oral contraceptives) appear to promote formation of liver cell tumors. Today, in the era of "minipills" that contain small amounts of estrogen, such hormone-induced tumors are rare. Furthermore, most of the reported tumors are benign liver cell adenomas.

ALCOHOLIC LIVER DISEASE

Alcohol is an important cause of liver diseases. Chronic alcohol abuse may cause the following hepatic lesions:

- **Fatty liver** (an accumulation of triglycerides in the liver)
- Alcoholic hepatitis
- Cirrhosis

Ethyl alcohol is imbibed in large quantities in most Western countries, primarily because of its mind-altering effects. However, it is also an important source of calories (7 calories per gram) and has complex metabolic and potentially toxic effects on many cells in the body. Alcohol affects the liver, inhibiting some enzymes and stimulating others, as discussed in Chapter 1. It also alters the fluidity and function of cell membranes, as well as the intracellular transport of organelles and metabolites. Because of increased fatty acid synthesis, decreased fatty acid oxidation, and decreased export of fats in the form of lipoproteins, alcohol invariably produces fatty changes in liver cells in a dose-dependent manner. The liver becomes enlarged, but without any metabolic consequences or symptoms. These changes are completely reversible, disappearing after the patient stops drinking.

A small number of patients with alcoholic fatty liver (10% to 15%) develop signs of **alcoholic hepatitis.** These signs usually include fever, leukocytosis, abdominal pain, and jaundice. Histologic examination of the liver shows fatty change of hepatocytes and focal necrosis of liver cells associated with leukocytic infiltrates and bile stasis. The cytoplasm of hepatocytes often contains eosinophilic aggregates of intermediate cytoskeletal filaments, which form so-called Mallory's hyaline (Figure 11-13). Special stains show pericellular fibrosis especially around the central venule. Although highly suggestive of alcohol abuse, none of these histologic findings is diagnostic of alcoholic hepatitis. Similar findings can be seen in some obese persons, in persons with diabetes, and occasionally even without any obvious causes. This disease is called **steatohepatitis,** and if no reasons for the fatty change and other pathologic findings are discovered, the disease is called *idiopathic steatohepatitis.* Like alcoholic hepatitis, steatohepatitis can progress to cirrhosis in some cases.

Cirrhosis is the most serious complication of alcohol abuse. It is not known why some alcoholic patients develop

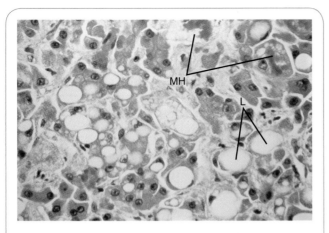

Figure 11-13 Alcoholic hepatitis. Hepatocytes contain lipid (L) droplets and eosinophilic Mallory's hyaline (MH).

cirrhosis and others do not. In some cases it is preceded by alcoholic hepatitis. In others it may be attributable to the additive effects of alcohol and other toxins or viruses. In most instances it is not possible to sort out all the factors that contribute to the progression of the disease, particularly if the cirrhosis evolves insidiously over a long period.

HEREDITARY DISEASES OF THE LIVER

Essentially all hereditary metabolic diseases affect the liver. However, the symptoms of liver cell injury are in most metabolic genetic diseases usually overshadowed by symptoms pertaining to other organs. Only a few examples of hereditary diseases that present primarily as hepatic disorders or induce significant changes in the liver are presented here. These hepatic lesions may vary from mild to severe.

GILBERT'S DISEASE

Gilbert's disease is an autosomal dominant disorder of bilirubin metabolism that affects about 5% of the total population. The disease causes intermittent jaundice that usually begins after puberty and that is most common in male subjects. Unconjugated hyperbilirubinemia, which is typical of this disorder, reflects a defect in the uptake of bilirubin from blood into liver cells. The nature of the enzyme defect that causes this hereditary jaundice is unknown. Except for jaundice, these patients have no other symptoms and thus require no treatment.

HEMOCHROMATOSIS

Hereditary **hemochromatosis** is an autosomal recessive defect of iron absorption that results in excessive accumulation of iron in the liver and several other organs. This accumulation of iron stores, which can be increased by up to 50 times the normal level, damages liver cells and induces cirrhosis. The

cirrhotic liver is typically enlarged, heavy, and micronodular. Because of the rusty red-brown appearance of the tissue, it is often called *pigmentary cirrhosis.* Excess amounts of the iron pigment hemosiderin can be demonstrated in the liver by the Prussian blue histochemical reaction.

The gene for the hereditary hemochromatosis (called *HFE gene*) has been identified, and its mutations have been found to be extremely prevalent. Approximately 10% of the persons of northern European origin are heterozygous and 0.4% are homozygous for these gene mutations and could develop the disease. However, the symptoms occur in only a small proportion of homozygous persons. In addition to cirrhosis, they show pigmentation of the skin and diabetes mellitus, a combination of symptoms referred to as *bronze diabetes.* Other endocrine organs may also be affected, and congestive heart failure is a common cause of death. The diagnosis of hemochromatosis is established by demonstrating a high concentration of iron in the blood, high saturation of *transferrin* (the main iron transport protein of the plasma), and the presence of iron deposits in the cirrhotic liver. Therapy for hereditary hemochromatosis is directed at reducing the iron stores, which is best accomplished by bloodletting. Weekly phlebotomies have a most beneficial effect and significantly prolong the lives of these patients.

WILSON'S DISEASE

Wilson's disease, also known as *hepatolenticular degeneration,* is an autosomal recessive disorder of copper metabolism that produces lesions in the liver, brain, and eye. Heterozygotes are found at a relatively high rate (1:200), but the disease, which occurs only in some homozygotic persons, has a much lower prevalence (1 per 40,000 persons).

The mutated gene for Wilson's disease (called *ATP7B gene*) has been identified, but the mechanisms underlying the disease remain obscure. It is thought that the defect lies in the inability of liver cells to excrete copper in bile. Because this is the primary means for preventing copper overload, the defect results in excessive copper storage in the liver. The concentration of the copper carrier protein ceruloplasmin is also decreased in serum, which leads to compensatory binding of copper to albumin. This albumin-bound copper has a tendency to precipitate in the brain and the eyes.

The symptoms of Wilson's disease may be related to the toxic effect of copper, which is deposited in the liver, the eyes, or the brain. In the liver, excess copper causes cirrhosis. This form of cirrhosis has an early onset and may even be diagnosed in children. Additional findings include Kayser-Fleischer ring of the eye, which appears as a brownish discoloration of the iris; reddish-brown discoloration and degeneration of striatum and closely related basal ganglia of the brain; and acute hemolytic episodes. Wilson's disease can be treated with chelating (metal-binding) agents, such as D-penicillamine, which bind copper and remove it from the body. Chelating agents can be used not only to prevent the disease but also to alleviate symptoms in patients who have already developed signs of copper toxicity.

277

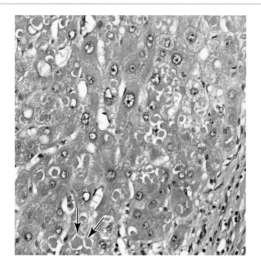

Figure 11-14 Alpha₁-antitrypsin deficiency. The liver cells contain cytoplasmic globules (arrows) composed of α_1-antitrypsin.

TABLE 11-4 Liver Diseases of Presumptive Immune Origin

	Autoimmune Hepatitis	Primary Biliary Cirrhosis	Primary Sclerosing Cholangitis
Sex predominance	Females	Females	Males
Age (years)	20–30	30–60	20–40
Bile duct lesions			
Intrahepatic	+/−	++	+
Extrahepatic	−	−	++
Hepatitis (intralobular)	+/−	+/−	−
Antibodies to:			
Mitochondria	−/+	++	−
Nuclear antigens	++	+/−	−
Smooth muscle	++	−	−
Steroid therapy	++	−	−

ALPHA₁-ANTITRYPSIN DEFICIENCY

Alpha₁-antitrypsin deficiency (AAT) is an autosomal recessive disorder that is related to the presence of the PiZ allele of the gene that encodes for AAT. As mentioned in Chapter 8, this mutation of the Pi gene is found in about 5% of the population, and in homozygous PiZ mutants it may cause emphysema and cirrhosis of the liver. AAT is synthesized in the liver; in PiZ homozygotes it accumulates in the form of cytoplasmic globules inside the liver cells (Figure 11-14). The exact mechanism for liver cell injury is unknown.

A significant number of affected persons develop childhood cholestasis and chronic hepatitis, which progress to cirrhosis in about 20% of affected individuals. AAT deficiency is one of the most common causes of childhood cirrhosis. The disease may be latent until puberty or adulthood, when it usually presents with clinical signs of cirrhosis, which may also give rise to liver cancer.

IMMUNE DISORDERS

An immunologic origin has been proposed for several liver diseases, including autoimmune hepatitis, primary biliary cirrhosis, and primary sclerosing cholangitis, although it has not been conclusively proven that any liver disease is primarily an immune disorder. The features of these three diseases are summarized in Table 11-4.

AUTOIMMUNE HEPATITIS

Autoimmune hepatitis is a form of chronic hepatitis. It is thought to be immune mediated because, like systemic lupus erythematosus, it is associated with other autoimmune phenomena. The disease predominantly affects young women and is serologically characterized by high concentration of immunoglobulin in serums and by high titer of antinuclear antibodies and other autoantibodies. The most important among the various antibodies are antibodies to smooth muscle (ASM). Liver biopsy usually shows signs of inflammation in the portal areas extending into the lobules. The inflammatory infiltrates typically contain numerous plasma cells and lymphocytes. Clinically the disease resembles other forms of chronic hepatitis but has a more favorable diagnosis. It responds very well to steroid treatment.

PRIMARY BILIARY CIRRHOSIS

Primary biliary cirrhosis (PBC) is a disease of unknown etiology that is characterized by destruction of intrahepatic bile ducts and progression to cirrhosis. This "nonsuppurative destructive cholangitis," as it is also known, resembles the T-cell–mediated destruction of bile ducts associated with hepatic transplants and the graft-versus-host disease that often follows bone marrow transplantation. Hence it has been proposed that PBC is an immune disease mediated by type IV hypersensitivity reactions. The appearance of T lymphocytes within the lesions and the formation of granulomas also suggest that the disease is a cellular immune response, but the nature of the antigen evoking this response remains unknown. Most patients also have antibodies to mitochondria. Although this could mean that the humoral immune system is involved, the appearance of antibodies could be secondary to tissue destruction and therefore of limited pathogenetic significance.

PBC predominantly affects women (the ratio of females to males is 9:1). The disease begins as an inflammation of the intrahepatic bile ducts. Infiltrates of lymphocytes and macrophages subsequently destroy the bile ducts (Figure 11-15). Occasionally the portal tracts also contain granulomas. The destruction of bile ducts is accompanied by intrahepatic cholestasis and fibrosis, which ultimately leads to cirrhosis.

Clinically, biliary cirrhosis has an insidious onset. It affects middle-aged women who present with nonspecific symptoms, such as fatigue and loss of appetite. Itching related to jaundice, enlargement of the liver, and biochemical signs of liver disease are prominent features. The diagnosis is confirmed based on the ability to demonstrate antimitochondrial antibodies and on liver biopsy findings. Other immunologic findings may also be present, and many women have signs of some other immune disorder, such as mild hemolytic anemia, atrophic gastritis, and thyroiditis. As the bile duct destruction proceeds, obstructive jaundice becomes more pronounced, the stools become acholic, and steatorrhea develops. Biliary obstruction impedes the excretion of cholesterol, which is often deposited in the subcutaneous connective tissue in the form of small yellow nodules called *xanthomas* (from the Greek *xanthos*, meaning "yellow"). These are not true neoplasms but rather are infiltrates of macrophages loaded with lipid. Ultimately, affected patients develop cirrhosis, which is lethal unless a suitable donor is found for liver transplantation.

PRIMARY SCLEROSING CHOLANGITIS

Primary sclerosing cholangitis is a disease of unknown origin that also may have an immune pathogenesis. In contrast to PCB, it primarily affects adult men younger than 40 years. The associated destruction of intrahepatic and extrahepatic bile ducts by lymphocytes and macrophages is consistent with a cell-mediated immune reaction, but the original antigen inciting the cellular infiltrates remains obscure. The cellular phase of the disease is followed by fibrosis that obliterates the bile ducts inside and outside the liver (see Figure 11-15). The disease is typically segmental; therefore the larger bile ducts appear to be beaded and composed of alternating narrowed fibrotic and dilated segments. In approximately 60% of cases, the patients have a preexisting inflammatory bowel disease—more often ulcerative colitis than Crohn's disease. Many patients show evidence of other immune disorders and may have various autoantibodies in their blood. In all cases the liver disease is progressive, causing obstructive jaundice and secondary biliary cirrhosis. Cholangiocellular carcinoma develops in these patients with cirrhotic livers at an increased rate, considered to be approximately 10%. The overall prognosis of primary sclerosing cholangitis is unfavorable, but liver transplantation may save the life of an affected patient.

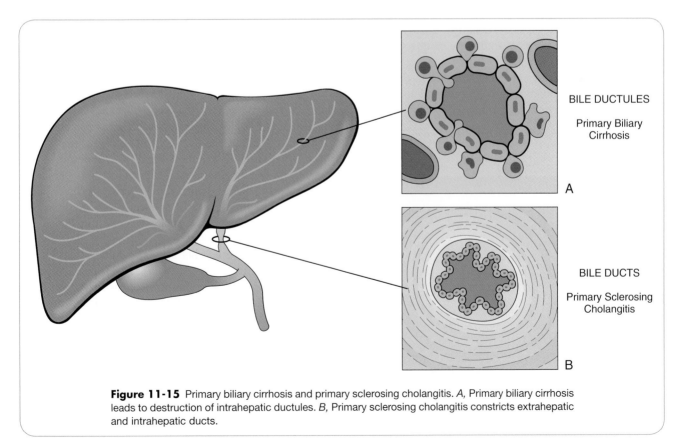

Figure 11-15 Primary biliary cirrhosis and primary sclerosing cholangitis. *A,* Primary biliary cirrhosis leads to destruction of intrahepatic ductules. *B,* Primary sclerosing cholangitis constricts extrahepatic and intrahepatic ducts.

BACTERIAL, PROTOZOAL, AND PARASITIC INFECTIONS

The liver is resistant to bacterial infections, presumably because of the protective role of phagocytic Kupffer cells. Thus all infections except viral hepatitis are rare in the United States. Bacterial, protozoal, and parasitic pathogens may reach the liver by the following methods:

- *An ascending route,* via the bile ducts, from the duodenum (typical of ascending bacterial cholangitis)
- *Blood flowing to the hepatic artery or portal vein,* causing portal vein infection, also known as *pylephlebitis*
- *Direct inoculation* (as in wounds)
- *Extension* from adjacent abdominal organs or from a perihepatic or subphrenic (subdiaphragmatic) abscess

Ascending cholangitis is the most important form of bacterial liver infection. It is usually caused by gram-negative enteric organisms, such as *Escherichia coli, Proteus mirabilis,* and *Streptococcus fecalis.* These cholangitic abscesses of the liver may be solitary or multiple. Most are associated with biliary obstruction caused by ascending infection with enteric bacteria. *E. coli* and other aerobic and anaerobic bacteria are easily cultured from the pus, but in 25% of patients the fluid appears sterile and no bacteria can be isolated, presumably because of their removal by phagocytic liver cells.

Pylephlebitic abscesses (i.e., those that develop as a result of the entry of bacteria into the liver through the portal vein) may be solitary or multiple. Before the antibiotic era, pylephlebitic abscess of the liver was a common complication of acute appendicitis. Today it is less common, usually affecting patients with inflammatory bowel disease or infected diverticula of the sigmoid colon.

Protozoal and parasitic infections are rare in the United States but are more common in the tropics and countries of Asia and Africa. For example, *Entamoeba histolytica* may infect the liver in persons who travel to Central America and Mexico. For reasons that are not entirely clear, all such infections occur more commonly in males than in females. Infections usually promote suppuration, but the pus remains localized to bile ducts or encapsulated within hepatic parenchyma in the form of abscesses (Figure 11-16). *S. mansoni* or *Schistosoma japonicum* may infect the liver during travels to Southeast Asia. *Clonorchis sinensis* is endemic in China.

GALLSTONES

Gallstones (cholelithiasis) are concretions composed of chemicals normally formed in bile. They are extremely common and in the United States more than half a million people undergo biliary surgery for gallstones each year. An estimated 20% of people older than 65 years have gallstones. Women are especially at risk; the incidence of gallstones is three times higher in women than in men. Because of a metabolic deficiency, Native Americans, such as Pima Indians, are at an extremely high risk for developing gallstones. Indeed, 75% of the women in this population develop gallstones by the age of 25 years. The incidence of gallstones is higher in whites than in blacks, which further underscores the genetic predisposition for this disease.

Pathogenesis

There are two types of gallstones: cholesterol stones and pigmentary stones. More than 75% of the gallstones that develop in patients in the United States are cholesterol stones; the remainder are either brown or black pigmentary stones. Each of these stones is formed as a result of a distinct mechanism, although it is not uncommon to have mixed stones, which shows that these pathogenetic mechanisms may be interrelated.

Cholesterol stones are formed in bile that is supersaturated with cholesterol and at the same time contain decreased amounts of bile acids and lecithin. Bile acids and lecithin are secreted together by the liver cells but independently of cholesterol. In the gallbladder these substances form water-soluble micelles with cholesterol. These micelles form only if the three substances are present in appropriate concentrations. If the normal ratio of bile components is altered, the bile becomes *lithogenic* (i.e., capable of stone formation). This occurs typically in obese persons who excrete large amounts of cholesterol in the bile but also may occur in patients with certain metabolic disorders, such as diabetes. Pregnancy, estrogen therapy, use of oral contraceptives, and use of certain drugs used for the treatment of hypercholesterolemia (e.g., clofibrate) also promote cholesterol excretion in the bile. Such bile is prone to accelerated nucleation of cholesterol crystals, which is most apparent during the concentration of bile in the gallbladder. The slower bile flow that occurs with age also predisposes such individuals to gallstone formation. It is thus understandable that most cholesterol gallstones are located in the gallbladder and that the typical risk factors include the so-called four Fs: *f*emale, older than *f*orty, *f*ertile, and *f*at.

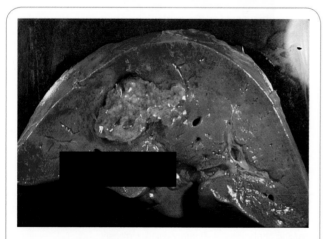

Figure 11-16 Amebic abscess. This cavitary lesion contains yellow, pastelike material.

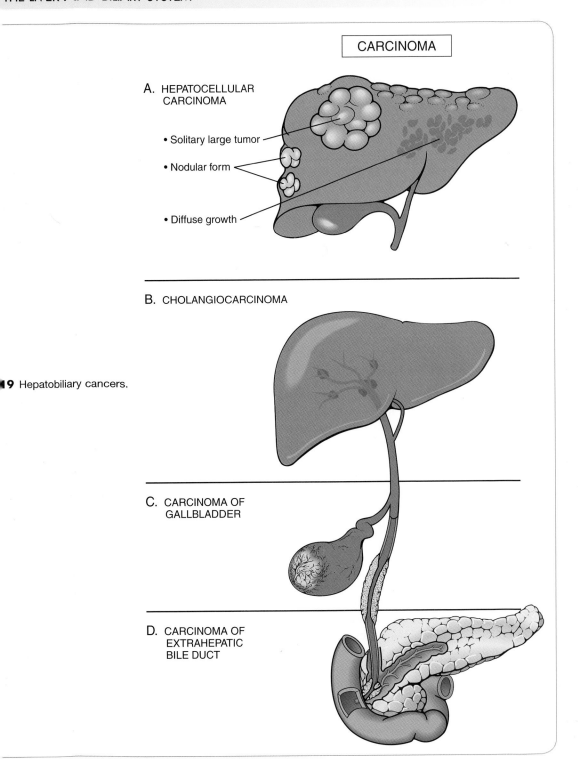

CARCINOMA

A. HEPATOCELLULAR CARCINOMA

• Solitary large tumor

• Nodular form

• Diffuse growth

B. CHOLANGIOCARCINOMA

19 Hepatobiliary cancers.

C. CARCINOMA OF GALLBLADDER

D. CARCINOMA OF EXTRAHEPATIC BILE DUCT

the highest incidence of gallbladder cancer d.

is initially localized to the gallbladder, even-
ugh the wall of the gallbladder, infiltrating
stages of disease the tumor may invade the
ducts and cause jaundice, or it may infiltrate
d cause intestinal obstruction. Metastases are

most prominent in local lymph nodes and adjacent abdominal organs.

Clinical Features

Gallbladder carcinoma produces few symptoms, and most of those, such as local discomfort or pain in the gallbladder area, may remain unnoticed or may be overshadowed by symptoms of cholelithiasis. Because of the delay in diagnosis, most tumors are discovered too late for surgical resection. By the

Pigmentary stones are composed of calcium bilirubinate and are either black or brown. The *black stones,* which are most common in Western countries, form in the gallbladders of patients with chronic hemolytic anemia (e.g., sickle cell anemia) and those with cirrhosis. In such patients the stones form presumably because of supersaturation of bile with bilirubin. *Brown stones* are often laminated and consist of alternating layers of calcium bilirubinate and cholesterol admixed with calcium. These stones occur more commonly in individuals living in the Far East than in those from the West and are often associated with biliary infections or infestations with liver flukes, such as Clonorchis sinensis. Brown stones are most often located in the extrahepatic bile ducts and tend to recur after removal. It is believed that these stones form as a result of the action of bacteria and parasites, which change the biochemical composition of bile.

Pathology

Cholesterol stones are typically solitary; measure 1 to 5 cm in diameter; and are round, yellow, and firm. On cross-sectioning, they have a glistening, radiating, crystalline appearance. Black pigmentary stones, which measure 5 to 10 mm in diameter, are multiple, jet black, ovoid or polygonal, and often faceted (Figure 11-17). They are soft and can be crushed between the fingers. Brown pigmentary stones are irregularly shaped and vary in size from 1 to 3 cm. On cross-sectioning, they are often laminated (i.e., they show darker and lighter layers around a central core).

The gallbladder harboring the stones usually shows signs of inflammation (**cholecystitis**). This develops because the gallstones may mechanically injure the mucosa, allowing entry of enteric bacteria into the wall of the gallbladder. Acute cholecystitis may evolve into a chronic inflammation. Severe infection, especially if associated with obstruction of the biliary outflow tract, may cause gangrene of the gallbladder. The necrotic wall of the gangrenous gallbladder may then rupture, leading to bacterial peritonitis. Alternatively, the inflamed serosa of the gallbladder may stimulate adhesion with the intestinal loops and the formation of a cholecystoenteric fistula. This fistula may serve as a conduit through which the gallstones may be

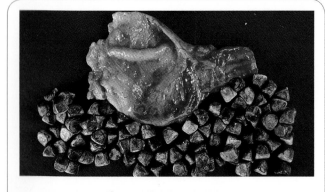

Figure 11-17 Gallstones.

discharged into the intestine. Obstruction of the intestine with gallstones causes *gallstone ileus.*

Chronic obstruction of the cystic duct interrupts the normal circulation of bile through the gallbladder. Bile in an obstructed gallbladder may become resorbed and may be replaced with clear, watery fluid by a process called *hydrops of the gallbladder.* If the hydrops persists, the wall of the nonfunctioning gallbladder may become thickened and fibrotic and ultimately will undergo dystrophic calcification (also called *porcelain gallbladder*).

The obstruction of the cystic duct prevents normal flow of bile into and out of the gallbladder but does not affect the flow of hepatic bile into the intestine. Gallstones forming in the common bile duct or small gallbladder stones that are discharged through the cystic duct may obstruct the common bile duct and produce obstructive jaundice. Approximately 50% of all cases of extrahepatic jaundice are attributable to gallstones in the common bile duct. Long-standing obstruction of the common bile duct may cause secondary biliary cirrhosis. Gallstones also predispose individuals to ascending infections of the biliary tract and are well-known causes of ascending bacterial cholangitis. Gallbladders that are removed to treat cholelithiasis occasionally contain cancerous lesions, but these are rare and there is no proof of a pathogenetic link between gallstones and cancer.

Clinical Features

Most gallstones are asymptomatic or produce minor nonspecific symptoms that require no treatment. Many gallstones are incidentally discovered during routine x-ray examination; indeed, only 20% of all patients with gallstones present with clinical symptoms, which are usually related to cholecystitis or obstruction of the cystic duct or the common bile duct (Figure 11-18).

Histologic signs of chronic cholecystitis are found in almost all gallbladders that contain stones. Such cases of chronic cholecystitis usually are associated with only minor discomfort. Obstruction of the cystic duct is typically associated with smooth muscle cell contraction and bouts of excruciating spasmodic pain *(biliary colic).* Obstruction of the cystic duct may lead to exacerbation of cholecystitis and also to reinfection. Such cases of superimposed acute cholecystitis usually present with fever.

The gallstones released into the common bile duct or those formed in the major ducts may obstruct the bile flow from the liver and cause jaundice. These stones also predispose the affected individual to ascending cholangitis.

The diagnosis of gallstones, suggested by the typical symptoms of obstruction of bile flow and biliary colic, is usually confirmed by x-ray studies. Gallstones that contain radiopaque calcium salts can be seen on plain x-ray films. Approximately 30% of cholesterol stones and more than 50% of black stones can be seen on plain x-ray studies. The remaining gallstones cannot be seen on routine radiographs and are best visualized by ultrasonography.

The treatment of gallstones may take several forms. Asymptomatic gallstones usually do not require treatment,

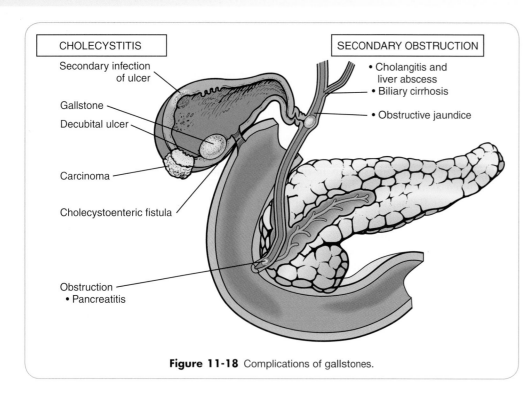

CHOLECYSTITIS

Secondary infection of ulcer

Gallstone

Decubital ulcer

Carcinoma

Cholecystoenteric fistula

Obstruction
• Pancreatitis

SECONDARY OBSTRUCTION

• Cholangitis and liver abscess
• Biliary cirrhosis

• Obstructive jaundice

Figure 11-18 Complications of gallstones.

whereas acute impaction and biliary colic require prompt treatment with antispasmodic and analgesic drugs. Biliary stones may be removed surgically or dissolved by extracorporeal shock wave therapy *(lithotripsy)*. Recently, good results have been reported for the chemical dissolution of stones with appropriate drugs.

HEPATOBILIARY NEOPLASMS

The primary tumors of the liver may be benign or malignant (Table 11-5). Benign tumors of the liver and the biliary tract are of limited clinical significance. The most common tumor

is *cavernous hemangioma,* which is present in 5% of livers at autopsy. These hemangiomas are usually small (less than 2 cm in diameter) and cause no symptoms.

Benign hepatocellular adenomas are rare tumors composed of cells resembling normal hepatocytes. These tumors appear almost exclusively in women, which suggests that the female sex hormones may play an important pathogenetic role. Indeed, almost all hepatocellular adenomas have been diagnosed in women who are pregnant or are taking oral contraceptives. In view of the widespread use of oral contraceptives and the fact that only 1 in 40,000 of these women will develop a benign liver tumor, one must postulate that some additional factors play a role in tumorigenesis. For unknown

reasons, these hepatocellular adenomas are highly vascular and tend to bleed, sometimes profusely, into the peritoneal cavity.

Malignant tumors can originate from epithelial cells of the liver, bile ducts, gallbladder, and rarely even from Kupffer cells.

- *Hepatocellular carcinomas* are the most important primary liver tumors, causing more than 1 million deaths worldwide. In the United States and Western countries, these tumors have an incidence of 5 per 100,000 and account for 2% of cancer deaths, but the incidence of this cancer is on the rise. By contrast, the incidence is 100 per 100,000 in Far East Asia, Africa, and other parts of the world in which HBV is endemic.
- *Cholangiocarcinomas* (i.e., tumors involving the intrahepatic or extrahepatic bile ducts) are less common, representing only 1% of all hepatobiliary tumors.
- *Gallbladder cancer* is less common than liver cancers, with an incidence of 1 in 50,000 persons, accounting for less than 1% of all cancer deaths.

HEPATOCELLULAR CARCINOMA

Hepatocellular carcinoma is a highly malignant tumor composed of neoplastic liver cells. The tumor occurs in adults and has a male predominance. The male-to-female ratio is 4:1. Most tumors originate in cirrhotic livers.

In the Far East and sub-Saharan Africa, where HBV is endemic, such tumors often appear in adults 30 to 50 years of age. In the United States and other nonendemic areas, these tumors occur most often in elderly persons. Hepatoblastoma, a liver cell cancer affecting children, develops in noncirrhotic livers but is rare worldwide.

Pathology

Hepatocellular carcinoma presents in three forms: (1) as a diffuse infiltrative lesion, (2) as a solitary mass limited to one lobe of the liver, or (3) as multiple nodules (Figure 11-19). These lesions may be yellow because they contain glycogen and lipid, brown like normal liver, or green because of discoloration with bile. On histologic examination, the tumor is composed of cells resembling, to some extent, normal liver cells. Well-differentiated tumors may even produce bile, whereas the poorly differentiated tumors are composed of small epithelial cells that show few signs of differentiation. Tumor cells often synthesize **alpha-fetoprotein (AFP),** a protein that can be demonstrated in the cytoplasm by immunohistochemical methods and in the serum by biochemical means. AFP is useful for early diagnosis of primary malignant liver cell tumors, even though it is found in the serum of only 50% of all patients.

Clinical Features

Clinical symptoms of hepatocellular cancer include nonspecific signs of malignant disease, such as weight loss, loss of appetite, and nausea, and symptoms that are directly related to tumor growth within the liver. The enlarged liver is tender

and even painful, comp[...]
Portal hypertension with [...]
common and often devel[...]
tal vein by tumor or tum[...]
vein. Tumors may obstru[...]
nous thrombosis, and im[...]
from the liver. This is cal[...]
typically associated with [...]
ary to venous congestion[...]

Hepatocellular carcino[...]
paraneoplastic syndromes[...]
functions of tumor cells. [...]
secrete insulin-like grow[...]
mors that produce erythr[...]
perestrinism, hypercholes[...]
noted in some patients. [...]

Metastases of hepato[...]
local lymph nodes in [...]
organs or lungs. Overa[...]
poor prognosis and the [...]

BILE DUCT CANC[...]

*Cholangiocarcinoma is [...]
In the United States the[...]
common in other parts [...]
duct cancer with infecti[...]
been noticed in China. [...]
but well-known risk fac[...]

Pathology

**Bile ductal carcinom[...]
special histologic fe[...]
other gastrointestinal [...]
originate from intrah[...]
Figure 11-19).

Clinical Features [...]

Intrahepatic tumors c[...]
and are incurable by [...]
extrahepatic duct proc[...]
development and can [...]
tumors have a some[...]
while still operable. T[...]
angiocarcinoma is 1[...]
better (35%) for thos[...]
the papilla of Vater.

CARCINOMA C[...]

Carcinoma of the [...]
epithelium of the g[...]
patients and is two [...]
males. This correla[...]
stones in females an[...]
in gallbladders harb[...]
the Pima Indians, a[...]

Figure

gallstones—ha[...]
in the entire w[...]

Pathology

The tumor, wh[...]
tually grows t[...]
the liver. In la[...]
extrahepatic b[...]
the duodenum

TABLE 11-5 Primary Hepatobiliary Neoplasms

Tumor	Incidence	Risk Factors	Markers
Liver cell adenoma	F:M = 9:1 Rare	Oral contraceptive use	—
Hepatocellular carcinoma	M:F = 4:1 Rare in United States and Europe Common in Asia and Africa	Cirrhosis of any type, HBV, HCV, hemochromatosis, AAT deficiency	AFP
Cholangiocellular carcinoma	M:F = 5:1 Rare in United States Common in China	*Clonorchis sinensis* infection Primary sclerosing cholangitis	NS (CEA)
Gallbladder carcinoma	F:M = 2:1 Rare in United States Common in Pima Indians and Mexicans	Cholelithiasis	NS (CEA)

AAT, alpha₁-antitrypsin; AFP, alpha-fetoprotein; CEA, carcinoembryonic antigen; F:M, female-to-male ratio; HBV, hepatitis B virus; HCV, hepatitis C virus; M:F, male-to-female ratio; NS, nonspecific.

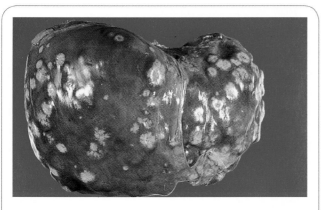

Figure 11-20 Metastatic carcinoma of the liver. The liver contains multiple nodules that have a depressed central area. This umbilicated appearance (resembling the belly button) is typical of metastatic tumor nodules.

Transplantation of the liver is a complicated operation, but it has become routine in many medical centers throughout the world. Because of antigenic differences between the host and the donor, however, the liver will invariably show some signs of transplant rejection. This immune response of the host can be suppressed by corticosteroids and immunosuppressive cytotoxic drugs. Despite treatment, the host's T cells may damage the transplant and ruin its function. The most important consequences of immune rejection are the destruction of the bile ducts and intrahepatic blood vessels. Recurrence of HBV or HCV infection in patients suffering from chronic viral hepatitis is also common. Liver transplant recipients are at increased risk for various nosocomial diseases, such as cytomegalovirus, herpesvirus, or fungal infections. Nevertheless, most liver transplant patients survive with appropriate treatment for at least 5 to 10 years and often much longer.

time a tumor has caused jaundice or intestinal obstruction, it is usually too advanced to be resected. Therefore the prognosis for these lesions is abysmal, and the 5-year survival rate is only 5%.

METASTASES TO THE LIVER

Secondary liver tumors (i.e., metastases) are much more common in the United States than are primary liver tumors. These metastases, which reach the liver through the portal or arterial circulation, are most often related to primary tumors of the gastrointestinal tract, lungs, and breast. The metastases are typically multiple and appear as round nodules with a central softened or indented necrotic area (Figure 11-20).

Clinical Features

Metastases are the most common causes of hepatic enlargement. The liver is tender and may extend several fingerbreadths below the right costal margin. Jaundice, ascites, and splenomegaly are common symptoms. The diagnosis is typically made by computed tomography (CT) studies and is confirmed by liver biopsy. The appearance of liver metastases is an ominous sign; most patients die within months after these metastases have been identified.

LIVER TRANSPLANTATION

End-stage liver disease (cirrhosis) invariably proved fatal until recently, when it became possible to replace a terminally damaged liver with a new liver from a healthy donor. Today thousands of **liver transplantations** are performed worldwide, and the results are most encouraging.

The indications for liver transplantation are broad and include all forms of cirrhosis, as well as acute liver necrosis caused by viruses, toxins, or drugs. Liver transplantation is the treatment of choice for cirrhosis secondary to metabolic disorders, such as α_1-AT deficiency, Wilson's disease, or hemochromatosis.

REVIEW QUESTIONS

1. How is the liver connected to the intestine and the great vessels?
2. Which cells form liver lobules?
3. What are the main functions of the liver?
4. What are the consequences of portal hypertension?
5. How is bilirubin formed and excreted?
6. Which enzymes are released into the circulation from damaged liver cells?
7. What are three principal forms of jaundice, and what causes each of them?
8. Compare the biochemical laboratory findings in prehepatic, hepatic, and posthepatic jaundice.
9. What are the causes of viral hepatitis?
10. Compare viral hepatitis A with viral hepatitis B and C.
11. Explain the significance of serologic tests for the diagnosis of viral hepatitis.
12. Compare the findings in acute and chronic hepatitis.
13. What is cirrhosis, and how does this disease present clinically?
14. What are the most common causes of cirrhosis?
15. Compare portal and biliary cirrhosis.
16. Describe the gross and microscopic features of a cirrhotic liver.
17. Why are some cirrhotic livers yellow and some others are rusty brown?
18. What is the pathogenesis of ascites and splenomegaly in chronic liver disease?
19. What is the pathogenesis of hepatic encephalopathy, and how does it present clinically?
20. What is hepatorenal syndrome?

21. Which endocrine abnormalities are found in patients with cirrhosis?

22. Why do patients with cirrhosis bleed?

23. Compare predictable and unpredictable liver injury caused by drugs.

24. How does alcohol affect the liver?

25. What is Gilbert's disease?

26. Compare hereditary hemochromatosis and Wilson's disease.

27. How does alpha$_1$-antitrypsin deficiency affect the liver?

28. What is autoimmune hepatitis?

29. Compare primary biliary cirrhosis and primary sclerosing cholangitis.

30. How do bacteria, protozoa, and parasites infect the liver?

31. What is the difference between cholangitic and pylephlebitic abscesses?

32. How are gallstones formed?

33. Compare cholesterol stones with pigmentary gallstones.

34. What is the pathogenesis of cholecystitis?

35. List the most important complications of cholelithiasis and cholecystitis.

36. List the most important primary tumors of the hepatobiliary tract.

37. Compare hepatocellular carcinoma with cholangiocarcinoma.

38. Compare cholangiocarcinoma with gallbladder carcinoma.

39. Compare the pathology of primary and metastatic liver tumors.

40. What are the indications for liver transplantation?

The Pancreas

Chapter Outline

NORMAL ANATOMY AND PHYSIOLOGY
OVERVIEW OF MAJOR DISEASES
  Pancreatitis
    Acute Edematous Pancreatitis
    Acute Pancreatitis

  Chronic Pancreatitis
Pancreatic Neoplasms
  Adenocarcinoma of the Pancreas
  Tumors of the Endocrine Pancreas
Diabetes Mellitus

Key Terms and Concepts

Alcohol abuse
Amylase
Diabetes mellitus
Diarrhea

Gallstone
Gastrinoma
Insulinoma
Islet cell tumor

Lipase
Malabsorption
Pancreatic pseudocyst
Peptidases

Learning Objectives

After reading this chapter, the student should be able to:

1. Describe the gross and microscopic anatomy of the pancreas.
2. Describe the main functions of the exocrine pancreas and list the main components of pancreatic juice.
3. List two main hormones produced by the islets of Langerhans and describe their function.
4. Discuss the pathogenesis of acute pancreatitis.
5. List three biochemical changes and three symptoms caused by acute pancreatitis.
6. List three main complications of acute pancreatitis.
7. Explain the pathogenesis of chronic pancreatitis.
8. List the main clinical symptoms of chronic pancreatitis and relate them to the pathologic changes in the pancreas.
9. Discuss the gross and microscopic features of pancreatic carcinoma.
10. Compare the clinical symptoms of carcinoma involving the head and the tail of the pancreas.
11. List two syndromes caused by islet cell tumors.
12. Describe the gross and microscopic features of islet cell tumors and relate these to the clinical course of the disease.
13. Discuss the pathogenesis of type 1 and type 2 diabetes.
14. Compare the essential features of type 1 and type 2 diabetes.
15. List the main complications of diabetes.

NORMAL ANATOMY AND PHYSIOLOGY

The pancreas is an endocrine and exocrine gland composed of an exocrine and an endocrine part (Figure 12-1). It is located in the retroperitoneal space of the upper abdomen and is closely attached to other retroperitoneal structures, most notably the ganglia and nerves of the celiac plexus. Because of this close relationship between the pancreas and the retroperitoneal nerves, pain radiating into the back is one of the common features of pancreatic diseases.

The pancreas can be divided into three parts: the head, which lies within the loop of duodenum; the midportion, which is called the *body*; and the tail, which extends laterally and left to the hilus of the spleen (see Figure 12-1). More than 98% of the entire pancreas consists of exocrine tissue—acini, ductules, and ducts. The endocrine cells are arranged into islets of Langerhans that are scattered through the entire organ but are most prominent in the tail.

The digestive juices produced by the exocrine pancreatic cells drain through the main pancreatic duct into the duodenum. The terminal part of the main pancreatic duct is confluent with the common bile duct, forming the ampulla of Vater. The distal part of the ampulla, encased in the smooth muscle of the sphincter of Oddi, enters into the lumen of the duodenum, protruding in the form of a small nubbin called the *papilla of Vater*. There is often an accessory duct entering the duodenum as well, which is unrelated to the bile duct. This close relationship of the head of the pancreas and the duodenum, as well as the common bile duct, is important for an understanding of the obstructive symptoms caused by tumors of the head of the pancreas. Reflux of bile into the pancreatic duct as a result of obstruction of the papilla of Vater may be important in the pathogenesis of pancreatitis, as explained later. Hormones produced by the endocrine cells are released into the blood circulation; therefore there is no need for endocrine excretory ducts.

The exocrine pancreas is the main source of digestive enzymes, the most important of which include the following:
- **Amylase,** which is essential for the digestion of starch
- **Lipase,** which is essential for the digestion of lipids
- **Peptidases,** such as trypsin and chymotrypsin, which are essential for the digestion of proteins

All these enzymes are synthesized in the acinar cells and released into the ductal system in an inactive form (i.e., like proenzymes). Pancreatic juice also contains bicarbonate and small amounts of mucin, which are released from the ductal cells.

The secretion of pancreatic juices is controlled by the vagus nerve and the polypeptide hormones cholecystokinin and secretin. These hormones are released from the duodenum in response to the entry of acidic and fat-rich food into its lumen from the stomach. Cholecystokinin stimulates the secretion of enzymes, whereas secretin stimulates the release of bicarbonate. The pancreatic juices that contain proenzymes and bicarbonates are mixed with the duodenal content. This results in activation of enzymes through the action of intestinal enteropeptidase and the alkalization of the luminal content

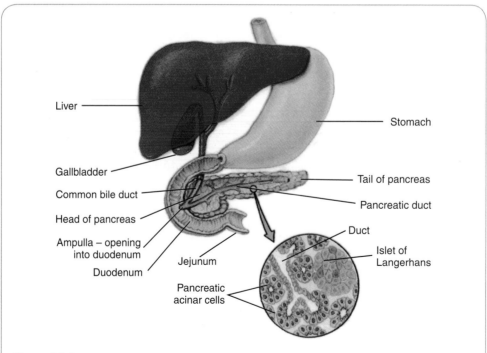

Figure 12-1 The pancreas in relation to the liver, duodenum, and stomach. The inset shows the acini, ducts, and islet. (From Applegate EJ: The Anatomy and Physiology Learning System, 4th ed, St. Louis, 2011, Saunders.)

through the action of bicarbonates. Bicarbonates act as buffers to neutralize the gastric hydrochloric acid, and by raising the pH in the intestine they provide optimal conditions for the action of pancreatic digestive enzymes. It should be noted that cholecystokinin also stimulates contraction of the gallbladder and secretin stimulates production of bile in the liver. Because bile and pancreatic juices have a common terminal outflow tract, it is easy to see how heavy meals, especially those rich in lipids, can overburden the pancreaticobiliary ductal system and cause potentially harmful consequences.

 Did You Know?

Islets of Langerhans were discovered in 1868 by a German medical student, Paul Langerhans. In addition, he described the phagocytic cells of the epidermis, which also bear his name. Not bad for a young man who proved that one does not have to have a doctoral degree to make great discoveries!

The endocrine pancreatic cells secrete several polypeptide hormones, the most important of which are insulin and glucagon. The excess or deficiency of these hormones produces distinct clinical symptoms, which are discussed later.

OVERVIEW OF MAJOR DISEASES

The most important diseases affecting the exocrine pancreas are the following:

- Pancreatitis
- Tumors
- Diabetes mellitus (DM)

The most important disease caused by dysfunction of the endocrine pancreas is **diabetes mellitus (DM)**. Tumors of the endocrine pancreas are relatively rare and thus receive only brief mention.

Several facts important to an understanding of pancreatic diseases are presented here, before a discussion of specific pathologic entities.

1. *The pancreas is anatomically and functionally a part of the digestive tract.* Pancreatic juice is produced at a rate of 100 mL per hour, or 2 to 3 L per day. The production of pancreatic juice is hormonally controlled and is coordinated with the production of other digestive enzymes. Improper diet, overeating, consumption of a fat-rich diet, and **alcohol abuse** strain the pancreas and biliary system. A loss of pancreatic parenchymal cells or inadequate drainage of juices into the duodenum profoundly affects digestion. Incomplete absorption of digested food results in **malabsorption** and **diarrhea** (loose and frequent stools), which are the most important consequences of pancreatic diseases.

2. *Many symptoms of pancreatic diseases can be understood in terms of basic anatomic facts.* In this context it is essential to remember that the pancreas is in close contact with the duodenum, the common bile duct, and the retroperitoneal nerves of the celiac plexus. Because tumors of the head of pancreas often occlude the common bile duct, obstructive jaundice is a common symptom. Duodenal obstruction is usually found in more advanced cases. Invasion of the retroperitoneal nerves is a common cause of back pain in patients with pancreatic cancer, but nerve involvement can also occur in those with chronic pancreatitis as well.

3. *Pancreatic juice contains inactive proenzymes that are activated in the intestine.* Proenzymes, such as trypsinogen or prolipase, are kinetically inactive while passing through the pancreas and are therefore innocuous to ductal cells. Premature activation of proteolytic or lipolytic enzymes in the ducts or, even worse, in the parenchyma of the pancreas may result in enzymatic tissue destruction secondary to enzyme action. Once released into the tissue, the enzymes act as autocatalysts and it is very difficult to interrupt their destructive action. This process may result in large tissue defects known as **pancreatic pseudocysts.** Pancreatic enzymes can be activated inside the pancreas chemically or by trauma (even by surgical scalpel or needle). It is no wonder, then, that surgeons do not like to operate near the pancreas or perform pancreatic biopsies.

4. *Under normal circumstances, pancreatic enzymes are found in trace amounts in the circulating blood.* Pancreatic necrosis, typical of acute pancreatitis, results in a release of enzymes from damaged acini and disrupted ducts. Proteolytic enzymes, such as elastase, further destroy not only the pancreatic parenchyma but also the vessel wall, which makes it possible for enzymes to enter the circulation. Because pancreatic enzymes can be detected in blood, blood tests are useful in the diagnosis of pancreatic disease. Likewise, because these enzymes pass from the blood into the urine, urinalysis is also a valuable source of diagnostic data.

5. *The anatomic location of the pancreas accounts for most symptoms and, largely, for the poor prognosis of pancreatic cancer.* Carcinoma of the pancreas is the fourth most common cause of cancer-related death in males and the fifth most common cause in females. This tumor is essentially incurable because in most cases it is detected too late to allow surgical resection. Because of their location, pancreatic tumors are clinically silent for extended periods and produce no early warning signs. There are presently no screening techniques that allow early detection of these tumors at a stage when they are still operable.

6. *Endocrine tumors are composed of slowly dividing endocrine cells that are biologically less aggressive than exocrine malignant lesions.* For reasons that are unknown, endocrine tumors of the pancreas grow slowly. In this respect these tumors resemble carcinoids, the neuroendocrine tumors of the intestines. Histologically, too, pancreatic islet cell tumors and carcinoids resemble one another. Endocrine tumors produce hormone-related symptoms, permitting earlier detection. Unfortunately, endocrine tumors account for only 2% of all pancreatic neoplasms.

7. *Insulin is the most important hormone secreted by the pancreas.* Insulin regulates the intermediary metabolism

of carbohydrates and lipids. A deficiency of insulin results in DM. Diabetes is the most prevalent endocrine disease, affecting millions of people worldwide. In the past it was a lethal disease. Even today—at a time when the disease can be treated with animal insulin and drugs that stimulate release of insulin from islet cells—its long-term prognosis is unfavorable. Diabetes is one of the most important risk factors for atherosclerosis.

PANCREATITIS

Pancreatitis is an inflammation of the pancreas. It can occur in acute or chronic form. In contrast to the inflammations in other organs, which are typically caused by infectious agents, pancreatitis is in most cases a sterile chemical inflammation. The inflammation is a secondary reaction to tissue destruction caused by digestive enzymes released from damaged exocrine pancreatic cells.

There are three important forms of pancreatitis:

- Acute edematous pancreatitis
- Acute hemorrhagic pancreatitis (acute pancreatic necrosis)
- Chronic pancreatitis

ACUTE EDEMATOUS PANCREATITIS

Acute edematous pancreatitis is a mild form of pancreatic injury; its incidence cannot be determined because most patients do not require hospitalization and the disease is not registered for statistical purposes. Histologic evidence of mild pancreatic inflammation is found in 0.5% of autopsies, indicating that such pancreatitis occurs more often than it is clinically diagnosed. *Acute hemorrhagic pancreatitis* is a serious disease that still has a high mortality and can have serious sequelae. It is encountered in 1 of every 500 hospital admissions. The incidence of *chronic pancreatitis* has been estimated to be 3 to 5 per 100,000 adults.

ACUTE PANCREATITIS

Acute pancreatitis is an acute response to tissue necrosis caused by digestive enzymes released from exocrine pancreatic cells. Because acute edematous pancreatitis is rarely diagnosed clinically, here we concentrate on acute hemorrhagic pancreatitis, a medical emergency characterized by typical symptoms and laboratory findings.

Etiology and Pathogenesis

Pancreatic exocrine cells forming the acinus secrete digestive enzymes into the ductules, where the enzymes enter the larger ducts. In the pancreatic ducts the enzymes are mixed with bicarbonates and mucins secreted by the ductal cells. From the ducts the pancreatic juices reach the duodenum through the papilla of Vater. Within the pancreas the enzymes remain in an inactive form (i.e., as proenzymes), becoming activated only on entry into the duodenum. Premature activation of

proenzymes within the pancreas results in *autodigestion:* tissue lysis caused by the action of pancreatic enzymes.

Experimental data show that pancreatic autodigestion can be induced in a number of ways, including the following:

- Obstruction of the main pancreatic duct
- Injection of bile or other chemicals into the pancreatic duct
- Mechanical disruption of the pancreatic acinar cells
- Chemical injury of pancreatic acinar cells
- Overstimulation of pancreatic acinar cells

In all these experimental models of acute pancreatitis in animals, it is possible to provoke an acute pancreatic cell necrosis, typically followed by acute inflammation. However, the clinical relevance of experimental data remains questionable and our understanding of the human disease is still incomplete. Nevertheless, good arguments have been advanced that the experimental models have their clinical equivalents, as illustrated in Figure 12-2.

Obstruction of the main pancreatic duct is a potentially important cause of pancreatitis, and it can occur in association with biliary disease. As noted before, the main pancreatic duct and the common bile duct are confluent in their terminal part, and both discharge their contents into the duodenum through the papilla of Vater. Obstruction of the papilla of Vater or the pancreatobiliary duct by **gallstones** is an important factor in the pathogenesis of acute pancreatitis; at least 50% of patients have gallstones. The obstruction could also lead to the reflux of bile into the pancreas. Bile normally activates pancreatic proenzymes in the intestine, and presumably it could activate the enzymes prematurely in the pancreatic ducts as well.

Mechanical disruption of pancreatic cells has been documented in patients who develop acute pancreatitis after abdominal trauma, such as seat belt trauma in car accidents. Chemical injury of pancreatic cells can be induced by various drugs, such as cytotoxic anticancer drugs. However, drugs rarely precipitate acute pancreatic necrosis. Overstimulation of pancreatic cells by secretin could be the cause of pancreatitis in obese persons indulging in fatty foods. It is believed that alcohol also stimulates pancreatic secretion. An increased incidence of acute pancreatitis has been reported in alcoholics.

Clinically, acute pancreatitis is related to gallstones and alcohol abuse in about 80% of cases. Other rare causes account for 5%, and the remaining 15% are idiopathic (i.e., without an obvious external cause) (Box 12-1). Reflux of bile into the pancreas can also increase intrapancreatic pressure and can activate the proenzymes, thus causing autodigestion. Alcohol can cause spasm of the sphincter of Oddi in the papilla of Vater, likewise increasing intrapancreatic pressure. Although alcohol is known to be toxic to cells and could presumably damage and disrupt acinar cells directly, the exact mechanism for alcoholic injury of the pancreas is still unknown. Alcohol could also stimulate pancreatic acinar cells, directly or through its effects on the intestine and the action of secretin, which is the primary stimulant (secretagogue) for release of enzymes from the acinar cells.

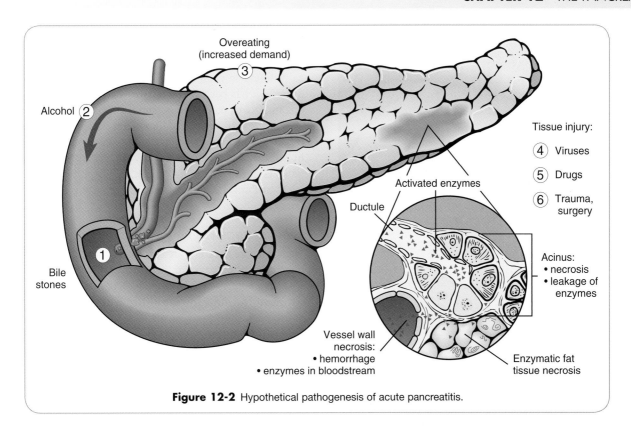

Figure 12-2 Hypothetical pathogenesis of acute pancreatitis.

<table>
<tr><td colspan="2">BOX 12-1   Causes of Acute Pancreatitis</td></tr>
<tr>
<td valign="top">
Common (95%)
Alcohol   } 80%
Bile stones
Unknown: 15%
</td>
<td valign="top">
Rare (5%)
Trauma (as from a car accident)
Surgery
  Partial resection of pancreas
  Biopsy of pancreas
Drug-induced
  Diuretics
  Oral contraceptives
Metabolic
  Hyperlipidemia
Infection
  Mumps
</td>
</tr>
</table>

Regardless of the precipitating cause of acute pancreatitis, the tissue damage occurs in a predictable manner and is always mediated by pancreatic digestive enzymes. Proteolysis caused by activation of trypsinogen, the inactive form of trypsin, leads to necrosis of tissues. Elastase acts on the elastic tissue, forming large gaps in the blood vessel wall that result in massive hemorrhage. The action of lipase on fat cells inside the pancreas and the peripancreatic fat tissues results in fat necrosis. Other hydrolytic enzymes, more than 100 of which are present in the pancreatic juice, act on other tissue components, including carbohydrates, DNA, and RNA.

Enzymatic tissue destruction is accompanied by liquefaction of the digested pancreas. This fluid also accumulates in cystic spaces within the pancreas. These spaces are called *pseudocysts* because they are not lined by an internal epithelial cell layer, as are regular cysts. Necrotic tissue foci tend to attract calcium salts and undergo dystrophic calcification. Free fatty acids formed through the hydrolysis of triglycerides also bind calcium ions, thus forming calcium soaps, which can be seen as whitish specks underneath the peritoneum and wherever the fat cells have undergone enzymatic necrosis.

Pathology

Acute pancreatitis is marked by massive edema, hemorrhage, and necrosis of the pancreas (Figure 12-3). The pancreas appears swollen and is permeated with blood. Yellow or smudgy brownish-yellow areas of necrosis appear 2 to 3 days after the onset of the attack. The leakage of digestive enzymes into the abdominal cavity may cause peritoneal irritation, and a chemical peritonitis may ensue. Areas of fat necrosis appear as grayish-yellow discolorations that gradually calcify and become whitish. By the end of the first week, pseudocysts appear as small cavities filled with liquefied tissue and pancreatic enzymes. These small cavities coalesce into larger pseudocysts, which are typically found in patients who survive the initial attack.

Histologically, the hallmarks of normal pancreatic tissue are lost as a result of necrosis. The necrotic pancreatic cells are transformed into amorphous granular material. The fat cells, which are normally vacuolated and filled with fat, lose their outlines and transform into washed-out "ghosts" composed of collapsed cell membranes.

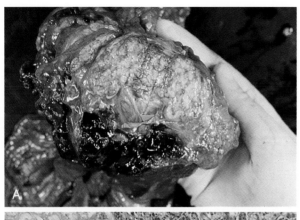

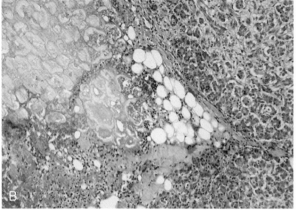

Figure 12-3 Acute pancreatitis. *A,* Gross appearance of the pancreas. Note the massive hemorrhage into the pancreas, which appears swollen. *B,* Necrotic foci are scattered throughout the parenchyma.

Complications

Acute pancreatitis commonly causes complications (Figure 12-4). As already mentioned, the spilling of digestive enzymes into the peritoneal cavity causes peritonitis. Small cystic spaces resulting from the destruction of the parenchyma of the pancreas may become confluent, resulting in large pseudocysts that resemble bags filled with fluid. These pseudocysts may replace large portions of the pancreatic parenchyma or may distend the pancreas, compressing and displacing the duodenum or the stomach. The content of pseudocysts, as well as the remaining necrotic pancreatic parenchyma, may become infected by enteric bacteria. This bacterial infection leads to the formation of abscesses. In contrast to pseudocysts, which contain liquefied tissue debris and enzymes, pancreatic abscesses contain pus. However, the capsule of the pseudocyst resembles the wall of an abscess. In both these structures the capsule is composed of fibrotic granulation tissues formed in an attempt to delimit the spread of tissue destruction and inflammation. Such granulation tissue becomes increasingly fibrotic until finally these cystic structures assume the appearance of leather bags (Figure 12-5).

Chronic pancreatitis is a late complication of acute pancreatitis. Destruction of pancreatic tissue in acute pancreatitis may result in exocrine pancreatic insufficiency, which is typically found in persons who have had recurrent bouts of the disease. It has been estimated that chronic pancreatitis develops in 20% of patients who survive acute pancreatitis.

Diabetes is an uncommon consequence of pancreatic tissue destruction associated with acute pancreatitis. Acute hyperglycemia, which is usually mild, may be seen in many patients during the initial attack. Massive destruction of the islets of Langerhans, resulting in permanent diabetes, is less common.

Clinical Features

Acute pancreatitis is a disease of sudden onset. Typically it occurs in patients with a history of gallstones or alcoholism. Characteristic symptoms include abdominal pain and distention, nausea, and vomiting. Affected patients display apprehensiveness, are in great distress, and sweat profusely. The pain is often uncontrollable. Syncope and rapidly developing shock are typical of severe disease. Peritoneal rigidity signals the onset of peritonitis, which is usually accompanied by paralytic ileus.

The diagnosis of acute pancreatitis can be corroborated by laboratory data. In addition to leukocytosis, which develops in response to acute inflammation, serum tests typically reveal a marked elevation in amylase and lipase levels. Pancreatic enzymes are also found in the urine. Peritoneal fluid may contain the same enzyme. Biochemical signs of pancreatitis appear 24 to 72 hours after the onset of the attack.

Radiographic findings are also useful. Computed tomography (CT) scans may be used to demonstrate swelling in the pancreas. In patients with rapidly developing peritonitis, x-ray studies can help rule out other catastrophic abdominal events, such as perforation of the intestines. In later stages of disease, radiographs may demonstrate calcification.

> **? Did You Know?**
>
> Pseudocysts that form in the pancreas after an attack of acute pancreatitis contain digestive enzymes that prevent healing of the pseudocyst. To allow tissues to heal, surgeons drain the pancreatic juices through a pouch made by attaching the opened pseudocyst to the external abdominal wall. The name for this procedure, *marsupialization,* is derived from the Latin word for "pouch." The same word is used for the animal order *Marsupialia,* which includes kangaroos and opossums. To most patients, marsupialization probably sounds less intimidating than kangaroozation or possumization!

There is no effective treatment for acute pancreatitis; however, efforts should be directed at containing the damage and preventing the systemic consequences of shock. The overall mortality rate of acute pancreatitis is still in the range of 20%. Death is usually the consequence of circulatory shock. Elderly patients with acute respiratory failure, hypotension,

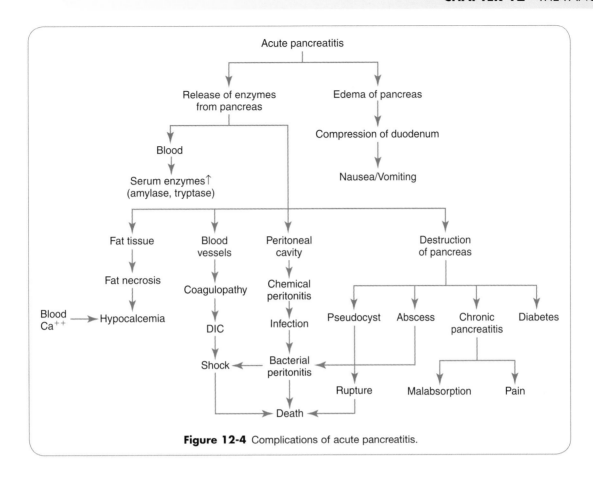

Figure 12-4 Complications of acute pancreatitis.

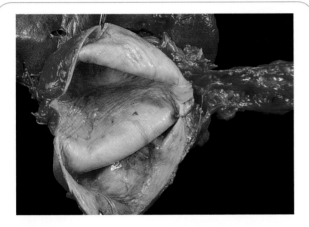

Figure 12-5 Pancreatic pseudocyst. After drainage of its content, the pseudocyst in the tail of the pancreas appears as a fibrous sac. (From Damjanov I, Linder J: Pathology: A Color Atlas, St. Louis, 2000, Mosby.)

and peritonitis have the highest risk of all populations, with a mortality rate near 50%.

Patients who survive the acute attack are at a risk for recurrence. This can be prevented by removing gallstones, eliminating alcohol, and avoiding a high-fat diet. Symptoms of chronic pancreatitis occur in about 20% of surviving patients.

CHRONIC PANCREATITIS

Chronic pancreatitis is characterized by irregular fibrosis replacing portions of the normal pancreatic parenchyma. These changes are progressive and irreversible and produce exocrine and endocrine pancreatic insufficiency. The disease is found in 4 per 100,000 adults and is more common in males than in females; the male-to-female ratio is 3:1.

Chronic pancreatitis has an insidious onset; thus it is very difficult to determine either its cause or pathogenesis. However, a history of alcohol abuse can be elicited in most patients. Therefore it is believed that alcohol accounts for more than 70% of cases. Because chronic alcoholism is much more widespread than chronic pancreatitis, it is difficult to explain why only some patients with chronic alcoholism develop this disease and others are spared. In a few cases, chronic pancreatitis is preceded by acute pancreatitis, but in most instances the onset of the disease is slow and imperceptible. In a few patients, chronic pancreatic insufficiency follows trauma or pancreatic surgery or occurs during the course of systemic metabolic and endocrine diseases. It is most puzzling that 20% of patients have no risk factors or preexisting disease and present with idiopathic chronic pancreatitis.

Pathology

On gross examination, the pancreas does not show the typical lobulation but appears fibrotic and firm. The main pancreatic duct is usually dilated and often contains stones (Figure 12-6).

293

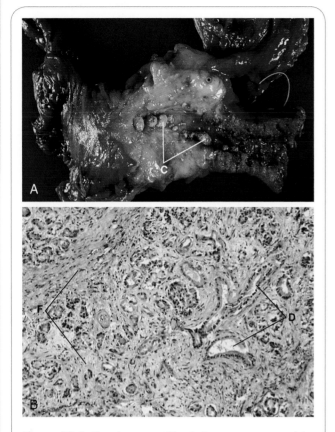

Figure 12-6 Chronic pancreatitis. *A,* Gross appearance of the atrophic pancreas. Note the calculi (C) in the dilated duct. *B,* Histologic examination reveals that the acini have been replaced by fibrous tissue (F) surrounding the remaining ducts (D).

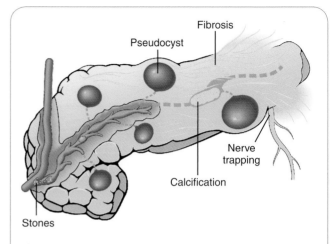

Figure 12-7 Chronic pancreatitis may lead to the formation of ductal stones, pseudocysts, calcification, or fibrosis that entraps nerves, causing pain.

Fibrous tissues may extend from the pancreas into the surrounding structures and cause constriction of the common bile duct, duodenum, or pylorus. Histologically there is marked fibrosis, with scattered foci of chronic inflammation replacing the acini. The ducts and islets of Langerhans tend to persist longer, but in advanced cases they too are destroyed and obliterated by fibrosis. Calcifications of the fibrous tissue are common.

Clinical Features

The symptoms of chronic pancreatitis develop insidiously. These symptoms are due to the various anatomic changes that might occur with chronic pancreatitis, as shown in Figure 12-7. Typically the symptoms and clinical signs include the following:

- *Pain.* This is related to the entrapment of nerves in the fibrous tissue, which often extends into the celiac plexus. Fibrosis may cause stenosis of the duodenum, which impedes the passage of food from the stomach into the duodenum, causing pain after eating.
- *Exocrine pancreatic insufficiency.* Destruction of acinar cells reduces the capacity of the pancreas to produce digestive enzymes, which results in malabsorption and steatorrhea. Lack of trypsin and chymotrypsin results in

malabsorption of proteins. Lipase deficiency accounts for the fatty stools and inappropriate absorption of fat and fat-soluble vitamins (A, D, K, and E). Most patients lose weight and feel weak. Signs of vitamin deficiency, such as night blindness secondary to avitaminosis A or a bleeding tendency secondary to avitaminosis K, are seen in severe cases.

- *Endocrine insufficiency.* Destruction of the islets of Langerhans occurs at a slower rate than does the loss of exocrine pancreatic cells. Nevertheless, in later stages of the disease more than 70% of patients have signs of diabetes mellitus.

The diagnosis of chronic pancreatitis is based on a typical history, which usually includes alcohol abuse, and the typical complaints. Pain, which is usually epigastric, tends to radiate into the back and is commonly exacerbated by drinking and the ingestion of fatty meals. Bulky, fatty stools are an important telltale sign. Weight loss is common.

The workup of the patient must include abdominal x-ray studies, which will usually show numerous calcifications in the pancreas. Laboratory findings may disclose mild elevations in amylase and lipase levels in serum, but they often yield normal values and are noncontributory. Most patients with advanced disease show hyperglycemia and other features of diabetes. The course of pancreatitis is relentless. It cannot be stopped or reversed, but some improvement may be noticed if the patient stops drinking. Malabsorption can be treated symptomatically by enzyme supplementation, but the commercial enzyme preparations are of low potency. Most patients compensate for low absorption by eating increased amounts of high-calorie food. With such adjustments, quality of life may not be normal but it is not shortened substantially. These patients tend to be at an increased risk for developing pancreatic cancer, which is approximately three times more common in this population than in age-matched controls.

PANCREATIC NEOPLASMS

Neoplasms of the pancreas can be classified clinically as benign or malignant. On gross examination, they may appear solid or cystic. On the basis of their origin, the tumors may be classified as being derived from either exocrine or endocrine cells. The tumors may show secretory activity, or they may be functionally inactive.

It is important to remember that most—more than 95%—pancreatic tumors have the following characteristics:

- *Adenocarcinomas* (i.e., malignant epithelial neoplasms)
- Solid, rather than cystic; *cystic tumors* such as cystadenomas and cystadenocarcinomas may occur but are very uncommon (2% of all tumors)
- Derived from the pancreatic ducts (i.e., originating from the exocrine part of the pancreas)
- Functionally silent (i.e., arising from ductal cells and secreting neither hormones nor enzymes)

ADENOCARCINOMA OF THE PANCREAS

Carcinoma of the pancreas, the most important tumor involving this organ, is the fourth major cause of cancer-related deaths in males and the fifth in females in the United States. Approximately 37,000 new cases are recorded every year in the United States, and nearly all patients die within 12 to 24 months of diagnosis.

The risk factors for pancreatic tumors have not been clearly delineated. The strongest epidemiologic association noted has been smoking, which increases the risk threefold. It has been proposed that dietary factors, such as a high-fat diet and alcohol abuse, predispose individuals to pancreatic cancer, but this hypothesis has not been definitively proven. Chronic pancreatitis has been associated with a twofold to threefold higher incidence of pancreatic cancer. However, this disease is relatively rare and can be implicated as a possible cause for only a minority of pancreatic carcinomas.

For all practical purposes, carcinoma of the pancreas is a disease of old age. The tumors rarely occur before the age of 40 years, but thereafter their incidence increases steadily. The incidence of tumors in males equals that in females, except in the group younger than 50 years, in which males outnumber females 3 to 1.

Pathology

Adenocarcinoma of the pancreas is an epithelial malignant lesion originating from ducts. Among the tumors diagnosed clinically, approximately 60% are located in the head of the pancreas (Figure 12-8). This is understandable because the head forms the bulk of the pancreas and contains most of the ducts. Furthermore, because these tumors of the pancreatic head tend to obstruct the bile ducts and cause jaundice, they are diagnosed more readily than are tumors of the body or the tail of the pancreas, which account for 15% of all pancreatic carcinomas. Approximately 25% of cancers involve the pancreas diffusely.

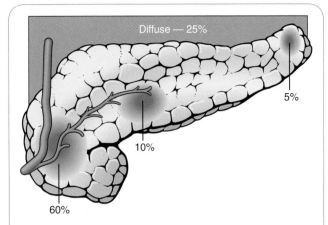

Figure 12-8 Carcinoma of the pancreas. The tumor is located in the head of the pancreas in 60% of cases but may also involve the body (10%) or the tail (5%). Diffuse infiltration of the entire organ by tumor occurs in 25% of cases.

Microscopic examination reveals that most tumors are adenocarcinomas that may be well differentiated, moderately differentiated, or undifferentiated (Figure 12-9). Well-differentiated tumors are composed of cells that resemble cells lining the duct, whereas undifferentiated tumors are more anaplastic and usually desmoplastic (i.e., they show prominent dense connective tissue stroma). Adenocarcinomas displaying unique histologic features, such as acinar cell carcinomas or cystadenocarcinomas, are rare.

Metastases occur early in the course of the disease. At the time of diagnosis, grossly visible metastases are found in the local lymph nodes of 40% of patients, and distant metastases are noted in yet another 40%. These metastatic lesions are most often in the liver but also occur commonly in the lungs and bones. Only 20% of affected patients have cancer that is strictly limited to the pancreas.

Clinical Features

Symptoms of pancreatic carcinoma depend on the location of the tumor, its size, and the extent of spread. Most often the symptoms are nonspecific and include weight loss, loss of appetite, nausea, and vomiting. Upper abdominal pain may suggest the pancreas as the cause of these cancer-related symptoms. Tumors located in the head of the pancreas tend to obstruct the common bile duct and cause jaundice. The gallbladder may be dilated and may even be palpable on physical examination *(Courvoisier's sign)*. Tumors of the body and tail of the pancreas do not cause jaundice but tend to invade the celiac plexus and cause pain. Splenomegaly may occur as a result of obstruction of the splenic vein. Migratory thrombophlebitis *(Trousseau's syndrome)* is a well-known paraneoplastic syndrome found in some patients.

Metastases and local spread of the tumor into the duodenum cause intestinal obstruction. Liver metastases cause enlargement of the liver. Peritoneal seeding is associated with ascites and a protruding abdomen, which are the presenting

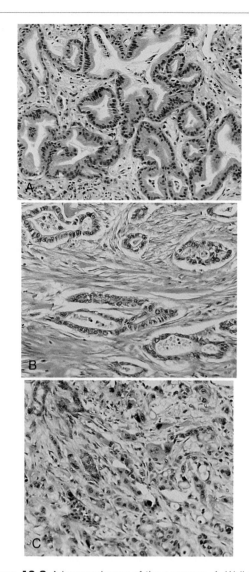

Figure 12-9 Adenocarcinoma of the pancreas. *A,* Well differentiated; *B,* moderately differentiated; *C,* poorly differentiated. (From Damjanov I, Linder J: Pathology: A Color Atlas, St. Louis, 2000, Mosby.)

Carcinoma of the pancreas is an incurable disease. Surgical resection may be attempted, but the results are not encouraging. Radiation therapy and chemotherapy are also ineffectual. The 5-year survival rate is less than 5%. Most patients die within the first year of diagnosis.

 Did You Know?

French physician Armand Trousseau noticed that patients with abdominal cancers, and especially carcinoma of the pancreas, may have thrombi of major veins. Appropriately, this tumor-related syndrome was named after Trousseau. It is interesting to note that the aging Dr. Trousseau himself developed the syndrome he described as a young physician.

TUMORS OF THE ENDOCRINE PANCREAS

Tumors of the endocrine pancreas are called **islet cell tumors,** because all of them originate from the endocrine cells in the islets of Langerhans. Endocrine tumors are rare; they are 10 times less common than carcinomas of the exocrine pancreas and have an incidence of 1 per 100,000 per year. Nevertheless, it is important to distinguish endocrine tumors from the more common adenocarcinomas for several reasons:

■ Endocrine pancreatic tumors are benign or low-grade malignant lesions, with a better prognosis than exocrine adenocarcinomas.

■ Endocrine pancreatic tumors are usually hormonally active and cause systemic symptoms that vary depending on the cell of origin and the predominant hormone released from the neoplastic cells. Hormones produced by these tumors are useful in establishing the diagnosis.

■ Endocrine tumors may be multiple and are also associated with tumors of other organs, as in multiple endocrine neoplasia syndrome type I (MEN1).

Endocrine tumors may originate from any of the four cell types in the normal islets of Langerhans. The most common tumors are *insulinomas,* which are composed of insulin-secreting beta cells. Glucagonomas, somatostatinomas, and VIPomas are less common.

Insulinomas, or beta-cell tumors, are typically small, solitary, benign tumors measuring 1 to 3 cm in diameter. These tumors secrete insulin, which can be detected in blood by radioimmunoassay. Hyperinsulinemia may cause hypoglycemia, syncope, and profuse sweating, especially after prolonged fasting. These symptoms can be reversed promptly by infusion of glucose. Insulinomas can be easily resected, which results in a permanent cure of the patient's hypoglycemic episodes.

The pancreas is also the most common site of gastrinomas, which constitute 25% of pancreatic endocrine tumors. The normal pancreatic islets of Langerhans do not contain gastrin-secreting cells, and it is believed that **gastrinomas** originate from developmentally pluripotent cells that are the common

findings in one third of patients. Distant metastases are also common and are usually found in the lungs.

The diagnosis of carcinoma of the pancreas is based on a combination of physical findings and radiologic findings. The CT scan is the most reliable technique for visualizing pancreatic tumors. Many tumors are diagnosed during laparoscopy performed to relieve intestinal or biliary obstruction. Endoscopic retrograde cholangiopancreatography or percutaneous transhepatic cholangiography are special radiographic techniques sometimes used to distinguish carcinoma from chronic pancreatitis. During these procedures, it is also possible to obtain cells for cytopathologic analysis. Pancreatic tumors can also be sampled by thin-needle aspiration biopsy or incisional biopsy during surgical exploration.

fetal precursors of pancreatic islet cells and normal gastric and intestinal G cells. Clinically, gastrinomas present as *Zollinger-Ellison syndrome,* which is marked by gastric hypersecretion and intractable peptic ulcers. Ulcers may be multiple, located in unusual sites, and resistant to standard medical therapy. Gastrinomas are usually malignant, and they may be multiple; in some families affected by MEN1, gastrinomas are associated with tumors of the pituitary and parathyroid glands.

DIABETES MELLITUS

The islets of Langerhans contain several endocrine cell types. Alpha cells, which secrete glucagon, account for 20%; beta cells, which secrete insulin, account for 70%; and the remaining 10% are delta cells, which secrete somatostatin or pancreatic polypeptide (PP).

Functional insufficiency of the islets of Langerhans, caused by a destruction of islets or a selective loss of beta cells, results in diabetes mellitus (DM). However, an anatomic or functional defect in the endocrine pancreas is only one of the causes of diabetes. Other causes of diabetes, which are unrelated to the pancreas, are also discussed here.

Definition and Classification

The term *diabetes* is derived from a Greek term meaning "to pass through." It was coined to denote *polyuria*—the production of large amounts of urine—which is the most common sign of the disease. The adjective *mellitus* was added to indicate that the urine was sweet (i.e., contained sugar), in contrast to diabetes insipidus, a pituitary polyuria caused by deficiency of antidiuretic hormone (ADH) in which the urine is insipid (i.e., tasteless). Because pituitary polyuria is rare and polyuria of DM is common, it has become customary to call the more common disease simply diabetes. The adjective diabetic has come to refer exclusively to DM and thus does not need to be followed by the adjective mellitus.

DM is a heterogeneous group of systemic disorders characterized by hyperglycemia; complex disturbances of carbohydrate, lipid, and protein metabolism; and a variety of organic changes resulting primarily from blood vessel pathology. Diabetes is a consequence of absolute or relative insulin deficiency or an abnormal response of target tissues to insulin.

Diabetes is very common, affecting between 1% and 2% of people worldwide. The symptoms vary from mild to severe, and although most have a mild form of the disease, the cumulative effects of long-standing diabetes account for approximately 35,000 deaths per year in the United States.

The classification of diabetes is based on pathogenetic principles. Various forms of DM are listed in Box 12-2. The two most common forms of diabetes are type 1 DM, and type 2 DM. Approximately 90% to 95% of all patients have type 2; 5% to 10% have type 1. Other forms of diabetes listed in Box 12-2 are relatively rare.

BOX 12-2   Classification of Diabetes Mellitus (DM)

1. Type 1 DM
2. Type 2 DM
3. Genetic defects of beta-cell function
4. Genetic defects resulting in abnormal insulin action
5. Secondary DM related to diseases of the exocrine pancreas
6. Secondary DM related to other endocrine disorders
7. DM caused by infection destroying the islets
8. Drug-induced DM
9. Genetic/chromosomal syndromes associated with DM
10. Gestational diabetes

Modified from the Position Statement of the American Diabetes Association, 2008.
All types of diabetes except type 1 DM and type 2 DM are rare.

 Did You Know?

The common form of diabetes characterized by elevated blood sugar and sugar in urine is called *diabetes mellitus,* in contrast to diabetes insipidus, which is caused by pituitary diseases. Ancient physicians tested urine by wetting a finger and licking it. If the urine was sweet, the disease was called *diabetes mellitus;* if the urine had no taste, the disease was called *diabetes insipidus,* from the Latin word *insipid,* meaning "tasteless."

Type 2 diabetes accounts for the vast majority of all cases of diabetes. In the United States approximately 20 million people have type 2 diabetes, and most of them are overweight. The incidence of type 1 diabetes is much lower (50 persons per 1 million), accounting for the disease in about 150,000 Americans. However, it occurs more often in children and adolescents. In persons younger than 20 years, the incidence of type 1 diabetes is three times higher than in the general population (i.e., 150 per 1 million). The incidence of new cases of type 1 DM has been steady over many years; approximately 15,000 persons develop this type of diabetes every year in the United States.

The salient features of type 1 and type 2 diabetes are presented in Table 12-1.

Pathogenesis

Diabetes may develop in the presence of several conditions, all of which are characterized by abnormal regulation of the intermediary metabolism of carbohydrates, lipids, and protein by insulin (Figure 12-10). The most important causes of these metabolic disturbances are the following:

- An absolute deficiency of insulin (e.g., lack of beta cells secondary to islet cell destruction)
- A relative deficiency of insulin (e.g., when the demand for insulin exceeds the supply)
- Interference with insulin binding to target tissues (e.g., tissue resistance to insulin as a result of faulty insulin receptors or antibodies to insulin or insulin receptors)

TABLE 12-1 Typical Features of Type 1 and Type 2 Diabetes

Characteristic	Type 1	Type 2
Age of onset (years)	Usually <30	Usually >30
Speed of onset	Sudden	Gradual
Body build	Normal	Obese (90%)
Family history	<20%	60%
Twin concordance	Low	High
Antibodies to islet cells	+	−
Histology of islets	Loss of beta cells	Normal, may be hyalinized
Serum insulin level	Low	Normal
Treatment	Insulin	Diet Oral hypoglycemics or insulin

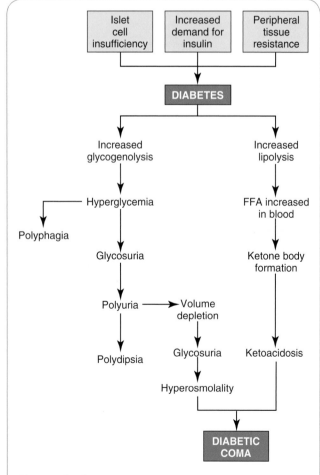

Figure 12-10 Pathogenesis of hyperglycemia and other metabolic and pathologic changes associated with diabetes mellitus. FFA, free fatty acids.

To understand the pathogenesis of DM, it is important to realize that insulin plays a crucial role in the intermediary metabolism of carbohydrates, lipids, and amino acids. Insulin is produced by the beta cells in the islets of Langerhans. Normal beta cells store insulin in neurosecretory cytoplasmic granules, which are released into the circulation after appropriate stimulation. The major stimulus for insulin secretion is *hyperglycemia* (i.e., high serum glucose level). Insulin reduces the level of serum glucose by promoting its influx into hepatocytes in the liver, where it is catabolized *(glycolysis)* and stored as glycogen *(glycogenesis)*. Insulin also decreases serum glucose concentration by stimulating the influx of glucose into the striated muscle cells, where it is used as a source of energy. Insulin deficiency results in hyperglycemia, whereas an excess of insulin causes hypoglycemia. Insulin has other functions as well. It stimulates the synthesis of proteins from amino acids, mainly in striated muscles, and fat formation from triglycerides in fat cells *(lipogenesis).* All these effects of insulin are mediated through the activation of the cellular insulin receptors, expressed on liver, muscle, and fat cells, as well as several other cell types. Insulin bound to the receptor triggers several cytoplasmic responses, in addition to glucose influx.

The effects of insulin are partially counteracted by glucagon (a polypeptide hormone secreted by the alpha cells in the islets of Langerhans), pituitary growth hormone, steroid hormones, and epinephrine. Lack of insulin, inhibition of its action (e.g., by antibodies to insulin), blockade of insulin receptors (e.g., by antibodies to insulin receptors), or inadequate cell response to insulin (the so-called postreceptor defect) can result in hyperglycemia, the first and foremost sign of DM. Excess glucose in the blood spills over into the urine, causing glucosuria. Glucose leads to osmotic diuresis and causes polyuria.

The utilization of glucose in striated muscle cells, including the heart, is impaired in DM. Anaerobic glycolysis, instead of oxidative aerobic glycolysis, is used for energy production, resulting in the formation of excessive amounts of lactic acid. This may cause lactic acidosis, a serious complication of untreated diabetes. Inadequate utilization of fats and reduced lipogenesis lead to the accumulation of free fatty acids, which are oxidized into ketones. Ketogenesis is another cause of acidosis in advanced diabetes *(ketoacidosis).*

Hyperglycemia also leads to the deposition of glucose in tissues that do not require insulin receptors for the uptake of glucose, such as the blood vessels, nerves, lens, and kidney tubules. In these tissues, glucose is metabolized to osmotically active compounds (sorbitol and fructose). This stimulates the influx of fluids into the affected tissue. Sorbitol is a polyol, or alcohol, that inhibits enzymes involved in the maintenance of cell homeostasis and probably has direct toxic effects on cells in various tissues.

The pathogenesis of the various forms of diabetes has not been fully explained. Overall, however, there is agreement about the following:

- *Diabetes has a genetic predisposition.* This hereditary predisposition is stronger for type 2 than for type 1 diabetes.

For example, type 1 is concordant in 50% of monozygotic twins, whereas the concordance of type 2 is much higher (more than 90%). The inheritance does not follow the rules of Mendelian genetics, and the disease is probably polygenic.

■ *Diabetes develops under the influence of some environmental factors.* In some cases of type 1 diabetes, sudden onset of the disease may be related to viral infection, such as measles or coxsackievirus B infection. Seasonal occurrences of type 1 diabetes, suggestive of "mini-epidemics," are also consistent with an infectious pathogenesis, although the suspected virus has not yet been isolated.

Antibodies to beta cells can be detected in the blood of patients with type 1 diabetes. In early stages of the disease, the islets of Langerhans are infiltrated with lymphocytes and macrophages, which apparently destroy the endocrine pancreatic tissue. In later stages of type 1 diabetes, the islets show a depletion of beta cells, which are replaced by hyalinized fibrous tissue. All this suggests an autoimmune reaction, which may be triggered by a virus or some other exogenous stimulus. However, in most instances the causative agent remains unidentified, and the pathogenesis of the disease is unknown.

Exogenous factors contributing to type 2 diabetes are obscure. Because type 2 diabetes occurs often in obese persons, a pathogenetic link between these two conditions has been postulated. However, not all obese persons have diabetes and not all diabetic patients are obese, which indicates that other factors may be important as well.

Pathology

The pathologic basis of diabetes is highly variable. In type 1 diabetes there is ample evidence of islet destruction and beta-cell loss. In early stages of type 1 diabetes, *insulitis* is present (i.e., mononuclear cell infiltration of the islets of Langerhans). Most of the cells involved in the destruction of islets are cytotoxic T lymphocytes and macrophages. This insulitis is short lived, but the damage is irreparable. The damaged islets show interstitial fibrosis and hyalinization (Figure 12-11). The hypoinsulinemia that ensues correlates directly with the extent of islet cell destruction.

In patients with type 2 diabetes, the islets of Langerhans are usually of normal size and contain a normal or even an increased number of beta cells. This probably reflects the body's attempt to compensate for the relative deficiency of insulin under conditions in which the demand is not met by the output. The same happens when the target tissues are resistant to the action of insulin.

Metabolic changes caused by diabetes affect many organs. Many, if not most, of these changes are a consequence of hyperglycemia, which adversely alters the metabolism of basement membranes and damages the small blood vessels. Diabetes also accelerates the development of atherosclerosis. Thus microangiopathy and atherosclerosis could be considered common denominators for most of the pathologic changes in diabetes. Diabetic patients are prone to infection, which is yet another cause of pathologic changes.

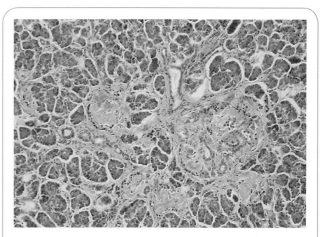

Figure 12-11 Histologic appearance of the islets of Langerhans in a patient with type 1 diabetes mellitus. Fibrous tissue replaces islet cells that have been lost. (From Damjanov I, Linder J: Pathology: A Color Atlas, St. Louis, 2000, Mosby.)

The extent of pathologic changes in diabetes depends on the type of diabetes, the duration of disease, and the coexistence of other diseases, but it primarily reflects the degree and duration of hyperglycemia. Patients whose disease is well controlled show fewer pathologic changes than those who have uncontrollable disease or those who have not been treated adequately.

Complications

The most prominent changes caused by uncontrolled or inadequately controlled diabetes involve the following organs or organ systems:

■ Cardiovascular system
■ Kidneys
■ Eyes
■ Nervous system

The main complications of diabetes are outlined in Figure 12-12.

Cardiovascular complications account for most of the morbidity and mortality of diabetes. Diabetes promotes the development of atherosclerosis in the aorta and its branches. The most important consequences of atherosclerosis include coronary heart disease, cerebrovascular diseases, and formation of aortic aneurysms. The arteries of the lower extremities are often affected, and their narrowing or occlusion results in *gangrene* of the toes or of the entire foot.

The renal complications of diabetes include glomerulosclerosis, pyelonephritis, and papillary necrosis. The glomerular capillaries show signs of diabetic microangiopathy and appear to be thickened. The mesangial areas are widened by the increased amounts of basement membranes, and the entire glomerulus ultimately becomes hyalinized and afunctional. Microangiopathy involving the arterioles (hyaline arteriosclerosis) causes renal ischemia, which results in tubular atrophy and interstitial fibrosis, and contributes to hypertension. Affected kidneys are also prone to infections,

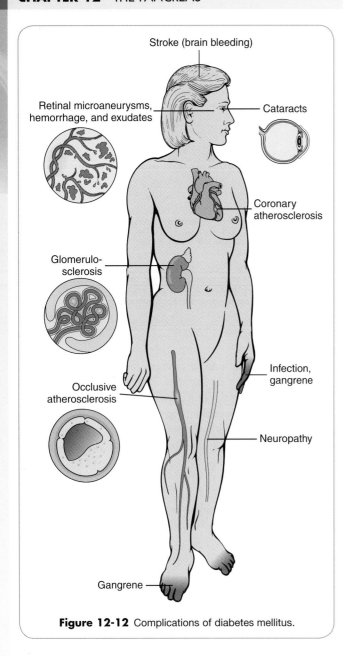

Stroke (brain bleeding)

Retinal microaneurysms, hemorrhage, and exudates

Cataracts

Coronary atherosclerosis

Glomerulo-sclerosis

Infection, gangrene

Occlusive atherosclerosis

Neuropathy

Gangrene

Figure 12-12 Complications of diabetes mellitus.

Both the central and peripheral nervous systems are often affected by diabetes. Most of the pathologic changes are related to diabetic microangiopathy, which leads to widespread focal ischemia. Diabetes usually affects the autonomic nerves, causing symptoms that vary from mild to severe urinary incontinence or impotence. Peripheral neuropathy, a common complication of diabetes, is partially a consequence of diabetic microangiopathy and partially related to the deposition of sorbitol and fructose in the axons and myelin sheaths. Clinically it presents with both sensory and motor deficits.

Clinical Features

The symptoms and clinical findings of diabetes are related to the following:

- Hyperglycemia and abnormalities of intermediate metabolism related to insulin deficiency
- Vascular changes caused by diabetes
- Increased susceptibility to infection

The most common symptoms of diabetes are polyuria and *polydipsia* (excessive thirst). Because of an excessive loss of water in urine, the patients feel thirsty and tend to drink a lot of fluids. Abnormal utilization of carbohydrates, proteins, and lipids generates a negative energy balance that results in muscle wasting, which is compensated for by an increased appetite. Affected patients tend to eat large amounts of food *(polyphagia).* Hyperglycemia predisposes individuals to bacterial infections, probably because high sugar content of blood and interstitial tissue fluids facilitates the growth of bacteria. Cardiovascular and cerebrovascular changes account for the fact that people with diabetes have a shorter life span (by 7 to 9 years) than their age-matched peers.

Treatment of diabetes depends on the type of disease, its duration and severity, and the presence or absence of complications. Patients with type 1 DM require insulin for the rest of their lives. Type 2 DM, when associated with obesity, may improve with weight loss and appropriate dietary modifications. Hypoglycemic drugs or insulin are prescribed for those who do not respond to dietary measures. Education plays an important role in the fight against diabetes, and in many cases the disease could be prevented by lifestyle and diet changes. Balanced diet, exercise, and weight control represent the best preventive measures and should be encouraged to combat the "diabesity epidemic," which is a major health problem in the United States today.

and bacterial pyelonephritis occurs frequently. Ischemic changes in the renal papilla (the part of the renal medulla that protrudes into the renal pelvis) may cause infarcts, which typically result in papillary necrosis. Necrotic papillae are sloughed off and discharged in the urine, usually obstructing the urethra and ultimately causing renal colic.

The eyes are often affected by diabetes, which is the leading cause of blindness in the United States. Diabetic microangiopathy affects the retinal vessels, causing microaneurysmal dilations, microinfarcts with hemorrhage, and (in most severe cases) reactive proliferation of vascular sprouts. Vascular changes may also obstruct the outflow of aqueous fluid and cause glaucoma. Diabetes also causes cataracts. These opacities of the lens are related to the deposition of sorbitol and fructose in the lens matrix and subsequent swelling caused by the osmotic action of these carbohydrates.

REVIEW QUESTIONS

1. How is the pancreas related to the small intestine?

2. Compare and contrast the features of the exocrine portion and the endocrine portion of the pancreas.

3. List the main secretory products of the pancreas.

4. List the main causes of acute pancreatitis.

5. Correlate the pathologic findings in acute pancreatitis with the clinical features of this disease.

6. What are the most common complications of acute pancreatitis?

7. What is chronic pancreatitis, and how does this disease present clinically?

8. How common are tumors of the pancreas?

9. Compare adenocarcinoma of the pancreas with tumors of the endocrine pancreas.

10. How common is diabetes mellitus?

11. Classify diabetes mellitus according to the pathogenesis of this disease.

12. Compare and contrast type 1 and type 2 (non–insulin-dependent) diabetes mellitus.

13. Explain the pathogenesis of hyperglycemia in diabetes mellitus.

14. Explain the pathogenesis of diabetic ketoacidosis.

15. Explain how the cardiovascular, renal, ocular, and neurologic complications of diabetes mellitus develop.

16. What is the pathogenesis of polydipsia, polyphagia, and polyuria in diabetes mellitus?

13 The Urinary Tract

Chapter Outline

NORMAL ANATOMY AND PHYSIOLOGY
OVERVIEW OF MAJOR DISEASES
    Localized Symptoms
    Systemic Symptoms
  Developmental Disorders
    Polycystic Kidney Disease
  Glomerular Diseases
    Classification
    Multiple Mechanisms
    Acute Glomerulonephritis
    Crescentic Glomerulonephritis
    Membranous Nephropathy
    Lipoid Nephrosis
    Focal Segmental Glomerulosclerosis
    Chronic Proliferative Glomerulonephritis

End-Stage Glomerulopathy
Metabolic Diseases
    Diabetes Mellitus
    Urinary Stones
    Urinary Tract Infections
Circulatory Disturbances
    Acute Tubular Necrosis
    Nephroangiosclerosis
    Hypertension
Neoplasms
    Renal Cell Carcinoma
    Urothelial Carcinoma of the Renal Pelvis
    Wilms' Tumor
    Carcinoma of the Urinary Bladder

Key Terms and Concepts

Anuria	Hematuria	Renal cell carcinoma (RCC)
Cystitis, chronic	Lipoid nephrosis	Renal failure
Diabetic nephropathy	Malignant hypertension	Renin
Dysuria	Membranous nephropathy	Systemic lupus erythematosus (SLE)
Erythropoietin	Multicystic renal dysplasia	Tubular necrosis
Focal segmental glomerulosclerosis (FSG)	Nephroangiosclerosis	Uremia
Glomerulonephritis	Oliguria	Urinary tract infection (UTI)
Glomerulosclerosis	Polycystic kidney disease	Urolithiasis
Glucosuria	Proteinuria	Urothelial carcinoma
Goodpasture's syndrome	Rapidly progressive glomerulonephritis (RPGN)	Wegener's granulomatosis
		Wilms' tumor

Learning Objectives

After reading this chapter, the student should be able to:

1. Describe the gross and microscopic anatomy of the urinary tract and the principal functions of the kidneys and the urinary bladder.
2. List two congenital renal malformations and explain the significance of adult polycystic kidney disease.
3. Discuss the pathogenesis, clinical course, and outcome of poststreptococcal and crescentic glomerulonephritis.
4. Discuss three causes of nephrotic syndrome.
5. Compare the pathogenesis of acute and chronic renal failure.
6. Describe the pathologic changes in the kidney caused by diabetes.
7. List four types of renal stones, explain their pathogenesis, and describe the clinical symptoms they produce.
8. List five causes of urinary obstruction.
9. Compare the pathology and clinical symptoms of acute and chronic pyelonephritis.
10. Discuss the etiology and pathogenesis of cystitis in men and women.
11. Define acute tubular necrosis and describe its pathogenesis and outcome.
12. Describe the pathology and clinical features of renal cell carcinoma, Wilms' tumor, and urothelial carcinoma of the renal pelvis.
13. Describe the pathology and clinical features of bladder cancer.

The urinary tract comprises the kidneys, the ureters, the urinary bladder, and the urethra (Figure 13-1). Diseases affecting the kidneys are usually treated by *nephrologists,* whereas *urologists* generally treat renal tumors and most diseases of the lower urinary tract. Nephrologists are among the busiest internal medicine consultants in most hospitals because they assist other doctors in dealing with electrolyte disturbances, which occur in the course of many diseases and especially in the postoperative period after major surgery.

NORMAL ANATOMY AND PHYSIOLOGY

The primary function of the urinary tract is the formation and excretion of urine. Urine is formed by ultrafiltration of blood in the kidneys. From the kidneys, the urine flows into the renal collecting system (renal calices and pelvis) and passes through the ureters before it reaches the urinary bladder. The urinary bladder serves as a receptacle for the urine. The urine is stored in the urinary bladder for several hours and then discharged from the body through the urethra.

The formation of urine in the kidneys is accomplished in the *nephron,* which represents the basic functional unit of each kidney. The kidneys contain approximately 2.5 million nephrons, each of which consists of a glomerulus, tubules, and collecting ducts (Figure 13-2). The glomerulus consists of specialized capillaries that are modified so that they allow selective passage of fluids and solutes from the blood into the lumen of the nephron. This "primary filtrate" is modified during its passage through the tubular parts of the nephron, which are known as the *proximal* and *distal tubules, loop of Henle,* and *collecting ducts.* The contents of the primary filtrate are partially resorbed and partially enriched by substances that are secreted into the nephron. Most of the fluid filtered in the glomeruli is actually resorbed and returned to the circulation. Because the primary filtrate is concentrated in the tubules, only a small portion of it is excreted as urine. Approximately 1.5 L of urine is excreted daily, which represents less than 10% of the blood volume filtered through the glomeruli.

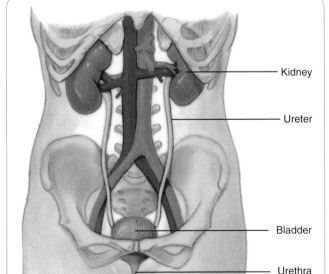

Figure 13-1 The urinary tract consists of the kidneys, ureters, urinary bladder, and urethra. (From Applegate EJ: The Anatomy and Physiology Learning System, 4th ed, St. Louis, 2011, Saunders.)

Labels: Kidney, Ureter, Bladder, Urethra

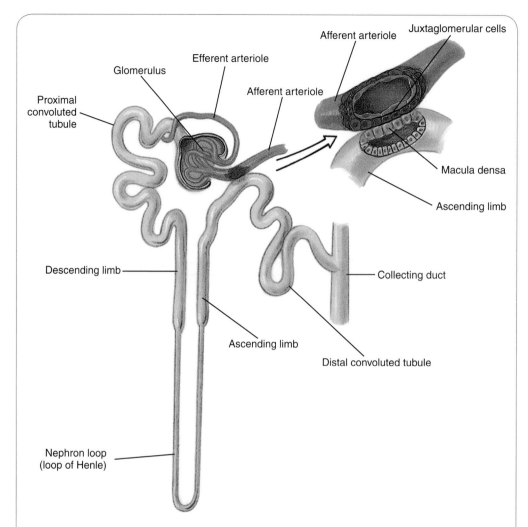

Figure 13-2 The nephron is the functional unit of the kidney. It consists of the glomerulus, convoluted tubules, and collecting ducts. The close positioning of blood vessels allows concentration of urine and selective excretion of minerals and water. (From Applegate EJ: The Anatomy and Physiology Learning System, 4th ed, St. Louis, 2011, Saunders.)

In contrast to the complex histology of the kidneys, the excretory portion of the urinary tract is relatively simple, reflecting its simple function. The calices, pelves, ureters, urinary bladder, and most of the urethra are lined by transitional epithelium. The transitional epithelium is "waterproof" and can withstand prolonged exposure to urine. External to this epithelial layer, these organs consist of connective tissue and smooth muscle cells. Transitional epithelium and the smooth muscular wall can expand, allowing the bladder to store urine. The smooth muscle in the bladder wall is important for extrusion of urine during voiding (*micturition,* or urination).

As mentioned, the urinary tract primarily has an excretory function. In addition, the kidney has secretory functions: It secretes **renin,** a hormone that raises blood pressure, and **erythropoietin,** the growth factor that stimulates the production of red blood cells (RBCs) in the bone marrow.

OVERVIEW OF MAJOR DISEASES

The most important diseases of the urinary tract are the following:
- Immunologic disorders (e.g., glomerulonephritis)
- Metabolic disorders (e.g., diabetic nephropathy)
- Circulatory disturbances (e.g., prerenal renal failure secondary to shock)
- Bacterial infections (e.g., cystitis, pyelonephritis)
- Tumors

Several facts important for the understanding of urinary tract pathology are presented here, before a discussion of specific pathologic entities.

1. *The primary function of the urinary tract is to form and excrete urine.* The kidneys must be anatomically normal to perform their normal function. However, the formation of urine also depends on sufficient blood flow and adequate

hydration of the body. Several polypeptide and steroid hormones also regulate renal function. The most important hormones are antidiuretic hormone (ADH), which is secreted by the posterior pituitary; atrial natriuretic hormone (ANH), which is derived from the atria of the heart; and aldosterone, which is from the zona glomerulosa of the adrenal cortex. Once the urine is formed, it can be discharged only if the urinary passages are patent. Any obstruction of the ureters (e.g., as a result of urinary stones) or of the urinary bladder (e.g., because of an enlarged prostate secondary to hyperplasia) will result in retention of urine.

Failure of the urinary tract to produce normal amounts of urine is called **renal failure,** which may be classified as prerenal, renal, or postrenal. Prerenal renal failure is most often caused by shock or heart insufficiency (e.g., myocardial infarction). Prerenal failure is usually reversible, and if its cause is cured, normal renal function can be restored. Intrarenal causes of acute renal failure, such as **tubular necrosis**, are also reversible. Although chronic renal failure previously was lethal, modern technology has made it feasible to treat even irreversible renal failure with dialysis machines or through renal transplantation. Postrenal causes of renal failure, such as prostatic disease or stones in the bladder, can be treated surgically.

2. *The urinary tract is extremely sensitive to bacterial infections.* The kidneys are perfused constantly by a high volume of blood, which is filtered in the glomeruli. Bacteria found in the circulation thus have a good chance of entering and colonizing the kidneys and causing a **urinary tract infection (UTI).** Moreover, because the urethral opening lies external to the body, bacteria may easily enter the urinary tract through it as well. UTIs that are acquired from bacteremia are called *descending* or *hematogenous infections,* whereas those attributable to upstream bacterial spread are called *ascending infections.*

3. *The specialized capillaries of the glomeruli are a ready target for bloodborne antibodies.* The glomeruli filter large amounts of blood. During this process, their basement membranes are exposed to potentially noxious plasma components—most notably, antibodies and antigen-antibody complexes. Glomeruli are thus often involved in many systemic autoimmune diseases mediated by antibodies. Antibody-mediated disease of the glomeruli is known as **glomerulonephritis.**

4. *Glomerular capillaries, although they are highly specialized, are nevertheless part of the circulatory system.* The glomeruli are affected by many diseases that involve the vasculature. Although atherosclerosis, which is a disease involving the larger arteries, does not affect the glomeruli directly, the narrowing within atherosclerotic renal arteries and their branches produces secondary changes in the glomeruli and their obsolescence **(glomerulosclerosis).** Renal arterioles and glomeruli are often pathologically altered by hypertension, which may damage the kidneys irreparably. Diabetes mellitus, a common metabolic disorder of the intermediate metabolism, affects the capillaries and arterioles in many organs. Hence, it is no surprise that this microangiopathy often damages the glomeruli as well *(diabetic glomerulosclerosis).*

5. *Renal tubules are composed of highly specialized cells that are very sensitive to a lack of oxygen and to the adverse action of toxins.* Like all other highly specialized cells, such as neurons, renal tubular cells require a constant supply of oxygen and nutrients. Even a short interruption of blood supply or a hypoperfusion of the kidneys, as typically occurs in *shock* or heart failure, results in *tubular necrosis.* Because the proximal tubular cells have the most complex function and require the most oxygen, they are most susceptible to hypoxia or anoxia. Many drugs, poisons, heavy metals, and endogenous waste products that are filtered through the glomeruli are taken up by the proximal tubular cells and may adversely affect them. For example, mercury salts inactivate the enzymes of the proximal tubules and, if ingested in large amounts (e.g., in suicidal mercury poisoning), can cause necrosis of the proximal tubules.

6. *The urinary tract consists of many mitotic or facultative mitotic cells that may undergo malignant transformation.* Tumors of the urinary tract develop most often in the urinary bladder, which is lined by regularly cycling (mitotic) cells. As with most other tumors, the causes of urogenital tumors are not known. However, because the urinary tract serves as a route for the excretion of chemicals, many of which are potential carcinogens, it is possible that some tumors are chemically induced. It has also been postulated that some tumors originate from the interaction of chemical carcinogens and endogenous proto-oncogenes. In support of this hypothesis is the finding of chromosomal changes in many renal cell and urinary bladder carcinomas. Wilms' tumor, the most common urinary tract tumor of infancy that shows a familial preponderance, has been linked to a deletion of a specific tumor suppressor gene in about 15% of cases (Wilms' tumor gene—*WT1*).

7. *Diseases of the urinary tract may present with local or systemic symptoms.* Diseases of the urinary tract produce a variety of symptoms that may be either localized to the urinary tract or systemic, affecting the entire body. The best-known local symptom is the flank pain that occurs with kidney infection *(pyelonephritis)* or renal tumors. Painful urination **(dysuria)** is the best-known symptom of cystitis. Urinary colic is a symptom associated with urinary stones impacted in the ureters. Colics are attacks of spasmodic pain that occur as the ureteral smooth muscles contract in an effort to propel the stone and relieve the urinary obstruction.

LOCALIZED SYMPTOMS

The local symptoms and findings are best exemplified by a variety of changes reflected in the urine itself. The *volume* of urine may be altered so that too much or too little urine is produced. Polyuria indicates an increased amount of urine, whereas **oliguria** means a decreased daily output of urine. **Anuria** is a state in which no urine is produced.

Did You Know?

The paintings of Cosmas and Damian, two Christian patron saints of physicians, can be seen in many fine art museums. One of these holy healers practiced what we would call today "internal medicine," and the other was a surgeon. The surgeon carries a scalpel and other instruments, whereas the internist is usually seen gazing at a bottle of urine. This type of "naked eye" urinalysis was widely used in the Middle Ages for diagnosing diseases. It is no wonder that almost nobody who was really sick was ever cured by medieval physicians.

The chemical composition of urine may be determined, and a microscopic analysis of urinary sediment is routinely performed in the clinical laboratory. **Proteinuria** and **glucosuria** refer to increased excretion of protein or glucose in the urine, respectively. **Hematuria,** which is blood in the urine, may present as a grossly visible change in the color of urine (e.g., the brown or red urine typical of macroscopic hematuria) or may be detectable only by microscopic analysis of urine (microscopic hematuria refers to RBCs in urine). *Pyuria* is the appearance of pus in urine. Such urine contains a large number of viable and dead polymorphonuclear leukocytes and appears turbid. Urine normally contains few bacteria, most of which are from the terminal urethra, which is normally colonized by bacteria. Infections of the urinary tract are associated with an increased number of bacteria in urine, which can be documented by quantitating bacteria in urine. Typically the results are expressed as the number of bacterial colonies per milliliter of urine. More than 100,000 colonies per milliliter is evidence of infection.

SYSTEMIC SYMPTOMS

Systemic symptoms and findings caused by urinary tract disease vary depending on the underlying pathologic condition. Bacterial infection affecting the kidneys, such as acute pyelonephritis, or acute cystitis affecting the urinary bladder may cause fever, shivering, and malaise, like any other infection. Renal failure may cause complex metabolic changes, mostly because of the accumulation of substances that cannot be excreted from the body through the urinary tract. This condition, called **uremia,** is, in simplified terms, equivalent to "poisoning with urine." It is characterized by retention of water; minerals (e.g., sodium, potassium, chloride, calcium, and phosphate); organic substances, such as creatinine or uric acid; and other nitrogen-rich substances, such as ammonia, which are measured in the clinical laboratory as blood urea nitrogen (BUN). Hypercalcemia or hyperkalemia endanger life because these metabolic changes may cause cardiac arrest. Chronic uremia is marked by profound neurologic changes and depression of the central nervous system, which initially presents as somnolence and fatigue and ultimately results in coma and death. Fortunately, by an act of Congress introduced in the 1970s, all Americans are entitled to free treatment of chronic renal failure; therefore, chronic uremia is a condition that is rarely seen today.

DEVELOPMENTAL DISORDERS

Developmental disorders of the urinary tract are very common. Fortunately, most of these anomalies do not produce symptoms and are often discovered only by chance. For example, 1 in 800 people is born with only one kidney *(one-sided renal agenesis)* or with a solitary horseshoe kidney formed by the fusion of the kidneys in the midline. Patients with such anomalies are usually asymptomatic, and the congenital defect is often noted on routine x-ray examination for some other disease or if the affected person is being considered for kidney donation. Clearly, these individuals cannot donate their solitary kidney for transplantation. *Bilateral renal agenesis* is incompatible with life, and death occurs soon after birth.

POLYCYSTIC KIDNEY DISEASE

The most important developmental disorder of the urinary tract is autosomal dominant **polycystic kidney disease** (ADPKD), which is inherited as a Mendelian trait at a rate of 1:1000. In 85% of all cases the disease is related to the mutation of a gene encoding *polycystin-1,* a cell-to-cell adhesion molecule holding cells together. ADPKD affects the kidneys bilaterally. Both kidneys are enlarged, contain numerous cysts, and weigh 3000 to 4000 g, which is 20 times more than the normal weight of 150 to 200 g. These cysts, which are derived from obstructed tubules, contain fluid (Figure 13-3). The reasons for the obstruction of tubules are unknown. Cystic change in the tubules gradually impairs renal function. Most affected patients develop renal failure by the age of 40 to 50 years.

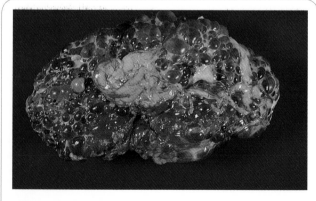

Figure 13-3 Autosomal dominant polycystic kidney disease. Note the numerous cysts.

ADPKD must be distinguished from several other congenital kidney diseases, most of which present during infancy and childhood. The most important of these is **multicystic renal dysplasia.** In contrast to ADPKD, multicystic renal dysplasia is usually unilateral. The enlarged abnormal kidney may be palpated by either a parent or the pediatrician. Unilateral renal lesions can easily be removed without consequences, and if the kidney is normal, the patient has an excellent chance for complete recovery.

 Did You Know?

Three most common palpable posterior abdominal masses in infants and small children are as follows : multicystic renal dysplasia, Wilms' tumor of the kidney, and neuroblastoma of the adrenal gland.

GLOMERULAR DISEASES

CLASSIFICATION

The classification of glomerular diseases may be based on morphology, pathogenesis, or clinical presentation of the diseases. On the basis of pathogenesis, glomerular diseases can be classified into the following categories (Figure 13-4):

- Immunologic diseases
- Metabolic disorders
- Circulatory disturbances

IMMUNOLOGIC DISEASES

Immunologic injury is most often mediated by antibodies and can be classified as a type II (cytotoxic) or type III (immune complex) hypersensitivity reaction. Pathologic studies reveal that such injury is marked by deposits of immunoglobulins in the glomeruli. If the deposition of immunoglobulins evokes an inflammatory reaction, the disease is classified as glomerulonephritis. Those glomerulopathies that have an immunologic pathogenesis or a presumptive immunologic pathogenesis but that do not show signs of inflammation carry names without the suffix -*itis* (which is reserved for inflammatory disease). Within this category, the most important diseases are lipoid nephrosis, membranous nephropathy, and *immunoglobulin A (IgA)* nephropathy *(Berger's disease).*

Immune-mediated glomerulonephritis can occur in an isolated form (primary) or in the course of a systemic disease (secondary), as in systemic lupus erythematosus or **Wegener's granulomatosis.** Primary glomerulonephritis is often limited to the glomeruli, whereas secondary glomerulonephritis is usually associated with tubulointerstitial renal inflammation.

METABOLIC DISORDERS

Metabolic glomerulopathy occurs in the course of systemic metabolic disorders. The best example is diabetes mellitus, which typically presents with polyuria and glycosuria and leads to chronic renal failure in about 5% to 10% of affected

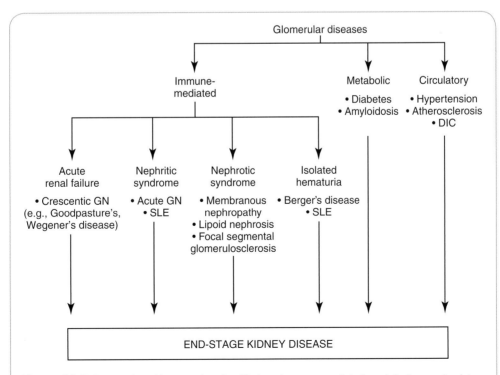

Figure 13-4 Glomerulopathies can be classified as immune-mediated, metabolic, or circulatory diseases. All of these diseases may terminate in end-stage kidney disease. DIC, disseminated intravascular coagulation; GN, glomerulonephritis; SLE, systemic lupus erythematosus.

patients. Diabetes causes biochemical changes in the composition of the basement membranes, which become thickened and glomerulosclerotic and lose their semipermeability. Diabetic glomerulosclerosis, like other metabolic glomerulopathies, is also associated with pathologic changes involving other parts of the kidney.

CIRCULATORY DISTURBANCES

Circulatory disturbances affect glomeruli in several ways. Atherosclerosis of the renal arteries is typically associated with hypoperfusion, which leads to involution and hyalinization of glomeruli. The sudden onset of hypertension may cause fibrinoid necrosis of the glomerular capillaries. Shock is often associated with disseminated intravascular coagulation (DIC) and the formation of microthrombi in the glomerular capillaries.

MULTIPLE MECHANISMS

The border between immunologic, metabolic, and circulatory glomerular diseases is not always sharp. This is best illustrated by diabetes. The metabolic changes of diabetes cause thickening of the glomerular basement membranes. Diabetes is also a systemic *microangiopathy* (i.e., disease of small vessels) and is often associated with atherosclerosis and hypertension, both of which affect the glomeruli, producing additional changes.

Clinical Features

Glomerular diseases can present clinically with a set of symptoms, which collectively are recognized as particular syndromes. The most important of these syndromes are as follows:

- Acute renal failure (rapidly progressive *glomerulonephritis*)
- Nephritic syndrome
- Nephrotic syndrome
- Isolated hematuria and/or proteinuria

Acute renal failure, or rapidly progressive glomerulonephritis, is characterized by a loss of renal excretory functions over a period of several weeks. The destruction of glomeruli presents initially with hematuria, progressing fast to oliguria and finally anuria. Acute renal failure is typically caused by crescentic glomerulonephritis.

Nephritic syndrome is diagnosed on the basis of typical clinical and laboratory findings. These include generalized edema, hypertension, hematuria, proteinuria, and hypoalbuminemia. Acute nephritis syndrome is usually caused by acute poststreptococcal or postinfectious glomerulonephritis. The most common cause of chronic nephritic syndrome is systemic lupus erythematosus.

Nephrotic syndrome is characterized by generalized edema, proteinuria, hypoalbuminemia, and often hyperlipidemia and lipiduria. The most common causes of nephrotic syndrome in adults are focal glomerulosclerosis, membranous nephropathy, and diabetes. Lipoid nephrosis is the most common cause of nephrotic syndrome in children.

Isolated glomerular hematuria, with or without proteinuria, is usually not accompanied by constant clinical symptoms and generally can be diagnosed only on the basis of abnormal urinary findings. This syndrome, as typically seen in IgA nephropathy (Berger's disease), may progress to chronic renal failure like any other immune-mediated glomerulonephritis.

ACUTE GLOMERULONEPHRITIS

Acute glomerulonephritis is an immune-mediated inflammatory glomerulopathy that occurs 1 to 2 weeks after an acute infection, most often a streptococcal upper respiratory disease ("strep throat"). The disease typically affects children. Before the era of antibiotics, poststreptococcal glomerulonephritis was very common. Today it is uncommon in the United States but is still prevalent in underdeveloped countries and even some countries as close to the United States as the Caribbean islands.

Acute poststreptococcal glomerulonephritis is caused by the antibodies produced in response to infection with certain streptococcal strains. The antigen-antibody complexes are trapped in the glomerular basement membranes, where they activate complement and thus attract inflammatory cells into the kidney (Figure 13-5). On histologic examination the glomeruli appear hypercellular because they contain an increased number of mesangial cells and numerous inflammatory cells (Figure 13-6). These cells compress or occlude the capillaries, thereby preventing blood flow through the glomeruli.

Clinical Features

Acute glomerulonephritis presents with nephritic syndrome. The damaged basement membranes of the inflamed glomeruli become permeable, which accounts for the proteinuria and hematuria. Reduced glomerular blood flow through the inflamed glomeruli results in reduced glomerular filtration rate and consequently reduced urinary output (oliguria). The urine of these patients typically appears murky brown, resembling "bouillon soup," a color resulting from the entry of broken red blood cells into the urine. Loss of proteins, mostly albumin, in the urine causes hypoalbuminemia, which, together with retention of sodium, results in edema. This edema is thus in part due to the loss of oncotic pressure of the plasma secondary to a loss of albumin in urine, and in part due to increased volume of extracellular fluids as a result of sodium retention in oliguria. Edema is most pronounced on the face, and especially in the loose subcutaneous tissue around the eyes. Edema of the brain and hypertension typically cause headaches and somnolence. The hypertension is caused by reduced blood flow through the arterioles leading to the inflamed glomeruli, which elicits a release of renin from the juxtaglomerular apparatus in the afferent arteriole.

The glomerular inflammation is usually short lived, and most patients recover completely. In 1% to 2% of affected patients, however, the disease may cause acute renal failure

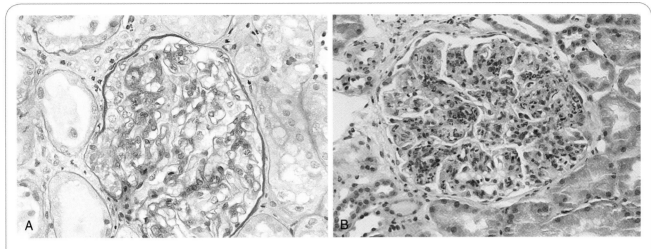

Figure 13-5 Acute glomerulonephritis. *A,* Normal glomerulus. *B,* This affected glomerulus appears hypercellular. This hypercellularity is mostly attributable to inflammatory cells and, in part, to the proliferation of mesangial cells responding to injury. Deposits of immune complexes on the epithelial side of the basement membrane form "humps."

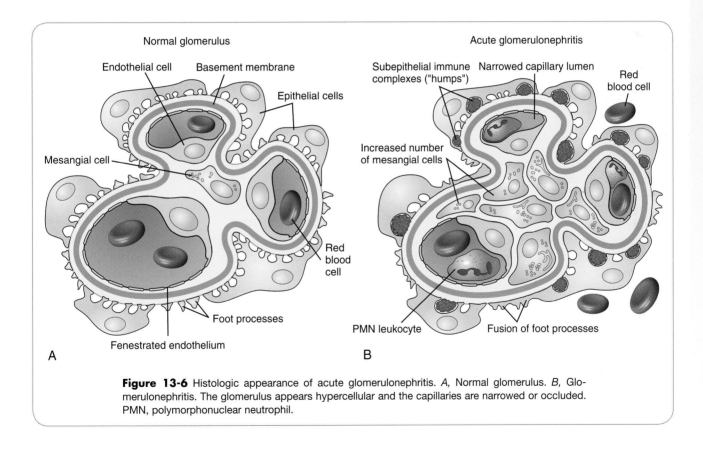

Figure 13-6 Histologic appearance of acute glomerulonephritis. *A,* Normal glomerulus. *B,* Glomerulonephritis. The glomerulus appears hypercellular and the capillaries are narrowed or occluded. PMN, polymorphonuclear neutrophil.

leading to chronic glomerulonephritis and end-stage kidney disease.

CRESCENTIC GLOMERULONEPHRITIS

Crescentic glomerulonephritis is a term used to describe severe glomerular injury accompanied by the formation of an exudate in the glomerular urinary space. The exudate consists predominantly of macrophages that have crossed through the damaged glomerular capillaries into the urinary space between the capillary tufts and Bowman's capsule (Figure 13-7). The term derives from the fact that the inflammatory cells surround the compressed capillary loops in the form of a crescent moon. Macrophages are gradually replaced by fibroblasts, which secrete collagen, leading to the scarring and complete obliteration of glomeruli.

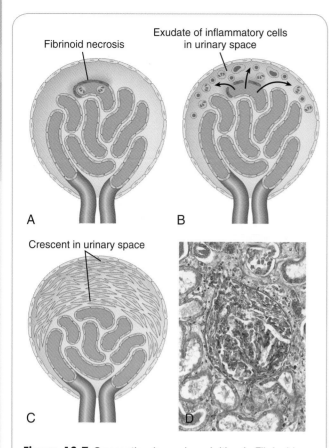

Figure 13-7 Crescentic glomerulonephritis. *A,* Fibrinoid necrosis. *B,* Artist's rendition of the crescent correlates with the changes seen microscopically. *C,* Crescent in urinary space. *D,* The urinary space contains a "crescent" composed of macrophages and some proliferated epithelial cells derived from the lining of Bowman's capsule.

Crescentic glomerulonephritis usually occurs after focal necrosis of the glomerular capillaries. Such focal necrotizing glomerulonephritis is typically found in **Goodpasture's syndrome,** an autoimmune disease characterized by the formation of antibodies to the body's own basement membrane component—collagen type IV. Injury of collagen type IV in the lungs causes intra-alveolar hemorrhage. In the glomeruli the antibodies cause rupture of the basement membranes. Macrophages exit through the holes in the basement membrane and accumulate in the urinary space, forming the crescents that compress the capillary loops. Because no blood flows through the compressed capillary loops, glomerular filtration ceases and anuria (i.e., acute renal failure) ensues. Clinically the disease is known as **rapidly progressive glomerulonephritis (RPGN).** Most patients never recover, and their survival depends on continuous dialysis or kidney transplantation.

Crescentic glomerulonephritis is a descriptive diagnosis. In addition to Goodpasture's syndrome, it may be caused by Wegener's granulomatosis and, less often, by other diseases, such as polyarteritis nodosa or severe poststreptococcal glomerulonephritis. Once the diagnosis of crescentic glomerulonephritis is

made by kidney biopsy, it is important to test the patient serologically to determine whether the blood contains antibodies of diagnostic significance. Finding of antibodies to collagen type IV will confirm the diagnosis of Goodpasture's syndrome. Antibodies to neutrophil cytoplasmic antigens (ANCA) are found in Wegener's granulomatosis.

MEMBRANOUS NEPHROPATHY

Membranous nephropathy is an immune-mediated glomerulopathy characterized by diffuse ("membranous") thickening of the glomerular basement membranes secondary to massive deposition of immune complexes. In contrast to acute glomerulonephritis, which causes nephritic syndrome, membranous nephropathy presents with a typical nephrotic syndrome. There is no evidence of inflammation. The glomeruli do not contain any inflammatory cells, and the urine is devoid of RBCs and inflammatory cells.

Membranous nephropathy is one of the most common immune nephrotic syndromes of adults. In 85% of the cases its etiology remains unknown. In addition to these idiopathic cases, a secondary disease of the same morphology can affect patients who have developed antibodies to tumors, drugs, or infectious agents, such as hepatitis B virus or *Treponema pallidum.*

Light microscopy reveals that the glomeruli have thick basement membranes but are normocellular—that is, they show no proliferative or inflammatory changes (Figure 13-8, *A*). Immunofluorescence microscopy demonstrates the granularity of these deposits (see Figure 13-8, *B*). On electron microscopy, one may see that the thickening of the basement membrane is attributable to the deposition of dense immune complexes (see Figure 13-8, *C*).

Clinical Features

Membranous nephropathy presents with the typical symptoms of nephrotic syndrome and does not respond to therapy. Proteinuria persists in most patients for years, but the disease progresses in only 40% of patients. These patients eventually develop chronic renal failure and require dialysis or renal transplantation.

LIPOID NEPHROSIS

Lipoid nephrosis, also known as *minimal change disease* or *nil disease,* is a disease of unknown etiology that also presents as nephrotic syndrome. It is the most common cause of nephrotic syndrome in children. The descriptive terms used for this disease reflect our ignorance about its pathogenesis. Lipoid nephrosis indicates only that the nephrotic syndrome is associated with hyperlipidemia and lipiduria. The other terms used as synonyms—minimal change disease or nil disease (from the Latin term *nihil,* meaning "nothing")—indicate that the glomeruli show no changes on light microscopy. On immunofluorescence microscopy, the glomeruli are seen not to contain any deposits of immunoglobulins. The only remarkable findings are seen on electron microscopy, which usually shows fusion of

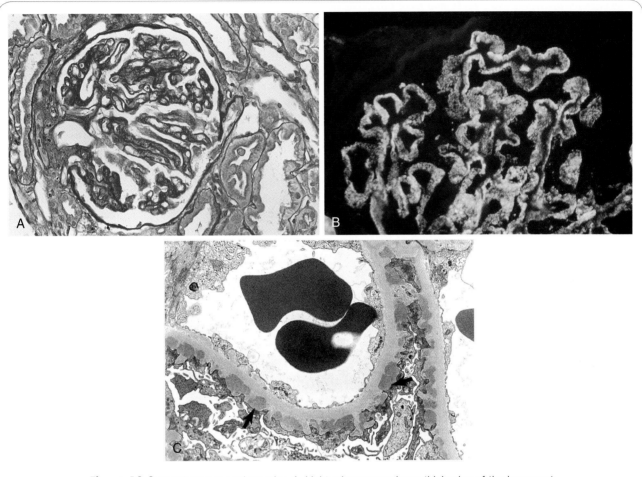

Figure 13-8 Membranous nephropathy. *A,* Light microscopy shows thickening of the basement membranes but no inflammatory cells. *B,* Immunofluorescence microscopy shows granular deposits along the basement membrane. *C,* Electron microscopy shows immune deposits (arrows) along the basement membrane.

the foot processes of the podocytes (which are also known as the *epithelial cells of the glomerulus*). Such changes can readily be distinguished from those of membranous nephropathy (Figure 13-9). Lipoid nephrosis responds favorably to corticosteroid treatment.

FOCAL SEGMENTAL GLOMERULOSCLEROSIS

Focal segmental glomerulosclerosis (FSG) is currently the most common cause of nephrotic syndrome in adults. However, it may occur in children as well. It is not a single clinicopathologic entity but rather a group of diseases that share some common features and present with partial scarring of glomerular loops. *Focal* means that some but not all glomeruli are affected, whereas *segmental* means that only some capillary loops in an affected glomerulus are scarred.

FSG can be classified as primary or secondary. In both forms the disease presents with proteinuria and nephrotic syndrome, which is unresponsive to corticosteroid therapy. The primary form of FSG occurs most often in children, and

the cause of it remains unknown. Often the physician thinks that the child has lipoid nephrosis, but the proper diagnosis becomes evident when the child does not respond to steroid treatment or when nephrotic syndrome recurs after steroid therapy. Secondary FSG occurs in a variety of diseases and is encountered in overtly obese persons, in persons infected with human immunodeficiency virus (HIV), in those with sickle cell anemia, after intravenous drug abuse, and in other conditions.

FSG usually does not respond to treatment, although some obese patients may respond well to weight reduction and treatment of their hypertension. FSG caused by HIV infection has a particularly bad prognosis and tends to progress quickly to end-stage kidney disease.

CHRONIC PROLIFERATIVE GLOMERULONEPHRITIS

Kidneys may be affected by several variants of primary immune-mediated glomerulonephropathies, which carry names such as *IgA nephropathy (Berger's disease), membranoproliferative glomerulonephritis type I* and *type II,* and *focal proliferative glomerulonephritis.* Common to all these diseases is that they have a chronic course, they do not respond to treatment, and they slowly but inexorably progress to end-stage kidney disease.

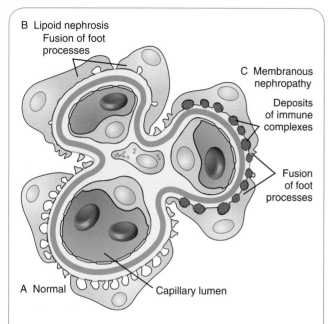

Figure 13-9 Schematic drawing of the glomerular changes in two forms of nephrotic syndrome as seen by electron microscopy. *A,* Normal appearance. *B,* Lipoid nephrosis does not cause any visible basement membrane changes, but fusion of the foot processes of epithelial cells is noted. *C,* Membranous nephropathy is characterized by subepithelial dense deposits of immune complexes.

Clinical Features

Chronic glomerulopathies listed earlier may present as nephrotic syndrome or nephritic syndrome with some hematuria, or they may be associated with only mild urinary findings, such as microscopic hematuria and proteinuria, and no clinical symptoms. There is no effective treatment for these diseases.

Chronic proliferative glomerulonephritis may occur in the course of systemic autoimmune diseases, most notably in **systemic lupus erythematosus (SLE).** Approximately 60% to 70% of patients with SLE develop some renal manifestations. The glomerular changes vary from mild to severe, and histologic findings indicate glomerulonephritis or membranous nephropathy with no proliferative changes. The glomerulonephritis of SLE responds well to corticosteroid treatment.

END-STAGE GLOMERULOPATHY

Most, if not all, immune-mediated glomerulopathies can progress to end-stage kidney disease. These immune-mediated diseases terminating in uremia have traditionally been called *chronic glomerulonephritis.* However, by the time chronic renal failure has developed, there has been no evidence of inflammation; hence, the term *glomerulonephritis* seems unjustified. Furthermore, all chronic glomerulopathies—be they immune, metabolic, or circulatory—appear ultimately identical. Because the morphologic study of terminally insufficient kidneys does not indicate the nature of the preexisting disease, it is best to be noncommittal and characterize such kidney diseases as end-stage glomerulopathy.

On gross examination the kidneys appear to be shrunken symmetrically (Figure 13-10, *A*). Their surface is finely

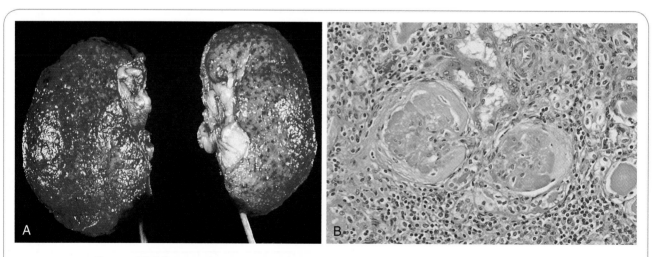

Figure 13-10 End-stage glomerulopathy—chronic glomerulonephritis. *A,* The kidneys appear small, are uniformly shrunken, and have a finely granular external surface. *B,* Histologic examination of the kidneys shows hyalinization of glomeruli and tubular atrophy. Fibrous tissue in the dilated interstitium surrounds atrophic tubules.

granular because of the loss of tubules. The fine granules are the remaining tubules surrounded by fibrous tissue. Histologic examination reveals that the glomeruli have undergone hyalinization and appear like solid globules composed of homogenized matrix (see Figure 13-10, *B*).

METABOLIC DISEASES

Many systemic metabolic diseases affect the kidneys. For example, in gout, which is characterized by *hyperuricemia*, there are deposits of uric acid crystals in the kidneys. In multiple myeloma, renal failure develops from deposits of light chains of immunoglobulins secreted by neoplastic plasma cells. The most important of the metabolic diseases is diabetes mellitus.

DIABETES MELLITUS

Diabetes mellitus is the most prevalent metabolic disease affecting the kidneys. Diabetic kidney disease is very common; indeed, of the 20 million Americans who have diabetes, 5% to 10% have some renal problems.

Diabetic nephropathy may present in several forms depending on which portion of the kidney is affected. Pathologic changes can be seen in the glomeruli, in the arteries and arterioles, and in the interstitium. The glomerular changes include thickening of the basement membranes and an increased amount of mesangial matrix. This pathologic change is known as diffuse glomerulosclerosis. The mesangial matrix expansion may lead to the formation of nodules, which is typical of nodular glomerulosclerosis or Kimmelstiel-Wilson disease (Figure 13-11). Regardless of the form of glomerulopathy, the basement membranes of the altered glomeruli show increased permeability, which typically results in proteinuria. Proteinuria usually develops 10 to 20 years after the

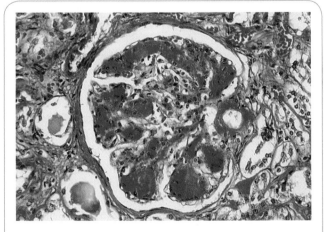

Figure 13-11 Nodular glomerulosclerosis of diabetes (Kimmelstiel-Wilson syndrome). The glomerulus shows mesangial nodules, a change associated with the nephrotic syndrome.

onset of diabetes. Proteinuria may be massive, and if it exceeds 3 g of protein per day (called *nephrotic-range proteinuria*), it causes nephrotic syndrome. Severe proteinuria heralds deterioration of renal function, and chronic renal insufficiency usually develops over a period of 5 years.

The vascular changes caused by diabetes are most prominent in the arterioles, which typically show hyalinosis, accompanied by thickening of the vessel wall and narrowing of the vascular lumen. These changes lead to ischemia and tubular atrophy. The most prominent chronic changes are seen in the papillary part of the medulla. Ischemic papillae may become infected and slough off onto the renal pelvis. This *papillary necrosis* is a serious complication of diabetes and can cause urinary obstruction and colic as the necrotic papillae detach and occlude the ureter.

The kidneys of diabetic patients are prone to bacterial infections, and pyelonephritis is an important complication. Recurrent bouts of bacterial pyelonephritis may ultimately destroy the kidneys. Such patients develop uremia and require dialysis or renal transplantation.

URINARY STONES

The formation of urinary stones or calculi (**urolithiasis**) is common. At least 5% of all adults in the United States will experience this condition at some point in their lives.

Based on their chemical structure, urinary stones can be classified into four main groups:

- Calcium stones
- Struvite stones
- Uric acid stones
- Cystine stones

Calcium stones, composed of either calcium oxalate or calcium phosphate, account for 75% of all stones. These stones are often associated with hyperexcretion of calcium in patients who have abnormal calcium metabolism (e.g., hyperabsorptive hypercalciuria). Such patients absorb too much calcium in the intestines. The tendency to form calcium stones may be inherited. *Struvite stones,* composed of magnesium ammonia phosphate or sulfate, account for 15% of urinary calculi. These stones are typically a complication of UTIs, which lead to formation of ammonia from the urea in the urine. Uric acid stones account for about 5% of all urinary stones. About 50% of patients with this type of stone have hyperuricemia, or gout, whereas others do not have an obvious metabolic disorder predisposing them to stone formation. *Cystine stones* account for 1% of urinary calculi. These rare stones are found in patients with inborn errors of amino acid metabolism, such as cystinosis.

Urinary stones are most often found in the renal pelvis or the urinary bladder. With the exception of struvite stones, which may be relatively large, most other stones are smaller than 3 mm in diameter. The stones may resemble crystals, or they may be small, round, or elongated grains or irregular masses. Struvite stones, also known as *staghorn calculi,* are larger and more irregular than the other types of stones. They grow progressively by the apposition of minerals and can fill the entire pelvis (Figure 13-12).

Clinical Features

Urinary stones are more common in men than in women, and in those 20 to 30 years of age. Typical symptoms of upper urinary tract stones include hematuria and urinary colics (i.e., spasmodic pain caused by the contraction of an obstructed ureter). Stones in the bladder tend to occur in older patients and are often associated with chronic infection.

Small stones can be voided spontaneously, whereupon the urinary symptoms resolve. However, the treatment of larger urinary stones requires surgery or mechanical extraction. This is often achieved only after the stones have been broken into smaller pieces by a process called *lithotripsy*. New techniques for the removal of urinary stones include ultrasonic targeting, which is used to fragment the stones into small pieces so that they can be voided spontaneously.

URINARY TRACT INFECTIONS

Among the various infections of the urinary tract (UTI), the most important are those caused by gram-negative bacteria, such as *Escherichia coli, Klebsiella,* and *Pseudomonas aerogunisa.* These bacteria are often called *uropathogens.* Viral and fungal infections are less common. Parasitic infections, such as cystitis caused by *Schistosoma haematobium,* reportedly affect 50 million people worldwide but are rare in the United States.

Bacterial infection of the kidney is called *pyelonephritis,* whereas infection of the urinary bladder is called *cystitis.* Both conditions can occur simultaneously or in succession. Clinically and pathologically, both pyelonephritis and cystitis can occur in an acute and a chronic form. Bacteria may reach the urinary tract either from blood *(hematogenous infection)* or, more often, through the urethra and the lower urinary tract *(ascending infection)* (Figure 13-13).

Hematogenous infection is typically preceded by septicemia. In such cases the urinary tract is secondarily infected from a primary focus in another organ from which the bacteria

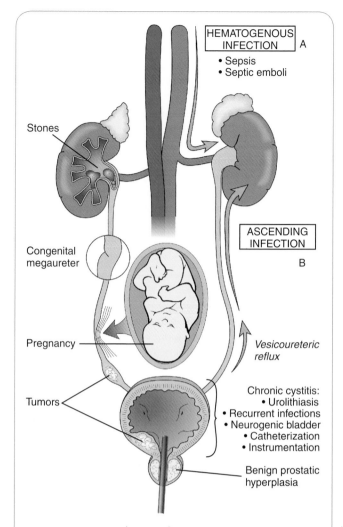

Figure 13-13 Routes of renal infection. *A,* Hematogenous infection. *B,* Ascending infection—causes of urinary tract obstruction that predispose individuals to urinary tract infection.

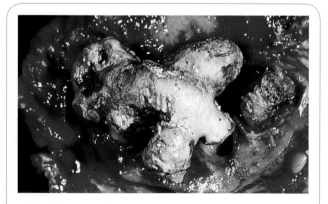

Figure 13-12 Irregularly shaped struvite stone in the renal pelvis.

spread into the blood. The primary infection may be in the endocardium, lungs, or gastrointestinal tract. Ascending infection, which is more common, may be acquired during sexual intercourse ("honeymoon cystitis"), but it also may occur without any obvious causes. It is a common complication of indwelling catheters inserted during surgery, after urinary bladder catheterization, or after urologic surgical procedures (e.g., removal of urinary bladder tumors). UTI is more common in women than in men, partially because of the shorter urethra in women, which allows easier bacterial colonization of the urinary bladder. Pregnancy also predisposes women to UTI, in part because of the mechanical effects of the enlarged uterus on the urinary bladder and the ureters and in part because of the relaxing effects of estrogen and progesterone on the smooth muscles of the urethra, urinary bladder, and ureter. Other conditions that predispose individuals to UTI are presented in Figure 13-13.

UTIs may involve the entire urinary tract, or they may present as localized infections (e.g., pyelonephritis and cystitis). Acute pyelonephritis is a suppurative infection of the kidneys.

On gross examination the kidneys contain foci of pus *(abscesses)*. In severe cases the pus may permeate the entire kidney and fill the renal pelvis *(pyonephrosis)*.

Chronic pyelonephritis may evolve from acute pyelonephritis, especially if there are recurrent attacks of acute infection. Persistent infection leads to destruction of the renal parenchyma and broad parenchymal scar formation. Ultimately, because of the loss of renal tissue, the affected kidney becomes small and irregularly scarred (Figure 13-14). Because the bacteria do not grow at the same rate in both kidneys and the infection is often unilateral, kidneys affected by chronic pyelonephritis are typically asymmetric. Indeed, it is not uncommon for one kidney to be completely shrunken and the other one to be spared.

Cystitis is an infection of the bladder that may occur in an acute or chronic form. Acute cystitis is characterized by grossly visible congestion and mucosal hemorrhages (Figure 13-15). These changes are best visualized with cystoscopy, a procedure in which the urologist observes the inside of the bladder with an instrument that has been introduced through the urethra. In severe cases the mucosa may be covered with pus or be ulcerated. Bladder biopsy specimens usually show the typical histologic features of acute inflammation. In

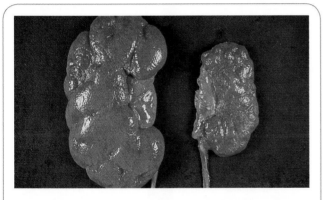

Figure 13-14 Small, shrunken, irregularly scarred kidney of a patient with chronic pyelonephritis. The other kidney is of normal size but also shows scarring on the upper pole.

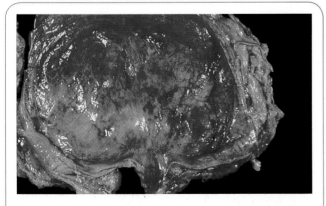

Figure 13-15 Acute cystitis. The mucosa of the bladder is red and swollen.

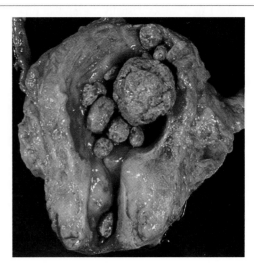

Figure 13-16 Chronic cystitis. Note the thickening in the wall of the urinary bladder. The bladder contains stones.

chronic cystitis the appearance of the mucosa varies considerably and includes foci of hemorrhage, ulceration, or thickening. The wall of the bladder is often thick, especially if cystitis is caused by chronic obstruction, as in urolithiasis or prostatic hyperplasia (Figure 13-16).

UTIs are treated with antibiotics and/or sulfa drugs. The infections are often resistant and, in many patients, tend to recur. UTIs that are associated with diabetes, calculi, or prostatic hyperplasia are especially resistant to treatment.

CIRCULATORY DISTURBANCES

Circulatory disturbances and vascular diseases affect the kidneys in many forms. Such disturbances may cause acute or chronic renal insufficiency.

ACUTE TUBULAR NECROSIS

A sudden decrease in arterial pressure will result in acute hypoperfusion of the kidneys. This typically occurs after myocardial infarction, any form of cardiac arrest, and all forms of hypotensive shock (e.g., massive bleeding). The reduction of blood flow is more prominent in the cortex than in the medulla. Cortical tubules, especially the highly specialized proximal convoluted tubules, are most affected. However, in severe hypotensive shock, the entire cortex may undergo necrosis *(renal cortical necrosis)*.

Renal failure that begins as prerenal becomes *renal* once ischemia has destroyed all the tubules. Such failure persists even after cardiac function has been restored or blood volume has been restored after massive blood loss. Patients who have tubular necrosis usually require support with an artificial kidney machine *(renal dialysis)* to survive. However, because the renal tubules may regenerate, the disrupted nephrons will heal spontaneously if one gives them time. Renal dialysis is usually continued for 1 to 2 weeks. Usually during that time, enough tubules regenerate to allow the kidneys to become functional again.

NEPHROANGIOSCLEROSIS

Atherosclerosis of the aorta, the renal artery, and its major branches may cause narrowing of the vascular lumen, which will significantly reduce blood flow through the kidneys. This leads to ischemic glomerulosclerosis and a loss of glomeruli, known collectively as **nephroangiosclerosis.** Loss of glomeruli is accompanied by tubular atrophy. The kidneys become small and show marked scarring. These scars actually represent multiple small infarcts in which the lost tubules have been replaced by fibrosis. Severe glomerulosclerosis may result in chronic renal insufficiency.

HYPERTENSION

Arterial hypertension often affects the intrarenal arteries and arterioles. Hypertension stimulates renal arterial and arteriolar contraction. Sustained arterial and arteriolar contraction ultimately leads to the thickening of the vessel walls. The arterial walls become fibrotic and multilayered, whereas the arterioles undergo hyalinization, similar to that seen in patients with diabetes. In patients who have **malignant hypertension,** as is typically seen in young black men who experience a sudden onset of high blood pressure, the arterioles do not have time to adjust. Such arterioles may undergo fibrinoid necrosis. Sustained malignant hypertension will cause hyperplasia of the smooth muscle cells in the vessel wall. These smooth muscle cells form crescentic layers around the narrower lumen of the arteriole, forming so-called onion ring–like lesions.

Arterial and arteriolar changes induced by hypertension result in ischemia of the renal parenchyma, causing histologic changes that may be similar to those induced by atherosclerosis or diabetes. Clinically such changes result in reduced renal function and ultimately may cause renal failure.

In most instances, hypertension is idiopathic; that is, it has no obvious cause. However, renal ischemia secondary to hypertensive arterial and arteriolar changes stimulates the renal juxtaglomerular apparatus to release renin. Renin may aggravate hypertension. In clinical terms, idiopathic hypertension could thus acquire features of secondary renal hypertension. This illustrates the important relationship of the kidneys and arterial hypertension. Clearly the kidney can be both the "victim" and the cause of hypertension.

NEOPLASMS

Tumors of the urinary tract are an important cause of morbidity and mortality. These tumors tend to have the following characteristics:

- They are malignant more often than benign.
- They affect older people.

- They are more common in men than in women.

For practical purposes, tumors of the urinary tract may be divided into four groups: (1) tumors of the kidney and renal pelvis, (2) tumors of the ureter, (3) tumors of the urinary bladder, and (4) tumors of the urethra (Figure 13-17). The first group comprises renal cell carcinoma (85%), urothelial carcinoma of the renal pelvis (8%), and Wilms' tumor (5%). The remaining 2% of the tumors in this group are extremely rare variants that do not warrant mention. Likewise, tumors of the ureter and urethra are not discussed because of their rarity.

Bladder tumors are the most common neoplasms of the urinary tract. In more than 90% of cases these tumors are transitional cell carcinomas. Benign tumors of transitional epithelium (transitional cell papilloma) are rare and of limited clinical significance.

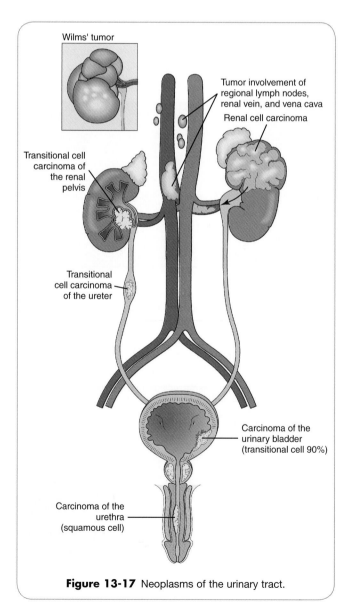

Figure 13-17 Neoplasms of the urinary tract.

RENAL CELL CARCINOMA

Renal cell carcinoma (RCC) is the most common kidney neoplasm, accounting for 85% of all tumors involving this organ. Almost 27,000 RCCs are diagnosed every year in the United States, and 11,000 deaths are attributed to this disease annually. RCC occurs in adults, and the median age of patients is 55 years. Males are affected two times more often than females.

Etiology

The causes of RCC are not known, and the risk factors for this tumor have not been defined. Epidemiologic data indicate a link with smoking, but this association is not as strong as that between smoking and lung cancer. The tumor has been found to occur more often in some families and tumor syndromes, such as von Hippel–Lindau *(VHL)* syndrome. This rare syndrome, typically associated with a loss of the *VHL* tumor suppressor gene, is characterized by the appearance of cerebellar hemangioblastomas and retinal angiomas; the syndrome has provided an unusual insight into the pathogenesis of renal cell tumors. RCC develops in approximately 40% of patients with VHL. It is even more remarkable that almost all (more than 95%) patients with RCC show a loss of the *VHL* tumor suppressor gene. It is thus believed that the *VHL* gene plays an important role in the pathogenesis of RCC.

Pathology

On gross examination, RCCs appear as nodules or masses that are sharply demarcated from the remaining renal parenchyma. On cross section they tend to be yellow and encapsulated (Figure 13-18); larger tumors extend through the renal capsule into the peritoneal fat and adjacent organs. It is common for RCC to invade the renal vein. Distant metastases often occur, but their distribution is unpredictable.

Histologic examination reveals that RCC is composed of cuboidal cells reminiscent of the renal tubules. In 80% of cases, tumors are classified as clear cell carcinomas. These tumors are composed of cells that have a clear cytoplasm, which is filled with glycogen and lipids. This accounts for the yellow color of the tumors on gross examination. The remaining 15% of tumors are classified as papillary carcinomas. Rare histologic variants such as chromophobe or collecting duct carcinoma account for 5% of tumors.

Clinical Features

The clinical presentation of RCC is highly variable. The typical triad of symptoms—flank pain, blood in the urine, and a palpable abdominal mass—is found in only 10% of patients. More than 50% of RCCs today are discovered accidentally on computed tomography (CT) scans performed for unrelated reasons. Microscopic hematuria, found in one third of all diagnosed cases, is the most common clinical finding. A significant number of tumors present with nonspecific symptoms, such as weight loss, fever, or hypertension. Metabolic paraneoplastic findings, such as hypercalcemia, erythrocytosis, and other abnormalities, are found in 20% of patients. These variegated clinical and biochemical findings account for the moniker "internist's tumor," as RCC is known colloquially; most of these tumors are diagnosed by internists examining patients for presumably nonrenal complaints. The tumors are treated surgically, but the overall 5-year survival is only 45%. In patients with small asymptomatic tumors limited to the kidney, however, the 5-year survival is much higher, exceeding 70%.

? **Did You Know?**

Most renal carcinomas do not produce clinical symptoms and are discovered accidentally by CT scanning while the doctors are examining the patient for something else. The tumor is seen protruding from the surface of the kidney.

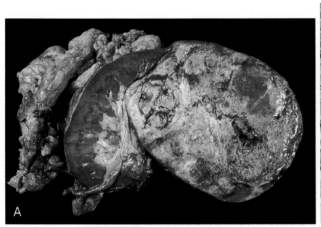
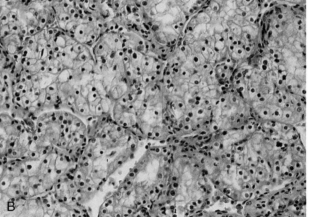

Figure 13-18 Renal cell carcinoma. *A,* Gross appearance of the tumor. *B,* Histologic examination reveals that the tissue consists of clear cells arranged into tubules.

UROTHELIAL CARCINOMA OF THE RENAL PELVIS

Urothelial carcinoma of the renal pelvis are papillary neoplasms that resemble transitional carcinoma of the urinary bladder. Like bladder tumors, they are classified as low-grade or high-grade neoplasms, with or without signs of invasion. Most tumors of the renal pelvis present with hematuria or urinary obstruction and colics early in the course of clinical disease. These symptoms provide clues for early diagnosis and early surgical intervention. Low-grade tumors have a better prognosis than high-grade invasive tumors, but the overall 5-year survival is 70%.

WILMS' TUMOR

Wilms' tumor, or *nephroblastoma,* is the most common of all solid tumors in infants and young children, affecting 1 in 10,000 children. Many, if not most, Wilms' tumors are present at the time of birth but become clinically apparent only between the second and fourth years of life. At least two distinct tumor supressor genes, appropriately named *WT1* and *WT2,* have been implicated in the pathogenesis of Wilms' tumor. *WT1* appears to be a transcription factor that probably plays an important role in normal development of the kidney and other organs. Deletion of *WT1* may result not only in tumorigenesis but also in multiple congenital malformations involving the eye, the brain, and parts of the urogenital system. Wilms' tumors that develop in children with those malformations are often bilateral.

Pathology

Wilms' tumor typically presents as a renal mass that can be either solitary or multinodular and that replaces the kidney to a large extent. In about 5% of cases the tumors are bilateral. On histologic examination the tumor is composed of immature cells, similar to those in the developing fetal kidney. These cells may form structures resembling fetal tubules and glomeruli, or they may be arranged into bundles of spindle cells without any evidence of differentiation, resembling renal blastema (fetal primordium of the kidney).

Clinical Features

Most tumors are discovered accidentally by a parent who has palpated the infant's abdominal mass or by a pediatrician during the course of a routine examination. Wilms' tumors are highly malignant neoplasms. Previously, when the only treatment of such tumors was surgery, the mortality was greater than 70%. Current therapy, based on surgery and chemotherapy with new cancer drugs, has improved the prognosis for Wilms' tumor such that more than 85% of the children with this tumor can now be cured.

CARCINOMA OF THE URINARY BLADDER

Carcinoma of the urinary bladder represents the most common urinary tract neoplasm. It has a peak incidence in those 60 to 80 years of age, and it is three times more common in males than in females. In the United States, 52,000 new cases are recorded yearly, and 10,000 deaths are attributed to this form of cancer annually. Thus, although bladder cancer is two times more common than RCCs, it accounts for approximately the same number of deaths. This discrepancy can be explained in part by the following facts:

- Bladder cancer has a tendency for papillary, exophytic growth into the lumen of the bladder. Bladder cancer is less invasive and less prone to metastasize than RCC. Almost 70% of all bladder carcinomas are low-grade exophytic tumors that have a favorable prognosis.
- Bladder tumors present with symptoms early in the course of their development. Intravesical growth causes urinary irritation and hematuria. Tumor cells may be readily identified in cytologic masses prepared from the urine. All these factors make early diagnosis feasible.
- Bladder tumors respond better than RCCs to combined surgical and chemotherapeutic treatment.

In most instances the etiology of bladder carcinomas is unknown. The most important risk factor in the United States is cigarette smoking, which increases the likelihood of bladder cancer proportionate to the total number of cigarettes smoked over the life span. Industrial carcinogens, such as azodyes and chemicals used in the rubber industry and textile printing, have been linked to bladder cancer, but with improved industrial hygiene, such chemicals have become less important. In Egypt and other parts of the world in which infection with *S. haematobium* is endemic, the high incidence of bladder cancer is related to the chronic cystitis caused by this parasite.

Pathology

Most bladder cancers (90%) are urothelial carcinomas. The remaining tumors comprise squamous cell carcinomas (5%), adenocarcinomas (2%), and sarcomas or metastases.

On gross examination the tumors are either papillary or flat. Papillary tumors appear as wartlike protrusions of the bladder mucosa (Figure 13-19). Flat tumors appear as mucosal plaques or thickenings. In either case the tumors may be invasive or noninvasive (Figure 13-20). The extent of invasion can be determined only by histologic examination of biopsy specimens or the surgically resected bladder.

Papillary urothelial carcinomas are graded histologically as low-grade or high-grade tumors. Papillae of low-grade tumors are lined by uniform cells, whereas those of high-grade tumors are lined by mitotically active hyperchromatic cells, showing considerable pleomorphism and high mitotic activity. Both low-grade and high-grade tumors may be invasive, but such an invasion of the muscle layer is more common in high-grade tumors. Low-grade tumors tend to recur for many years, and occasionally they may progress to a higher grade invasive carcinoma. Flat urothelial tumors may present in two forms: as carcinoma *in situ* or as invasive urothelial carcinoma. These tumors are composed of anaplastic cells that show only superficial resemblance to urethelial mucosa from which they have originated. Noninvasive and invasive forms of cancer can

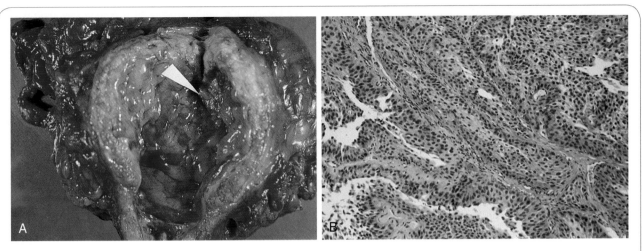

Figure 13-19 Bladder cancer. *A,* Gross appearance of an intraluminal mass. *B,* Histologic examination reveals that the mass is a papillary transitional cell carcinoma.

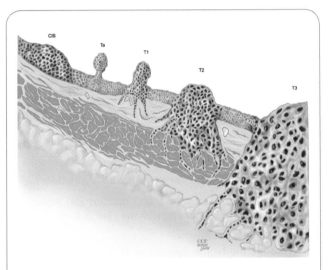

Figure 13-20 Bladder cancer. Urinary bladder cancer can occur in several forms: as a flat high-grade malignancy, carcinoma in situ (CIS), papillary tumor confined to the urothelium (Ta), papillary tumor invading the lamina propria (T1), papillary and invasive tumor involving the muscle layer of the bladder (T2), or invasive tumor extending through the wall into the perivesical fat tissue (T3). (From Wein AJ et al., eds: Campbell-Walsh Urology, 9th ed, Philadelphia, 2007, Saunders.)

coexist, and in many cases urothelial carcinomas are actually multifocal.

Squamous cell carcinoma and adenocarcinoma resemble histologically similar tumors originating in other parts of the body. Because the normal urinary bladder does not contain squamous and glandular cells we assume that these tumors must be preceded by squamous or glandular metaplasia, which usually occurs in foci of chronic inflammation. Adenocarcinomas may also originate from embryonic rests, especially the remnants of the fetal urachal duct connecting the fetal urinary bladder with the umbilicus. Sarcomas most often originate from the smooth muscular bladder wall and are classified as leiomyosarcomas.

Metastases of all urinary bladder carcinomas are initially found in the pelvic lymph nodes, but in later stages of disease the tumor may invade other pelvic organs and metastasize to distant sites, such as the lungs.

Clinical Features

Bladder cancer presents with urinary symptoms, such as hematuria, dysuria, or lower abdominal pain. The diagnosis made by cystoscopy must be confirmed by histologic examination of the tumor biopsy specimen. Cytologic examination of urinary sediment is also useful, especially in the case of early lesions, such as *carcinoma in situ* or multifocal flat lesions.

Treatment

Treatment of bladder cancer is based on surgical resection of tumors and chemotherapy. Good results have also been achieved with immunotherapy, specifically by intravesical instillation of adjuvants and immunopotentiators, such as an attenuated *Mycobacterium tuberculosis* known as *bacille Calmette-Guérin* (BCG). BCG stimulates granuloma formation and delayed hypersensitivity, thus destroying tumors locally.

Prognosis

The final prognosis depends on the histologic grade, histologic type (urothelial, squamous, adenocarcinoma), and clinical stage (i.e., spread of the tumor), which is usually determined according to the tumor-node-metastasis (TNM) system. Even low-grade localized tumors tend to recur, so lifelong urologic follow-up is mandatory. Recurrent tumors or new lesions can usually be resected with the aid of a cutting device attached to the cystoscope. Large tumors and invasive tumors require complete urinary bladder resection (cystectomy), whereupon a urinary receptacle is formed from the bowel loops and the ureters are implanted into it. Stage 1 low grade showing no invasion have a 95% 10-year survival, and only 10% of these tumors will progress to higher grade invasive cancer. Tumors invading the muscle layer of the bladder have an overall mortality of 25% to 30%, but the final prognosis in each case depends on the stage of the tumor.

REVIEW QUESTIONS

1. Explain how urine is formed and excreted.
2. Describe the principal portions of the nephron and explain how they function.
3. What is the functional significance of transitional epithelium?
4. Describe the effects of various hormones on the kidney.
5. Which hormones and growth factors does the kidney produce?
6. List the most important symptoms of kidney disease.
7. How common are renal developmental disorders, and which one of them is the most common?
8. Correlate the pathology of autosomal dominant polycystic kidney disease with the clinical features of this disease.
9. Classify glomerular diseases.
10. List the most important immunologic glomerular diseases.
11. List the most important metabolic glomerulopathies.
12. Explain how circulatory disorders affect glomeruli.
13. List the four most important syndromes related to glomerular diseases.
14. Compare nephrotic and nephritic syndrome.
15. Explain the pathogenesis of acute glomerulonephritis and correlate the pathologic and clinical findings in this disease.
16. Explain the pathogenesis of crescentic glomerulonephritis and relate the pathologic and clinical findings in this disease.
17. Explain the pathogenesis of membranous nephropathy and relate the pathologic and clinical findings in this disease.
18. What is lipoid nephrosis, and how is it diagnosed?
19. What do most forms of chronic proliferative glomerulonephritis have in common?
20. What is the cause of end-stage kidney disease, and how does it present clinically?
21. How does diabetes mellitus affect the kidneys?
22. List the four most common forms of kidney stones.
23. Compare ascending and descending urinary tract infections and list the most common predisposing conditions for these infections.
24. Compare the pathologic and clinical features of acute and chronic pyelonephritis.
25. Compare the causes of cystitis in men and women and in young and old people.
26. Compare the pathologic and clinical features of acute and chronic cystitis.
27. Explain how circulatory collapse causes renal tubular necrosis.
28. Explain the effects of hypertension on the kidneys.
29. List three common tumors of the urinary tract.
30. Compare renal cell carcinoma and Wilms' tumor.
31. Compare urothelial carcinoma of the renal pelvis and renal cell carcinoma.
32. How common is carcinoma of the urinary bladder?
33. Correlate the macroscopic and microscopic features of urinary bladder carcinoma with the clinical features of this tumor.
34. What are the typical symptoms of urinary bladder carcinoma?
35. What is the outcome of treatment of urinary bladder carcinoma?

The Male Reproductive System

14

Chapter Outline

NORMAL ANATOMY AND PHYSIOLOGY
OVERVIEW OF MAJOR DISEASES
    Infertility
    Infections
    Tumors
  Congenital Abnormalities
    Cryptorchidism

Infections
    Sexually Transmitted Diseases
Neoplasms
    Tumors of the Testis
    Prostatic Hyperplasia and Neoplasms
    Carcinoma of the Prostate
    Carcinoma of the Penis

Key Terms and Concepts

Alkaline phosphatase
Alpha-fetoprotein (AFP)
Androgens
Balanitis
Benign prostatic hyperplasia (BPH)
Carcinoma of the penis
Carcinoma of the prostate
Chancre
Chlamydia trachomatis
Chorionic gonadotropin
Condyloma acuminatum
Condyloma latum

Cryptorchidism
Epididymitis
Genital herpes
Gonorrhea
Infertility
Intratubular germ cell neoplasia
  (ITGCN)
Leydig cell tumor
Mycoplasma
Nonseminomatous germ cell tumors
  (NSGCTs)
Orchitis

Prostate-specific antigen (PSA)
Prostatitis
Seminoma
Sertoli cell tumor
Sexually transmitted diseases
Syphilis
Ureaplasma urealyticum
Urethritis
Yolk sac tumor

NORMAL ANATOMY AND PHYSIOLOGY

The male reproductive system comprises the *gonads* (testes), seminal excretory ducts (epididymis and vas deferens), accessory glands (seminal vesicles and prostate), and copulatory organ (penis) (Figure 14-1). The testes are localized in a specialized outpouching of the peritoneum, called the *scrotum,* which is covered on the outside with corrugated skin. The testes are linked with the rest of the reproductive system by the excretory ducts (epididymis and vas deferens). These excretory ducts are confluent with the ducts of the prostate, seminal vesicles, and urethra (i.e., the terminal portion of the lower urinary tract). The urethra is located within the shaft of the penis and thus has the double function of conducting and discharging both urine and seminal fluid.

On histologic examination, the testes are composed of seminiferous tubules and supporting structures, which include the blood vessels, stromal cells, and connective tissue (Figure 14-2). The stroma contains hormone-secreting Leydig cells. The seminiferous tubules are lined by germ cells in various stages of maturation and the supporting sex-cord cells, the Sertoli cells. The epididymal ducts are lined by secretory cells that produce a protein- and carbohydrate-rich fluid that bathes the sperm.

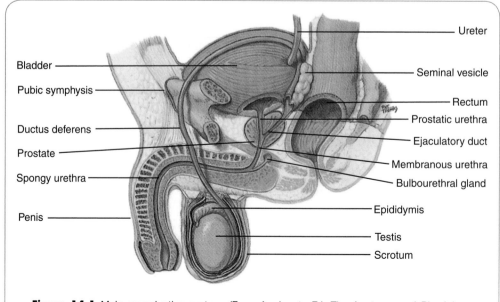

Figure 14-1 Male reproductive system. (From Applegate EJ: The Anatomy and Physiology Learning System, 4th ed, St. Louis, 2011, Saunders.)

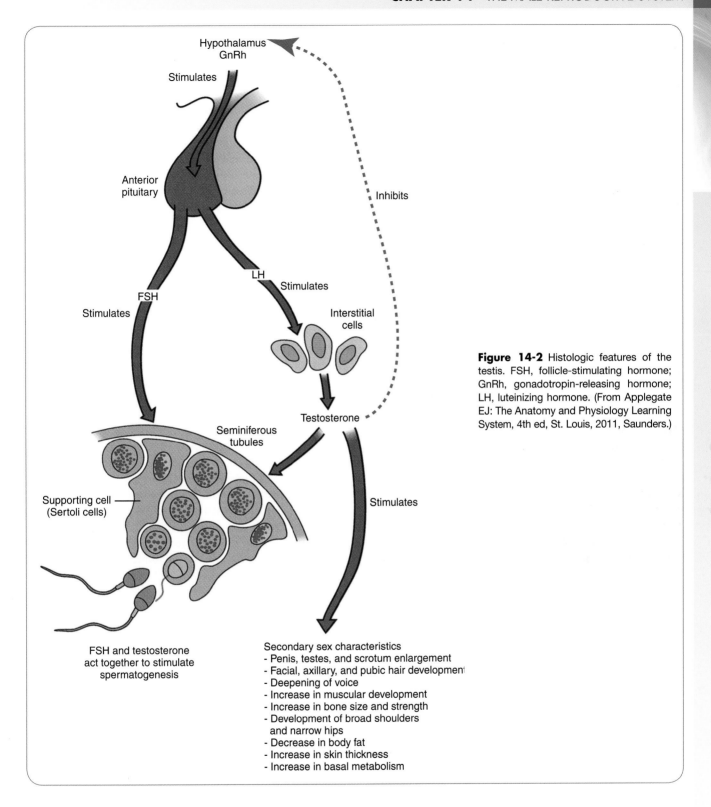

Hypothalamus
GnRh

Stimulates

Anterior
pituitary

Inhibits

LH

Stimulates

FSH

Stimulates

Interstitial
cells

Testosterone

Seminiferous
tubules

Supporting cell
(Sertoli cells)

Stimulates

FSH and testosterone
act together to stimulate
spermatogenesis

Secondary sex characteristics
- Penis, testes, and scrotum enlargement
- Facial, axillary, and pubic hair development
- Deepening of voice
- Increase in muscular development
- Increase in bone size and strength
- Development of broad shoulders
  and narrow hips
- Decrease in body fat
- Increase in skin thickness
- Increase in basal metabolism

Figure 14-2 Histologic features of the testis. FSH, follicle-stimulating hormone; GnRh, gonadotropin-releasing hormone; LH, luteinizing hormone. (From Applegate EJ: The Anatomy and Physiology Learning System, 4th ed, St. Louis, 2011, Saunders.)

During ejaculation, the epididymal sperm enter the seminal ampule, where they are mixed with the seminal fluid from the seminal vesicles and the prostatic fluid. This mixture is called the *ejaculate.* Ejaculate, once formed, enters the urethra and is discharged through the tip of the penile urethra outside the body. This fluid provides a vehicle for export of sperm from the testis.

The primary function of the male genital system is the production of sperm. The testes also secrete male hormones, **androgens,** which are the products of testicular interstitial cells called *Leydig cells.* The most important of the androgenic hormones is testosterone. Testosterone secretion is controlled by the pituitary gonadotropins.

OVERVIEW OF MAJOR DISEASES

In comparison with the diseases of the female reproductive organs, the diseases affecting the male reproductive organs generally receive less public attention. For instance, most adult women in civilized societies see their gynecologist at least once a year, whereas most males almost never consult a urologist during their lifetime. Few people even know that the real counterpart of a gynecologist is technically called an *andrologist* (in Greek, *andros* means "man"). In practice, "male problems" are treated by urologists, whereas andrologists deal only with male infertility. Pathologists specializing in diseases of the male reproductive organs are called *urogenital pathologists.*

The most important diseases of the male reproductive system are as follows:

- Infertility
- Infections
- Tumors

INFERTILITY

Fertility—the ability to produce offspring—is essential for the propagation of all species, including humans. Infertility can threaten families, tribes, nations, and ultimately all of humankind with extinction. Problems of fertility have been among the major concerns of humans since time immemorial and have important medical implications.

Infertility is defined as an inability to have children. Although the cause may lie with either the male or female partner, it is customary to treat the reproductive unit as a whole and thus refer not to infertile individuals but to infertile couples. Statistics show that the causes of infertility are split equally between females and males. It has been estimated that 1 in 6 couples in the United States is infertile and that the treatment of infertility costs society millions of dollars per year. Considerable advances have been made in the treatment of infertility among women, especially with the introduction of *in vitro* fertilization. However, no progress has been made in treating male infertility.

INFECTIONS

The male reproductive organs are prone to infection for several reasons, two of the most important being the following:

- Sexual intercourse between two persons brings into most intimate contact their genital organs, thus facilitating the transmission of pathogens.
- The ascent of microbial pathogens through the urethra occurs easily because the urethra is an open-ended tube, and although it is subdivided into several anatomic segments by distinct sphincters, these act more like hurdles than tight valves against ascending bacteria.

Most genital infections are sexually acquired; thus they have the highest prevalence among men in their prime. With age the pattern of infection changes, so in older men most infections are related to urinary retention caused by prostatic enlargement.

TUMORS

Among the tumors affecting the male reproductive organs, two deserve special attention: tumors of the prostate and tumors of the testis. Tumors of the prostate are important because they are very common and because they have a high mortality. Tumors of the testis are considerably less common. Malignant tumors of the testis are important because they affect men at the height of their productive life (25 to 45 years of age). These tumors can be treated very successfully.

Several facts important for an understanding of diseases of the male reproductive system are presented here, before a discussion of the most common pathologic entities.

1. *Abnormalities of male reproductive organs result from genetic and developmental disorders.* The genetic sex of every individual depends on a normal complement of sex chromosomes. As described in Chapter 5, trisomy of sex chromosomes (47,XXY) results in Klinefelter's syndrome. Affected persons have atrophic testes and are infertile. **Cryptorchidism** is a developmental defect that results in incomplete descent of the testis into its normal scrotal position.

2. *Male genital organs are in direct contact with the outside world; therefore most infections are acquired through an ascending route (i.e., through the urethra).* Infections in young and middle-aged men are typically acute and are often sexually acquired. Infections in older men tend to be chronic and are often related to urinary tract obstruction secondary to prostatic enlargement.

3. *The testes produce male sex hormones that act on all other reproductive organs.* Abnormalities in testosterone secretion during fetal life result in incomplete development of the reproductive organs, which require testosterone to develop normally. After birth and until puberty, the testes produce little testosterone. However, at puberty, under the influence of pituitary gonadotropins, a major surge in testosterone production occurs, determining the maturation of all male sex organs and secondary sexual characteristics. Premature activation of Leydig cells results in precocious puberty. The opposite is delayed puberty. Both conditions are usually related to hypothalamic and pituitary disturbances. If puberty does not occur and the testes remain infantile, the condition is called *hypogonadism*. These men are infertile and have eunuchoid body features, without body or pubic hair.

4. *The testis consists of spermatogenic cells, Sertoli cells, and Leydig cells, all of which can give rise to tumors.* Although the testes are small organs, they can give rise to a variety of histologically distinct tumors. This variety of tumors can be accounted for, in part, by the fact that such tumors arise from three distinct cell lineages: germ cells, Sertoli cells, and Leydig cells. Furthermore, neoplastic germ cells can differentiate into embryonic cells, as normally occurs after fertilization (the fusion of male and female germ cells).

These embryonic cells can form tumors that are histologically distinct from the normal cells in the testis and consist of tissues normally found in fetal or adult organs not related to the testis. Such tumors are called *teratomas,* or *teratocarcinomas* if malignant.

5. *The prostate is composed of epithelial and stromal cells that express receptors for sex hormones.* The development and function of the prostate depend on male sex hormones. Persons who have accidentally lost testes before puberty and those who were castrated before puberty have very small prostates because the prostate does not develop unless properly stimulated by androgens during puberty. Prostatic hyperplasia, commonly found in older men, is a hormonally induced lesion, although its pathogenesis is still unknown. It is thought to be related to an imbalance of male and female hormones that occurs as a result of a decrease in testosterone production with advancing age. The role of sex hormones in the pathogenesis of **carcinoma of the prostate** has been studied extensively but without any definitive conclusions.

CONGENITAL ABNORMALITIES

The most important abnormality of the male reproductive system is *cryptorchidism.* Other congenital defects of the testes, such as anorchia (absence of testes) or *polyorchidism* (three or more testes), are rare. Abnormalities of the penis are also rare. The most common is *hypospadias,* an abnormal opening of the urethra on the lower side of the shaft of the penis.

CRYPTORCHIDISM

Cryptorchidism is a congenital malpositioning of the testes outside their normal scrotal location (Figure 14-3).

Pathogenesis

The fetal testes, which develop from the genital ridge, are originally located in the abdominal cavity. During intrauterine life, the testes slowly descend toward the inguinal canal and through it, ultimately reaching the scrotum. The inguinal canal is obliterated, thus preventing the testes from retracting into the abdominal cavity. They remain permanently fixed in the scrotum.

In most boys the descent of the testes is fully completed by the time of birth. In 3% to 4% of newborn male infants, however, the inguinal canal remains open, allowing the cremasteric muscle that is attached to the testes to pull the testes back into the inguinal canal or even into the abdominal cavity. These are called *retractile testes.* In most cases the inguinal canal closes, and by the end of the first year of life, less than 1% of all male infants do not have one or both testes in the scrotum. These truly *cryptorchid* testes must be fixed in the scrotum surgically, and the inguinal canal must be closed surgically to prevent formation of a *hernia,* an outpouching of the abdominal organs (usually the intestines) into the scrotum.

The cause of cryptorchidism may be evident, as in the case of connective tissue adhesions within the fetal inguinal

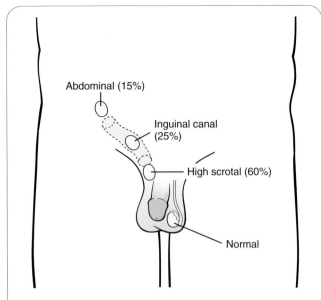

Figure 14-3 In cryptorchidism the testis is not in the scrotum but may be found in the inguinal canal or the abdominal cavity.

canal. In most instances, however, the cause remains unknown.

Pathology

Most cryptorchid testes that are surgically repositioned in the scrotum in early infancy develop normally. However, signs of atrophy and hypospermatogenesis are common.

Clinical Features

Infertility can result if both testes are cryptorchid, but if only one testis is affected, the other normal one will suffice to maintain fertility. Cryptorchid testes have a 10-fold greater risk of undergoing malignant transformation than do normal testes. Surgical correction at an early age reduces this risk but does not eliminate it completely. Apparently, many cryptorchid testes are abnormally developed and, even if repositioned, will retain a predisposition to form tumors.

INFECTIONS

Acute and chronic infections may involve the entire male reproductive system, but most often they are limited to a particular organ or two closely adjacent organs. The most important among these localized infections are **orchitis** (inflammation of the testes), epididymitis, prostatitis, urethritis, and balanitis (inflammation of the glans penis) (Figure 14-4). As mentioned earlier, in adult sexually active males, most infections are sexually acquired.

Clinical Features

Balanitis, which may present as localized or diffuse redness, swelling, or ulceration of the mucosa of the glans penis, is usually caused by viruses or bacteria. Herpesvirus typically

325

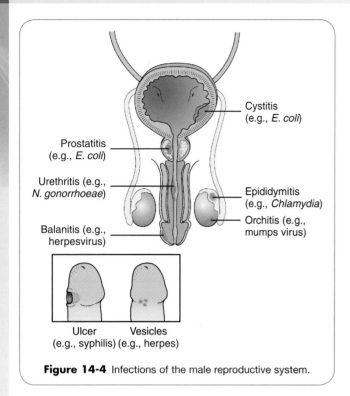

Prostatitis
(e.g., *E. coli*)

Cystitis
(e.g., *E. coli*)

Urethritis (e.g.,
N. gonorrhoeae)

Epididymitis
(e.g., *Chlamydia*)

Orchitis (e.g.,
mumps virus)

Balanitis (e.g.,
herpesvirus)

Ulcer   Vesicles
(e.g., syphilis) (e.g., herpes)

Figure 14-4 Infections of the male reproductive system.

causes vesicles that rupture, giving rise to shallow ulcers. Infection with *Treponema pallidum* causes ulcerations (called *syphilitic chancre*) of the glans or even the skin or the shaft of the penis.

Urethritis with purulent exudate is typical of infection with *Neisseria gonorrhoeae,* diplococci that can be readily demonstrated by microscopic examination of the inflammatory cells expressed from the urethra. If no bacteria are evident and there is no purulent exudate, it is customary to label the condition as *nonbacterial urethritis.* **Ureaplasma urealyticum,** a bacterialike microbe of the **Mycoplasma** species, accounts for about 20% of these cases. *Chlamydia trachomatis* is considered the cause of nongonococcal urethritis in about 50% of all cases. Chlamydial infection may cause production of antibodies that cross-react with human antigens expressed on several organs, including the urethra, uvea of the eye, and joints. The triad of urethritis, uveitis, and arthritis is called *Reiter's syndrome.* Some strains of *C. trachomatis* that are prevalent in tropical countries cause *lymphogranuloma venereum (LGV),* a disfiguring disease including suppurative inguinal lymphadenitis and multiple pus-draining sinuses in the genital area. Fortunately, these LGV strains are rare in the United States.

 Did You Know?

A commonly used mnemonic for symptoms of Reiter syndrome (urethritis, arthritis, and eye inflammation) is: *The patient cannot pee, cannot see, and cannot bend the knee.* Because Dr. Reiter committed crimes against humanity in Nazi Germany, there is a push to replace the eponym carrying his name with the term *reactive arthritis.*

Prostatitis is a disease affecting older men and is usually related to stagnation of urine. The infections are caused by uropathogens, a heterogeneous group of gram-negative bacteria such as *Escherichia coli* and *Proteus mirabilis.* The disease presents with pain during urination, urgency, and fever, and it has a tendency to recur.

Epididymitis is caused by ascending infection, and it is usually a complication of urethritis or prostatitis. In young men it is most often a complication of sexually acquired infections caused by pathogens, such as *N. gonorrhoeae* and *C. trachomatis.* In older patients it is caused by uropathogens, and typically it is a complication of urinary obstruction or prostatic surgery.

Orchitis may occur as an isolated infection, but more often it is combined with epididymitis *(epididymo-orchitis)* and is a complication of lower urogenital tract infection. Isolated orchitis is a typical complication of hematogenous spread, such as occurs in secondary syphilis, or in certain viral diseases, such as mumps. Before the introduction of immunization of infants against mumps, orchitis was found in about 20% of all cases and was an important cause of testicular injury.

SEXUALLY TRANSMITTED DISEASES

The most common **sexually transmitted diseases** are the following:

- Genital herpes
- Gonorrhea
- Chlamydial infections
- Syphilis

GENITAL HERPES

Genital herpes is caused by herpes simplex virus (HSV) type 2. This virus is closely related to HSV type 1, the cause of cold sores or blisters *(herpes labialis).* Both viruses invade the skin and mucosal cells, disrupting the epithelial layer and producing vesicles filled with clear fluid. The genital lesions are located on the glans or the skin of the shaft of the penis or the scrotum. The vesicles rupture and transform into shallow, painful ulcers that heal without scarring. The vesicles are typical enough to enable one to establish the diagnosis, but it may be confirmed by sampling cells from the vesicles for microscopic examination or virologic culture.

Genital herpes has a tendency to recur. Following the acute disease, the HSV travels along the axons of the peripheral nerves and invades the ganglion cells that innervate the genital area. In the ganglion cells, the virus remains in a balance with the host, causing no clinical symptoms. However, once this balance is disturbed—for example, by another infection or in immunosuppressed persons (e.g., those with acquired immunodeficiency syndrome [AIDS])—the virus is activated and it descends along the nerves into the genital area, producing new vesicular eruptions.

Individuals with active herpetic lesions are contagious, but even asymptomatic carriers or those with atypical nonvesicular lesions may transmit the disease. Permanent cure is not feasible, although antiviral drugs (e.g., acyclovir) provide some relief.

GONORRHEA

Infection with the diplococcus *N. gonorrhoeae* (also known as *gonococcus*) results in purulent urethritis. Typically, this sexually transmitted disease presents with burning on urination and a yellow urethral discharge 2 to 5 days after exposure.

Gonococcus invades the mucosa of the penile urethra and the adjacent periurethral glands. The inflamed mucosa is red, moist, and covered with purulent exudate, which on microscopic examination consists predominantly of polymorphonuclear neutrophils. Gonococci can be seen in the cytoplasm of inflammatory cells. Molecular biology probes are currently used as the methods of choice for the final diagnosis of gonococcal infections. Penicillin usually cures most infections, although recently more penicillin-resistant strains of bacteria have been reported.

The complications of gonococcal urethritis can be classified as local or distant. Ascending infection may lead to prostatitis and epididymitis. Connective tissue strictures that develop as a consequence of such infection cause narrowing of the urethra and can obliterate the epididymis. Typical consequences of inadequately treated **gonorrhea** include pain during urination or infertility secondary to obstructed sperm outflow. Gonococci may also disseminate by blood to distant sites. Gonococcal arthritis is the most common complication of such hematogenous spread.

CHLAMYDIAL INFECTIONS

Chlamydia are minuscule obligate intracellular pathogens that can survive only inside infected cells. ***Chlamydia trachomatis,*** the most important of these gram-negative bacteria, may be sexually transmitted and is actually the most common cause of bacterial urethritis in men. It can also infect women and cause urethritis, endometritis, and pelvic inflammatory disease (PID).

Chlamydial urethritis occurs most often in sexually active men. Previously it was called nonspecific or nongonococcal urethritis, because it often presented with urethral pain without any of the discharge that is so typical of gonorrhea. Many infected men have no symptoms; however, they are still infectious and may transmit the infection to their sexual partners. In other men the infection may spread to the prostate and epididymis and cause chronic inflammation and pain. The infection is best diagnosed by molecular biology tests performed on genital swabs or cells obtained from the urine specimen. Treatment includes broad-spectrum antibiotics.

SYPHILIS

Syphilis is a sexually acquired disease caused by the spirochete *T. pallidum.* Three stages of the disease—primary, secondary, and tertiary syphilis—are recognized.

Primary Stage

The primary lesion—a painless, indurated ulcer—develops 1 to 12 weeks after exposure. This ulcer, known as the primary **chancre,** develops most often on the glans penis, but it may appear on the inner side of the prepuce in uncircumcised men or on and around the anus in male homosexuals. The ulcer is accompanied by local, usually inguinal, lymph node enlargement. Histologic examination reveals that the infected tissue contains numerous spirochetes. *T. pallidum* can be identified by dark-field microscopy of samples obtained by swabbing the ulcer. However, this is rarely done, and in practice every ulcer of the penis is treated as syphilitic unless proved otherwise. The primary chancre heals spontaneously in about 4 to 6 weeks. With appropriate antibiotic treatment, it heals in a few days.

Secondary Stage

Symptoms that develop in secondary syphilis are manifestations of systemic spread of spirochetes and an immune reaction to the pathogen. The secondary stage occurs approximately 2 months to 2 years after the primary infection. Clinically it is marked by systemic symptoms, such as fever, malaise, macular rash, lymph node enlargement, and the appearance of slightly elevated skin lesions (papules) called **condyloma latum** (Figure 14-5). Many other symptoms and findings also may be present, such as mucosal ulcerations, central nervous system irritation (probably secondary to meningitis), hepatitis, and kidney symptoms. However, all these symptoms have a self-limited course and disappear spontaneously.

Tertiary Stage

After remission of the symptoms of secondary syphilis, the disease may enter a latent phase for an extended period. The symptoms of tertiary syphilis occur in a small number of untreated or incompletely treated patients 2 to 20 years after the

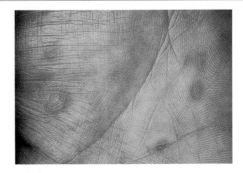

Figure 14-5 Condyloma latum. The lesions typically appear on the palms and soles. (From Habif TP et al: Skin Diseases, Diagnosis and Treatment, 2nd ed, St. Louis, 2005, Mosby.)

primary infection. The most important symptoms are related to the pathologic lesions of the cardiovascular and central nervous systems.

Histologic hallmarks of tertiary syphilis include chronic perivasculitis involving the small blood vessels and typical syphilitic granulomas called *gumma*. Lymphocytic and plasma cellular infiltrates around the vasa vasorum of the aorta, the small nutrient arteries in the wall of the aorta, cause destruction of the arterial wall with widening of the lumen *(aneurysm)*. Gummas of the cardiac valves also cause destruction and insufficiency of the valves, most often at the aortic orifice. Meningovascular syphilis causes destruction of the posterior columns of the spinal cord, evidenced as *tabes dorsalis*. As a result of destruction of sensory nerve axons in the posterior columns, these patients lose proprioception and have difficulty coordinating their movements. In the brain the loss of neurons secondary to syphilis results in dementia, known as *general paralysis of the insane*. These persons lose all mental faculties and are often paralyzed because of destruction of motor neurons.

The diagnosis of syphilis is based on serologic tests, which include the detection of *Treponema*-specific and nontreponemal antibodies in blood. Nontreponemal antibodies are best for screening purposes and are based on measuring antibodies to cardiolipin. The most widely used test in this category is called *VDRL*, named after the Venereal Disease Research Laboratory in which it was first developed. This test becomes positive 4 to 6 weeks after infection and is not specific for syphilis. Thus it may give false positive results in various other diseases such as systemic lupus erythematosus (SLE) and leprosy, and even in normal pregnancy. *Treponema*-specific tests are more precise, but they also become positive only after a 4- to 6-week interval following infection. These tests remain positive forever and are thus useful for the diagnosis of advanced stages of syphilis. In contrast to the effectiveness of antibiotics in the treatment of primary and secondary syphilis, tertiary syphilis is incurable. Therefore it is most important to diagnose the disease while it is curable and to treat it appropriately.

NEOPLASMS

TUMORS OF THE TESTIS

Testicular tumors account for only 1% of all neoplasms in men. Nevertheless, these tumors are clinically important because they occur at a relatively early age; indeed, the peak incidence occurs in men 25 to 45 years of age (Figure 14-6). The most important aspects of testicular cancer can be summarized by the "rule of nineties" as follows:

- Ninety percent of tumors occur in adulthood in the age group between 25 and 45 years. These tumors are rare before puberty and in older men. If a testicular tumor develops in an older man, most likely it represents a disseminated

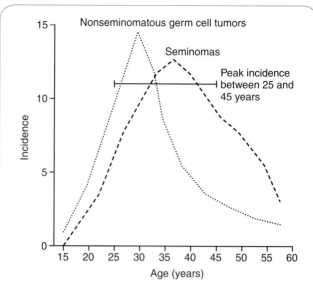

Figure 14-6 Incidence of testicular cancer according to age. Testicular tumors have a peak incidence in men 25 to 45 years old.

lymphoma or a metastasis from an abdominal primary lesion and not a primary testicular tumor.
- Ninety percent of tumors are of germ cell origin.
- Ninety percent of tumors are malignant. All testicular tumors follow the same metastatic pathway. Typically the tumors spread to periaortic lymph nodes in the abdomen. From this site, the tumors metastasize to the upper abdomen and may spread hematogenously to the liver, lungs, and brain.
- Ninety percent are curable with modern treatment. Previously, testicular tumors were associated with considerable mortality, but recent advances in chemotherapy have markedly improved the outlook for the vast majority of patients.

Etiology and Pathogenesis

More than 90% of testicular tumors develop from germ cells. Of the remaining, 5% are derived from Sertoli and Leydig cells and 5% represent metastases (Box 14-1). The etiology of testicular tumors is unknown. It has been noted that tumors develop more often in developmentally abnormal testes and in cryptorchid testes. Cryptorchidism is the most important predisposing condition. Such testes are at a 10-fold higher risk for neoplastic disease than normal testes. Surgical repositioning of the testis into the scrotum (orchidopexy) does not reduce the risk of neoplasia.

Malignant transformation of germ cells results in an intratubular tumor known as *carcinoma in situ* or **intratubular germ cell neoplasia (ITGCN)**. After a latent period, which can last 5 to 20 years, ITGCN cells cross the basement membrane and an invasive malignant disease develops. As shown

BOX 14-1 Testicular Tumors

Germ Cell Tumors
Seminoma (40%)
Malignant nonseminomatous germ cell (renal, prostatic, colonic)
    tumors (NSGCTs)
    Embryonal carcinoma (10%)
    Teratocarcinomas (25%)
    Choriocarcinoma (<1%)
Mixed tumors (seminoma and NSGCT) (10%)
Teratoma (3%)
Yolk sac tumor of infancy (2%)

Metastases
Lymphoma (2%)
Carcinoma (3%)

Sex Cord Cell Tumors
Leydig cell tumor (3%)
Sertoli cell tumor (2%)

should be remembered that the germ cells in the testis, like those in the ovary, are the precursors of embryonic cells. Embryonic cells are normally formed only from zygotes; that is, they form only after fusion of the male and female gametes. In contrast, EC cells are descendants of spontaneously activated male germ cells. It is not known why or how these germ cells give rise to EC cells. Clearly they must skip a few developmental steps, because they never mature into sperm or fuse with the female gamete, but they evolve into embryonic cells. Like normal embryonic cells, EC cells can differentiate into various fetal and adult tissues and even form components that resemble extraembryonic membranes (i.e., trophoblast of the placenta and yolk sac).

If all the embryonic cells differentiate into mature tissues, a teratoma forms. This is a benign tumor composed of somatic tissues (in Greek, *soma* means "body") derived from all three embryonic germ layers: ectoderm, endoderm, and mesoderm. In contrast, the malignant tumor that is composed of EC cells and somatic tissues is called a *teratocarcinoma*. Note that both teratomas and teratocarcinomas contain haphazardly arranged and intermixed tissues, such as skin, brain, muscle, and cartilage intestine. Teratocarcinomas also contain malignant stem cells (EC cells) and scattered trophoblastic and yolk sac epithelium. Trophoblastic cells, like the normal placental cells, secrete human chorionic gonadotropin (hCG) into the blood. Because hCG is not normally found in the serum or urine of males (or in females unless they are pregnant), the presence of hCG in a male is strong evidence of a germ cell tumor. Yolk sac cells secrete

in Figure 14-7, the tumors can develop in two directions. If the tumor cells retain the features of primitive gonocytes, forming a neoplasm composed of a single cell type, the resulting malignant lesion is called a *seminoma* (i.e., tumor of seminal epithelium–like cells). However, if the tumor cells acquire the characteristics of embryonic cells, the resulting malignant lesion is called *embryonal carcinoma* (EC). It

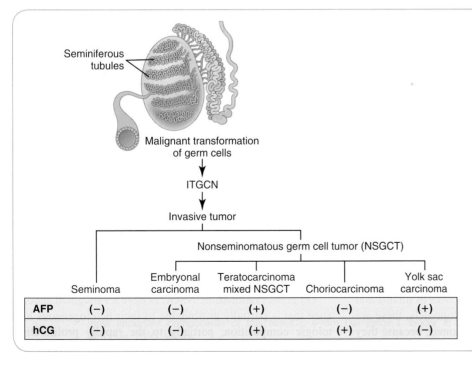

	Seminoma	Embryonal carcinoma	Teratocarcinoma mixed NSGCT	Choriocarcinoma	Yolk sac carcinoma
AFP	(−)	(−)	(+)	(−)	(+)
hCG	(−)	(−)	(+)	(+)	(−)

Figure 14-7 Histogenesis of malignant testicular germ cell tumors. The tumors originate from intratubular germ cells that form *carcinoma in situ,* also known as *intratubular germ cell neoplasia* (ITGCN). Tumors derived from ITGCN are divided into two major groups: seminomas and nonseminomatous germ cell tumors (NS-GCTs), the latter of which include several subtypes.

be detected in the serum of tumor-bearing patients; thus these tumors can be monitored by serologic means using AFP and hCG as tumor markers. After removal of the tumor, the elevated serum hCG and AFP levels usually decrease to undetectable levels, as one would expect in normal males. However, if the patient has metastases that have not been removed, serum hCG and AFP levels will remain elevated. Similarly, the initial decline in serum AFP and hCG levels will be reversed if there is tumor recurrence (Figure 14-10).

Until the 1970s, when the new treatment protocols based on platinum salts were introduced into clinical medicine, NSGCTs had a bad prognosis. Today's treatment of NSGCTs includes surgical resection of the primary tumor, resection of lymph nodes involved with metastases, and an intensive course of chemotherapy with several cytotoxic drugs in combination. A second-look operation is sometimes indicated, at which time residual tumor masses may be resected. With this therapeutic course, it is possible to achieve complete tumor eradication and a 5-year survival in excess of 90%.

OTHER TUMORS

As indicated in Box 14-1, seminomas and malignant NSGCTs of adulthood account for 90% of all testicular tumors. Because of their rarity other testicular tumors are of lesser importance.

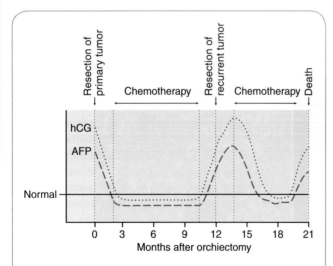

Figure 14-10 Alpha-fetoprotein (AFP) and human **chorionic gonadotropin** (hCG) are good serum markers for testicular nonseminomatous germ cell tumors (NSGCTs). Initial high serum levels of AFP and hCG drop to undetectable levels after resection of the primary tumor. The recurrence of the tumor is marked by rising serum levels of these tumor markers. As the tumor load increases, so does the serum concentration of AFP and hCG.

Yolk Sac Tumors

Yolk sac tumors occur in infancy and childhood, typically before the end of the fourth year of life. These tumors secrete AFP. Although potentially malignant, if removed in time, they have an excellent prognosis.

Leydig Cell Tumors

Leydig cell tumors, like the normal cells from which they originate, are hormonally active. These tumors produce either testosterone or estrogens and can occur at any age; although most are benign, 10% can present as low-grade malignant lesions, and some may even metastasize. Excess testosterone is usually not clinically apparent unless it occurs before puberty. In this age group, Leydig cell tumors may cause precocious puberty. In adult males, some Leydig cell tumors produce estrogen, which may cause gynecomastia, loss of libido, and feminization.

Sertoli Cell Tumors

Sertoli cell tumors are usually benign. Although these tumors may secrete inhibin and sex hormones, the symptoms are typically related to the testicular mass rather than to the small amounts of hormones produced by the tumor.

PROSTATIC HYPERPLASIA AND NEOPLASMS

Enlargement of the prostate may occur as a result of benign prostatic hyperplasia or carcinoma of the prostate. Benign prostatic hyperplasia is a reactive, benign hyperplastic lesion related to the hormonal changes in the body that occur with aging, whereas carcinoma of the prostate is a truly malignant tumor. It should be noted that prostatic carcinoma does not have a benign neoplastic equivalent; thus the diagnosis of "adenoma of the prostate" is never made. This does not mean that benign adenomas do not occur in the prostate. Actually, there is no good reason why such benign tumors would not happen in the prostate, but histologically such benign lesions cannot be distinguished from benign prostatic hyperplasia.

BENIGN PROSTATIC HYPERPLASIA

Benign prostatic hyperplasia (BPH) is a reactive enlargement of the periurethral portion of the prostate and the so-called median bar (median lobe), a part of the prostate located at the neck of the urinary bladder (Figure 14-11). As the prostate undergoes nodular hyperplasia, it compresses the urethra, and the median lobe may even act as a valve impeding urination. The centrally located hyperplastic nodules compress and expand the peripheral tissue. This is called the *surgical capsule of the prostate* because it loosely envelopes the abnormal tissue. BPH nodules can be surgically "shelled out" from the capsule, which is usually done by inserting a finger between the nodules and the cleavage plane formed underneath the capsule.

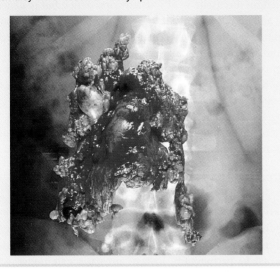

Pathogenesis

The pathogenesis of BPH is not fully understood. All theories proposed so far invoke a hormonal mechanism, implying that testosterone plays a crucial role. It is known that the development of the prostate at puberty occurs only in the presence of male sex hormones. Young men who are castrated before the onset of puberty have a small, nonfunctioning prostate. Experimental studies in dogs (which have a humanlike prostate and are typically used for prostate cancer research) reveal that the small prostates resulting from prepubertal castration can be made hyperplastic with exogenous testosterone and even more so with simultaneous administration of estrogen. It is possible that estrogen sensitizes the prostatic cells to the action of testosterone or that the male and female hormones act synergistically.

A similar interaction of estrogen and testosterone probably accounts for the BPH that occurs in older men; even though older men produce less testosterone than younger men, the relative increase of estrogen that occurs with age probably facilitates and augments the action of testosterone on the periurethral portion of the prostate. This part is apparently most sensitive to estrogens. Metabolic inhibitors of testosterone,

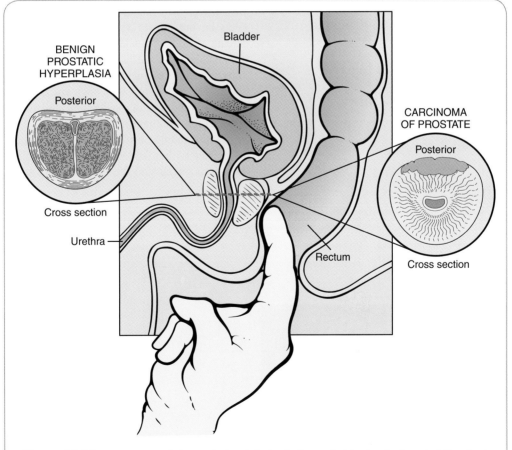

Figure 14-11 Benign prostatic hyperplasia originates in the central (periurethral) part of the gland and often involves the median lobe. In contrast, carcinoma of the prostate originates preferentially in the peripheral portion of the gland and often in the posterior lobe, which is readily accessible to digital palpation through the rectum.

which counteract the effects of male sex hormones, are often used instead of surgery to treat prostatic hyperplasia.

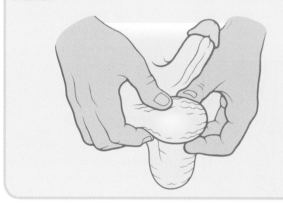
Pathology

On gross examination, prostates that are enlarged as a result of BPH appear nodular (Figure 14-12). The enlarged prostate may distort the urethra and compress the peripheral portions of the glands into a fibrous capsule ("surgical capsule"). On palpation the tissue is of uneven consistency but is generally soft and pliable. On histologic examination the tissue consists of numerous hyperplastic glands surrounded by an increased amount of fibromuscular stroma. The ratio of glandular to stromal hyperplasia varies from one case to another, and even within a single prostate there is considerable variation from one area to another. The proliferated glands may dilate cystically and accumulate prostatic secretions (Figure 14-13). This may predispose the affected individual to infection, which is common with BPH.

Clinical Features

The clinical symptoms of BPH are related to urethral compression and retention of urine. It should be noted that the periurethral location of hyperplastic nodules is associated with urinary symptoms early in the course of the disease, in contrast to peripherally located prostatic carcinoma, which produces such symptoms only in later stages of the disease. BPH causes distortion and elongation of the urethra, which also affect the sphincters regulating urination. The patient feels an urgency to void but cannot begin urinating. The stream of urine is weak, and the patient must strain to empty the bladder. At the end of micturition, the urine keeps dribbling and the patient often experiences loss of control and incontinence. Urinary frequency and dysuria (painful urination) are common and usually indicate a superseding infection that develops in the residual urine.

Long-standing obstruction of the bladder neck is typically associated with infections of the urinary bladder. Such infection may spread into the upper urinary tract. The increased

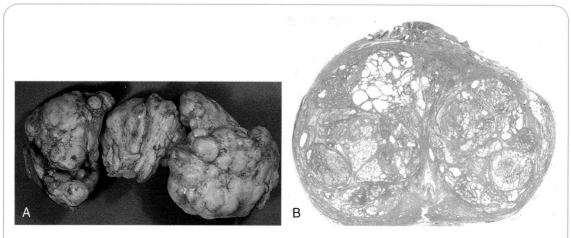

Figure 14-12 Hyperplasia of the prostate. *A,* The prostate is enlarged and nodular. B, On microscopic examination the cross section of a prostate shows cystic dilation of benign hyperplastic glands. (From Damjanov I, Linder J: Pathology: A Color Atlas, St. Louis, 2000, Mosby.)

The overall age-adjusted incidence of prostatic cancer is approximately 70 per 100,000, but these figures are misleading because such statistics take into consideration men of all ages. If the data are stratified by age, the incidence is more than 500 cases per 100,000 in the group 70 to 75 years of age and more than 1000 per 100,000 in those older than 80 years.

Etiology and Pathogenesis

The etiology and pathogenesis of prostatic carcinoma are poorly understood, and no definitive risk factors have been identified so far. As with BPH, the hormonal theories have the most proponents, and it is widely believed that testosterone stimulates the growth of prostatic cancer. There are several lines of evidence supporting this view, including the following:

- Prostatic carcinoma does not develop in persons who are castrated before puberty.
- Testosterone receptors have been demonstrated on prostatic carcinoma cells.
- Castration of patients with prostatic cancer usually retards the growth of the tumor.
- Antitestosterone drugs retard tumor growth.

Hormonal theories have been refuted by proponents of other explanations. Typically patients with prostatic carcinoma do not have elevated serum testosterone levels. Actually, most of them show an age-related decrease in testosterone output. Many urologists do not believe that castration improves the survival of such patients, and orchidectomy is rarely performed today in the course of treatment of prostate cancer.

Another puzzling aspect of prostatic cancer relates to the enormous racial differences noted in the incidence of this tumor. For example, the incidence of prostatic cancer in East Asians is more than 10 times lower than that among whites. Some of these differences may be related to environment, diet, and lifestyles, because Americans of Asian origin have a greater incidence of prostatic cancer than do their relatives living in Asia. Epidemiologists hope that these racial and environmental differences may also hold some clues about the causes of prostatic cancer.

Pathology

Carcinoma of the prostate originates in the peripheral (posterior lobe) glands. The initial tumor is limited to the glands, but it gives rise to locally invasive lesions (Fig. 14-13). Cancer spreads through the lymphatics and into the adjacent organs, primarily the rectum, urinary bladder, and other pelvic structures. Perineural invasion is particularly common. Pelvic lymph nodes and, subsequently, retroperitoneal abdominal lymph nodes are involved relatively early in the course of the disease.

Distant metastases occur via the lymphatics or blood (Figure 14-14). Among the most common distant organs involved are the vertebral bones, lungs, and liver. The lumbosacral vertebral and sacral bones are most often involved, presumably as a result of retrograde spread through the vertebral venous plexus, which drains venous blood from both the prostate and lower vertebrae and sacrum.

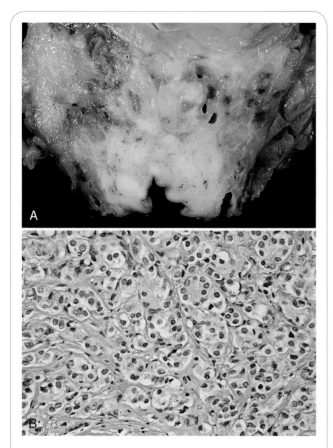

Figure 14-13 Carcinoma of the prostate. *A,* Cross section through the prostate at the bladder neck shows carcinoma—that is, a grayish white mass of indistinct borders replacing the normal prostate. *B,* Microscopically the tumor is composed of confluent neoplastic glands. (From Damjanov I, Linder J: Pathology: A Color Atlas, St. Louis, 2000, Mosby.)

pressure of urine in the bladder may cause reflux of urine into the ureters, dilation of ureters *(hydroureters)*, and dilation of the renal collecting system *(hydronephrosis)*.

CARCINOMA OF THE PROSTATE

The significance of prostatic carcinoma can be summarized as follows:

- It is the most common cancer in males.
- It is the third most common cause of cancer-related deaths in males.
- It is a tumor of older men, and as the longevity of the population increases, there is a constant increase in the incidence of prostatic cancer.
- There is still no adequate treatment for tumors that have extended beyond the confines of the prostate. More than 75% of all patients are diagnosed with such advanced tumors. The American Cancer Society estimates that more than 220,000 men will be diagnosed as having prostatic cancer this year and that approximately 30,000 will die of this disease.

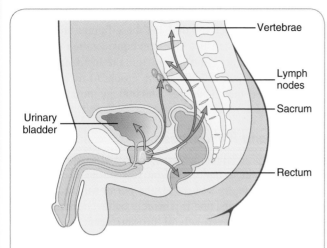

Figure 14-14 Carcinoma of the prostate invades locally into the rectum and the urinary bladder. It metastasizes to the lymph nodes and bones, most often the sacrum and vertebrae.

Labels: Vertebrae, Lymph nodes, Sacrum, Rectum, Urinary bladder

Histologic studies reveal that most prostatic malignant lesions are adenocarcinomas. Some tumors are well differentiated, whereas others are less well differentiated. Histologic grading of tumors is clinically important and is therefore done routinely by pathologists. The grading system developed by Gleason is widely used because it is easily mastered by all pathologists and is readily reproducible.

From a diagnostic point of view, it is important to note that prostatic cells produce **prostate-specific antigen (PSA),** a serine protease that is secreted normally into the semen. Its physiologic role is to liquefy the coagulum that forms from ejaculated sperm. PSA is normally present in prostatic secretions, and only a small fraction of it enters the blood. In healthy men, blood contains less than 4 ng/mL of PSA. Prostate cancer cells also produce PSA. However, because tumor cells are not arranged normally, considerable amounts of PSA secreted by prostate carcinoma cells will enter the blood. Blood levels of PSA exceeding 10 ng/mL are typically found in cancer patients. Unfortunately, about 30% to 40% of all patients with prostate cancer have only mild elevation of PSA levels, in the range from 4 to 6 ng/mL. Furthermore, other prostatic diseases, such as prostatitis and prostatic hyperplasia, can also cause PSA elevations in blood. Clearly a "positive PSA test" must be interpreted judiciously and in the context of other clinical findings.

Alkaline phosphatase is another blood enzyme that deserves to be mentioned in this context. In contrast to prostatic acid phosphatase (PAP) and PSA, alkaline phosphatase is not expressed or produced by prostatic cells. However, it is abundant in osteoblasts. When the prostatic carcinoma cells metastasize to the bone and evoke an osteoblastic reaction, the proliferation of osteoblasts results in an increase of alkaline phosphatase in the blood. Clearly, any tumor that causes osteoblastic metastases will cause elevation of serum alkaline phosphatase levels. However, elevated serum alkaline and PSA levels in an older man are

virtually diagnostic of prostatic carcinoma that has metastasized to the bones.

Clinical Features

The clinical presentation of prostatic cancer has few diagnostic features. This is primarily attributable to two factors:

- The tumor usually occurs in older men who already have some prostatic problems, usually BPH. Thus gradual worsening of the symptoms may go unnoticed.
- Prostatic carcinoma originates in the peripheral parts of the prostate; therefore it does not cause compression of the urethra or urinary problems until late in the course of the disease.

Early tumors—that is, those that are limited to the prostate—are the only form of prostatic cancer amenable to successful treatment. These tumors are typically asymptomatic and may be detected only by measuring the serum PSA levels and taking a biopsy specimen in those men who have elevated serum PSA. Symptoms begin when the tumor enlarges and extends beyond the confines of the prostate. Tumor extension into the surrounding organs usually is associated with pain (nerve invasion), dysuria or hematuria (urinary tract invasion), or constipation and intestinal obstruction (rectal invasion). Bone metastases cause dull and persistent pain. Bone fractures are uncommon but may occur, especially in patients with advanced disease.

Currently the only feasible approach to combating prostatic cancer is early detection and surgical resection before the tumor has spread beyond the prostate. The good news is that the prostate can readily be palpated using a finger inserted into the rectum. Indeed, no physical examination should be considered complete without a rectal examination, which is an absolute must in all men older than 50 years. If palpation reveals suspicious areas, those can be further evaluated with use of ultrasound. The ultrasound probe is introduced into the rectum, from which location even small tumors can be efficiently localized. This technique is very useful in delineating the extent of tumor spread in patients with more advanced disease. Finally, any suspicious lesions can readily be sampled for cytologic examination by thin-needle (or larger) cytologic aspiration or for a "through-cut" tissue biopsy using a thicker needle.

Prostatic cancer is best treated surgically, but extensive tumors usually are also treated with radiation therapy and, occasionally, with chemotherapy. Palliative radiation therapy is used to relieve pain in advanced cases, usually after the tumor has spread beyond the confines of the prostate or has metastasized to bones and other organs.

The prognosis depends to some degree on the histologic grade of the tumor, but the most significant prognostic factor is the extent of the tumor. Tumors of low grade (i.e., those that are well differentiated) grow more slowly and have the best prognosis. The histologic grade often correlates closely with the extent of tumor spread (i.e., the stage of tumor). Nevertheless, wide variations have been reported in the survival of patients, even when they have the same stage of disease. This is presumably because many of them have clinically inapparent metastases. It has been estimated that one third of all patients with tumors presumed to be confined to the prostate have lymph node metastases. The 5-year survival of patients with tumor limited to the prostate is 75%. Patients with tumors that have spread beyond the confines of the prostate have a 35% to 50% 5-year survival rate, depending on the exact stage of the tumor.

Did You Know?

Thousands of prostatectomies (surgical removal of the prostate) are performed every year for prostatic carcinoma or benign prostatic hyperplasia. During this rather complicated operation, it is not uncommon for the urologist to sever the nerves innervating the urinary bladder sphincters or the penis, and some patients become either incontinent, impotent, or both. To avoid these complications, many modern urologists perform so-called nerve-sparing operations. Satisfied patients are a major source of referral of new clients for these highly skilled surgeons.

CARCINOMA OF THE PENIS

Carcinoma of the penis is rare in the United States, where it affects only 1 to 2 men per 100,000. However, in parts of the world where neonatal circumcision is not practiced and genital hygiene is poor, this form of cancer is much more common. For example, in some countries of South America, such as Paraguay, it accounts for more than 10% of all cancers in men. Therefore carcinoma of the penis is considered an environmentally induced cancer, probably related to poor general and genital hygiene. Smegma—the product of the penile coronal glands, admixed to desquamated cells, and bacteria—is considered a carcinogenic influence. Because this material accumulates under the prepuce of uncircumcised men, it is believed to play a role as a contact carcinogen for the mucosal cells of the glans. Indeed, almost all tumors are located on the glans of the penis (Figure 14-15). Histologic examination reveals the tumors to be squamous cell carcinomas.

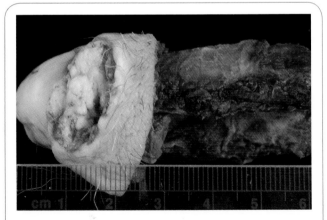

Figure 14-15 Carcinoma of the penis. An indurated and partially ulcerated mass is found at the border of the glans and the skin of the prepuce.

Treatment includes surgical amputation combined with radiation therapy. The prognosis depends on the stage of the disease: localized lesions have a good prognosis, whereas advanced lesions are less responsive to treatment.

REVIEW QUESTIONS

1. Describe how sperm is formed and excreted.
2. How are the functions of the testis regulated?
3. What is cryptorchidism, and how does it present clinically?
4. Explain the pathogenesis of infections, such as balanitis, urethritis, prostatitis, epididymitis, and orchitis.
5. Compare genital herpes simplex infection and gonorrhea with nongonococcal urethritis.
6. What are the pathologic and clinical features of primary, secondary, and tertiary syphilis?
7. How common are testicular tumors, and in which age group are they most often encountered?
8. Classify testicular germ cell tumors.
9. What is the difference between seminoma and nonseminomatous germ cell tumors?
10. What is the difference between teratoma and teratocarcinoma?
11. Which serologic tumor markers are useful for diagnosing testicular tumors?
12. How are testicular germ cell tumors treated, and what is the usual outcome of such treatment?
13. Compare Leydig cell tumors and Sertoli cell tumors.
14. What is benign prostatic hyperplasia, and what are its causes?
15. Correlate pathologic and clinical findings in benign prostatic hyperplasia.
16. How common is carcinoma of the prostate?
17. Discuss the possible role of hormones in the pathogenesis of prostatic carcinoma.
18. Correlate the pathologic and clinical findings in prostatic carcinoma.
19. What is the value of prostate-specific antigen in the diagnosis of prostatic carcinoma?
20. What is the outcome of treatment of prostatic carcinoma?
21. On what does the prognosis of prostatic carcinoma depend?
22. Correlate the pathologic and clinical features of carcinoma of the penis.

15

The Female Reproductive System

Chapter Outline

NORMAL ANATOMY AND PHYSIOLOGY
OVERVIEW OF MAJOR DISEASES
  Developmental Abnormalities
  Inflammatory Diseases
    Clinically Important Infections
  Hormonally Induced Lesions
    Endometrial Hyperplasia
  Neoplasia and Related Disorders
    Carcinoma of the Vulva
    Carcinoma of the Vagina

Carcinoma of the Cervix
Tumors of the Uterus
Tumors and Tumor-like Conditions of the Ovary
PATHOLOGY OF PREGNANCY
  Pathology of Fertilization
  Pathology of Implantation
    Ectopic Pregnancy
  Pathology of Placentation
    Placental Anomalies

Key Terms and Concepts

Abortion
Amenorrhea
Anovulatory cycle
Carcinoma of the cervix
Carcinoma of the endometrium
Carcinoma of the vagina
Carcinoma of the vulva
Cervicitis
Chlamydial infections
Choriocarcinoma
Chorionic gonadotropin (hCG)
Colposcopy
Cystadenocarcinoma
Cystadenoma
Dermoid cyst
Dysgerminoma
Eclampsia
Embryonal carcinoma
Endometrial biopsy
Endometrial carcinoma
Endometrial hyperplasia

Endometrioid adenocarcinoma
Endometriosis
Endometritis
Erythroplasia
Extrauterine pregnancy
Genital herpes
Germ cell tumors
Gestational trophoblastic disease
Gonorrhea
Granulosa cell tumor
Hermaphroditism
Human papillomavirus (HPV)
Hydatidiform mole
Hyperestrinism
Infertility
Krukenberg tumors
Leiomyoma
Leukoplakia
Menopause
Menorrhagia
Oocyte

Ovarian cysts
Ovarian tumors
Pap smear
Pelvic inflammatory disease (PID)
Placenta accreta
Placenta previa
Polycystic ovary syndrome (POS)
Preeclampsia
Salpingitis
Sertoli-Leydig cell tumor
Sex cord stromal tumors
Sexually transmitted diseases (STDs)
Syphilis
Teratocarcinoma
Teratoma
Toxemia of pregnancy
Tubo-ovarian abscess
Vaginitis
Virilization
Vulvitis
Yolk sac carcinoma

After reading this chapter, the student should be able to:

1. Describe the normal external and internal female organs.
2. Discuss the physiologic events at the time of menarche, during the normal menstrual cycle, and at the time of menopause.
3. Briefly describe the critical events of pregnancy: fertilization, implantation, placentation, and delivery.
4. List the most important causes and consequences of infection of the female genital tract.
5. List the most common causes of vaginal bleeding.
6. List the important causes and consequences of hyperestrinism.
7. List the risk factors for various forms of cancer in the female genital tract.
8. Name the most common tumors of the female genital tract and discuss their symptoms.
9. List and explain the procedures used to diagnose cancers of the cervix, uterus, and ovary.
10. Discuss the symptoms and consequences of endometriosis.
11. List the most common causes of abortion.
12. Explain ectopic pregnancy, including its causes, and list the most common sites where it occurs.
13. Describe gestational trophoblastic disease, with special emphasis on hydatidiform mole and choriocarcinoma.
14. Discuss toxemia of pregnancy and eclampsia.

NORMAL ANATOMY AND PHYSIOLOGY

The female reproductive system consists of both external and internal genital organs. The external genitalia can be seen on physical examination; in contrast, the internal genitalia, which are located in the pelvis, cannot be seen without special instruments, such as a vaginal speculum or laparoscope.

The principal parts of the female reproductive system are the vulva, vagina, uterus, fallopian tubes, and ovaries (Figure 15-1). The vulva includes the labia majora and minora, the clitoris, and the urethral orifice. In adult women it is surrounded by the hairy skin of the mons pubis. The vulva is the entrance into the vagina, a tube-like organ connecting the external and internal genital organs. The upper end of the vagina is occluded by the *cervix* of the uterus. However, because the cervix has a central

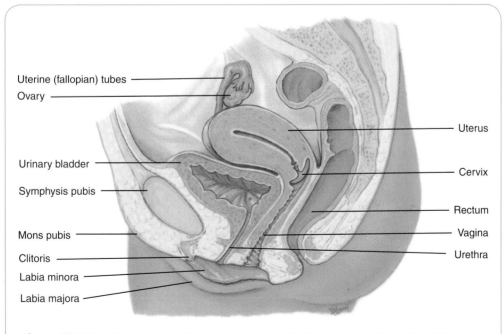

Figure 15-1 The female reproductive system consists of both external and internal genital organs, including the vulva, vagina, uterus, fallopian tubes, and ovaries. (From Applegate EJ: The Anatomy and Physiology Learning System, 4th ed, St. Louis, 2011, Saunders.)

canal, the vagina is not sealed shut, and its lumen is in direct continuity with the cavity of the uterus. The uterus extends into two tubelike structures, the fallopian tubes, which reach laterally from the top portion of the uterus to the ovaries. The fallopian tubes open freely into the abdominal cavity and are not attached to the ovary.

Histologically there are several important features of the female genital organs that deserve mention. The vulva, vagina, and external surface of the cervix are covered with squamous epithelium. The cervical canal, the uterine cavity, and the fallopian tubes are lined by glandular tissue. Squamous epithelium is more resistant to minor trauma and friction during intercourse and to bacterial invasion than is the glandular epithelium. As discussed later in the chapter, this factor is important to an understanding of infections of the genital tract. It is also worth remembering that the glandular epithelium of the uterus—called the *endometrium*—changes during the menstrual cycle.

The uterus and the fallopian tubes have two additional layers. On the outside these organs are covered with *serosa*, which is equivalent to the peritoneum enveloping other abdominal organs. The wall of the uterus and fallopian tubes consists of smooth muscle. The muscle layer of the uterus is called the *myometrium.*

The ovaries are almond-shaped organs composed of a connective tissue stroma, sex cord cells, and **oocytes.** The ovarian surface is covered with peritoneal cells. Below the surface are oocytes surrounded by specialized sex cord cells: granulosa and theca cells, that secrete female sex hormones. Oocytes and sex cords form functional units known as *follicles,* which enlarge under the influence of estrogens and then rupture around the fourteenth day of the menstrual cycle. This event is called *ovulation.*

The functions of the female reproductive organs are regulated by hormones of the hypothalamic-pituitary-ovarian axis (Figure 15-2). In adult women the hypothalamus cyclically secretes *gonadotropin-releasing hormone (GnRH),* which stimulates the pituitary to produce gonadotropins—*follicle-stimulating hormone (FSH)* and *luteinizing hormone (LH).* FSH and LH stimulate the ovary to produce estrogen or progesterone, which in turn act on the endometrium, promoting either proliferation of glands and stroma or glandular secretion, typical of the proliferative and secretory phase of the menstrual cycle, respectively (Figure 15-3). Ovarian hormones prime the endometrium for the implantation of the fertilized ovum in pregnancy. If pregnancy does not occur, the endometrium is shed and menstrual bleeding occurs.

The primary function of the female reproductive system is reproduction. The vagina serves for copulation and as a receptacle for ejaculated sperm. Fertilization of the oocytes released from the ovaries at the time of ovulation takes place in the fallopian tubes. The fertilized ovum *(zygote)* travels to the uterus, where it implants. Implantation of the zygote occurs only if the uterus is properly primed by hormones. The implantation is mediated by trophoblastic cells that form the outer layer of the embryo and are the precursors of the placenta. These cells, like the placenta, secrete human **chorionic**

gonadotropin (hCG), a hormone essential for the maintenance of pregnancy. Serum levels of hCG rise in pregnancy and also spill over into the urine, where hCG can be detected biochemically with a pregnancy test.

OVERVIEW OF MAJOR DISEASES

The physicians treating the diseases of female reproductive organs are called *gynecologists* (derived from the Greek word *gyne,* meaning "woman"). The most important diseases of the female reproductive system are the following:

- Infections
- Hormonal disorders
- Benign and malignant tumors
- Disorders related to pregnancy

Several facts important to an understanding of gynecologic pathology are presented here, before a discussion of specific pathologic entities.

1. *The female reproductive system is in direct contact with the external world.* Because of this direct contact, the female reproductive system is extremely prone to infections. Clinically these infections range in severity from being asymptomatic to producing only minor irritation and discomfort to causing major problems, especially if the infection is recurrent, as in chronic **pelvic inflammatory disease (PID).** PID is a major cause of pain and suffering in women of the reproductive age.

2. *Many infections of the female reproductive system are venereal in nature.* Venus was the Roman goddess of love, and the term *venereal infections* is a synonym for **sexually transmitted diseases (STDs).** The sexually active female, particularly if she has multiple partners or a single promiscuous partner, is at risk for infection. If infected, she may transmit the disease to her future sexual partners, or the infection may be spread transplacentally or during vaginal delivery of her offspring. Clearly, then, infectious diseases affect not only the health of the infected person but also that of other individuals; thus they have major social consequences.

3. *Infections of the female genital system are an important cause of infertility.* It is estimated that 50% of infertile women have, or have had in the past, a genital infection. PID is the most common cause of infertility. PID is also an important cause of **extrauterine pregnancies,** most of which result from abnormal implantation of the zygotes in the tubes.

4. *Hormonal disorders are another common cause of reproductive tract pathology.* Abnormal secretion of estrogen and progesterone from the ovary may cause menstrual abnormalities, such as **amenorrhea** (no bleeding at all) or **menorrhagia** (profuse bleeding). Estrogen may cause endometrial hyperplasia, and it is thought to contribute to the development of endometrial cancer. Hormones have a less pronounced effect on the fallopian tubes. Predictably, carcinomas of the fallopian tubes occur much less frequently than carcinoma of the endometrium.

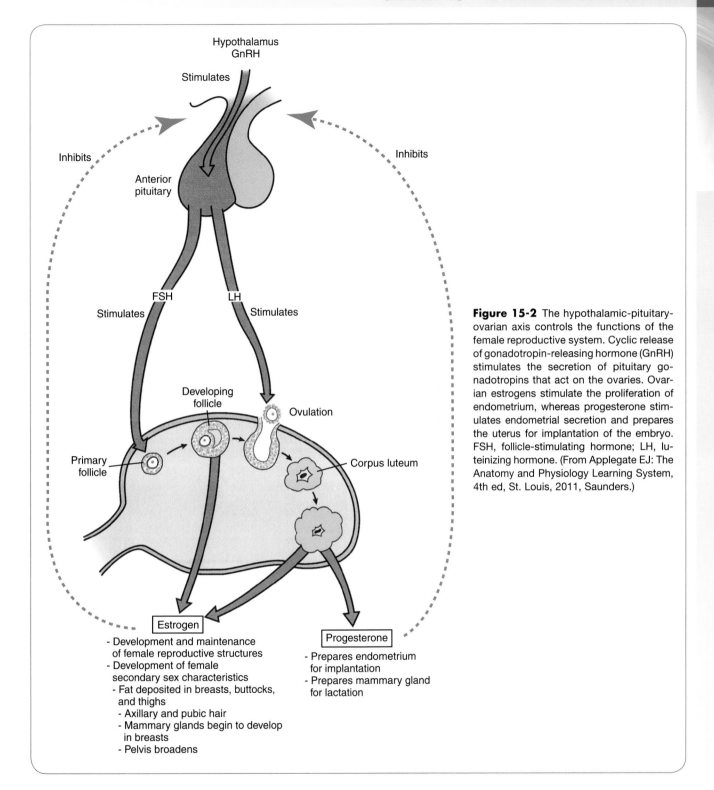

Figure 15-2 The hypothalamic-pituitary-ovarian axis controls the functions of the female reproductive system. Cyclic release of gonadotropin-releasing hormone (GnRH) stimulates the secretion of pituitary gonadotropins that act on the ovaries. Ovarian estrogens stimulate the proliferation of endometrium, whereas progesterone stimulates endometrial secretion and prepares the uterus for implantation of the embryo. FSH, follicle-stimulating hormone; LH, luteinizing hormone. (From Applegate EJ: The Anatomy and Physiology Learning System, 4th ed, St. Louis, 2011, Saunders.)

5. *Tumors of the reproductive tract are related to STDs or hormonal influences.* The causes of gynecologic tumors, like those in other organs, are not fully understood. Nevertheless, **carcinoma of the cervix** and **carcinoma of the vulva** often contain **human papillomavirus (HPV).** The incidence of this cancer correlates with exposure to other sexually transmitted viruses. **Carcinoma**

of the endometrium and many **ovarian tumors** appear to have a hormonal basis.

6. *Preventive screening has reduced the mortality from some forms of cancer such as cervical carcinoma.* Before the midpoint of the twentieth century, squamous carcinoma of the cervix was one of the most common fatal cancers of women. It is a tribute to the preventive efforts of the health

341

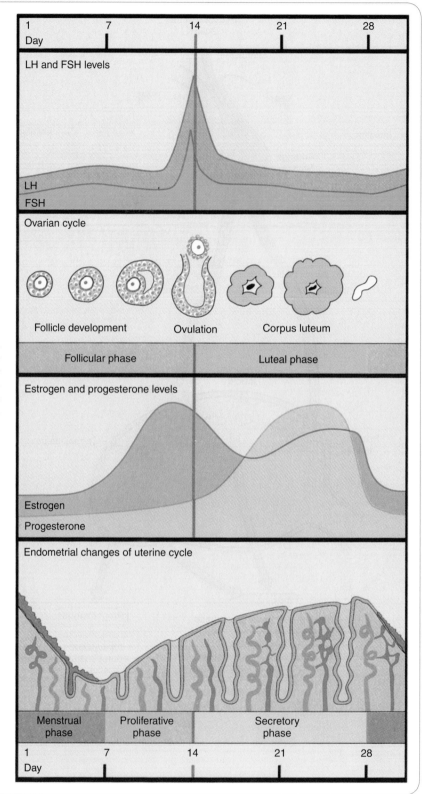

Figure 15-3 The normal menstrual cycle consists of a proliferative (follicular) and a secretory (luteal) phase. Menstrual bleeding occurs after the luteal phase. FSH, follicle-stimulating hormone; LH, luteinizing hormone. (From Applegate EJ: The Anatomy and Physiology Learning System, 4th ed, St. Louis, 2011, Saunders.)

care system that death secondary to cervical carcinoma is less common today. This in large part is a result of screening with the Papanicolaou test **(Pap smear),** which detects premalignant cervical abnormalities and allows efficient treatment. Uterine tumors are also readily detectable because

they present as abnormal bleeding. This accounts for the good treatment results of both cervical and uterine cancer. Unfortunately, malignant diseases of the ovary are not so easily detected, and these tumors still claim many lives. New techniques of molecular biology will probably contribute even more to the fight against gynecologic cancer. Vaccination against HPV, an important cause of cervical carcinoma, will presumably reduce the incidence of this form of cancer.

7. *Pathology of pregnancy occurs as a result of disturbances in critical events essential for the maintenance of pregnancy.* Considering the complexities of human reproduction, it is a minor miracle that pregnancy occurs at all. The inability to conceive **(infertility)** has been recorded in every sixth couple trying to conceive a child. Pregnancy may be abnormal from the beginning. For example, the embryo may implant in the wrong place, such as in a fallopian tube that cannot support embryonic development *(extrauterine pregnancy).* The placenta may develop abnormally and give rise to hydatidiform mole and choriocarcinoma. The adverse effects of pregnancy are best exemplified by **toxemia of pregnancy,** a systemic disease that affects all major organs.

? Did You Know?

A Papanicolaou smear is a painless procedure. It is the best and most efficient way of detecting early cervical neoplasia. The procedure is performed during a vaginal gynecologic examination. The examiner inserts a swab or spatula and scrapes the cervix to obtain cells for cytopathologic examination.

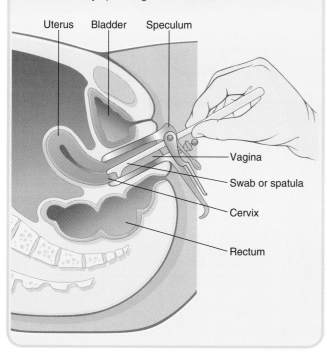

DEVELOPMENTAL ABNORMALITIES

Developmental anomalies of the female genital organs are rare, which is surprising considering the complexity of their formation during fetal life. *Agenesis of the vagina or uterus, duplication of the uterus,* and *bicornuate uterus* are mentioned

here as possible, albeit rare, causes of sexual dysfunction and infertility.

Discordance between the genetic sex and the phenotypic sex of an individual may result in developmental abnormalities known as *hermaphroditism.* Such intersexual individuals have both male and female features or something in between. The historic term **hermaphroditism** (derived from the names of two Greek gods, one male [Hermes] and one female [Aphrodite]) has been replaced by three more specific terms:

- *True hermaphroditism* is diagnosed when the gonads are both male and female. For example, one gonad may be a testis and the other an ovary, or they may be fused into an *ovotestis.*

- *Male pseudohermaphroditism* occurs when a person is genetically male but has female features. For example, in testicular feminization syndrome, the genetic males have a vulva, vagina, and well-developed breasts. However, the gonad is a testis, usually located inside the abdomen. Testes secrete male hormones, but the tissues have no receptors for testosterone and cannot respond to androgenic stimulation. Hence the external genitalia become female.

- *Female pseudohermaphroditism* is the correct term when a person is genetically female but has male features. For example, in congenital adrenal hyperplasia, the genetic females show virilization of the vulva. The clitoris enlarges and transforms into a micropenis. Congenital adrenal hyperplasia, the most common form of intersexualism, affects 1 in 4000 female neonates.

The most important chromosomal anomaly associated with abnormal genital development is Turner's syndrome, usually related to monosomy X (discussed in Chapter 5). This congenital disorder affects 1 in 3000 newborn babies. Clinically it presents with a lack of menstruation and infertility.

INFLAMMATORY DISEASES

Inflammatory diseases of the female genital system may be considered from several points of view and classified accordingly:

1. *Anatomic classification.* This classification system is based on the clinical or pathologic assessment of inflammation. The inflammation may be localized, or it may diffusely involve the entire female reproductive system and even spread to adjacent structures, such as the urethra, bladder, or rectum. Terms such as **vulvitis, vaginitis,** and **cervicitis,** are self-explanatory designations for the inflammation of these organs, although often more than one adjacent anatomic site is involved. It is thus common to diagnose vulvovaginitis or cervicovaginal infection. Infection of the body of the uterus is usually limited to the endometrium and is thus called **endometritis.** Inflammation of the fallopian tubes is called **salpingitis,** and inflammation of the ovaries is termed *oophoritis.* Inflammation of the entire female reproductive tract is known as *PID.*

2. *Chronologic classification.* With regard to the duration of the disease, the inflammations can be classified as acute,

chronic, or recurrent. Recurrent infections may be caused by a new pathogen or represent an exacerbation of latent, clinically dormant infections.

3. *Pathogenetic classification.* On the basis of pathogenesis, genital infections can be classified as ascending or descending, depending on the route by which the pathogens have reached the reproductive system. Descending infections typically occur as a result of hematogenous or lymphatic spread of pathogens from some other organ in the body (Figure 15-4). For example, tuberculosis of the genital organs is always a descending infection secondary to a focus of primary infection elsewhere, such as the lungs. Ascending infections are acquired mostly through sexual contact and are thus classified as STDs. The vagina is in direct continuity with the upper genital organs; thus any microbe introduced into the vagina can ascend upstream into the uterus and the fallopian tubes. Pregnancy is yet another risk factor, and approximately 5% of all pregnancies are accompanied by endometrial infection, which may spread to the fallopian tubes. Previously, illegal *abortions* were a major cause of endometrial infection and subsequent PID. Overall, ascending infections are usually polymicrobial and are more common than descending infections.

According to their pathogenesis, the symptoms of genital infections can be classified as local or systemic. Local symptoms predominate, but they may also be associated with systemic symptoms, such as fever, malaise, and general uneasiness. Entry of pathogens into the circulation may cause septicemia and widespread infection of other organs. Entry of bacteria into the peritoneal cavity, usually through the open, fimbriated end of the fallopian tubes, may result in *peritonitis*.

4. *Etiologic classification.* On the basis of etiology, genital tract infections may be classified as bacterial, chlamydial, viral, fungal, or protozoal. Many cases are caused by more than one pathogen and are classified as polymicrobial.

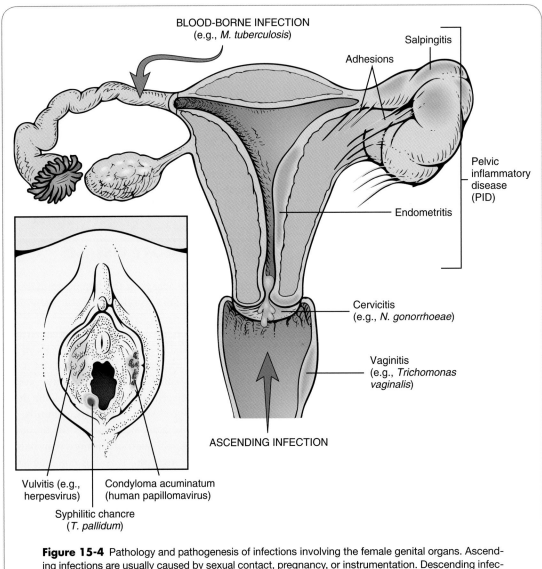

Figure 15-4 Pathology and pathogenesis of infections involving the female genital organs. Ascending infections are usually caused by sexual contact, pregnancy, or instrumentation. Descending infections are hematogenous or lymphogenous.

Bacterial Infections

Bacterial infections are common causes of STDs. Neisseria gonorrhoeae is the cause of gonorrhea and *Treponema pallidum* is the cause of syphilis. *Streptococcus* and *Staphylococcus* are widespread bacteria that may cause infection of the genital organs by an ascending or descending route. Mixed bacterial infections are commonly found in patients with PID.

Chlamydial Infections

Chlamydial infections are caused by sexually transmitted *Chlamydia trachomatis*. These bacteria are obligate intracellular organisms (i.e., they cannot live or reproduce outside the cells). *Chlamydiae* may cause cervicitis and urethritis and are important pathogens in PID. Chlamydia is the most common sexually transmitted pathogen in the United States, with more than a million new cases diagnosed yearly in this country. Estimates are that another 2 million women have chronic chlamydial genital infections.

Viral Infections

Viral infections are also commonly acquired by sexual contact. The most important pathogens are herpesvirus and HPV, which typically affect the vulva, vagina, and cervix.

Fungal Infections

Fungal infections typically cause vulvovaginitis. The most common fungal pathogen is *Candida albicans,* which lives on moist surfaces (e.g., the vagina) and does not invade deeper into the tissues.

Protozoal Infections

Protozoal infections are typically limited to the vagina. The most important pathogen is *Trichomonas vaginalis,* a common cause of vaginal discharge in women of reproductive age.

CLINICALLY IMPORTANT INFECTIONS

The most important genital infections are listed in Table 15-1.

Genital Viral Infections

Most important viral pathogens are herpes simplex virus (HSV) and HPV. **Genital herpes** is most often caused by HSV-2 infection, but in some instances it may be caused by HSV-1, the virus that typically causes lip lesions. Genital herpes typically presents with grouped blisters on the vulva or the perineal skin. Infection with HPV can result in the formation of warts on the vulva, called *condyloma acuminatum.* HPV infection of the cervix or the vagina results in plaques known as *flat condyloma,* but, as we will see later, it may also cause squamous cell carcinoma.

? **Did You Know?**

HPV infection may cause genital warts called condyloma accuminatum. As seen here, these warts are often multiple because the virus can easily spread all over the vulva.

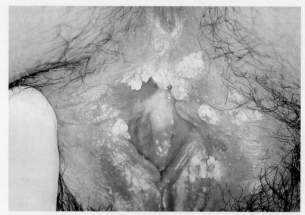

(From Damjanov I, Linder J: Pathology: A Color Atlas, St. Louis, 2000, Mosby.)

TABLE 15-1 Common Genital Infections

Disease	Organism	Estimated Yearly Occurrence*	Typical Genital Pathology
Genital herpes	Herpes simplex virus type 2	300,000	Painful, recurrent, genital blisters
Human papillomavirus (HPV) infection	HPV	6 million	Labial, vaginal, and cervical warts (condyloma); carcinoma
Infectious vaginitis	*Trichomonas vaginalis, Gardnerella vaginalis,* or *Candida albicans*	7 million (mostly undiagnosed)	Vaginitis with discharge
Chlamydial infection	*Chlamydia trachomatis*	1,200,000	Urethritis or cervicitis with discharge; pelvic inflammatory disease (PID)
Gonorrhea	*Neisseria gonorrhoeae*	330,000	Urethritis or cervicitis with discharge; PID
Syphilis	*Treponema pallidum*	13,500	Vulvar ulcers

* Estimates in rounded numbers based on the data compiled by the Centers for Disease Control and Prevention (CDC), U.S. Statistics, 2008.

Infectious Vaginitis

The vagina is lined by squamous epithelium, which prevents the entry of pathogens into the wall of the vagina. Hence most pathogens causing vaginitis remain in the lumen. The most important causes of vaginitis are the protozoon *T. vaginalis,* the bacterium *Gardnerella vaginalis,* and the fungus *C. albicans.* Such infections are associated with copious discharge. The discharge may be clear or turbid and yellow and mucinous or frothy; it often has a foul smell. Infectious vaginitis can be treated with drugs; metronidazole is administered for Trichomonas, antibiotics for bacteria, and fungicides for Candida infection.

Chlamydial Infections

Chlamydial infections present as nonspecific inflammation of the vulva, internal female genital organs, and urethra. Because urethritis is common, dysuria is an important symptom. Vaginal discharge accompanies vaginitis and cervicitis. The infection may enter the uterus and fallopian tube and is thus an important cause of PID. Such PID causes lower abdominal pain and tenderness and is often accompanied by fever and systemic symptoms. Infertility is a common complication. Babies born to women infected with Chlamydia are at risk for developing neonatal conjunctivitis, which must be prevented by preventive application of eye drops to all newborns. Infected neonates are at risk for developing neonatal pneumonia, estimated to occur in 20% of all infected newborns.

Gonorrhea

Gonorrhea, a prevalent STD, affects the lower and the upper genital system. It also causes urethritis (dysuria) and may even cause proctitis (infection of the rectum). PID and infertility are important and common complications. Septicemia and arthritis are found in a significant number of affected patients. Infants born to infected mothers can develop purulent conjunctivitis, which may seriously damage the eyes and cause loss of vision.

Syphilis

Primary **syphilis** presents in females as vulvar ulcers, chancre, or cervicitis and vaginal lesions. These lesions develop usually 3 to 4 weeks after infection. If untreated, the disease may progress to secondary and even tertiary syphilis.

 Did You Know?

Gonococcal conjunctivitis was so common among neonates that it was considered one of the major public health problems in many American cities of the nineteenth century. The solution to this problem was proposed by Dr. Barnes, who found out that silver nitrate droplets could prevent eye infection of neonates. He patented his medicine under the name Argyrol. The widespread preventive use of Argyrol eye droplets made Dr. Barnes both rich and famous. The world renowned Barnes Foundation, located near Philadelphia, housing an invaluable collection of French Impressionist paintings, is an enduring monument to both Argyrol and its inventor.

Pelvic Inflammatory Disease

Pelvic inflammatory disease (PID) is the most important complication of all lower genital tract infections, which occurs when the pathogens ascend into the uterine cavity. PID is most often caused by STDs such as those related to infection with Chlamydia and *N. gonorrhoeae*. In one third of women with PID there is no preexisting STD; their disease is caused by mixed bacterial infection related to the endogenous bacterial flora of the vulva and perineum.

The fallopian tubes bear the brunt of the infection, becoming red, swollen, filled with pus, and adherent to other organs. An abscess involving the fallopian tube and ovary **(tubo-ovarian abscess)** may form. The patient typically has severe lower abdominal pain, fever, nausea, and vaginal discharge or bleeding. Diffuse inflammation of the peritoneum *(peritonitis),* a rare but very serious complication, may result from the entry of bacteria into the peritoneal cavity.

As the infection progresses, other bacteria of vaginal origin may invade the fallopian tubes, which accounts for the fact that multiple bacteria can be isolated from older lesions. During the healing phase of inflammation, the fallopian tubes may become scarred and obstructed. If blockage is complete, infertility ensues. PID also predisposes individuals to ectopic pregnancy because the inflamed folds of the fallopian tube may entrap the fertilized ovum and not allow it to pass to the uterus.

HORMONALLY INDUCED LESIONS

The normal function of the female reproductive system depends on the proper output of ovarian hormones, which, in turn, depends on the normal function of the hypothalamic-pituitary-ovarian axis. Lesions can be caused by an excess or a lack of hormones.

ENDOMETRIAL HYPERPLASIA

The normal menstrual cycle that typically lasts 28 days is divided into three phases (see Figure 15-3). The pivotal moment of the normal cycle is ovulation, which occurs on the 14th day. If ovulation does not occur, the proliferative phase of the menstrual cycle will continue and the secretory phase will never be initiated. This is called an **anovulatory cycle.** The endometrium will continue to proliferate because of continuous estrogenic stimulation unopposed by progesterone, resulting in marked thickening of the endometrial mucosa **(endometrial hyperplasia).** However, because the endometrium cannot proliferate indefinitely, it finally outgrows its own blood supply. The superficial layers that do not receive enough blood become ischemic and necrotize. The endometrium then begins to shed, resulting in uterine bleeding. This occurs typically 2 to 3 weeks after the expected time of menstruation.

The causes of anovulation may be organic or functional. The functional disturbances are more common than the organic lesions, which are rare. For example, anovulation is common in pubertal girls in whom the normal cycle of the hypothalamus has not yet been established. Psychological factors, such as anxiety induced by examination or imagined pregnancy, can also cause anovulation. Anorexia nervosa and bulimia are typically associated with anovulation, and it may persist for a long time. Anovulation is also common in athletes. It is important to remember that the ovary contains a finite number of oocytes, and once all the oocytes have been exhausted, at the time of **menopause,** anovulation will ensue. This typically occurs between the ages of 48 and 55 years. However, some women enter early menopause and stop having menstruation in midlife.

Endometrial hyperplasia can be caused by an excess of estrogen. **Hyperestrinism** may be exogenous (e.g., induced by hormone pills or injections). Endogenous hyperestrinism reflects ovarian dysfunction or, less commonly, may be related to estrogen-producing tumors (e.g., thecoma of the ovary).

The hyperplastic endometrium contains an increased number of glands. These glands may be cystic, as in simple or cystic hyperplasia (Figure 15-5). Alternatively the glands may be more crowded, producing complex hyperplasia. Complex hyperplasia is classified by pathologists into two categories: complex hyperplasia without atypia and complex hyperplasia with atypia.

Simple hyperplasia is an innocuous change, whereas the other forms of hyperplasia should be considered as possible precursors of cancer. Approximately 2% to 3% of patients with complex hyperplasia without atypia develop cancer. As many as 25% to 30% of the women who have complex hyperplasia with atypia develop endometrial adenocarcinoma. These women should be watched carefully, and those who have completed their reproductive function may choose to have their uterus removed prophylactically.

NEOPLASIA AND RELATED DISORDERS

Tumors of the female tract are common and are an important cause of morbidity in women. Tumors can occur at any age but are most common in women older than age 35 years. The following facts illustrate the magnitude of this problem:
- Gynecologic malignant lesions account for 15% of all malignant tumors and for 10% of all cancer deaths in women.
- An estimated 78,000 to 80,000 new cases of gynecologic cancer and 28,000 to 30,000 cancer-related deaths are expected each year. The most common malignant tumors are listed by anatomic site in Table 15-2.
- For every malignant tumor, there are approximately five benign tumors diagnosed and even more tumorlike conditions, such as cysts and endometriosis. It has been estimated that 25% of women older than 30 years have uterine leiomyomas. **Ovarian cysts** are found in two thirds of women of reproductive age, although most of these are non-neoplastic, small, and clinically insignificant.

CARCINOMA OF THE VULVA

Carcinoma of the vulva is relatively rare, accounting for 3% of all gynecologic cancers. The most important facts about vulvar malignant disease are as follows:
- Carcinoma of the vulva is a carcinoma of older women. The median age at the time of diagnosis is 60 years.
- The tumor can be recognized by gross inspection of the external genitalia. It presents as a wartlike or slightly raised (macular) mucosal lesion or ulceration (Figure 15-6). Invasive carcinoma is preceded by carcinoma *in situ* (CIS) and by preneoplastic lesions that can be diagnosed on the basis of histologic findings following biopsy. Clinically, many of these precursors of cancer present as **leukoplakia** or **erythroplasia** (i.e., white or red patches, respectively).
- Clinical symptoms include itching, discomfort, frank pain, and bleeding, but a significant number of patients, at least 1 in 5, are asymptomatic.
- Histologically the tumor is usually a squamous cell carcinoma.

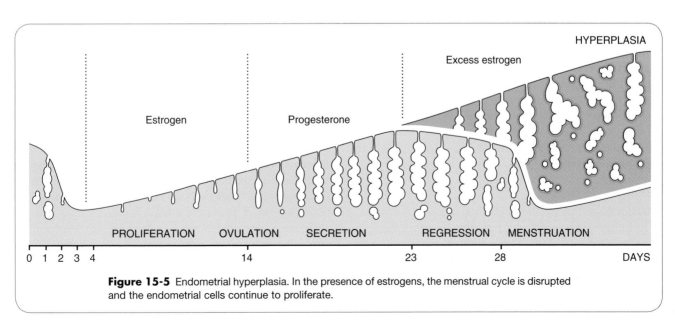

Figure 15-5 Endometrial hyperplasia. In the presence of estrogens, the menstrual cycle is disrupted and the endometrial cells continue to proliferate.

TABLE 15-2 Gynecologic Cancer Statistics in the United States

Site	New Cases	Deaths
Cervix uteri	12,200	4,200
Body of the uterus	43,500	8,000
Ovary	21,800	14,000
Vulva	3,900	900
Vagina and other sites	2,300	800
Total	83,700	27,900

Data rounded up to the nearest hundred from the original report of the American Cancer Society, 2010.

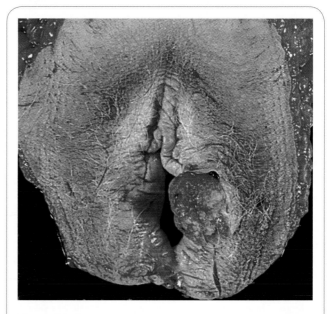

Figure 15-6 Carcinoma of the vulva. (From Damjanov I, Linder J: Pathology: A Color Atlas, St. Louis, 2000, Mosby.)

The tumor grows slowly, and if the diagnosis is made before it has metastasized to the lymph nodes, the patient has a 70% chance of surviving 5 years after surgical resection. Patients with tumors that have spread to the lymph nodes have a less favorable prognosis. Treatment includes surgical resection of the tumor and sometimes of the entire vulva *(vulvectomy),* supplemented by radiation therapy and chemotherapy in advanced cases.

CARCINOMA OF THE VAGINA

Carcinoma of the vagina is relatively uncommon, accounting for only 2% of all gynecologic cancers. In most aspects it resembles vulvar cancer, in that it is a disease of older women and is histologically a squamous cell carcinoma. It can be detected only on gynecologic examination. Vaginal Pap smears are also useful for diagnosis.

CARCINOMA OF THE CERVIX

Carcinoma of the cervix, once the most common form of gynecologic cancer, accounts for approximately 20% of all malignant tumors of the female reproductive tract. Nevertheless, it is still ranked as the eighth major cancer-related cause of death, and it causes more deaths than carcinoma of the body of the uterus, vagina, and vulva together. The reduced mortality achieved over the past 50 years is directly related to early detection of cervical cancer and related preneoplastic conditions by routine use of Pap smears by gynecologists. For each carcinoma reported to the cancer registry, the official statistics still show four CIS or dysplasias, confirming that the incidence of cervical cancer has not decreased but that detection in early stages has improved.

Etiology

Although the ultimate cause of cervical cancer is not known, the scientific evidence indicates that in most women this form of cancer is caused by HPV. Cervical carcinoma is most common in women with the following characteristics:

- Began having sexual intercourse at an early age
- Have multiple sexual partners (e.g., prostitutes are at increased risk)
- Have evidence of HPV infection, especially certain subtypes
- Have had other STDs such as genital herpes or syphilis
- Smoke tobacco

HPV infection plays the key role in the pathogenesis of cervical carcinoma. It should be noted that there are more than 80 types of HPV, but only some of these viruses cause cervical cancer. Hence it is important to perform viral studies and determine the type of virus causing the infection. Vaccine against the most common cancer-causing HPVs has been scientifically tested and proven to be effective in preventing cervical cancer. This vaccine can be given to both boys and girls in their teens, and scientists hope it will reduce the incidence of cervical carcinoma, especially in parts of the world (e.g., South America, Africa, and Asia) where this form of cancer is still a very common and apparently preventable disease.

Pathogenesis

Carcinoma of the cervix is a squamous cell carcinoma. As mentioned earlier, the outer surface of the cervix *(exocervix)* is covered with squamous epithelium, whereas the endocervical canal is lined by columnar epithelium. The point where these two epithelia meet is called the *transformation zone.* Most cervical carcinomas originate in this zone, which is marked by intense cell proliferation. It should be noted that this zone may widen after cervical trauma, which typically occurs during vaginal delivery of a baby when the cervix ruptures to allow birth. Chronic inflammation of the transformation zone also causes its widening. One could assume then that women who have had numerous vaginal deliveries or those who have genitourinary infections because of promiscuity have an altered transformation zone. Because proliferating cells are increasingly susceptible to viral infection, exposure to oncogenic HPV viruses could induce neoplastic transformation of the transformation zone. The transformed cells do not respond to normal regulatory stimuli operating in the tissue. They do not mature as the normal cervical cells do, but remain undifferentiated and proliferate uncontrollably.

The lack of normal maturation of squamous epithelium can be histologically recognized as dysplasia. It is customary to grade dysplasia as mild, moderate, or severe (Figure 15-7). Severe dysplasia may progress to carcinoma that initially is limited to the boundaries of the normal epithelium and is therefore called *CIS*. Carcinoma cells may cross the basal membrane and invade the underlying connective tissue stroma. At this point the carcinoma is considered invasive. Such tumors can further spread locally or can invade the lymphatics and the blood vessels and metastasize to distant sites.

The preinvasive neoplastic lesions—dysplasia and CIS—are also called *cervical intraepithelial neoplasia* (CIN) and are graded from I to III. Because the abnormal cells are shed into the vagina and can be scraped by the gynecologist, the diagnosis can also be made on the basis of cytologic studies. This painless procedure, the Pap smear, has saved many lives. Today this test is being replaced by tests that assay HPV because of the strong correlation between HPV and cervical carcinoma; however, the Pap test is still the most efficient way to detect cervical lesions.

Viral studies of cervical biopsy specimens show that most CIN lesions contain HPV. In cytologic smears, such lesions present with koilocytes, vacuolated cells typical of HPV infection. Only types 16 and 18 and, to a lesser extent, types 31, 33, 34, and 35 HPV are associated with cancer. Types 16 and 18 together account for about 70% of cervical cancers. Other HPV types (e.g., types 6 and 11) are found in benign lesions, such as condyloma acuminatum, and are not related to cancer.

Accordingly, it is important not only to identify HPV infection by recognizing the koilocytic cells but also to type the virus, because it may provide new data for risk assessment and the prognosis of cervical lesions.

Pathology

Carcinoma of the cervix is histologically a squamous cell carcinoma. The earliest lesions are barely recognizable by examination with the naked eye. **Colposcopy** may be used to identify the mucosal abnormalities. These changes are typically described as "mosaic" or "punctate." The cervix changes from a normal, smooth pattern to these pathologic patterns as a result of the presence of abnormal cells, irregular maturation of cells, and ingrowth of new blood vessels into the tumor zone.

Once an invasive tumor develops, it may take several forms, classified as exophytic or endophytic, depending on whether the predominant direction of growth is inside or outside the cervix. Exophytic tumors protrude into the vagina and are cauliflower-like fungating masses. Invasive tumors, called *endophytic* ("inside growing"), usually present as craterlike ulcerations. A variegated appearance is common in advanced cancers, which do not follow any prescribed mode but grow indiscriminately in all directions.

Because the clinical prognosis of cervical cancer depends primarily on the extent of tumor spread, staging is imperative. This is done according to the following criteria (Figure 15-8):

Stage 0—no gross lesions; **carcinoma** in situ microscopically limited to the mucosa (CIN III)

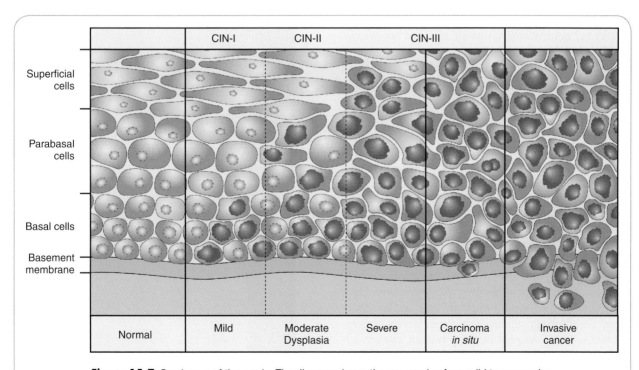

Figure 15-7 Carcinoma of the cervix. The diagram shows the progression from mild to severe dysplasia and invasive cancer. The preinvasive lesions may be graded as mild, moderate, or severe dysplasia, or as carcinoma *in situ* or cervical intraepithelial neoplasia (CIN I–III). Compare the lack of epithelial maturation in CIN with the normal epithelium that shows distinct basal, suprabasal, and superficial layers. Also, note that the basement membrane is intact in all forms of CIN but is breached in invasive cancer.

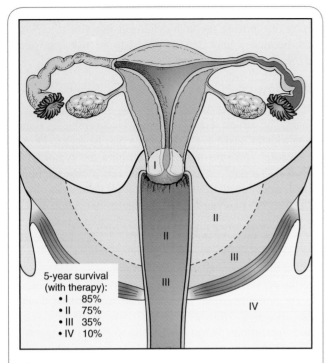

Figure 15-8 Staging of carcinoma of the cervix. Staging provides the most important data for determining prognosis in patients with cervical carcinoma.

5-year survival (with therapy):
- I 85%
- II 75%
- III 35%
- IV 10%

Stage I—invasive carcinoma confined to the cervix

Stage II—carcinoma extending beyond the confines of the cervix but not reaching the pelvic wall and not extending below the upper part of the vagina

Stage III—tumor reaching the pelvic wall and/or invading the lower third of the vagina

Stage IV—tumor that has spread beyond the pelvis or has infiltrated the adjacent organs; these tumors are also associated with metastases

Clinical Features

The median age of patients diagnosed with invasive carcinoma of the cervix is 50 years. In contrast, the median age of women diagnosed with CIN is 35 years. Because we know that CIN precedes invasive carcinoma in almost all cases, it is safe to conclude that it takes approximately 15 years for an invasive tumor to develop. During this period, most women have either no symptoms or only nonspecific minor symptoms, such as increased vaginal discharge or bleeding after intercourse. Once the tumor develops, all these symptoms may become more prominent. The discharge ultimately becomes bloody or purulent and foul-smelling. Vaginal bleeding is scant, even in advanced cases, and is not a common finding. Pain is not a feature of cervical cancer, and it occurs only after the tumor has spread extensively beyond the cervix. These symptoms are nonspecific, and it takes a long time for the symptoms to truly interfere with daily life. Without active surveillance, most women with cervical cancer would probably seek medical treatment only after the tumor had spread well beyond the treatable stages.

Advanced carcinoma invades the adjacent organs, most notably the urinary bladder and the rectum, causing urinary urgency or obstruction. Complete urinary tract obstruction causes slowly progressive renal failure, which is still the most common cause of death in these patients. The metastases tend to follow the lymph drainage of the cervix and typically involve the pelvic lymph nodes. Distant metastases to the abdominal and thoracic organs may occur in terminal stages.

CIN can be resected surgically with a scalpel (knife), with laser ablation, or by cryotherapy (freezing). *Loop electrosurgical excision procedure (LEEP)* is currently the most popular method for removing preinvasive cervical cancer (CIN II and CIN III). Advanced lesions are treated surgically, in combination with radiation therapy and chemotherapy.

The prognosis of carcinoma of the cervix depends primarily on the stage of the tumor. The preinvasive cancer (CIN) is curable, whereas stage IV cancer is almost always lethal and has a 5-year survival rate of 15%.

? Did You Know?

Colposcopy is performed with an instrument called a *colposcope*, which is inserted into the vagina and used to observe the external surface of the cervix. The top figure shows the colposcopic appearance of a normal cervix, whereas the bottom one shows a cervix altered by cervical intraepithelial neoplasia. The normal cervix is smooth, whereas the abnormal cervix shows irregularities that are readily identified.

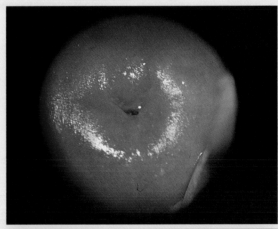

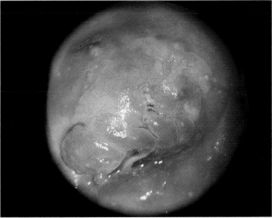

(Photographs courtesy Dr. Warren Lang.)

From all that you have learned so far about carcinoma of the cervix, the most important fact to remember is that this cancer can be recognized early and that a simple test (the Pap smear or HPV detection), performed on a regular basis, can save the lives of at least 7000 women annually in the United States. Recent studies of vaccination of girls and young women against HPV 16 and HPV 18 have shown that this active immunization can prevent essentially all cancers related to these two types of virus. The various diagnostic and therapeutic procedures used by gynecologists to treat cervical cancer are listed in Table 15-3.

TUMORS OF THE UTERUS

The body of the uterus consists of two tissues—endometrium and myometrium—both of which can give rise to uterine tumors. Theoretically these tumors can be benign or malignant. However, in practice most tumors originating from the myometrial smooth muscle cells are benign *(leiomyomas),* and the malignant ones, *leiomyosarcomas,* are very rare. In contrast, essentially all tumors originating from the endometrium are malignant. These include endometrial adenocarcinomas derived from endometrial glands, endometrial stromal sarcomas derived from stromal cells, and carcinosarcomas (also called *mixed mesodermal tumors* or *mixed müllerian tumors*) derived from both the glands and the stroma. Only the two most common tumors— endometrial adenocarcinomas and leiomyomas—are discussed here because all other neoplasms are rare.

ENDOMETRIAL CARCINOMA

Endometrial carcinoma is the most common malignant tumor of the female genital tract, accounting for approximately 50% of all gynecologic malignant disease (see Table 15-2).

Histologically the tumor is an adenocarcinoma, indicating that it arises from the epithelial cells lining the endometrial glands.

Benign endometrial tumors, which in other organs would be called *adenomas,* are not recognized clinically. As mentioned earlier, the endometrium is shed every month; in all likelihood, the benign tumors included in such endometrium are discarded in the menstrual blood. However, those benign glandular proliferations that persist are indistinguishable from endometrial hyperplasia, a hormonally induced lesion already discussed. Accordingly, although the endometrium does not have benign tumors, complex adenomatous hyperplasia could be considered the benign equivalent of adenocarcinoma. As mentioned before, complex adenomatous hyperplasia may evolve into atypical hyperplasia, and this can then progress to adenocarcinoma in a sequence reminiscent of the progression of cervical dysplasia to CIS and squamous cell carcinoma.

Etiology and Pathogenesis

In view of the fact that endometrial carcinoma originates in a hormonally sensitive tissue, it has traditionally been considered a sex hormone–induced malignant lesion. As mentioned earlier, estrogens stimulate endometrial proliferation in the proliferative phase. Several clinical studies have found an association between hyperestrinism and endometrial cancer, regardless of the source of estrogens. Thus endometrial cancer is more common in women with the following characteristics:

- They are taking exogenous estrogen in the form of pills or injections.
- They have estrogen-producing tumors.
- They are obese and form estrogen at an increased rate by peripheral (fat tissue) conversion of other endogenous

TABLE 15-3 Diagnostic Tests and Therapeutic Procedures for Carcinoma of the Cervix

Test/Procedure	Description	Objective
Pap smear	A wooden spatula is used to scrape cells from the exocervix. A brush is inserted into the endocervical canal to remove the cells.	To detect dysplastic and early neoplastic cells, HPV infection, *Trichomonas* infection
Colposcopy	The colposcope, a stereoscopic microscope, is used to examine the vagina and cervix to magnify and detect lesions invisible to the naked eye. With this instrument, one cannot see beyond the lower endocervical canal.	To detect dysplastic lesions; often used after routine screening with a Pap smear if dysplastic cells are detected
Punch biopsy	A surgical instrument is used to remove small portions of abnormal tissue for microscopic examination.	To provide tissue for pathologic examination; may be curative for small lesions
Cone biopsy	A cone-shaped portion of exocervical and endocervical tissue is surgically removed. (This technique removes a relatively large segment of tissue and may be associated with complications. Thus it is generally for noninvasive lesions and not used if the previous techniques can adequately characterize the lesion and guide treatment.)	To allow more extensive tissue sampling for pathologic evaluation; may be curative for noninvasive lesions
Hysterectomy	The uterus is surgically removed.	To treat advanced cancer
Pelvic exenteration	All pelvic organs are surgically removed.	Used as a last resort to reduce the tumor burden ("debulking")

HPV, human papillomavirus.

steroids. (Diabetes mellitus and hypertension are both known to be risk factors, but it is unclear whether these risk factors have a direct or an indirect effect. Because diabetes and hypertension are often associated with obesity, the potentiation of carcinogenic risk may be indirect.)

- They are nulliparous or have early menarche and late menopause. (These women have longer exposure to estrogens than women who have a shorter reproductive life—that is, those who have late menarche and early menopause.)

Because pregnancy is dominated by progesterone rather than estrogen and because it provides the endometrium a respite from proliferation, multiple pregnancies reduce the risk of endometrial cancer. Thus women who have many children have less endometrial cancer than nulliparous women do.

It has been postulated that estrogens stimulate the proliferation of endometrial glands, which ultimately undergo malignant transformation. Recent data indicate that estrogen-induced hyperplasia and neoplasia might be related to the inactivation of a tumor suppressor, known as *PTEN* (*p*hosphatase and *ten*sin homologue). This gene, which normally inhibits cell proliferation and promotes apoptosis, is inactivated or lost in estrogen-induced endometrial lesions and could be the key event in the histogenesis of endometrial cancers.

In animal experiments it is possible to induce endometrial cancer with prolonged estrogen treatment. Even more tumors can be induced by combining estrogen treatment with chemical carcinogens, suggesting that the estrogen effects could be potentiated by some chemical or viral carcinogens. These natural or human-made carcinogens remain unknown at the present time.

Exogenous estrogens are used extensively in clinical medicine, especially for replacement therapy in postmenopausal women whose ovaries have a reduced capacity for estrogen production. Estrogen has many beneficial effects; most notably, it prevents bone loss that occurs at an accelerated rate after menopause *(postmenopausal osteoporosis)*. On the other hand, estrogen increases the risk of endometrial cancer and therefore most doctors discourage older women from taking estrogens

Pathology

In early stages of development, endometrial tumors appear as small polyps or thickened mucosal lining prone to bleeding. Most tumors are exophytic—that is, they grow into the endometrial cavity—but if left untreated, they become endophytic and invade into the myometrium. On gross examination the fully developed tumor appears as an ulcerated or fungating mass protruding into the uterine lumen (Figure 15-9). The tissue is friable and soft because it consists predominantly of atypical glands and very little connective tissue stroma. It is prone to fragmentation, and bleeding is common. Because of their invasive growth, endometrial carcinomas penetrate into the myometrium and may extend all the way to the serosa. They also grow into the endocervix and may extend through the cervical canal into the vagina. Early metastases are found in pelvic lymph nodes, but later the tumor may involve higher

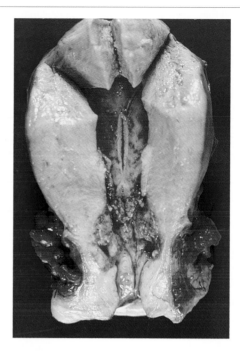

Figure 15-9 Endometrial carcinoma. The lower segment of the uterine cavity contains a tumor.

abdominal lymph nodes and metastasize hematogenously to distant sites.

Histologically these tumors are classified as adenocarcinomas. In most instances these tumors resemble endometrial glands and are called *endometrioid*. Less often, endometrial adenocarcinomas resemble ovarian serous or clear-cell adenocarcinomas. These nonendometrioid carcinomas are usually found in older women and are not related to hyperestrinism. They also have a worse prognosis than typical **endometrioid adenocarcinomas.**

The most important prognostic feature of endometrial carcinoma is the stage of the tumor (i.e., the size of the lesion and the extent of spread). The stage is determined as follows (Figure 15-10):

Stage I—carcinoma confined to the endometrium

Stage II—carcinoma extending into the cervix and invading the myometrium; depth of myometrial invasion is important for prognosis

Stage III—carcinoma extending through the wall of the uterus but not outside the true pelvis

Stage IV—carcinoma infiltrating the bladder or the rectum or extending outside the true pelvis

Clinical Features

Endometrial carcinoma is rare before age 35, but its incidence increases steadily thereafter. Most often it affects women entering menopause and those who are already postmenopausal. The most common presenting symptom of endometrial cancer is vaginal bleeding. It may occur as spotting between two menstruations or as prolonged and more pronounced menstrual bleeding *(menorrhagia).*

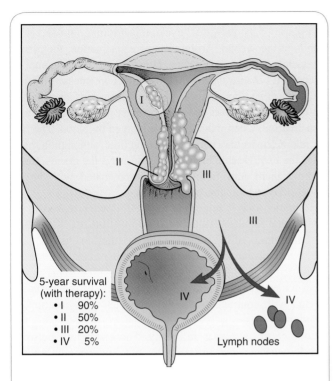

Figure 15-10 Staging of endometrial carcinoma is important for determining prognosis. Tumors detected in early stages have an excellent prognosis.

5-year survival
(with therapy):
• I   90%
• II 50%
• III 20%
• IV 5%

Lymph nodes

Many tumors remain clinically inapparent for prolonged periods, especially in younger premenopausal women. Any abnormal vaginal bleeding should prompt the gynecologist to find its causes, and that is how most endometrial cancers are diagnosed. Postmenopausal women should be scrutinized even more carefully. Final diagnosis is made by endometrial biopsy, which should be performed in all patients in whom the disease is suspected.

Endometrial biopsy is performed by gynecologists. It is a relatively minor procedure that is done in an office setting. The tissue may be sampled with an aspirator, a plastic tube that is introduced through the cervix into the uterine cavity. Additional tissue can be obtained by dilating the cervix and scraping the endometrium with a curette, a procedure commonly known as *dilation and curettage* (D&C).

The tissue obtained by these procedures is fixed in formalin and submitted to the pathology laboratory for histologic examination. Staging usually requires additional clinical examinations to determine the extent of tumor spread. In most instances, staging is performed by the gynecologist removing the tumor. Staging provides the most reliable data for the prognosis of each particular tumor (see Figure 15-10).

The treatment of endometrial cancer requires a *hysterectomy,* which is removal of the affected uterus (in Greek, *hysteron* means "uterus" and *ectomy* means "removal"). If the tumor has metastasized to the lymph nodes, the gynecologist will resect as many enlarged lymph nodes as can be identified. Such lymph nodes are examined histologically to determine

whether they are involved by cancer. Radiation therapy and adjuvant chemotherapy are prescribed for patients with advanced disease.

LEIOMYOMA

Leiomyomas are benign tumors originating from the smooth muscle cells of the myometrium. Most myometrial tumors are benign; only 1% to 2% are malignant. These are called *leiomyosarcomas.* It seems that leiomyosarcomas originate *de novo* and not from preexisting benign tumors. Thus leiomyomas are not premalignant lesions and have no predilection to malignant transformation.

Leiomyomas are the most common uterine tumors. Approximately 20% of all women of reproductive age have leiomyomas, although in most instances these are small and clinically inapparent. Leiomyomas are not seen in prepubertal girls, and they do not develop after menopause. Those tumors that originate during the reproductive years but persist after menopause shrink in size because of a loss of smooth muscle cells. Only the stromal fibroblasts surrounded by collagen fibers remain, imparting to the tumors their firm consistency and whitish color. For such tumors the term *fibroids* (often used in clinical practice) is truly justified.

The symptoms of leiomyomas vary, depending primarily on their size and location (Figure 15-11). Small tumors are asymptomatic. Large and multiple tumors (especially those that are subserosal) produce a "mass effect" (i.e., symptoms related to the compression of the rectum and urinary bladder). Abdominal heaviness, urinary urgency, and constipation are commonly encountered. On the other hand, tumors located underneath the mucosa tend to grow into the endometrial

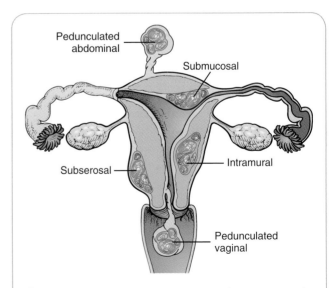

Pedunculated abdominal
Submucosal
Subserosal
Intramural
Pedunculated vaginal

Figure 15-11 Leiomyoma of the uterus. The tumors may be subserosal, intramural, or submucosal. Subserosal and submucosal tumors may be pedunculated and may protrude from the uterine surface or into the uterine cavity, respectively. The stalk of pedunculated tumors may also become twisted.

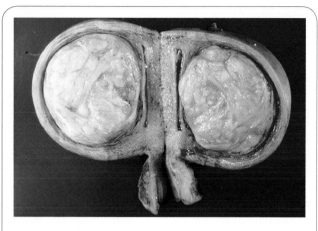

Figure 15-12 Leiomyoma of the uterus. The tumor fills the endometrial cavity and distends the uterus. On cross section the tumor has a whorled appearance.

cavity and cause menstrual irregularities and endometrial bleeding (Figure 15-12).

ENDOMETRIOSIS

The term **endometriosis** is used for foci of endometrial tissue that form tumorlike nodules outside the uterus. Currently most doctors think that these nodules of endometrium form from a retrograde menstrual flow, which brings the shedding endometrium into the peritoneal cavity. Endometriosis is most often located on the ovary or on the pelvic peritoneum, but occasionally it may be found outside the pelvis, even on the umbilicus (Figure 15-13).

The foci of endometriosis are composed of uterine glands and stroma. These glands respond to estrogenic stimulation and proliferate concomitantly with the normal endometrium in the first phase of the menstrual cycle, transforming into secretory glands in the second. At the time of menstruation, the glands degenerate and bleeding occurs. However, the blood cannot be discharged because the endometriotic foci are encased by normal connective tissue and peritoneum. The lesions grow during the proliferative phase and enlarge even more at the time of menstruation, when they become engorged by blood. The foci of endometriosis may persist for a long time, although in many cases the extravasated blood finally destroys the glands, transforming them into fibrotic scars impregnated with brown blood–derived pigment (hemosiderin).

Endometriosis is important for the following reasons:

- It is very common. It has been estimated that 15% to 20% of all women of reproductive age have endometriosis.
- The lesions expand during the menstrual cycle and are infiltrated with blood at the time of menstruation. This causes peritoneal irritation and pain. Suppression of menstruation (e.g., with contraceptive pills) alleviates the symptoms of endometriosis.
- Endometriosis causes infertility. The exact link between endometriosis and infertility is not understood, but the treatment of endometriosis may cure infertility in many women having both these problems.
- Endometriosis is a benign, self-limited disorder that does not progress to cancer. It is important to assure patients who have endometriosis that this is not a dangerous condition, although it may cause them considerable pain and discomfort.
- Ovarian endometriosis may present with relatively large cystic lesions measuring several centimeters in diameter. Typically cysts are filled with brownish-red viscous fluid derived from decomposed blood. These endometriotic cysts appear like tumors and are called *endometriomas,* or more colloquially, "chocolate cysts." Pain and discomfort are the

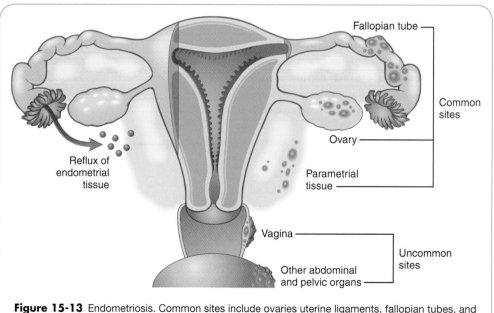

Figure 15-13 Endometriosis. Common sites include ovaries uterine ligaments, fallopian tubes, and pouch of Douglas; other sites are rarely involved.

most common reasons for their removal. The larger lesions resemble tumors on gynecologic examination.

TUMORS AND TUMOR-LIKE CONDITIONS OF THE OVARY

Neoplasms represent the most important pathologic lesions of the ovaries and deserve considerable attention. Nevertheless, we should not forget that there are other, non-neoplastic, conditions, such as cysts and endometriosis, that can enlarge the ovaries and that can be mistaken for tumors.

OVARIAN CYSTS

Cysts of the ovary are common. Remember that the ovarian follicles enlarge during the proliferative stage of the menstrual cycle and transform into graafian follicles. Only one graafian follicle ruptures at ovulation. Those follicles that have not ruptured may remain filled with follicular fluid and may further enlarge into fluid-filled follicular cysts. Similarly, if the ovulated follicle transforms into a corpus luteum but does not involute and transform into a fibrotic corpus albicans, its cavity could fill in with fluid and a corpus luteum cyst could form.

Most ovarian cysts are solitary. Ovaries that are bilaterally enlarged and studded with follicular cysts cause a functional disturbance known as **polycystic ovary syndrome (POS).** Originally it was thought that affected women did not ovulate because the cortical fibrous tissue did not allow the follicles to rupture. A surgical incision ("wedge resection of the ovary") was previously practiced under the assumption that it will allow the passage of oocytes through the fibrous cortical tissue. However, today we know that anovulation is not caused by anatomic abnormalities. Instead, these women have complex hormonal disturbances and do not ovulate, despite high output of gonadotropins from the pituitary. Furthermore, the persistent follicles also contribute to the hormonal imbalance.

Cortical stromal cells secrete androgens, causing masculinization (e.g., facial hair growth, acne, and body hirsutism). Infertility is the most important clinical complaint.

OVARIAN NEOPLASMS

Ovarian tumors form a complex group of benign and malignant lesions that belong to several subtypes. These can be divided on the basis of their cell of origin into four major groups, as follows (Figure 15-14):
- Tumors of the surface (germinal) epithelium
- Tumors of the germ cells
- Tumors of the sex cord stromal cells
- Nonspecific tumors of the ovarian stroma or metastases from other organs

The benign tumors are, fortunately, more common than the malignant ones. Nevertheless, a few important facts should be mentioned to understand the magnitude of the problem:
- Ovarian cancer is the second most common gynecologic cancer but is ranked first for death caused by gynecologic

cancer. It causes more deaths than all other tumors of the reproductive female tract.
- Ovarian cancer is the fourth most common cause of cancer in women.
- Approximately 22,000 new cases of ovarian cancer occur annually, and some 15,000 women die of ovarian cancer every year.

Etiology and Pathogenesis

Very little is known about the pathogenesis of ovarian tumors, especially the most common variety, which involve the surface epithelium. Nevertheless, from the available clinical data and the experimental models, it is possible to suggest several hypotheses that provide at least partial explanations for these neoplasms.

Surface epithelial cells, the most common progenitors of tumors in the ovary, are akin to the mesothelial cells lining the peritoneal surface of other abdominal organs. Nevertheless, ovarian cells are somewhat specialized and are probably developmentally distinct from other peritoneal lining cells. It is unknown how these cells become malignant. However, it is known that the surface epithelium of the ovary is ruptured at each ovulation and that this little wound heals by the proliferation of epithelial cells adjacent to the site of rupture. Apparently, these proliferating cells are at increased risk of becoming transformed into tumors than are the nonproliferating ones. Women who do not ovulate (e.g., those who have no oocytes, as in Turner's syndrome) do not develop ovarian cancer. Oral contraceptives suppress ovulation and reduce the risk of ovarian cancer. We should also mention that the best animal models for human ovarian cancer are hens. Egg-laying hens traumatize their ovarian surface epithelium in the same way that ovulating women do. If the hens are not slaughtered for human consumption but are allowed to age, many of them will develop ovarian cancer similar to human epithelial cancer.

Germ cell tumors originate from activated oocytes that have also undergone a neoplastic transformation. Tumors composed of cells that resemble gonocytes are called **dysgerminomas.** These malignant tumors are ovarian equivalents of testicular seminomas. Like their testicular counterparts, dysgerminomas occur most often in postpubertal young persons and are very radiosensitive.

Activated germ cells in the ovary may give rise to embryonic cells, which thereafter differentiate in various mature tissues and give rise to **teratomas.** There is considerable experimental evidence to show that this process corresponds to parthenogenetic activation of oocytes (in Greek, *parthenos* means "virgin" and *genesis* means "formation"). Recalling the information presented in most basic biology courses, you may remember that in many lower animals the female germ cell can become parthenogenetically activated without the fertilization that occurs following fusion with the sperm. Activated oocytes give rise to embryonic cells, which further develop, finally producing the entire organism. In mammals, parthenogenetically activated oocytes cannot progress so far and a fetus

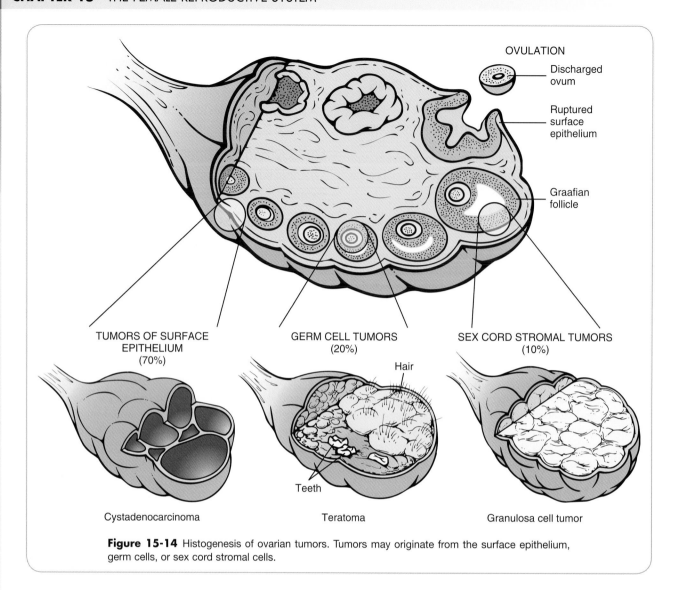

Figure 15-14 Histogenesis of ovarian tumors. Tumors may originate from the surface epithelium, germ cells, or sex cord stromal cells.

cannot be formed without the male gamete. Nevertheless, it has been shown in mice (and this probably occurs in women as well) that the parthenogenetically activated oocytes may form various normal embryonic structures that are found in ovarian teratomas.

If the embryonic cells formed from parthenogenetically activated oocytes become malignant, they will form malignant germ cell tumors. Such tumors are called **teratocarcinomas,** or *mixed germ cell tumors.* In most instances, the malignant stem cells of these malignant germ cell tumors are malignant embryonic cells—called **embryonal carcinoma** cells. In other instances, malignant germ cell tumors may contain malignant yolk sac epithelium or cells corresponding to placental trophoblasts, corresponding to cells found in the fetal membranes and placenta. These malignant cells can outgrow and destroy other tumor cells, and by the time such tumors are diagnosed, they are composed only of these extraembryonic structures. Tumors composed of yolk sac elements are called **yolk sac carcinomas.** Tumors composed of malignant trophoblastic cells (cytotrophoblastic and syncytiotrophoblastic cells) are called *choriocarcinomas.*

Sex cord stromal tumors are composed of cells resembling granulosa and theca cells of the graafian follicle or steroid-producing luteinized stromal cells. Under normal conditions, the function of these cells is controlled by pituitary gonadotropins. Tumors probably develop because of dysregulation of the hormonal conditions in the body. In experimental animals, granulosa and theca cell tumors can be induced by overstimulating the animals with gonadotropins or by combining the hormonal treatment with some chemical and viral carcinogens.

OVARIAN SURFACE EPITHELIAL TUMORS

Ovarian surface epithelial tumors are classified on the basis of their biologic features and whether they are benign or malignant. They can be further subclassified, on the basis of their histologic characteristics, into more specific categories (e.g., serous, mucinous, endometrioid). These classifications are rather complex and are usually hotly debated by pathologists and gynecologic oncologists. To simplify these complex issues, only the most salient features of epithelial ovarian tumors are presented here, as follows:

- Essentially almost all tumors of the surface epithelium of the ovary are adenomas or adenocarcinomas.
- On the basis of cell type and the nature of their secretion, the most common tumors are classified as serous, mucinous, or endometrioid. Serous tumors secrete clear fluid resembling serum, whereas those that are mucinous secrete mucin. Endometrioid tumors resemble endometrial glands and do not secrete anything. All other forms of ovarian epithelial tumors are rare.
- Serous and mucinous tumors are cystic, whereas endometrioid tumors are solid. From the gross appearance of the tumor and its content, one can tentatively classify most tumors. Histologic examination must be performed to determine whether the tumor is benign or malignant. If benign, the tumors are thus called serous or mucinous **cystadenoma**, and if malignant, **cystadenocarcinoma**.
- Serous and mucinous tumors are classified as benign, borderline malignant, or malignant. All endometrioid tumors are malignant.

If these facts are combined, then the tumors can be classified as seen in Table 15-4.

Serous tumors are the most common form. They often consist of several cysts lumped together within a common outer capsule. Serous tumors are benign in 60% of cases, borderline in 15%, and malignant in 25%. Approximately 30% of benign tumors and 60% of malignant tumors are bilateral. The malignant tumors often form papillae, and the cells tend to grow through the capsule of cysts (Figure 15-15). Malignant cells implant on the serosa of the peritoneal cavity and cause ascites.

Compared with serous tumors, mucinous tumors are more often benign and less commonly bilateral (10% to 30%). Most of these tumors are benign or borderline malignant; mucinous adenocarcinomas of the ovary are rare. The cavity of these tumors is filled with thick yellowish or white jellylike material (Figure 15-16).

Endometrioid carcinomas are solid malignant tumors. Histologically they are composed of glands that resemble endometrial glands. In about 20% of cases the clinical symptoms of ovarian surface epithelial tumors are relatively nonspecific. Because these small tumors do not produce symptoms, once they are recognized it is often too late for treatment. In about 20% of cases there is also a uterine tumor, suggesting that endometrial and ovarian tumors can arise at the same time or that a tumor involving one organ has metastasized to the other.

The prognosis of these tumors depends on the histologic diagnosis and the stage of disease (i.e., the extent of spread of the tumor). The primary role of the pathologist is to determine whether the tumor is benign, malignant, or of intermediate malignancy. Benign tumors have an excellent prognosis, and the 5-year survival is 100%. Borderline-malignant tumors also have a good prognosis, although their 5-year survival is somewhat lower than 85%.

Surgery and chemotherapy are of limited assistance, and the overall 5-year survival for malignant epithelial ovarian tumor is 10% to 40%, depending on the stage of the tumor.

GERM CELL TUMORS

Germ cell tumors account for 20% of all ovarian tumors. There are several histologic types (Table 15-5). The most important facts about ovarian tumors are as follows:

- Germ cell tumors occur predominantly in women younger than 25 years.
- The most common germ cell tumor of the ovary is benign cystic teratoma, which accounts for 95% of all these tumors.
- Overall, teratoma is the most common ovarian tumor in women younger than 25 years.
- Teratomas may contain teeth or calcified parts that can be recognized on radiographic studies.

However, they do not produce serologic markers. On the other hand, mixed germ cell tumors (teratocarcinomas) secrete alpha-fetoprotein (AFP) and hCG, which serve as serologic markers for these neoplasms and aid in their diagnosis. Pure yolk sac carcinomas secrete only AFP.

Teratoma presents as a cyst lined on the inside with hairy skin; thus they are often called **dermoid cysts.** The wall of the tumor contains other tissues, most often teeth and cartilage. The skin appendages, such as sebaceous and sweat glands, secrete sebum and sweat into the cavity. This remains there and decomposes into malodorous, mushy material. When the tumor is resected and the cavity is opened, the contents stink, the same way our skin would stink if it were not washed for a few years.

Teratomas are benign tumors that nevertheless should be resected. If they are left in place, the skin and the other tissues of its wall may gradually undergo malignant transformation. This usually occurs in older women; although it is rare, it should not occur at all if the woman is under appropriate gynecologic supervision.

SEX CORD STROMAL TUMORS

Sex cord stromal tumors originate from the specialized, ovarian stromal cells forming the follicles. They account for 5% of all ovarian tumors. Three tumor types are recognized: granulose cell tumors, theca cell tumors, and Sertoli-Leydig cell tumors.

TABLE 15-4 Ovarian Tumor Classification

Benign Lesions	Borderline-Malignant Lesions	Malignant Lesions
Serous cystadenoma	Serous tumor of borderline malignancy	Serous cystadenocarcinoma
Mucinous cystadenoma	Mucinous tumor of borderline malignancy	Mucinous cystadenocarcinoma
—	—	Endometrioid adenocarcinoma

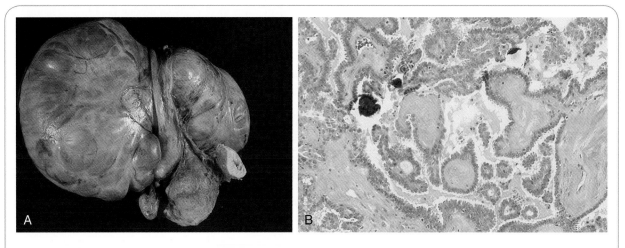

Figure 15-15 Serous cystadenocarcinoma of the ovary. *A,* External view of a bosselated tumor. The nodular surface corresponds to cysts filled with fluid. *B,* Histologic examination reveals that the cysts are lined by serous cuboidal epithelium. The same cells line the papillae that project into the lumen of the cavity. The dark material represents calcifications, which are common in these tumors.

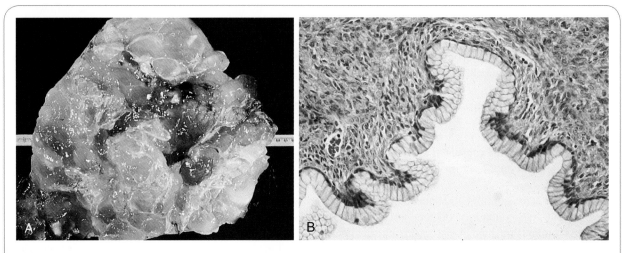

Figure 15-16 Mucinous cystadenoma of the ovary. *A,* The cysts are filled with mucin, a jellylike substance. *B,* Histologic examination reveals that the mucinous cells are filled with clear material (mucin) and have basally located nuclei.

TABLE 15-5 Germ Cell Tumors of the Ovary

Tumor Type	Gross Appearance	Histologic Findings	Serologic Markers
Teratoma	Cyst	Skin and other mature tissues, teeth, bones	None
Immature teratoma	Solid, soft mass	Neural tissue but may contain other fetal tissue as well	None
Teratocarcinoma (mixed germ cell tumor)	Solid	Embryonal carcinoma cells, various embryonic tissues, yolk sac, trophoblastic cells	AFP, hCG
Embryonal carcinoma	Solid	Embryonal carcinoma cells that do not differentiate	None; possibly AFP or hCG
Yolk sac carcinoma	Solid	Yolk sac–like structures	AFP
Choriocarcinoma	Solid, hemorrhagic	Cytotrophoblast and syncytiotrophoblast, like placental villi	hCG
Dysgerminoma	Solid	Clear cells surrounded by lymphocytes (like seminoma of testis)	None; slightly elevated hCG levels may be noted

AFP, alpha-fetoprotein; hCG, human chorionic gonadotropin.

Granulosa cell tumors are solid tumors composed of cells resembling the granulosa cells of the ovarian follicles. These tumors may be hormonally inactive or they may produce estrogens, thus causing menstrual irregularities. The small tumors are usually benign, but the larger ones may be malignant. However, even these grow slowly and are not too aggressive.

Thecomas, or theca cell tumors, are solid tumors that secrete estrogens. They are always benign and often cause menstrual irregularities and endometrial hyperplasia.

Sertoli-Leydig cell tumors are also solid tumors and are composed of hormonally active cells that secrete androgens and cause **virilization**. Typical signs are deepening of the voice, facial hair, male-pattern baldness, hairy chest and abdomen, and hypertrophy of the clitoris. Menstrual irregularities and infertility are signs of smaller tumors and those that are less active hormonally. Sertoli-Leydig cell tumors may be benign or malignant.

METASTASES

Metastases involving the ovaries originate most often from carcinomas of the endometrium and breast. These tumors often have estrogen receptors, which could explain their predilection for metastasizing to the ovaries. Tumors of the gastrointestinal tract also metastasize to the ovaries. Most notable among these is carcinoma of the stomach, which tends to produce bilateral enlargement of the ovaries. These are called **Krukenberg tumors** in honor of the pathologist who first described this form of metastasis.

Did You Know?

Did you ever her the term *jelly-belly*? This medical student term is used for a mucus-secreting tumor that has metastasized all over the peritoneum, filling the abdominal cavity with mucus ("jelly"). This condition, technically called pseudomyxoma peritonei, was thought to be a complication of ovarian mucinous tumors. Today we know that in most instances "jelly-belly" is actually caused by metastatic spread of tumors located in the appendix. Accordingly, all patients with malignant mucinous tumors of the ovary must be examined for a potential primary adenocarcinoma of the gastrointestinal tract.

PATHOLOGY OF PREGNANCY

Pregnancy may be disrupted or pathologically altered at several points in time. The pathology of pregnancy is discussed here in terms of abnormal fertilization, implantation, placentation, and maternofetal interaction.

PATHOLOGY OF FERTILIZATION

Fertilization marks the fusion of the sperm and ovum. The oocyte matures into an ovum in the graafian follicle and is expelled from the ovary into the abdominal cavity at the time

of ovulation. It then enters the fallopian tube, where it meets the spermatozoa. Normal fertilization occurs in the fallopian tube. The fertilized ovum (the zygote) travels to the uterus and implants into a receptive (i.e., properly hormonally primed) endometrium.

Four types of factors can prevent fertilization:
- Ovum-related factors
- Sperm-related factors
- Genital organ–related factors
- Systemic factors affecting the male or female partner

Did You Know?

Some ovarian germ cell tumors contain trophoblastic (placenta-like) cells that secrete human chorionic gonadotropin into the blood. Because this hormone of pregnancy is excreted in urine, the urine of women with such tumors will give a positive result on a commercial urinary pregnancy test. Similar testicular germ cell tumors can be a cause of a positive pregnancy test in men!

Ovum-Related Factors

Ovum-related factors are poorly understood. The ovum may be immature if meiotic division was incomplete. From the experience gained with *in vitro* fertilization, it is known that some women have "better" ova than others. The ova of older women are generally of inferior quality, but for unknown reasons, even mature, apparently normal ova of young women do not fertilize in 20% of cases.

Sperm-Related Factors

Sperm-related factors are also poorly understood. Sperm quality varies from one man to another. Some men produce no living spermatozoa *(azoospermia),* whereas others do not produce enough sperm *(oligospermia).* Still others have immotile spermatozoa or spermatozoa that do not swim fast enough and thus have a reduced capacity to penetrate the ovum.

Genital Organ Factors

Genital organ factors that prevent fertilization most often occur in women and are related to fallopian tube pathology and PID. It has been estimated that PID accounts for 30% of all causes of infertility in women. In such cases the fallopian tubes are occluded or deformed by chronic inflammation or adhesions, or they contain pus that prevents the normal union of the ovum and the spermatozoa. Even if fertilization does occur, many zygotes are killed by the inflammatory cells that permeate the tissues. Fortunately, women with PID usually have a normal capacity to produce oocytes. If these ova are surgically retrieved, they may be fertilized by the mate's sperm in a test tube. The zygotes thus formed *in vitro* are then transferred into the uterus, bypassing the abnormal fallopian tube.

Systemic Factors

Systemic factors causing infertility are poorly understood. The best known are immune mechanisms. Antibodies to spermatozoa or ova may prevent fertilization, implantation, or the development of the placenta.

PATHOLOGY OF IMPLANTATION

Following fertilization in the fallopian tube, the ovum travels into the uterus, where it implants approximately 6 days after ovulation. For this to happen, the uterus must be receptive—that is, it must be hormonally primed to accept the zygote. In women with hormonal problems, the uterus cannot accept the zygote and cannot provide support for the outgrowth and development of the embryo. Similarly, if there is chronic endometritis or intrauterine adhesions *(Asherman's syndrome),* implantation cannot take place. Endocrine defects are usually treated by hormonal replacement therapy, whereas intrauterine adhesions are generally removed by curettage or by intrauterine surgery with the guidance of a *hysteroscope* (an instrument used for inspection of the uterine cavity).

ECTOPIC PREGNANCY

Ectopic pregnancy is a term used to denote all forms of extrauterine pregnancies in which implantation occurs outside the uterus. This can occur in many locations, such as the ovary, fallopian tube, and even the abdominal cavity (Figure 15-17). Most ectopic pregnancies (95%) occur in the fallopian tubes;

less often they may involve the ovary or pelvic peritoneum. In most affected women the fallopian tube has been pathologically altered by PID, previous surgery, or foci of endometriosis. The intratubal adhesions located between the chronically inflamed mucosal folds form a barrier to normal passage of the zygote, and the zygote then implants at the site of obstruction. The trophoblast cells of the placenta that forms at the site of implantation penetrate the thin wall of the tube. It can erode the wall of some of the major vessels, causing bleeding, or it can destroy the muscle layer of the tube and rupture it. Rupture of a fallopian tube containing an ectopic pregnancy sac is a catastrophic event that requires immediate surgical intervention to prevent fatal hemorrhage.

PATHOLOGY OF PLACENTATION

The human placenta consists of a disk and chorionic amniotic membranes that together form the fetal sac. The fetus, which is attached to the placenta by the umbilical cord, floats within the sac in amniotic fluid.

PLACENTAL ANOMALIES

Placental anomalies include abnormalities in the size, shape, or function of the placenta and membranes, the placental cord, and the amniotic fluid. Most of these represent variations from normal that have no direct consequences on the outcome of pregnancy. For example, the placentae of twins are often multiple or segmented, but these variant forms are as efficient in supporting the fetuses as the classic placenta is.

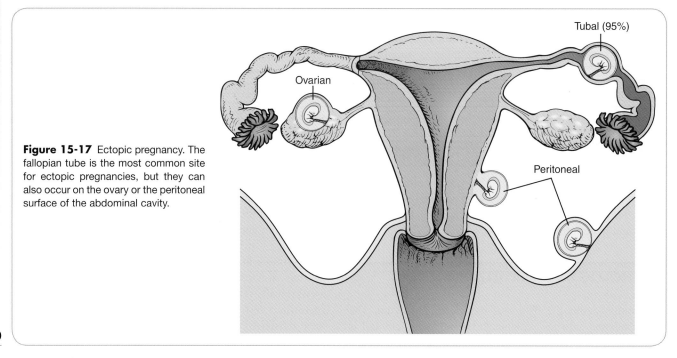

Figure 15-17 Ectopic pregnancy. The fallopian tube is the most common site for ectopic pregnancies, but they can also occur on the ovary or the peritoneal surface of the abdominal cavity.

PLACENTA ACCRETA

Placenta accreta is the result of deep penetration of the placental villi into the wall of the uterus. This usually occurs because the endometrial stroma does not undergo decidual transformation and does not form the so-called decidual membrane. This membrane provides the normal bedding for the placenta and limits the invasion of trophoblast into the uterus. In its absence the placenta extends into the muscularis. In such cases the placenta does not shell out spontaneously from the uterus at the time of birth, and this may cause extensive bleeding. Manual extraction of the placenta must be performed to remove it from the uterus after delivery.

PLACENTA PREVIA

Placenta previa is the result of implantation of the zygote in the lower segment of the uterus, with consequent positioning of the placental disk over the internal orifice of the cervix. Patients with this abnormality are prone to bleeding. Because the bleeding during vaginal delivery may endanger the fetus and the mother, cesarean section is usually performed.

ABORTION

Abortion is an interruption of pregnancy before the term of fetal viability, which, by convention, means a body weight of 500 g, or 20 weeks' gestation. *Spontaneous abortion* denotes abortions that do not have an identifiable cause; by contrast, *induced abortions* are those performed at the woman's request, usually by a gynecologist.

Spontaneous abortions may be further classified clinically as complete, threatened, incomplete, or missed. *Complete abortion* is when the fetus and placenta are expulsed and the woman resumes normal menstruation without any intervention. *Incomplete abortion* is one that is marked by cervical dilation and expulsion of some fetal parts and placenta, with others being retained. A *missed abortion* is characterized by the death of a fetus, which remains *in utero* for some time, usually several weeks. The macerated fetus must be evacuated surgically if it is not delivered spontaneously. *Threatened abortion* is a condition in which there is cervical bleeding but the cervix does not dilate, and the pregnancy may continue uneventfully.

It has been estimated that at least one third of all pregnancies end in spontaneous abortion. There are many possible causes of spontaneous abortion, but in most cases the real cause remains obscure. Developmental anomalies of the embryo and the placenta account for most cases.

GESTATIONAL TROPHOBLASTIC DISEASE

Abnormalities of placentation that lead to tumorlike changes in the placenta or placental malignant disease represent a spectrum of changes grouped together under the name of **gestational trophoblastic disease** (GTD). The trophoblast—the epithelium lining the placental villi—consists of two cell types: cytotrophoblastic and syncytiotrophoblastic cells. GTD is a disease that involves this epithelium, and it includes a spectrum of proliferative lesions. The benign form of GTD, marked by limited proliferation of the trophoblastic cells, is called **hydatidiform mole.** The malignant form of GTD is called *choriocarcinoma.*

HYDATIDIFORM MOLE

Hydatidiform mole is a placental abnormality that occurs in 1 of every 2000 pregnancies. It is marked by trophoblastic proliferation and hydropic degeneration of the chorionic villi. In the most common form—*complete mole*—the fetus cannot be identified in the amniotic sac. The *incomplete mole* usually has attached to it fetal parts and even partially preserved normal placental tissue.

It has been shown that complete hydatidiform moles result from abnormal fertilization (Figure 15-18). Normally the fetus and the placenta have 46 chromosomes, half of which have been inherited from the mother and the other half from the father. The cells of the complete mole have a 46,XX karyotype. However, all the chromosomes are of paternal origin. Apparently, at the time of fertilization, the maternal chromosomes are lost from the zygote on which the paternal 23,X set of chromosomes reduplicates, bringing the number of chromosomes to 46. This process is called *androgenesis.* Without the maternal chromosomes, the embryo proper cannot develop and the placenta undergoes hydropic degeneration.

The incomplete moles evolve from oocytes fertilized with two spermatozoa; therefore the cells have 69 chromosomes—one set from the mother and two sets from the father. This

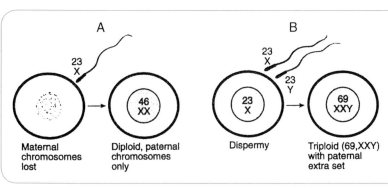

Figure 15-18 Pathogenesis of hydatidiform mole. *A,* Complete hydatidiform mole results from androgenesis, in which the maternal chromosomes are lost and all the chromosomes in the fertilized ovum are of paternal origin. *B,* Partial mole results from the entry of two sperms into the oocyte. (From Damjanov I: Pathology Secrets, 3rd ed, Philadelphia, 2008, Mosby.)

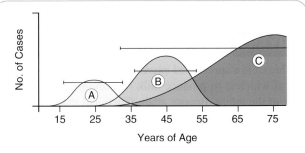

Figure 16-2 Age-related incidence of various breast diseases. *A,* Fibroadenoma is a disease of young women, with a peak incidence in the twenties. *B,* Fibrocystic change affects women of reproductive age, typically increasing in incidence after the age of 30 years. *C,* The incidence of breast cancer increases sharply after the age of 45 years and peaks in postmenopausal women.

OVERVIEW OF MAJOR DISEASES

The most important diseases affecting the breast can be categorized as follows:

- Tumors
- Hormonally induced changes
- Inflammatory diseases

Some hormonal and neoplastic diseases may be interrelated.

Several facts pertaining to diseases of the breast should be kept in mind:

1. *Breast diseases predominantly affect females.* This does not mean that males do not have breast diseases, but in comparison with females, such diseases are relatively rare. This point is best illustrated by the fact that for every breast cancer diagnosed in men, there are 100 such carcinomas diagnosed in women.

2. *The breast consists of cells and tissues that respond to hormones.* Normal female breasts swell and become tense or even painful before the onset of menstruation. Hormonal disturbances of the pituitary and ovary, including the effect of exogenous hormones injected into the body, also affect the breast and may even modify pathologic processes in the breast. Some breast cancers, like normal cells, express hormone receptors and respond to steroid hormones. Blocking the estrogen receptors on cancer cells may slow the growth of tumors.

3. *Each age group of women is affected by different breast diseases* (Figure 16-2). **Fibroadenomas,** which are benign tumors of the breast, occur mostly in postpubertal girls and young women. Fibrocystic disease is most prevalent in middle-aged women. Breast cancer is most common in older women.

4. *The functional status of the breast predisposes this organ to different diseases.* For example, acute inflammation (acute *mastitis*) is almost exclusively found in lactating women.

5. *Some breast diseases show racial differences.* For example, breast cancer is less common in Japanese women than in white women.

6. *Cancer is the most important disease affecting the breast.* Next to lung cancer, breast cancer is the most common malignant tumor in women. At present, 1 woman in 9 in the United States will develop breast cancer during her life span.

Because of the high incidence of breast cancer and the significant mortality of this malignant disease, it is important to take all possible measures to diagnose this tumor. However, one should remember that not all breast masses are cancerous. Malignant lesions must be distinguished from benign ones, which also produce breast lumps. The final distinction between benign and malignant lesions can be made only by cytologic or histologic examination of breast tissue. Many breast nodules turn out to be benign, but that does not mean that the biopsy should not have been performed. Benign lesions, such as fibrocystic disease and fibroadenoma, account for approximately 50% of all breast masses that are subjected to surgical biopsy; the remainder are malignant.

DEVELOPMENTAL ANOMALIES

Developmental anomalies of the breast are rare and are usually only of cosmetic significance. *Amastia* refers to congenital absence of the breast. *Polymastia* denotes conditions in which more than two breasts have developed. *Supernumerary breasts* can occur, usually along the milk line (as one would find in cats and dogs). *Polythelia* is a condition in which there are supernumerary nipples without glands. *Accessory breast tissue* without a nipple may occasionally be found in the axilla. Such nodules are composed of normal tissue and should not be confused with tumors.

INFLAMMATION OF THE BREAST

Like any other part of the body, breast tissue may be invaded by microbes that can cause infection, accompanied with typical signs of inflammation. Inflammation of the breast is called **mastitis.** It may be acute or chronic.

Acute mastitis is the most important and the most common inflammatory disease of the breast. It affects approximately 10% of women who are lactating. Typically, it is caused by purulent bacteria, such as *Staphylococcus* or *Streptococcus*. The microbes invade the breast through the dilated milk ducts or through skin lacerations or minor injuries acquired during suckling (Figure 16-3). Stagnant milk in breasts that have not been fully emptied by suckling provides a good growth medium for the bacteria.

Acute inflammation may spread through the entire breast or cause a localized abscess to form. In either case the lesion develops quickly and causes localized or diffuse swelling of the breast. The inflamed area appears red, is painful, and is sensitive to palpation.

The entire area is edematous and, histologically, is infiltrated with numerous acute inflammatory cells, mostly polymorphonuclear leukocytes (PMNs). The excretory ducts may contain pus, and if massive suppuration occurs in conjunction with destruction of tissue, an abscess will develop. However, this does not usually happen if acute mastitis is recognized early and the lesion is properly treated. Breast feeding should be continued because mastitis does not pose a health problem for the infant. In most cases, drainage of the inflammatory exudate can be achieved through the ducts, thereby alleviating the problem. If infection persists, antibiotics may be indicated. Only in the worst cases is a surgical incision required to release pus from an abscess.

Chronic mastitis is a rare disease, the causes of which are unknown. Because it produces small lumps in the breast and may mimic cancer, affected patients occasionally undergo biopsy. In such cases the biopsy sample is submitted for histologic diagnosis by pathologists. Chronic mastitis does not require any additional treatment.

HORMONALLY INDUCED CHANGES

The epithelial cells lining the ducts and acini of the breast, as well as the intralobular connective tissue, respond to sex hormones during the normal menstrual cycle. After menopause, when the ovaries cease secreting estrogens, the breasts undergo atrophy and shrivel. The fact that atrophy can be prevented by administering estrogen to older women shows that the breasts are sensitive to estrogens and progesterone throughout the life span.

PUBERTAL CHANGES

At the time of puberty the breasts enlarge under the influence of sex hormones. Excessive response of the breast tissue to estrogens causes enormous enlargement of the breast in some women. This usually affects only one breast, suggesting an abnormal local tissue response rather than an excess of hormones. This condition is called **juvenile hyperplasia** of the breast, or virginal hyperplasia. Reduction mammoplasty, a procedure designed to remove excess tissue, may be performed for cosmetic purposes to equalize the size of the breasts.

GYNECOMASTIA

Male breasts do not develop and do not enlarge at the time of puberty. However, in some boys, the hormonal changes associated with puberty may cause breast enlargement secondary

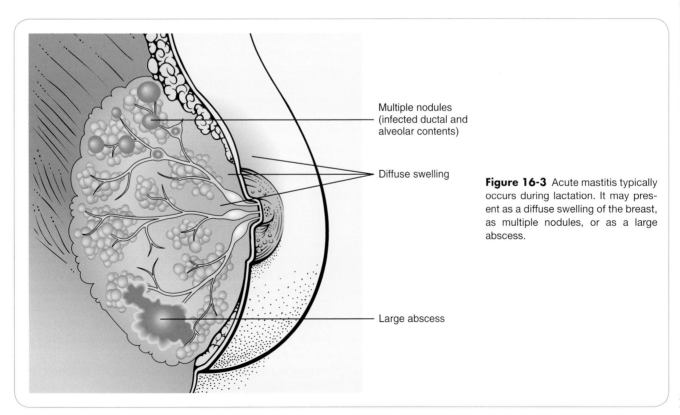

Multiple nodules (infected ductal and alveolar contents)

Diffuse swelling

Large abscess

Figure 16-3 Acute mastitis typically occurs during lactation. It may present as a diffuse swelling of the breast, as multiple nodules, or as a large abscess.

to an inordinate proliferation of the excretory ducts and the surrounding connective tissue. This is called **gynecomastia** (derived from the Greek words *gyne,* meaning "woman," and *mastos,* meaning "breast"). Female-like enlargement of the male breast may also occur in adult life, usually as a result of an excess of estrogens. Estrogen-secreting tumors, such as adrenal tumors or Leydig cell tumor of the testis, are a well-known cause of gynecomastia. The relative excess of estrogen that can accompany cirrhosis of the liver, especially in alcoholic patients, also may cause gynecomastia. Gynecomastia may be related to reduced testosterone production and is found in men with Klinefelter's syndrome or pituitary hypogonadism. Some drugs, such as cimetidine (used in the treatment of peptic ulcer), may cause male breast enlargement. In 25% of cases the cause of gynecomastia cannot be identified.

FIBROCYSTIC CHANGE

Fibrocystic change is a term used to describe fibrosis and cysts—that is, the reactive and degenerative changes that occur in the breasts of some adult women. Previously these changes were considered signs of a specific disease and were collectively referred to as *fibrocystic disease.* This term is no longer used for these changes, which are partially consequences of hormonal stimulation and inappropriate tissue reaction of the breast and partially the results of changes related to aging.

Histologic signs indicative of fibrocystic change are found in approximately 50% of all women whose breasts are examined at biopsy or autopsy. Clinical signs of fibrocystic change are less common; indeed, it is estimated that only 10% to 15% of women between 20 and 50 years of age have symptoms pertaining to fibrocystic change. Fibrocystic change does not occur before puberty, and it is unusual to diagnose the onset of fibrocystic change clinically in postmenopausal women. Women who have symptoms related to fibrocystic disease report gradual improvement after menopause and a flair up of symptoms if placed on estrogen replacement therapy. Even though oral contraceptives contain estrogens, many women of reproductive age notice fewer symptoms while taking oral contraceptives.

Pathogenesis

The exact pathogenesis of fibrocystic changes in the breasts is not known. Authorities agree that the changes are hormonally induced, and most believe that they result from an altered response of breast tissue to cyclical hormonal changes that normally occur during the menstrual cycle. As mentioned earlier, the TDLUs respond to estrogen and progesterone by enlarging toward the end of the menstrual cycle and decreasing in size at the time of menstruation, when the blood concentration of sex hormones decreases. Fibrocystic changes develop in the breast parenchyma if (1) the hormonal cyclicity is disturbed, (2) the proliferation of ducts continues unopposed and no involution occurs, or (3) the hormone-responsive intralobular stroma is replaced by hormone-insensitive dense collagenous fibrous tissue. The ensuing pathologic changes may include dense

fibrosis, cystic dilation of the ducts, and various ductal proliferative changes.

The most constant feature of fibrocystic change is fibrosis. In this condition the loose intralobular connective tissue of the breast is typically replaced by dense connective tissue that is rich in collagen but unresponsive to hormones (Figure 16-4). The border between the intralobular and interlobular connective tissue becomes indistinct. The breast consists of dense, broad sheets of collagenous tissue, and the loose connective tissue of the lobules is not visible.

The ductal epithelium, which retains its responsiveness to hormones, continues to proliferate even though the surrounding stroma is hormone insensitive. These dilated ducts may become entrapped by the connective tissue strands, leading to formation of *cysts.* The cells lining these cysts continue to secrete fluid that cannot be discharged because of fibrous tissue obstruction. This further enlarges the cysts. At the same time, the interruption of blood supply caused by fibrous strands causes degenerative changes, necrosis, and subsequent calcification of the stroma.

The epithelial cells of the breast ducts retain the capacity to respond to hormonal stimuli. Because the epithelium and the surrounding intralobular stroma are in a delicate balance and the stroma directly or indirectly regulates the proliferation and maturation of the epithelium, the ducts that are devoid of their normal surroundings may proliferate in an unregulated manner, giving rise to *sclerosing adenosis.* If the epithelial proliferation predominates, **proliferative breast disease** develops.

Pathology

As the name *fibrocystic change* implies, two constant features of this condition are fibrosis and cysts. The third component of this change, which is not reflected in the name but is almost always present, is *epithelial proliferation.* This proliferative breast disease includes ductal budding and crowding of ductules, known as **sclerosing adenosis,** and small papillary projections **(papillomatosis).**

Larger papillomas may form, protruding into the lumen of larger ducts. More than 80% of large duct papillomas produce a nipple discharge or bleeding.

Clinical Features

Fibrocystic changes usually affect both breasts. Because the changes are asymmetric, however, patients may complain mostly of one-sided pain, nodularity, and sensitivity on palpation. Careful palpation will usually reveal fine nodularity, which imparts a stringlike consistency to both breasts. Small lumps that fluctuate (corresponding to fluid-filled cysts) are also easily palpated. Mammography may reveal condensed areas, cysts, and even areas of calcification. Because calcific areas are occasionally indistinguishable from those seen in cancer, biopsy examination is the only safe way to establish a definitive diagnosis.

Typical fibrocystic change does not require treatment. Proliferative changes without atypia and papillomas are associated

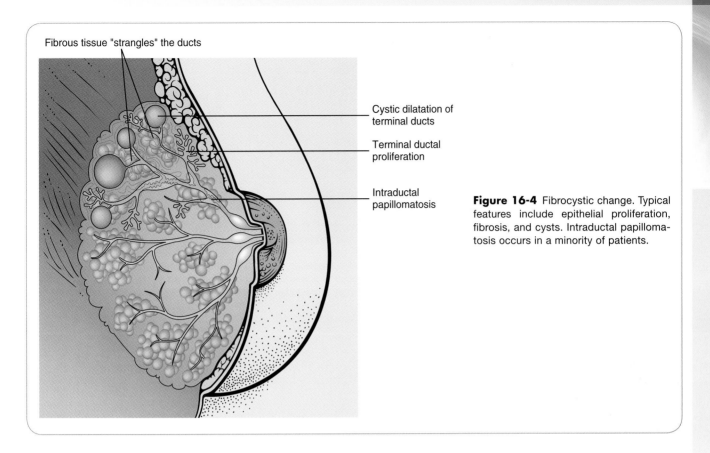

Fibrous tissue "strangles" the ducts

Cystic dilatation of terminal ducts

Terminal ductal proliferation

Intraductal papillomatosis

Figure 16-4 Fibrocystic change. Typical features include epithelial proliferation, fibrosis, and cysts. Intraductal papillomatosis occurs in a minority of patients.

with a 1.5- to 2-fold increase in risk for subsequent cancer. Thus if the woman is concerned or the lesion contains mammographically visible calcifications and other signs that are potentially of concern, a limited resection of the breast tissue in the form of a *lumpectomy* may be performed.

PROLIFERATIVE BREAST DISEASE WITH ATYPIA

In approximately 5% to 15% of women who have the characteristic palpatory features of fibrocystic change accompanied by calcifications on mammography, breast biopsy shows atypical ductal hyperplasia or atypical lobular hyperplasia. Overall these changes are relatively rare and are found only in 5% of all breast biopsies.

Pathology

Atypical ductal or lobular hyperplasia are changes that have some of the cellular and histologic features of carcinoma **in situ** but do not meet the strict criteria for making the definitive diagnosis of malignancy. For example, atypical ductal hyperplasia involves fewer ducts than ductal carcinoma *in situ*, and the ducts that are involved are not entirely filled with atypical cells. Likewise, the cells forming lobular atypical hyperplasia resemble those in lobular carcinoma *in situ* but do not fill more than 50% of lobules and, generally speaking, form only small groups.

Drugs, such as estrogen antagonist tamoxifen, or lumpectomy, may reduce the risk of cancer; even without treatment 80% of women will not develop cancer.

BENIGN TUMORS

Fibroadenoma is the most important and most common of the benign tumors of the breast. Typical tumors measure 2 to 5 cm in diameter and are well encapsulated, round, and lobulated. As the name implies, the tumor is composed of two components: fibrous stroma and glandular epithelium (Figure 16-5). The fibroblastic component of the tumor corresponds to the hormone-sensitive intralobular connective tissue, whereas the glands represent excretory ducts.

Fibroadenomas primarily affect young women (see Figure 16-2). Because they consist of hormonally sensitive cells, it has been hypothesized that the tumors represent an abnormal exaggerated response of breast tissue to sex hormones. These well-encapsulated and sharply demarcated tumors can be shelled out and are removed easily by surgeons without serious consequences. Fibroadenomas do not recur and do not undergo malignant transformation; therefore they have an excellent prognosis.

Another tumor composed of epithelial and stromal cells is **phyllodes tumor.** In contrast to fibroadenomas, the stroma of phyllodes tumors is hypercellular, and in 10% of cases it may

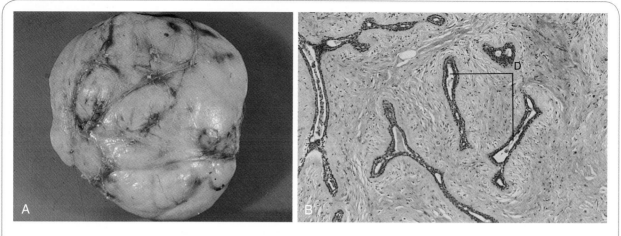

Figure 16-5 Fibroadenoma. *A,* This tumor, which was shelled out from the breast, appears to be well encapsulated and smooth. *B,* Histologic features of fibroadenoma include elongated ducts (D) surrounded by connective tissue stroma that is similar to the loose, intralobular connective tissue in the normal breast.

be overtly malignant. Phyllodes tumors may be diagnosed in women of any age, but most are found in women over 40 years of age. Typically, these tumors are well circumscribed and can be removed with ease. Malignant phyllosed tumors are rare. They require a more extensive resection to prevent local recurrence and even metastatic spread of such tumors.

MALIGNANT TUMORS

Carcinoma of the breast is the most important breast tumor. The following statistics illustrate the public health impact of breast cancer in the United States:

- Breast cancer is the most common cancer in women, surpassed in lethality only by lung cancer.
- Estimates are that 1 woman in 9 will develop breast cancer during her life span (Figure 16-6).
- At least 210,000 new cases of breast cancer are diagnosed each year. The number of new cases is increasing steadily.
- Approximately 40,000 women die of breast cancer every year.

Etiology and Pathogenesis

The cause of breast cancer is unknown. However, several important risk factors for breast cancer have been identified. The most significant leads point to hormonal and genetic etiologic influences. The search for these carcinogenic factors has led to discovery of tumor suppressor genes, which play a critical role in breast cancer. These genes, known as ***BRCA1*** and ***BRCA2,*** account for 20% of familial breast cancers, or 3% of all breast cancers. *BRCA1* and *BRCA2* mutations are found at a rate of 1 in 200 to 400 women and account for 30% of breast cancers in women under the age of 45 years. However, these tumor suppressor genes are not involved with nonfamilial breast cancer, the etiology of which remains enigmatic.

Breast cancer has been studied in experiments on animals, which have provided important clues to the pathogenesis of

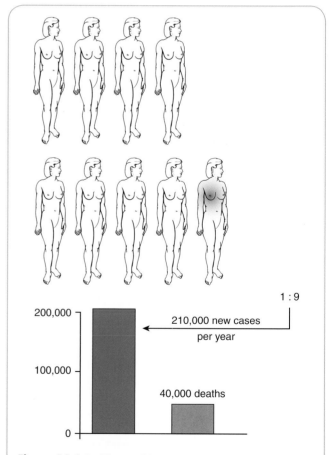

Figure 16-6 Incidence of breast cancer. Breast cancer is the second most common cancer in women. Approximately 210,000 new cases are diagnosed every year in the United States. Approximately 40,000 women die of breast cancer each year. One woman in nine will develop breast cancer during her lifetime.

human tumors. Breast cancer–inducing *viruses* have been identified in mice, and it is possible that similar viruses exist in humans, although none of them has been identified so far. Similarly, chemical carcinogens are known to induce breast cancer in rats, which makes it plausible that some human breast cancers are related to chemicals. *Hormonal factors* have also been found to be important in the pathogenesis of breast tumors in laboratory animals. In humans the evidence for the hormonal influences is based mostly on epidemiologic data, which indicate that estrogens promote breast cancer formation. Oral contraceptives do not change the risk.

Risk Factors

The most important risk factors of breast cancer identified thus far are as follows:

- *Sex.* Females are affected 100 times more often than males.
- *Age.* Breast cancer is very rare before puberty and unusual in young women under the age of 30 years. The incidence slowly rises after the age of 35 years and peaks in postmenopausal women who are about 60 years of age. Only 20% to 30% of women are less than 50 years at the time of diagnosis.
- *Race and ethnicity.* The risk of breast cancer varies among races. In the United States, for women ages 50 to 70, the risk is 1 in 15 for non-Hispanic whites, 1 in 20 for African Americans, 1 in 26 for Asians/Pacific Islanders, and 1 in 27 for Hispanics. The prevalence of *BRCA1* and *BRCA2* mutations also shows racial and ethnic differences.
- *Genetic predisposition.* Breast cancer occurs more often in some families. If a mother had or has breast cancer, all daughters have an increased risk, especially if the cancer was diagnosed at an early age and several first-degree relatives have breast cancer. Nevertheless, more than 85% of all women with a family history of breast cancer will not develop such tumors.
- *Hormonal factors.* Many clinical and epidemiologic data indicate that sex hormones play an important role in the pathogenesis of breast cancer. Thus women who are exposed to estrogen for prolonged periods are more likely to develop breast cancer than those who are not. It is well known that breast cancer is more common in women who have an early menarche and late menopause and are therefore under the influence of ovarian sex hormones for a prolonged period. Similarly, nulliparous women are at greater risk for breast cancer than those who have numerous children, presumably because pregnancy interrupts the cyclic secretion of ovarian estrogen. Resection of ovaries before the age of 35 years considerably lowers the risk of breast cancer; however, oophorectomy at a later age does not reduce the risk. Postmenopausal hormone supplementation, on the other hand, increases the risk. Finally, it should be noted that many breast tumors have estrogen receptors; the growth of these cells can be slowed by synthetic antiestrogens, which also points to an important role for hormones in breast cancer.

- *Presence of other cancers.* The incidence of breast cancer is increased in women who have cancer in the other breast and in those who have ovarian or endometrial cancer. It is possible that all these cancers are hormonally induced, occurring in women in whom there is hyperestrinism or dysregulation of the pituitary-ovarian axis. However, some ovarian cancers are related to *BRCA1* or *BRCA2* and occur in families that have mutations of these tumor suppressor genes. Approximately 1% of all breast cancers occur in women with the familial cancer Li-Fraumeni syndrome, characterized by the mutation of *TP53* tumor suppressor gene and multiple organ neoplasia.
- *Premalignant breast changes.* Papillomatosis and atypical intraductal or lobular hyperplasia are premalignant changes that occur in the breasts of some women. Some atypical intraductal or lobular lesions will progress to invasive carcinoma during a period of several years, but 80% of women will not develop cancer.

The most important risk factors are summarized in Table 16-1 and Table 16-2.

TABLE 16-1 Risk Factors for Breast Cancer

Risk Factor	Low Risk	High Risk
Sex	Male	Female
Age (years)	<30	>45
Race	East Asians	Whites (especially Jews)
Family history	—	Mother or sister with breast cancer
Reproductive history	Multiparity Breastfeeding Pregnancy at an early age	Early menarche Late menopause No children (nulliparity) Late age at first pregnancy

TABLE 16-2 Risk Factors for Breast Cancer Associated with Other Breast Lesions or Cancers of Other Organs*

Fibrocystic change	1x
Proliferative breast disease without atypia	1.2–2x
Atypical ductal and lobular hyperplasia	45x
Ductal carcinoma *in situ*	8–10x
Cancer of the contralateral breast	10x
Ovary	8–10x
Uterus	8–10x

*The average risk is 1, and the increased risk is given as multiples of this average (x).

Pathology

Most malignant breast tumors are of epithelial origin and are therefore classified as carcinomas. Histologically, there are several subtypes of **breast carcinoma,** but 80% are classified as **invasive ductal carcinomas.** Other histologic subtypes of ductal carcinoma, such as medullary, mucinous, or tubular carcinoma, are less common. This is unfortunate because these subtypes have a somewhat better prognosis than infiltrating duct carcinomas. In 10% of cases tumors originate from the intralobular epithelium and are called **invasive lobular carcinomas.**

Invasive (infiltrating) ductal and lobular carcinomas of the breast are preceded by a preinvasive stage called **ductal carcinoma *in situ*** (DCIS) and lobular carcinoma *in situ* (LCIS), respectively. Once the tumor cells invade across the basement membrane delimiting the normal ducts and acini from the stroma, they transform into invasive adenocarcinomas that are accompanied by a very strong desmoplastic reaction (*desmos* meaning "connection" in Greek, and *desmoplastic reaction* meaning "a connective tissue stromal reaction to the tumor"). Because of this dense connective tissue, the tumors appear firm and gritty on sectioning and are also called **scirrhous carcinomas** (Figure 16-7). The dense connective tissue pulls on the adjacent tissue, causing puckering of the skin and retraction of the nipple, which are typical signs of a malignant breast lesion. On palpation, these tumors are firm. They do not have sharp margins, because they infiltrate into the surrounding tissues.

Most breast carcinomas (50%) occur in the upper lateral quadrant and less commonly in other quadrants (Figure 16-8).

Approximately 20% of breast cancers are central, underneath the areola.

Breast cancer tends to metastasize via the lymphatics. Because most lymph ducts drain into the axillary lymph nodes, it is to be expected that most metastases are found in the axillary area. Medially or centrally located tumors may spread into the internal mammary lymph nodes. From the lymph nodes, the tumor cells enter the blood circulation and are carried away hematogenously to all major organs. Distant metastases are common in the lungs, liver, bones, brain, and adrenals (see Figure 16-8).

Clinical Features

Carcinoma of the breast presents as a mass lesion. Typically (in 80% to 90% of cases), the lump is detected by self-examination, by palpation in the doctor's office, or by mammography. It may be of any size, often measuring 1 cm to several centimeters in diameter. Occasionally it is associated with enlarged axillary lymph nodes. Other modes of presentation are less common (Table 16-3). Tumors spreading through the ducts may invade the epithelium of the nipple or cause dimpling of the skin, known under the French name *peau d'orange* (orange peel).

Breast self-examination is very important for breast cancer diagnosis. The American Cancer Society recommends the procedure of self-examination outlined in Figure 16-9 for all women.

A complete physical examination of females must, in all instances, include palpation of the breasts. The breasts must be inspected and palpated routinely, with special emphasis on the detection of minor and major irregularities in texture, consistency, and shape. Any patient with suspicious masses or nodules should undergo breast biopsy.

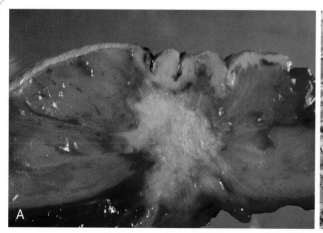
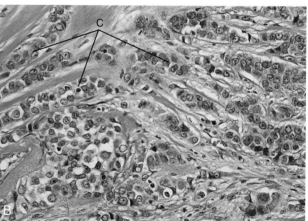

Figure 16-7 Breast carcinoma. *A,* On gross inspection, the tumor appears to be grayish-white as a result of the abundance of connective tissue between the tumor cells. Such desmoplastic tumors are firm and gritty on sectioning. *B,* Histologic appearance of an infiltrating duct carcinoma of the breast. Note the groups and strands of cancer cells (C) surrounded by abundant collagenous connective tissue that stains pink.

? Did You Know?

Despite all the attempts to make women more aware of breast cancer and to encourage them to seek medical assistance as soon as they note any abnormalities on breast self-examination, many women still ignore such advice. As shown in this photograph, some women present with advanced cancer.

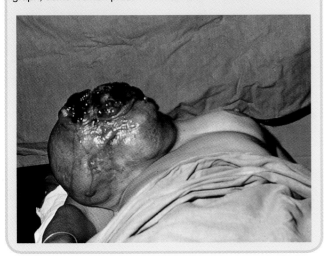

TABLE 16-3 Clinical Presentation of Breast Cancer

Mode of Diagnosis or Presentation	Incidence	
Breast mass discovered by palpation	+++	80%–90%
Asymptomatic tumor discovered by mammography	++	
Pain (mastodynia, or painful breast mass)	+	10%–20%
Nipple retraction, eczematoid reaction, or discharge	+	
Distant metastases	+	

+++, very common; ++, common; +, less common (10% or less).

Mammography is a specialized x-ray technique that allows detailed examination of the breast with low-density radiographs. Tumor masses can be detected in early stages of development, even before they have reached a size that can be palpated (Figure 16-10). Indeed, the smallest tumors that can be detected by palpation are 2 to 2.5 cm in diameter,

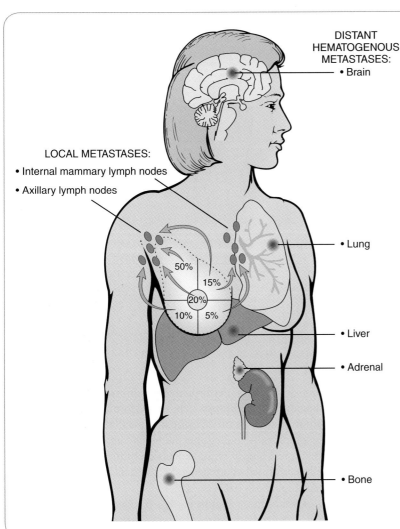

Figure 16-8 The distribution of breast carcinoma in the breast and the pathway of lymphatic metastasis. Most tumors are found in the upper lateral quadrant (50%). The next most common site is the subareolar region beneath the nipple (20%). Most tumors metastasize to the axillary lymph nodes. Medially located tumors may metastasize to the internal mammary lymph nodes. In addition to lymph node metastases, tumors tend to metastasize to the lungs, liver, brain, bones, and adrenals.

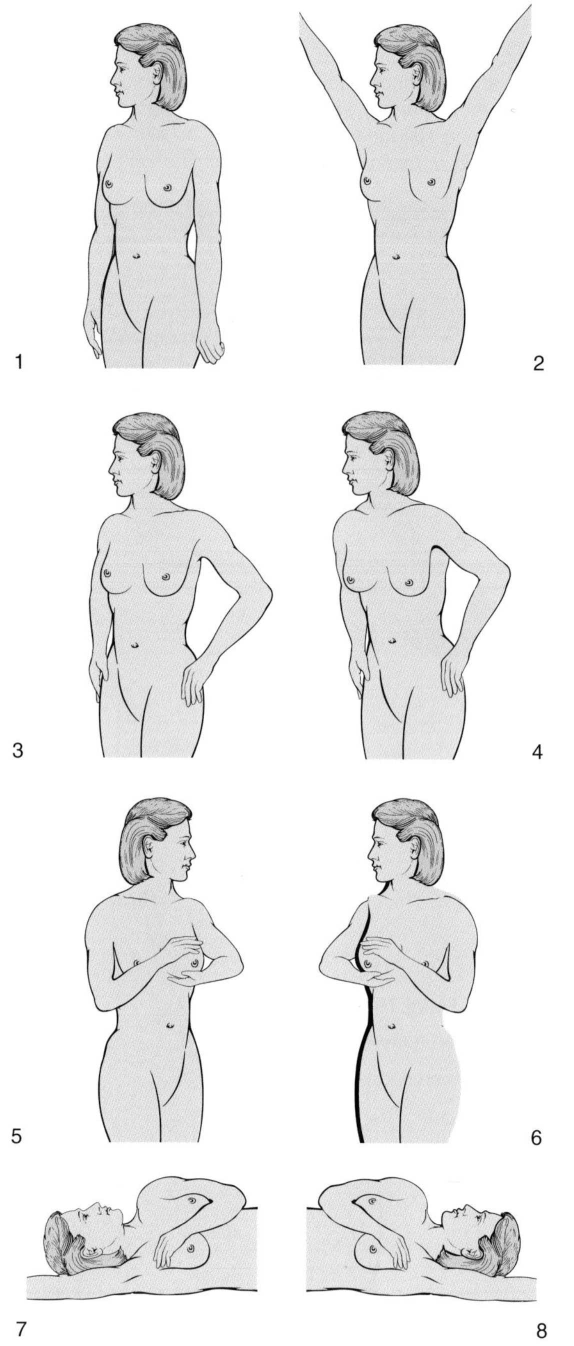

Figure 16-9 Breast self-examination. While in an upright position, stand in front of a mirror and inspects the breasts in the normal position.

1. Stand in front of the mirror and observe the breast for any lumps, swelling, irregularities, or marked asymmetry.
2. Raise your arms above your head.
3. Place your hands on your hips.
4. Flex your shoulders forward.
5. Then cradle the left breast and gently feel it with the fingers of the opposite hand.
6. Repeat this palpation on the right side.
7. While lying on your side, with your right hand stretched above your head, palpate the right breast with the fingers of your left hand.
8. Reverse your position and repeat this step, this time palpating the left breast.

whereas by mammography one can detect lesions measuring less than 0.5 cm. Such lesions are typically recognized as an area of increased density on the radiograph, and often, calcifications are detected within them. The American Cancer Society recommends that mammographies be performed at regular intervals in all women older than 40 years. Today mammography represents the best approach for early diagnosis of breast cancer.

If a lump is detected on self-examination or by a doctor or nurse or if an abnormality is seen on mammography, a breast biopsy should be performed to obtain material for pathologic diagnosis. The **biopsy** can be performed in an outpatient clinic or doctor's office using the so-called stereotactic (mammographically guided) needle biopsy under local anesthesia. A surgical biopsy requires incision of the skin; thus it is usually performed under general anesthesia in an operating room (see Figure 16-10).

Each of these approaches has its advantages and disadvantages. A needle biopsy specimen is relatively small, but even with this approach one can reach the diagnosis in almost all

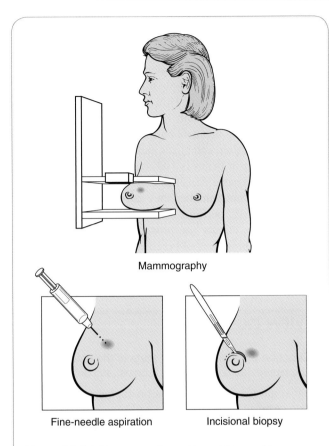

Mammography

Fine-needle aspiration   Incisional biopsy

Figure 16-10 Mammography and breast biopsy. Mammography is a noninvasive, usually painless procedure that is easily performed with a special x-ray machine. Fine-needle aspiration biopsy of the breast requires only local anesthesia and is simple to perform. Surgical breast biopsy is performed in the operating room, usually under general anesthesia.

lymph node does not find microscopic metastases, there is no need for further lymph node dissection. However, if the tumor has spread to the sentinel lymph node, additional lymph nodes must be removed from the axilla in an attempt to remove as much tumor tissue as possible. Final staging of the tumor is performed on the basis of the gross appearance of the tumor and the extent of its spread to local lymph nodes and distant organs, which are usually examined radiologically.

The prognosis of breast cancer depends on the stage of the disease (Figure 16-11).

- **Stage 0** which includes preinvasive cancers (DCIS), has a 92% 5-year survival rate.
- **Stage I** cancer includes relatively small, localized tumors (less than 2 cm in diameter) without any distant metastases. Surgical removal of the tumor is associated with an 87% 5-year survival rate.
- **Stage II** tumors measure more than 2 cm but less than 5 cm in diameter. There may be local metastases in one to three lymph nodes, but there is no evidence of distant spread. The 5-year survival rate in these patients is 75%.
- **Stage III** tumors measure more than 5 cm in diameter, with or without regional spread but without distant metastases. It also includes tumors smaller than 5 cm with more than four lymph node metastases and any tumor that has spread to the skin and the chest wall. The 5-year survival rate is 45%.
- **Stage IV** tumors may be of any size; they may or may not be associated with local metastases in the lymph nodes, but

cases. The biopsy provides enough tissue for proper classification and grading of tumors but cannot be used for the staging of the tumor.

The treatment of breast cancer includes surgical resection of the primary tumor and any metastases, radiation therapy, and chemotherapy. Tumors composed of cells that express estrogen receptors are also treated with synthetic antiestrogens. Many larger tumors require chemotherapy before surgery. Such treatment, known as **neodjuvant chemotherapy,** will typically shrink the size of most tumors and even eradicate some metastases from lymph nodes, making the surgical intervention more curative.

Several surgical procedures are currently in use. **Lumpectomy** is the most conservative surgical procedure, because it is limited to resection of the tumor. **Mastectomy** refers to removal of the entire breast, which is often associated with biopsy of the sentinel lymph node or axillary lymph node dissection. The sentinel lymph node is the first lymph node on the drainage path from the tumor to the axilla and can be identified intraoperatively by the surgeon. If the pathologist performing the frozen section analysis of the sentinel

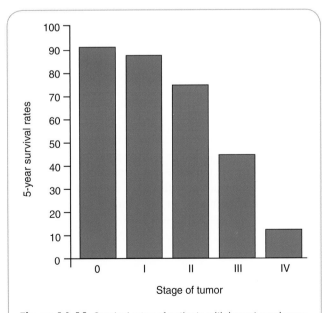

Figure 16-11 Survival rates of patients with breast carcinoma. The 5-year survival rate after mastectomy depends on the stage of the disease. Preinvasive (stage 0) and small tumors diagnosed before they have metastasized have a very good to excellent prognosis. Advanced tumors that have widely metastasized (stage IV) have a poor prognosis.

they are associated with distant metastases. The 5-year survival rate is only 13%.

Did You Know?

Breast carcinoma may present as eczema or rash of the nipple. Often the patient mistakenly assumes that she has a skin disease or allergy. Note the superficial lesion of the nipple in this surgical specimen. The underlying breast tissue was infiltrated with cancer. This superficial breast cancer, which has invaded the skin of the nipple, is called *Paget's disease*, named for the British surgeon who first recognized this lesion in the nineteenth century. Incidentally, Paget also described a bone disease that carries his name.

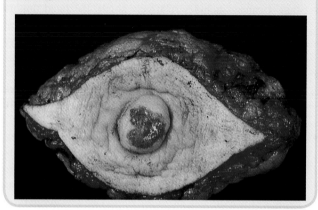

Although staging of breast tumors provides the most accurate prognostic data, other factors should also be taken into consideration. As mentioned before, the histologic subtype of the tumor is important, and there are several variants that have a relatively better prognosis. However, most breast carcinomas are infiltrating duct carcinomas, and the more favorable variants are less common. Histologic grading of the tumor is important and is usually performed on a scale from 1 to 3. Grade 3 tumors, which are less differentiated, show a more rapid growth rate and have a worse prognosis than slower growing, well-differentiated or moderately differentiated (grade 1 and grade 2) tumors. Estrogen and progesterone receptors are expressed on some tumors but not on others. If a tumor is receptor positive, it will respond to antiestrogens (e.g., tamoxifen). Pathologists can determine which tumors express the **epidermal growth factor receptor** (HER2/neu) by immunohistochemistry or by using molecular biology tests. Tumors that are HER2/neu positive have a poorer survival. These women, accounting for 10% to 30% of all breast carcinoma patients, are candidates for treatment with antibodies to this receptor, such as trastuzumab.

Numerous advances in early diagnosis and treatment of breast carcinoma have significantly contributed to the cure rate of this cancer. However, even though breast cancer is a curable disease in most instances, many women still die of this cancer. Most tumor recurrences happen within the first 5 years of diagnosis. Late recurrences—that is, those that occur more than 10 years after initial diagnosis—are uncommon, accounting for less than 5% of all recurrent cancers.

LESIONS OF THE MALE BREAST

The male breast is a rudimentary organ, smaller than the average female breast. It has a nipple from which the ducts extend into the subcutaneous tissue. However, lobules are not formed and fibrofatty tissue is scant. The most important pathologic conditions affecting the male breast are gynecomastia, which was discussed earlier, and breast cancer.

Breast cancer in males is 100 times less common than in females. In most cases it is diagnosed relatively late—mostly because men do not think that they can develop breast cancer and rarely, if ever, perform a breast self-examination. This delay adversely affects the prognosis, which is generally worse than the prognosis of breast cancer in females. Breast cancer in men has the same histologic features as cancers of the female breast.

REVIEW QUESTIONS

1. Describe the main anatomic parts of the breast, such as the nipple, lactiferous ducts, lobules, and acini.
2. What are the most important breast diseases in various age groups?
3. What is acute mastitis, and when does it usually occur?
4. How do hormones affect breasts in women and men?
5. What is gynecomastia?
6. How common is fibrocystic change of the breast, and how does it present clinically?
7. What are the pathologic features of fibrocystic change?
8. What is fibroadenoma, and how does it present clinically?
9. What are the risk factors for breast cancer?
10. What is the most common microscopic type of breast cancer?
11. Correlate the macroscopic and microscopic pathology of infiltrating duct carcinoma.
12. How does breast cancer metastasize?
13. How should the self-examination of breasts be performed?
14. How is breast cancer usually diagnosed?
15. What are the diagnosis and survival rates of breast carcinoma diagnosed in various clinical stages of the disease?

The Endocrine System

Chapter Outline

NORMAL ANATOMY AND PHYSIOLOGY
OVERVIEW OF MAJOR DISEASES
  Pituitary Diseases
    Syndromes of Pituitary Hyperfunction
    Pituitary Hypofunction
    Nonfunctioning Pituitary Tumors
  Thyroid Diseases
    Hyperthyroidism
    Hypothyroidism
    Nodular Goiter
    Thyroid Neoplasms

Diseases of the Parathyroid Glands
    Hyperparathyroidism
    Hypoparathyroidism
Diseases of the Adrenal Cortex
    Adrenocortical Hyperfunction
    Adrenocortical Hypofunction
Diseases of the Adrenal Medulla
    Neuroblastoma
    Pheochromocytoma

Key Terms and Concepts

Acromegaly
Addison's disease
Adrenocortical tumors
Adrenogenital syndrome
Cushing's syndrome
Diabetes insipidus
Exophthalmos
Gigantism
Goiter
Hashimoto's thyroiditis
Hyperaldosteronism
Hypercalcemia

Hyperparathyroidism
Hyperthyroidism
Hypocalcemia
Hypogonadism
Hypoparathyroidism
Hypothyroidism
Iodine deficiency
Multiple endocrine neoplasia (MEN)
Myxedema
Neuroblastoma
Panhypopituitarism
Parathyroid adenoma

Parathyroid hyperplasia, primary
  and secondary
Pheochromocytoma
Pituitary adenoma
Prolactinoma
Sella turcica
Sheehan's syndrome
Thyroid tumors
Trophic hormone
Vanillylmandelic acid (VMA)
Waterhouse-Friderichsen syndrome

Learning Objectives

After reading this chapter, the student should be able to:

1. Describe the normal anatomy and functions of the pituitary, thyroid, parathyroids, and adrenals.
2. Explain the pathogenesis of pituitary hormonal hyperactivity and list at least three syndromes that may develop under these conditions.
3. Describe the symptoms of pituitary insufficiency and explain its causes.
4. Define Graves' disease and explain its pathogenesis and main symptoms.
5. List three causes of hypothyroidism and five principal symptoms of this condition.
6. List the four most important thyroid tumors and their main features.
7. List three causes of hyperparathyroidism and explain the pathologic findings in this disease.
8. Explain the symptoms and laboratory abnormalities caused by hypoparathyroidism.
9. List the three most important syndromes of adrenocortical hyperfunction and explain the symptoms of these disorders.
10. List three causes of Addison's disease and the primary symptoms of this disease.
11. Describe the symptoms of pheochromocytoma and neuroblastoma and the typical laboratory findings found in patients with these tumors.

The endocrine system (a term derived from the Greek words *endo,* meaning "inside," and *krinein,* meaning "to secrete") comprises several glands (pituitary, thyroid, parathyroid, and adrenals) and scattered cells in the gonads, pancreas, intestine, and other organs (Figure 17-1).

The primary function of endocrine cells is to produce hormones—that is, chemical substances that regulate the function of other cells, tissues, or organs. In contrast to exocrine glands, which secrete their products into an external space through excretory ducts, the endocrine organs do not have ducts and so are called the *ductless* glands. Hormones are secreted into the blood or extracellular spaces. Hormones that are released into the circulation act on distant organs *(endocrine effect),* whereas hormones that are released locally into the tissue spaces act on adjacent cells *(paracrine effect).* For example, pituitary hormones exert an endocrine effect on the thyroid, adrenals, or gonads. Glucagon, secreted by the alpha cells of the islets of Langerhans, has a local paracrine effect on insulin-secreting beta cells.

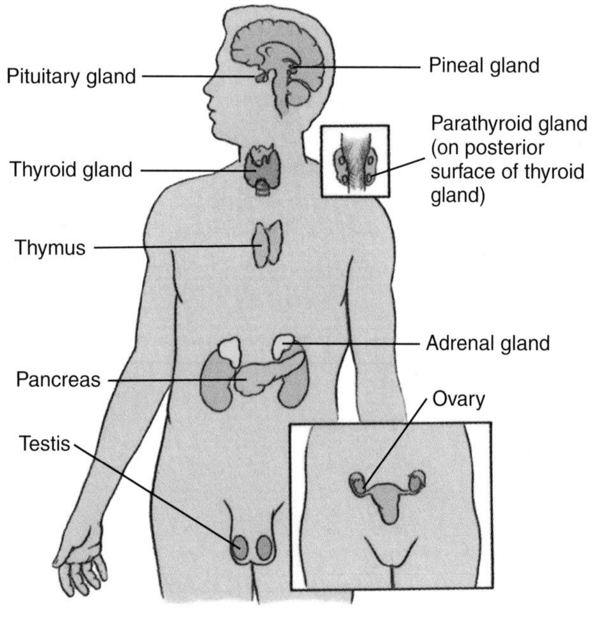

In this chapter, for practical reasons, discussion is limited to the four major endocrine glands: the pituitary, thyroid, parathyroid, and adrenals. The endocrine functions of the islets of Langerhans were discussed in Chapter 12, and the endocrine functions of the gonads have already been discussed in Chapters 14 and 15. Traditionally, diseases involving these organs are treated by *endocrinologists.* In this context it is worth noting that diabetes mellitus is the most important endocrine disorder. With the exception of diabetes, all other endocrine diseases are uncommon.

Figure 17-1 Endocrine glands. (From Applegate EJ: The Anatomy and Physiology Learning System, 4th ed, Philadelphia, 2011, Saunders.)

NORMAL ANATOMY AND PHYSIOLOGY

The pituitary, thyroid, parathyroids, and adrenals are unrelated to each other and have distinct anatomic locations (see Figure 17-1). The pituitary is located intracranially in an indentation of the base of the cranium called the **sella turcica** (a Latin term meaning "Turkish saddle"). The pituitary consists of two parts (anterior and posterior), which are connected to the hypothalamus via a stalk that contains extensions of neurons and the vessels of the pituitary portal system. These blood vessels transport—from the hypothalamus into the pituitary—the neuroendocrine releasing factors that regulate the function of the pituitary cells.

The anterior pituitary, or adenohypophysis, consists of five distinct cell types, each of which is named according to the hormone it secretes. These hormones are as follows:

- Growth hormone (GH)
- Prolactin (PRL)
- Adrenocorticotropic hormone (ACTH)
- Gonadotropins (luteinizing hormone [LH] and follicle-stimulating hormone [FSH])
- Thyrotropic hormone (thyroid-stimulating hormone [TSH])

The functions of pituitary hormones are summarized in Figure 17-2.

The secretion of hormones of the anterior pituitary is regulated by positive stimulation exerted by the cells in the hypothalamic centers and by the negative feedback inhibition created by the hormones produced by the target endocrine cells in the thyroid, adrenals, and gonads. Pituitary hormones do not have any influence on the parathyroid or the medulla of the adrenals, which therefore are not part of the hypothalamic-pituitary regulatory axis.

The posterior pituitary, or neurohypophysis, is composed of cytoplasmic processes of neural cells whose nuclei and perikaryons are located in the hypothalamus. These cells release oxytocin and antidiuretic hormone (ADH). In contrast to the hormones of the anterior pituitary, which are trophic and stimulate the functions of other endocrine glands, the hormones of the posterior pituitary have no trophic functions. These hormones act on nonendocrine cells; oxytocin stimulates the contraction of the gravid uterus and ADH promotes the resorption of water from the renal tubules.

The thyroid is an endocrine gland located in the neck. It consists of two types of cells: follicular cells and C cells. Follicular cells secrete thyroid hormones (*thyroxine,* or *tetraiodothyronine* [T_4], and *triiodothyronine* [T_3]), which are essential for maintaining the intermediate metabolism. The *C cells* secrete *calcitonin,* a polypeptide that is involved in the maintenance of calcium homeostasis. The secretion of T_3 and T_4 is regulated by TSH. The secretion of calcitonin is influenced by the concentration of calcium in serum.

The parathyroids are located in the neck, behind the thyroid. There are usually four glands, each of which is the size of a coffee bean. Parathyroid glands secrete *parathormone (PTH),* a polypeptide involved in regulating homeostasis of serum calcium and phosphate. PTH stimulates the release of calcium from bones and also resorption of calcium from the primary urine in the kidneys, thus causing an elevation of calcium concentration in blood. PTH has additional complex functions, primarily acting on the kidneys, where it promotes the formation of the active form of vitamin D, promotes diuresis by inhibiting the resorption of sodium and bicarbonate, and reduces the clearance of uric acid.

The adrenals are paired organs located in the retroperitoneal space of the abdominal cavity and attached to the upper pole of each kidney. Each adrenal consists of a cortex and a medulla, which, although anatomically fused into a single organ, embryologically and functionally represent two separate entities that are physiologically not related to one another.

The adrenal cortex consists of three zones:

- Zona glomerulosa, which secretes mineralocorticoids (e.g., aldosterone)

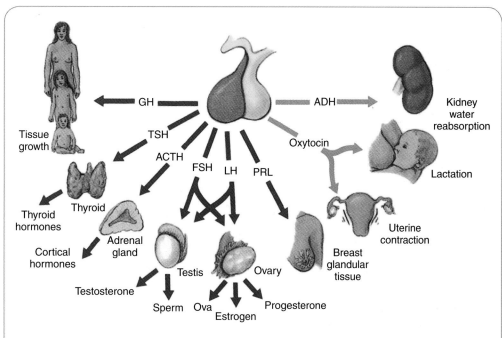

Figure 17-2 The effect of pituitary hormones on target tissues. ACTH, adrenocorticotropic hormone; ADH, antidiuretic hormone; FSH, follicle-stimulating hormone; GH, growth hormone; LH, luteinizing hormone; PRL, prolactin; TSH, thyroid-stimulating hormone. (Modified from Applegate EJ: The Anatomy and Physiology Learning System, 4th ed, St. Louis, 2011, Saunders.)

- Zona fasciculata, which secretes glucocorticoids (e.g., cortisone)
- Zona reticularis, which secretes sex steroids (e.g., estrogens and androgens)

Zona fasciculata and reticularis are under the control of pituitary ACTH, whereas zona glomerulosa responds to the stimuli of the renin-angiotensin system. The steroid hormones of the adrenal cortex regulate the homeostasis of potassium and sodium and the metabolism of carbohydrates; they also act on sex hormone–responsive tissues. In addition to these primary functions, the adrenal steroids are involved in many other metabolic processes. These hormones also modulate inflammation and somatic responses to external stimuli.

The adrenal medulla, which is embryologically derived from the neural crest and thus actually part of the autonomic sympathetic neural system, consists of cells that secrete epinephrine and norepinephrine. These biogenic amines act on smooth muscle cells, heart cells, and many other cells that have adrenergic receptors. In addition to providing sympathetic stimuli, epinephrine and norepinephrine also influence the intermediate metabolism of carbohydrates. Among other effects, epinephrine and norepinephrine cause elevation of blood pressure, tachycardia, and hyperglycemia.

OVERVIEW OF MAJOR DISEASES

The most important diseases involving the endocrine glands present as follows:
- Hyperfunction
- Hypofunction
- Tumors

Several facts important to an understanding of endocrine pathology are presented here, before a discussion of the most important pathologic entities.

1. *The function of the endocrine glands is tightly regulated by positive and negative stimuli.* The function of the thyroid, adrenals, and gonads is regulated by the anterior pituitary, which secretes the **trophic hormones** TSH, ACTH, LH, and FSH. The function of the pituitary is in turn regulated by the *hypothalamic releasing factors* (e.g., gonadotropin-releasing hormone [GnRH]). The hormones of the peripheral target glands released into the blood have a negative inhibitory influence on the hypothalamus and the pituitary (Figure 17-3). Lack of trophic stimuli leads to incomplete development or atrophy of peripheral endocrine glands. For example, congenital developmental disorders involving the hypothalamus result in **hypogonadism** (i.e., small testes or ovaries). A lack of response of the target peripheral endocrine organ and a decreased feedback inhibition leads to hypersecretion of pituitary trophic hormones. For example, destruction of the adrenals by tuberculosis in Addison's disease is accompanied by hypersecretion of ACTH.

2. *Prolonged hyperstimulation by trophic hormones or metabolic signals leads not only to hyperfunction but also to physical enlargement of the peripheral endocrine glands.*

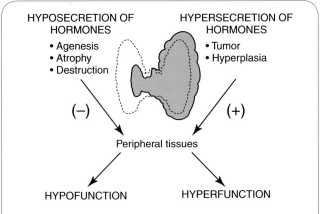

Figure 17-3 Hypofunction and hyperfunction of the endocrine glands.

The thyroid, when overstimulated by TSH, enlarges and becomes nodular. ACTH stimulation leads to adrenocortical hyperplasia.

3. *Hyperfunctioning endocrine glands may be hyperplastic or neoplastic.* Hyperfunctioning endocrine glands are usually enlarged (see Figure 17-3). The enlargement may be attributable to hyperplasia (i.e., a reactive increase in cell number) or to benign or malignant tumors. The distinction between hyperplasia and neoplasia is not always clear cut. For example, adenoma of the parathyroids is histologically indistinguishable from parathyroid hyperplasia. Because pathologists cannot differentiate between these two processes, they designate symmetric enlargement of all four parathyroid glands hyperplasia. If only one gland is enlarged and the others are of usual size, the enlarged gland is considered involved by an adenoma.

4. *Hypofunction of the endocrine glands is usually attributable to the incomplete development, atrophy, or destruction of secretory cells.* Agenesis of the thyroid is a relatively common cause of congenital hypothyroidism found in 1 in 4000 neonates. Atrophy, destruction, and loss of endocrine cells or the entire gland may be caused by several mechanisms, the most important of which are inflammation, tumors, and medical and surgical interventions. Inflammation may be caused by infectious organisms or autoimmune processes. Tumors, whether benign or malignant, primary or secondary, may destroy adjacent endocrine cells. For example, adrenal hypofunction may be secondary to adrenal destruction by tuberculosis, autoimmune adrenalitis, or metastatic carcinoma. Corticosteroid therapy suppresses the secretion of ACTH and causes adrenal atrophy. Inadvertent surgical removal of the parathyroid glands during neck surgery for cancer is the most common cause of hypoparathyroidism in adults.

5. *Neoplastic or hyperplastic enlargement of the endocrine glands results in mass lesions that compress adjacent structures.* Local symptoms caused by endocrine gland enlargement are most evident in diseases of the pituitary and the thyroid. Enlargement of the pituitary, which is in

close proximity to the optic nerve decussation, produces defects in the visual field (so-called bitemporal hemianopsia, or bilateral loss of peripheral [temporal] sight). Thyroid tumors may produce a bulge on the anterior side of the neck or compress the larynx, trachea, and the nerves or blood vessels of the neck. Neoplastic adrenal enlargement rarely presents with signs of compression unless the tumor has reached a considerable size or has invaded adjacent organs. Parathyroid adenomas are so small that they rarely, if ever, produce symptoms of local compression.

6. *Adenomas of the pituitary, parathyroids, and adrenals cannot always be distinguished from carcinomas on the basis of their histologic features.* Benign tumors of the anterior pituitary, parathyroid glands, and adrenals may have the same histologic features as carcinomas of these organs. The only definitive sign of malignancy of such tumors is the presence of metastases. The histologic diagnosis of thyroid malignant lesions is much easier to establish, because these tumors show clear and readily recognizable signs of malignancy.

7. *Tumors of one endocrine gland may be associated with neoplasia and/or hyperplasia of other glands.* **Multiple endocrine neoplasia (MEN)** is a name for at least three hereditary syndromes: MEN1, MEN2A, and MEN2B. In MEN1, an autosomal dominant condition caused by a mutation of the *MEN1* gene, the tumors originate from the pituitary, parathyroids, and pancreatic islets of Langerhans. In MEN2A, a condition caused by an activating mutation of the *RET* proto-oncogenes, the tumors include medullary carcinoma originating from C cells of the thyroid, pheochromocytoma originating from the medulla of the adrenal, and parathyroid adenoma or hyperplasia. Patients with this syndrome die of medullary carcinoma of the thyroid, a calcitonin-producing tumor. In family members affected by MEN2A, thyroid tumors can be recognized in early stages of their development and removed by thyroidectomy, thus preventing mortality. MEN2B, which resembles MEN2A and has the same endocrine lesions, also includes additional multiple skin and mucosal nerve tumors but lacks hyperparathyroidism.

8. *Endocrine symptoms may be paraneoplastic; that is, they may be caused by hormones secreted by tumors of non-endocrine glands.* Such symptoms may be indistinguishable from those caused by hyperfunction of the endocrine glands themselves. The best examples are lung tumors. Small-cell carcinomas of the lung may produce ACTH and thus cause *Cushing's syndrome,* much like pituitary ACTH-secreting tumors. Squamous cell carcinomas of the lung may produce signs of hyperparathyroidism by secreting a parathyroid hormone–related polypeptide (PTHrP). An excess of PTHrP, which is normally secreted by the squamous cells of the skin, causes hypercalcemia and produces clinical symptoms resembling those seen in patients with parathyroid tumors or parathyroid gland hyperplasia.

PITUITARY DISEASES

Diseases of the pituitary are uncommon but may present as follows:
- Pituitary hyperfunction
- Pituitary hypofunction
- Hormonally silent tumors, causing only a mass effect

SYNDROMES OF PITUITARY HYPERFUNCTION

Pituitary hyperfunction may present in the form of several syndromes depending on which one of the five cells is hyperfunctioning. The pituitary is usually enlarged (Figure 17-4). The enlargement may be attributable to macroscopic or microscopic **pituitary adenomas**, which are usually composed of a single cell type but may also contain several cell types. Most common are tumors composed of lactotropic cells. These adenomas, also known as *prolactinomas,* account for approximately 30% of all pituitary tumors. Less common are somatotropic, corticotropic, and gonadotropic adenomas. Tumors composed of TSH-secreting cells are extremely rare. Almost all these tumors are benign; malignant pituitary tumors are exceptionally rare.

? Did You Know?

Right, This patient has coarse facial features typical of acromegaly. *Left,* Compare the patient's face several years before she developed the pituitary tumor.

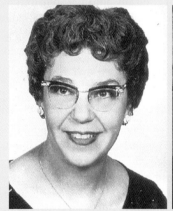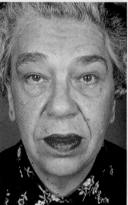

Courtesy of the Group for Research in Pathology Educations (GRIPE), Okalahoma City, Oklahoma.

Prolactinomas (lactotropic adenomas) are usually small, benign tumors measuring less than 10 mm in diameter *(microadenomas).* They are composed of prolactin-secreting cells and usually cause hyperprolactinemia. The typical symptoms of hyperprolactinemia are easily recognized in women of reproductive age and include amenorrhea (lack of menstruation), galactorrhea (spontaneous milk secretion unrelated to pregnancy), and infertility. Hyperprolactinemia inhibits the pulsatile secretion of LH, which is essential for

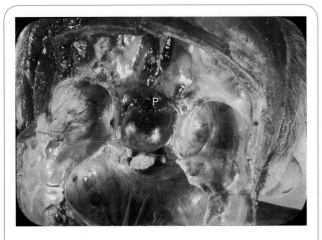

Figure 17-4 Pituitary adenoma. The enlarged pituitary (P) can be seen bulging from the sella turcica at the base of the skull.

normal ovulation to occur, thus causing the menstrual irregularities and infertility. In addition, prolactin stimulates milk production in the breast. In males the symptoms of prolactinomas are usually vague and may include impotence or loss of libido. The function of prolactinomas can be inhibited with bromocriptine, which acts like dopamine, the natural inhibitor of prolactin secretion. Surgery, performed through the nose (transnasal approach to the sella turcica), is reserved for larger tumors only.

Somatotropic adenomas are composed of cells synthesizing growth hormone. In contrast to prolactinomas, which are usually microscopic, 75% of clinically apparent somatotropic adenomas are visible by the naked eye or by modern radiologic techniques (e.g., computed tomography [CT] scanning). Because they measure more than 10 mm in diameter, they are classified as *macroadenomas.*

The clinical symptoms of hypersecretion of growth hormones depend on the age of the patient. In prepubertal patients—that is, before closure of the epiphyseal growth plate of the long bones—these tumors stimulate longitudinal skeletal growth, resulting in **gigantism.** Some of these pituitary giants are more than 8 feet tall. In postpubertal patients, somatotropic adenomas cause **acromegaly** (from the Greek words *acros,* meaning "end portion," and *megalos,* meaning "big"), which presents as enlargement of the acral parts of the extremities (fingers, hands, and toes), tongue, jaws, and nose. The internal organs are also enlarged (e.g., cardiomegaly). Excess growth hormone causes metabolic disturbances, such as hyperglycemia and hypercalcemia.

Surgical removal of the tumor is the treatment of choice. The metabolic symptoms improve, but the bone changes do not regress.

Corticotropic adenomas are composed of ACTH-secreting cells. Most tumors are microadenomas and are clinically recognized by the typical signs of *Cushing's disease.* These symptoms are similar to those caused by corticosteroid-producing adrenocortical lesions and are described under that heading

later. Removal of the pituitary tumor results in an improvement in clinical symptoms.

PITUITARY HYPOFUNCTION

Endocrine insufficiency of the pituitary causes hypofunction of secondary organs, which depend on trophic stimuli from the pituitary. Pituitary hypofunction is rare, but it may be encountered in any age group. It may involve all pituitary cells **(panhypopituitarism),** or it may be selective—that is, limited to one subset of anterior pituitary cells (e.g., hypogonadism secondary to the deficiency of gonadotropic cells) or posterior pituitary cells (e.g., diabetes insipidus).

The causes of pituitary hypofunction include the following:

- Congenital developmental defects, as in pituitary dwarfism or hypogonadism
- Tumors that compress the normal pituitary (e.g., nonfunctioning pituitary adenoma) or cerebral and meningeal tumors that destroy the hypothalamus and the pituitary stalk (e.g., craniopharyngioma, meningioma, or glioma)
- Circulatory disturbances such as ischemia, as in postpartum necrosis **(Sheehan's syndrome)** or pituitary apoplexy with bleeding into an enlarged pituitary or pituitary tumor, or subarachnoidal hemorrhage at the base of the brain
- Trauma of the base of the skull, or intracranial surgery

The diagnosis of pituitary insufficiency may be suspected clinically but must be confirmed by appropriate biochemical tests, which will show hormone deficiency.

Panhypopituitarism of adults is marked by general weakness, cold intolerance, poor appetite, weight loss, and hypotension. Women affected by this disease do not menstruate; affected men suffer from impotence and loss of libido. Childhood pituitary insufficiency results in dwarfism.

Diabetes insipidus is marked by a lack of ADH secondary to destructive lesions of the hypothalamus or pituitary stalk or tumors of the posterior pituitary. It may be caused by tumors, infection of the brain or meninges, intracranial hemorrhage, or trauma involving the bones of the base of the skull. Because ADH prevents the resorption of water from the fluid filtered in the renal glomeruli, patients with diabetes insipidus secrete large amounts (5 to 6 L/day) of hypotonic urine.

Pituitary insufficiency requires substitution therapy with appropriate hormones. The most spectacular results have been achieved in the treatment of congenital pituitary dwarfism; affected patients can achieve normal growth if treated appropriately. Substitution therapy with ADH is effective in the treatment of diabetes insipidus.

NONFUNCTIONING PITUITARY TUMORS

Approximately 25% of all pituitary tumors do not produce hormonal symptoms and are called hormonally silent adenomas. These tumors are composed of nonsecretory pituitary cells, pituitary cells showing no signs of hormone synthesis ("*null cells*"), or mitochondria-filled nonfunctioning pituitary cells *(oncocytes).* Clinically, such tumors may cause a mass effect and expand the sella turcica, as seen by x-ray examination.

The tumor mass may compress the normal pituitary, causing hypopituitarism or diabetes insipidus. Suprasellar growth of pituitary tumors may lead to compression of the optic chiasm and partial blindness. This loss of both temporal visual fields is known as bitemporal hemianopsia. Pituitary tumors also may cause signs of increased intracranial pressure, which requires prompt treatment.

It is worth remembering that pituitary tumors are intracranial and thus usually removed by neurosurgeons. They represent approximately 10% of all symptomatic intracranial tumors. Many pituitary tumors are small and asymptomatic; asymptomatic, usually microscopic pituitary tumors are found at autopsy in 20% of people 60 years and older.

THYROID DISEASES

Thyroid diseases are common, but fortunately they can be diagnosed readily and treated with very good results. Thyroid diseases present as functional disturbances (hyperfunction or hypofunction) or as mass lesions (neoplasms or non-neoplastic enlargement, known as *goiter*).

HYPERTHYROIDISM

Hyperthyroidism *(thyrotoxicosis)* is a hypermetabolic state that results from an excess of free thyroid hormones (T_3 and T_4) in blood. The most important causes of hyperthyroidism are the following (Figure 17-5):

- Autoimmunity, as in Graves' disease (85% of all cases)

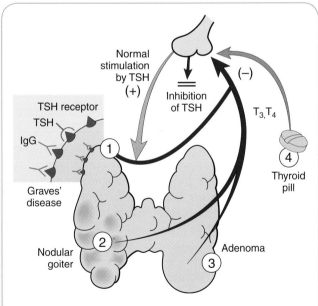

Figure 17-5 Hyperthyroidism may have several causes, among them *(1)* Graves' disease, *(2)* nodular goiter, *(3)* toxic adenoma of the thyroid, and *(4)* exogenous thyroid medication. Triiodothyronine (T_3) and thyroxine (T_4) normally inhibit secretion of thyroid-stimulating hormone (TSH), which accounts for the low concentration of TSH in these forms of hyperthyroidism. IgG, immunoglobulin G.

- Idiopathic nodular hyperplasia of the thyroid, as in toxic goiter
- Tumors, such as hyperfunctioning thyroid adenoma

Other causes, such as temporary thyroid hyperfunction in Hashimoto's disease, are less common. Uncontrolled intake of thyroid hormone pills, which are often used for the self-treatment of obesity, may cause self-inflicted hyperthyroidism (Figure 17-6).

Graves' disease is an autoimmune disorder resulting from the breakdown of self-tolerance to one or more thyroid components, which become autoantigenic. The disease is most often caused by antibodies to the TSH receptor on the surface

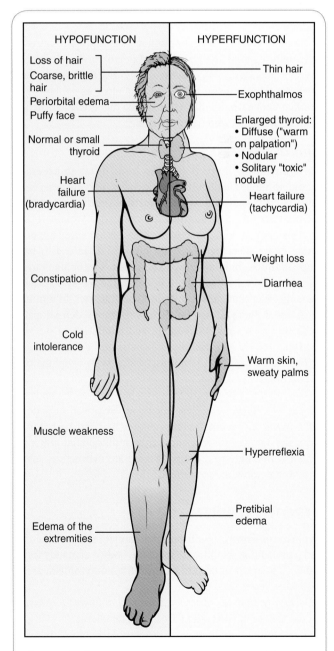

Figure 17-6 Comparison of hyperthyroidism and hypothyroidism.

of thyroid follicular cells that stimulate the production of thyroid hormones. In addition to antibodies to the TSH receptor, which are found in almost all patients with Graves' disease, some patients have thyroid growth–stimulating antibodies, which cause the proliferation of thyroid follicular cells. Some patients have TSH-binding inhibitor immunoglobulins, which may either stimulate or inhibit the function of thyroid cells. The disease occurs 10 times more often in women than in men and may be associated with other autoimmune disorders.

The thyroid affected by Graves' disease is diffusely enlarged. Histologically, the enlarged thyroid is composed of hyperplastic follicles lined with hyperactive, tall, cuboidal cells. The thyroid also contains lymphoid follicles, which are yet another sign that this disease is immune mediated.

Nodular goiter is a less common but important cause of hyperthyroidism. The thyroid gland is enlarged and nodular. Thyroid adenomas may occasionally be hyperactive and cause hyperthyroidism. Such tumors appear as solitary nodules that concentrate radioactive iodine and are diagnosed as "hot nodules" on radioactive scanning.

Clinical Features

The symptoms of hyperthyroidism result from an excess of thyroid hormones and include restlessness, nervousness, emotional lability, sweating, and tachycardia. Cardiac palpitation, muscular tremor, and diarrhea are common. Weight loss is often seen, even though the patient has an increased appetite. Furthermore, most patients with Graves' disease also have **exophthalmos** (bulging eyes). The cause of exophthalmos is not known, but it is thought to be related to the systemic immune disorder that causes thyroid hyperfunction. In a minority of cases, there is also localized infiltrative dermatopathy presenting as scaling, thickening, and induration of the skin overlying the shins. Hyperthyroidism caused by nodular goiter or thyroid adenoma is not associated with exophthalmos and pretibial myxedema.

The treatment of hyperthyroidism depends on the underlying pathologic process. Best results are achieved in patients with solitary hyperfunctioning nodules that can be removed surgically. Graves' disease and diffuse multinodular goiter are treated with antithyroid drugs; if these are ineffective, subtotal thyroidectomy is recommended.

HYPOTHYROIDISM

Hypothyroidism results from a functional failure of the thyroid gland and its inability to meet the body's demands for T_4 and T_3. The most important causes of hypothyroidism are as follows:

- *Developmental defects* (e.g., *congenital thyroid aplasia*). This condition is found in 1 of 4000 newborns.
- *Thyroiditis.* Inflammation of the thyroid is most often immune mediated and includes several disorders known as lymphocytic thyroiditis, Hashimoto's thyroiditis, and related diseases.
- *Hashimoto's thyroiditis* is the most common cause of hypothyroidism. It is 10 times more common in women than men. It has a genetic component and may be associated with other autoimmune disease. Nevertheless, it is usually diagnosed in elderly women over the age of 60 years.
- *Thyroidectomy* (surgical removal of the thyroid). Such iatrogenic hypothyroidism typically evolves postoperatively after resection of a thyroid that has been infiltrated by tumor.
- *Iodine deficiency.* The human body requires iodine, and if the food and water consumed do not contain adequate amounts of iodine, as occurs in some parts of the world (e.g., the Alps of Switzerland or the Andes of South America), hypothyroidism may ensue. Iodine is preventively added to the salt in most Western countries; thus iodine deficiency is rare in the United States.

Pathology

The pathologic basis of hypothyroidism varies depending on its causes. Children born with congenital thyroid aplasia do not have a thyroid. Thyroiditis leads to thyroid enlargement, which is usually symmetric. Histologically, such a gland is infiltrated with lymphocytes, which destroy thyroid follicles. Subsequent healing and fibrosis may actually reduce the size of the thyroid.

Deficiency of iodine in food and water is usually associated with nodular enlargement of the thyroid *(goiter).* Because the thyroid cannot synthesize enough T_3 and T_4, its follicles undergo compensatory hyperplasia in an attempt to increase the production of hormones. In many cases this compensatory mechanism is not sufficient and the serum levels of T_3 and T_4 are low. Low concentrations of T_3 and T_4 in serum do not provide feedback inhibition of the pituitary, which responds to low levels of thyroid hormones by overproducing TSH. TSH stimulation without adequate supplies of iodine further promotes the enlargement of the thyroid but cannot correct the hormone deficiency.

Clinical Features

The symptoms of hypothyroidism depend on the patient's age. In children the deficiency of thyroid hormones affects the growth of the entire body and, most specifically, development of the central nervous system. If the thyroid deficiency is not recognized, the child's growth is stunted *(thyroid dwarfism)* and mental development is retarded *(cretinism).* These children also have numerous other metabolic disturbances. The hypothyroidism of adults is also known as **myxedema,** named so because the skin of these patients appears edematous, doughlike, and puffy.

Deficiency of thyroid hormones affects essentially all organs in the body, slowing their function. The patient is sleepy, lacks mental alertness, tires easily, and lacks endurance. The heart beats slowly *(bradycardia);* the intestines lose mobility *(constipation);* and the skeletal muscles are weak, stiff, and aching.

The diagnosis of hypothyroidism is based on biochemical measurements of thyroid hormones in circulation. T_4 and T_3 levels are low, whereas the TSH level is elevated. Treatment with synthetic thyroid hormones yields excellent results in most cases, although such substitution therapy may then be required for the rest of the patient's life.

NODULAR GOITER

Enlargement of the thyroid is called **goiter** (from the Latin term *guttur*, meaning "throat") or *struma* (from the Latin verb *struo,* meaning "to pile up"). The term *goiter* is noncommittal and includes enlargements caused by a functional disturbance (as in Graves' disease), iodine deficiency, or neoplasia. Most often the cause of goiter is unknown *(idiopathic goiter).*

Pathology

The nodular goiter consists of nodules that enlarge and deform the thyroid (Figure 17-7). Histologically these nodules consist of thyroid follicles that vary in size and shape and are usually filled with colloid. Between the nodules, the struma consists of vessels and collagen fibers infiltrated with lymphocytes and macrophages. Secondary changes, such as calcification, hemorrhage, and atrophy of the compressed follicles in the surrounding parenchyma, are common.

Clinical Features

Most goiters are euthyroid; that is, they do not cause either hyperthyroidism or hypothyroidism. The symptoms are related to the compression of adjacent structures and include coughing and hoarseness secondary to the pressure of the enlarged thyroid on the larynx or recurrent laryngeal nerve. The treatment of goiter includes resection of the enlarged portions of the thyroid.

THYROID NEOPLASMS

Thyroid tumors may be benign or malignant. Benign thyroid tumors are very common. Although they are found in 3% to 4% of all adults, they are of limited clinical significance, primarily

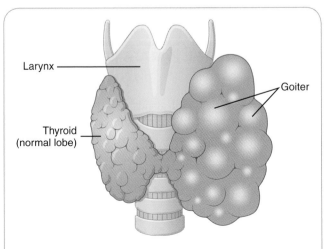

Figure 17-7 Goiter. One or both thyroid lobes may be enlarged and deformed by numerous hyperplastic nodules.

because such tumors are small. Malignant thyroid tumors are rare and are outnumbered by benign tumors by a ratio of 10:1. Thyroid tumors are more common in women than in men and thus every year there are approximately 15 malignant tumor diagnoses in 100,000 women and 5 per 100,000 men. The mortality is 0.1 per 100,000 men and women.

Adenomas

Follicular adenoma of the thyroid is the most common benign tumor. It presents as a nodule, which may vary in size. Most adenomas are small, well encapsulated with fibrous tissue, and composed of thyroid follicles. Typically, adenomas comprise cells that do not take up radioactive iodine more avidly than does normal thyroid. On radioscanning with radioactive iodine, such adenomas cannot be distinguished from normal tissue. Other tumors are composed of afunctional thyroid cells that form so-called cold nodules, which are unable to concentrate radioactive iodine. In this respect, such cold nodules resemble carcinomas, many of which cannot concentrate iodine either. The final diagnosis can be made only by microscopic examination of biopsy material. Thyroid adenomas are not premalignant; thus, most small nodules do not require any treatment. Larger tumors are usually removed for cosmetic reasons to correct the deformity in the contour of the neck.

Carcinoma

Carcinoma of the thyroid occurs in several histologic forms, including papillary, follicular, medullary, and anaplastic carcinoma (Figure 17-8). All these tumors except medullary carcinomas originate from follicular cells. Among the risk factors for developing thyroid tumors, the best documented are the effects of nuclear irradiation. After the explosion of the atomic bomb in Japan in 1945, as well as after the nuclear plant accident in Chernobyl in Ukraine in the 1980s, epidemiologists noticed an increase in the incidence of thyroid cancer. Thyroid tumors are, for unknown reasons, more common in females than in males.

PAPILLARY CARCINOMA

Papillary carcinoma accounts for 80% of all malignant thyroid tumors. It is a low-grade, hormonally inactive tumor that usually presents as a cold nodule on radioscans. The tumor tends to metastasize to the local lymph nodes; distant metastases are rarely found and usually only late in the course of the disease.

Papillary carcinoma is four times more common in women than in men. It occurs relatively early in life and has a peak incidence in the third to fifth decade. This tumor has a very favorable prognosis; indeed, 80% of patients are alive 10 years after diagnosis.

FOLLICULAR CARCINOMA

Follicular carcinoma is much less common than papillary carcinoma, accounting for only 15% of malignant thyroid diseases. Most patients are older than 40 years, and 75% are female. The tumor grows more aggressively than papillary carcinoma, but it still has a good prognosis. Overall, 65% of

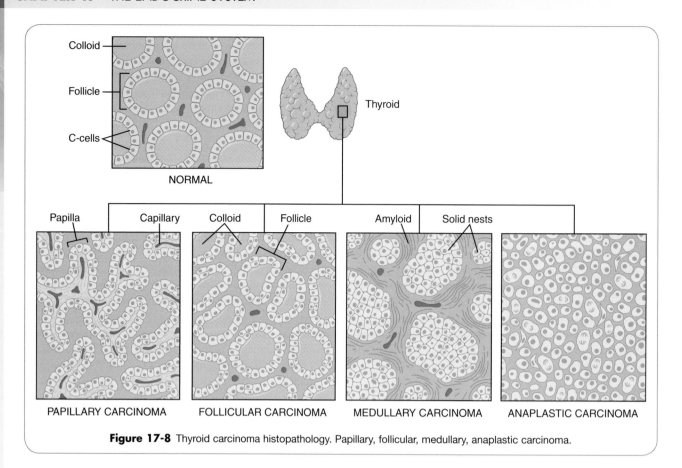

Figure 17-8 Thyroid carcinoma histopathology. Papillary, follicular, medullary, anaplastic carcinoma.

patients survive 10 years. The tumor cells resemble normal follicular cells of the thyroid and form colloid.

Clinically, follicular carcinoma presents as a slowly growing nodule. Most of these tumors do not concentrate radioactive iodine (cold nodules), but some of them take up radioactive iodine and produce thyroid hormones (hot nodules). Those tumors that do concentrate iodine can be treated with radioactive iodine, because accumulated radioactive iodine is a strong source of internal radiation and it kills cells. This treatment is especially suitable for patients who have widespread metastases.

MEDULLARY CARCINOMA

Medullary carcinoma differs from other thyroid tumors in that it is derived from C cells. Like the normal C cells, medullary carcinomas produce *calcitonin,* a hormone involved in regulating the homeostasis of calcium. Histologically, medullary carcinoma is composed of round or oval neuroendocrine cells arranged into groups and nests. The stroma of the tumor contains amyloid, which is derived from calcitonin.

Medullary carcinoma may be inherited, and it can occur concomitantly with pheochromocytoma in MEN2. MEN2 is related to germline mutations of the *RET* proto-oncogene, which are found in 95% of affected families. Familial medullary carcinomas are usually discovered in early adulthood and have a good prognosis if surgically removed. Sporadic tumors, which occur at 60 years of age and older, have a less

favorable prognosis, and only 50% of patients survive 5 years after diagnosis.

ANAPLASTIC CARCINOMA

Anaplastic (undifferentiated) carcinoma is a rare tumor, accounting for 1% to 2% of all thyroid neoplasms. It has an extremely unfavorable prognosis, and most patients die within 1 year of diagnosis. Histologically, such tumors are composed of undifferentiated large or small tumor cells that bear no resemblance to normal thyroid cells.

DISEASES OF THE PARATHYROID GLANDS

Diseases of the parathyroid glands present as either hyperfunction (oversecretion of parathyroid hormone [PTH]) or hypofunction. These diseases cause disturbances in the homeostasis of calcium and phosphate.

HYPERPARATHYROIDISM

Hyperparathyroidism is defined as parathyroid gland hyperfunction that results in increased levels of PTH in circulating blood. Hyperparathyroidism may be primary (i.e., caused by parathyroid hyperplasia or neoplasia) or secondary, in which case it is usually related to chronic renal failure. In less than

5% of all cases, hyperparathyroidism is part of a hereditary syndrome, most often MEN1.

In 80% of cases, primary hyperparathyroidism is caused by a benign parathyroid adenoma; in 18% it is the result of the hyperplasia of parathyroid glands. In 2% of cases it is caused by parathyroid carcinoma. There are normally four parathyroid glands. **Parathyroid adenomas** or *carcinomas* are characterized by enlargement of one gland, with the other glands being normal (Figure 17-9). Parathyroid adenomas are occasionally multiple, involving two or even three glands. In parathyroid hyperplasia, all four glands are enlarged. Because the diagnosis of adenoma or hyperplasia cannot be made preoperatively, it is essential that the surgeon explore all four glands. If adenomatous enlargement of one gland is identified, that gland is usually removed and the others left intact. If all four glands are enlarged, the surgeon usually removes three glands and leaves behind only one, which should suffice to maintain normal calcium-phosphate homeostasis.

Secondary parathyroid hyperplasia is indistinguishable from **primary parathyroid hyperplasia,** because all four glands are symmetrically enlarged. Enlargement of the parathyroid glands and their hyperfunction is a compensatory mechanism triggered by hypocalcemia caused by chronic renal disease. Hypovitaminosis D, as in osteomalacia or intestinal malabsorption syndromes, may have the same results.

Pathology

The histologic changes in the parathyroid glands are identical regardless of the cause of hyperparathyroidism. Parathyroid adenomas or carcinomas, as well as hyperplastic glands, are composed of parathyroid cells arranged into dense sheets. These cells replace the fat cells that are normally found inside the gland. In parathyroid adenomas, one may occasionally see remnants of the compressed preexisting gland, but this is not always evident. In hyperplastic glands, there is no evidence of normal parathyroid tissue. Parathyroid carcinomas may consist of invasive cells extending beyond the normal confines of the gland.

Hyperparathyroidism is characterized by an excess of PTH in the circulation. PTH acts primarily on the bones and kidneys. In the bones, it stimulates osteoclasts, leading to bone resorption and the release of calcium into the circulation. In the kidneys, PTH promotes resorption of calcium from the tubular lumen, thus diminishing excretion of calcium in urine. PTH also promotes the formation of the active form of vitamin D_3 in the kidneys, which in turn facilitates the uptake of calcium from food in the intestine (Figure 17-10). Hypercalcemia and compensatory hypophosphatemia are thus the primary biochemical abnormalities detected by blood analysis. PTH serum concentrations are also elevated.

Clinical Features

The clinical symptoms of hyperparathyroidism are related to increased PTH activity. The bones show signs of decalcification and are prone to fractures. **Hypercalcemia** leads to deposition of calcium salts in the kidney *(nephrocalcinosis)* and formation of urinary stones *(urolithiasis)*. Ocular and skin calcifications may be present. An excess of calcium produces lethargy, muscle weakness, and conduction defects in the heart.

The treatment of primary hyperparathyroidism includes surgical exploration of the neck and resection of the hyperfunctioning glands or the tumor. Secondary hyperparathyroidism can also be surgically treated, but in addition, it is important to correct the basic metabolic defect that caused PTH hypersecretion. However, there is no need to rush with parathyroid surgery. After renal transplantation, the glands may regress to normal size and the metabolic disturbances may disappear. If renal transplantation does not normalize calcium and phosphate balance, one can assume that the hyperfunction of the parathyroids has apparently taken an autonomous course. Such cases, which are called *tertiary hyperparathyroidism,* are rare. Surprisingly, chromosomal analysis of the enlarged parathyroids of patients with tertiary hyperparathyroidism has revealed chromosomal changes identical to those seen in parathyroid adenomas. This suggests that prolonged metabolic stimulation can cause irreversible neoplastic changes in the parathyroid cells. Because tertiary hyperparathyroidism represents a form of metabolically induced neoplasia, like any other tumor, it can be cured only through surgery.

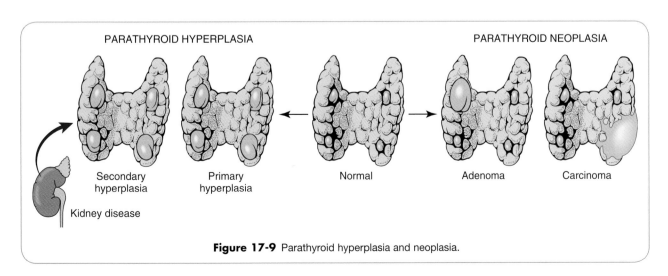

PARATHYROID HYPERPLASIA

PARATHYROID NEOPLASIA

Secondary hyperplasia

Primary hyperplasia

Kidney disease

Normal

Adenoma

Carcinoma

Figure 17-9 Parathyroid hyperplasia and neoplasia.

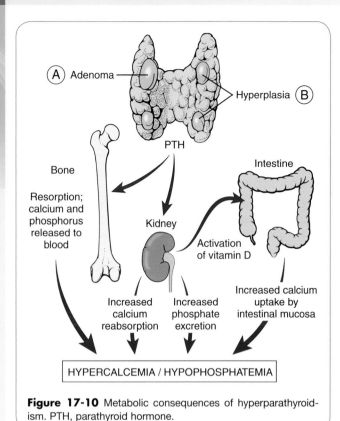

Figure 17-10 Metabolic consequences of hyperparathyroidism. PTH, parathyroid hormone.

HYPOPARATHYROIDISM

Hypoparathyroidism results from parathyroid hypofunction or a complete loss of function of the parathyroid glands. Overall, it is a rare condition that most commonly occurs after inadvertent removal of all four parathyroid glands during cancer surgery of the neck. Congenital, genetic, or autoimmune causes of hypoparathyroidism are extremely rare.

Clinical Features

The clinical symptoms of hypoparathyroidism reflect metabolic disturbances caused by a deficiency of PTH. The most important of these is **hypocalcemia,** which results in changes in neuromuscular excitability and muscular contraction. The skeletal muscles tend to become spastic *(hypocalcemic tetany).* The heart action becomes irregular, and in severe cases, cardiac arrest may occur. The activity of the nerves is also altered, fluctuating between hyperexcitability and depression. All the symptoms can be ameliorated by substitutional hormonal therapy with synthetic PTH.

DISEASES OF THE ADRENAL CORTEX

Diseases of the adrenal cortex cause metabolic disturbances that reflect an excess or a deficiency of adrenal steroids. Each of the three zones of the adrenal cortex—zona glomerulosa, zona fasciculata, and zona reticularis—may be affected, either separately or jointly. The secretion of mineralocorticoids,

glucocorticoids, or sex steroids may be altered; the excess or deficiency of these hormones will produce either disturbances in the metabolism of minerals (sodium, potassium, and chloride), carbohydrate metabolism, or sexual problems.

ADRENOCORTICAL HYPERFUNCTION

Adrenocortical hyperfunction results in three partially overlapping syndromes (Figure 17-11):

- **Hyperaldosteronism** (or Conn's syndrome), which is caused by hypersecretion of mineralocorticoids (aldosterone)
- Hypercortisolism (or **Cushing's syndrome**), which is caused by hypersecretion of glucocorticoids (cortisol)
- **Adrenogenital syndrome,** which is caused by hypersecretion of the adrenal sex steroids (androgens)

Cushing's syndrome is the most common of these three syndromes. Hypercortisolism is caused either by adrenal hyperplasia or neoplasia. In about 70% of cases, hypercortisolism occurs as a result of hypersecretion of ACTH from pituitary adenomas. This association was originally described by the Canadian neurosurgeon Harvey Cushing and is therefore called *Cushing's disease.* Subsequently, it was noticed that the same symptoms could occur as a result of hypersecretion of corticosteroids from **adrenocortical tumors,** a clinical entity that was called *Cushing's syndrome* to distinguish it from the disease caused by corticotropic adenomas of the pituitary. Adrenocortical tumors account for about 20% of the

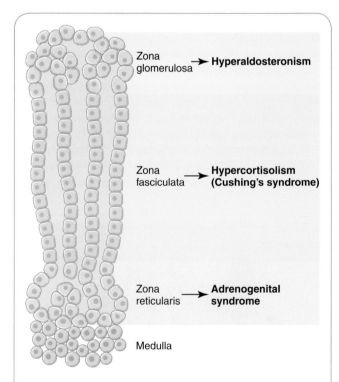

Figure 17-11 Adrenal cortical hyperfunction. Hyperfunction or tumors of the zona glomerulosa result in hyperaldosteronisms. Hyperfunction or tumors of the zona fasciculata result in hypercortisolism. Hyperfunction of the zona reticularis results in adrenogenital syndrome.

cases of hypercortisolism. Approximately 10% of cases are caused by extrapituitary tumors, such as small-cell carcinoma of the lung, which is the most common source of ectopically secreted ACTH (Figure 17-12). Hypercortisolism may also be found in patients treated with synthetic steroids for rheumatoid arthritis, systemic lupus erythematosus, and other autoimmune diseases.

Pathology

Hyperplasia of the adrenals leads to bilateral thickening of the adrenal cortex. Tumors of the adrenal appear as discrete nodules or marked irregular enlargement of the entire gland. These tumors may be benign adenomas or malignant lesions (carcinomas). Typically, adrenocortical tumors are yellow because of their high lipid content (Figure 17-13). Adenomas are usually well circumscribed, whereas carcinomas tend to extend into the adjacent tissues. Histologically, adenomas and well-differentiated carcinomas cannot always be distinguished from one another. However, invasive carcinomas show marked cellular pleomorphism.

Clinical Features

Symptoms of hypercortisolism include a peculiar "central" obesity that is most prominent on the face and trunk, resulting in a so-called moon face and buffalo hump (Figure 17-14).

The patients appear red in the face because of a plethora of blood, hypertension, and thinning of the skin. Glucose intolerance and overt diabetes are the most common biochemical disturbances. Typically, affected patients experience fatigue and weakness and are mentally unstable. They also have numerous other minor problems, reflecting abnormal intermediate metabolism of carbohydrates.

Endogenous Cushing's syndrome and Cushing's disease are rare. Under the term *endogenous* one includes the diseases caused by hyperfunctioning adrenals, with or without pituitary disease, in contrast to exogenous Cushing's syndrome, which results from administration of exogenous corticosteroids. In clinical practice the most common cause of Cushing's syndrome is corticosteroid therapy, which is widely used for the treatment of various immune disorders, such as rheumatoid arthritis or asthma; renal diseases, such as nephrotic syndrome; and many skin diseases. Exogenously induced Cushing's syndrome responds well to gradual tapering off and cessation of steroid treatment.

Hyperaldosteronism is a rare disease that is typically caused by an adenoma of the zona glomerulosa. Adenoma is found in 70% of cases, whereas the remaining 30% have cortical hyperplasia. Clinically, hyperaldosteronism presents with retention of sodium and loss of potassium. Changes in the concentration of minerals, accompanied by a retention of water, result in

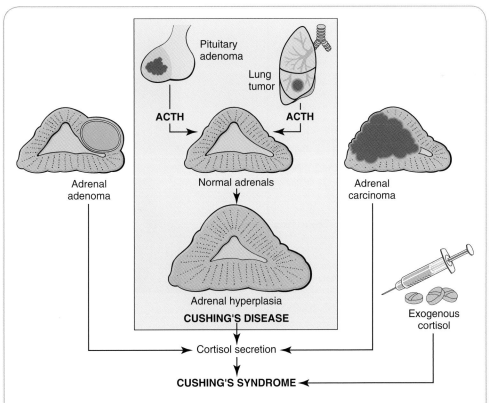

Figure 17-12 Hypercortisolism in Cushing's disease and Cushing's syndrome. Excessive production of cortisol is related to the overstimulation of adrenals by adrenocorticotropic hormone (ACTH). Cushing's syndrome can be caused by hormone-producing adrenocortical tumors or primary adrenocortical hyperplasia or exogenous corticosteroids.

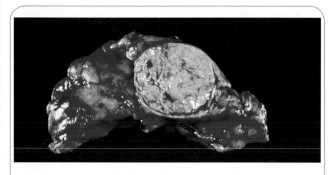

Figure 17-13 Adrenocortical adenoma. The neoplastic nodule is yellow because of increased lipid content.

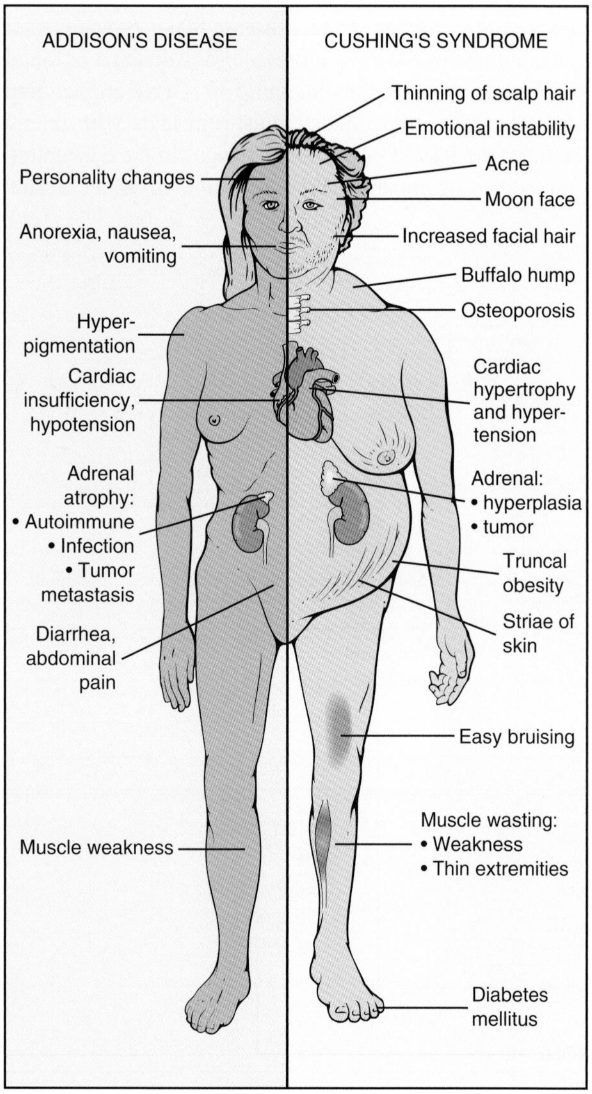

hypertension (*hypernatremic hypokalemic hypertension*). Although this adrenal disease is rare, occurring in less than 0.1% of hypertensive patients, it is important to bear in mind that it is surgically treatable. Removal of the pathologically altered adrenal gland results in complete cure of the hypertension.

Primary hyperaldosteronism must be clinically distinguished from secondary hyperaldosteronism, a much more common disease. The secretion of aldosterone is physiologically stimulated by angiotensin, which is formed from angiotensinogen under the influence of renin. Renin is secreted from the juxtaglomerular apparatus of the kidney, and elevated levels of renin are typically found in various renal diseases. Hence, secondary hyperaldosteronism is associated with hyper-reninemia, in contrast to primary hyperaldosteronism, which is renin independent and associated with normal levels of renin in circulation. Measurements of renin and aldosterone in blood are important in determining whether hyperaldosteronism is caused by a renal or adrenal disease.

? Did You Know?

Patients treated with corticosteroids develop the clinical features of Cushing's syndrome. As shown in the photograph, they have cushingoid features—"moon face," obesity, and cutaneous striae.

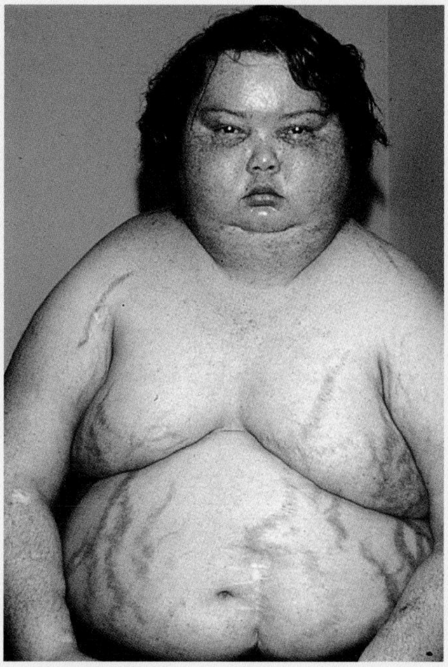

Figure 17-14 showing comparison:

ADDISON'S DISEASE	CUSHING'S SYNDROME
Personality changes	Thinning of scalp hair
Anorexia, nausea, vomiting	Emotional instability
Hyper-pigmentation	Acne
Cardiac insufficiency, hypotension	Moon face
Adrenal atrophy: • Autoimmune • Infection • Tumor metastasis	Increased facial hair
Diarrhea, abdominal pain	Buffalo hump
Muscle weakness	Osteoporosis
	Cardiac hypertrophy and hypertension
	Adrenal: • hyperplasia • tumor
	Truncal obesity
	Striae of skin
	Easy bruising
	Muscle wasting: • Weakness • Thin extremities
	Diabetes mellitus

Figure 17-14 Comparison of adrenocortical hyperfunction and hypofunction.

Adrenogenital syndrome, which is also known as *adrenal virilism,* is a rare disease that can affect neonates or adults. As the name implies, the disease is typically found in females who experience virilization as a result of an excess of androgenic hormones.

Adrenogenital syndrome may be congenital (i.e., present at birth), or it may develop in adulthood. In neonates this disease is related to one of several inborn errors of steroid metabolism (e.g., 21-hydroxylase deficiency). An excess of androgens results in partial virilization of the external female genitalia. The vulva in these patients shows partial fusion of the labio-scrotal folds, and the clitoris may be enlarged *(clitoromegaly).* Some of these female children are assigned the wrong sex. Although genetically female, they are reared as males. In adult women, adrenogenital syndrome is usually related to androgen-producing tumors, which cause virilization with hirsutism, deepening of the voice, and loss of menstruation.

The treatment of adrenocortical hyperfunction depends on the cause of the disease and usually involves either surgical resection of hyperfunctioning tumors or medical suppression of the abnormal endocrine stimulatory pathway. For example, in congenital deficiency of 21-hydroxylase, virilization of the female external genitalia can be reversed by treating the child with cortisol. Cortisol is not produced in these children. Exogenous cortisol will provide the negative feedback impulse to the pituitary, inhibiting the excessive release of ACTH that occurs because of the lack of a natural inhibitor (endogenous cortisol). Through reduction of ACTH secretion, the exogenous cortisol reduces the overproduction of androgen in the adrenal. Without androgenic stimulation, the external female genitalia lose their male features and resume normal development comparable to that of normal female children.

ADRENOCORTICAL HYPOFUNCTION

Adrenocortical hypofunction is usually a consequence of adrenal destruction. This can occur suddenly in an acute form, as in meningococcal septicemia (so-called **Waterhouse-Friderichsen syndrome**), or slowly as a result of the destruction of the adrenocortex by autoimmune disease *(autoimmune adrenalitis).* Infections, such as tuberculosis or histoplasmosis, or a primary or metastatic malignant tumor may also destroy the adrenals, causing adrenal insufficiency. Carcinomas of the breast and lungs are the most common tumors that metastasize to the adrenals, and if the metastases are bilateral, such tumors cause adrenal insufficiency.

Adrenal insufficiency results in a clinical syndrome known as **Addison's disease.** Today, 70% of the cases of Addison's disease are caused by an autoimmune adrenalitis, in contrast to previous times, when the disease was mostly caused by tuberculosis. However, infections, such as tuberculosis and fungal diseases, still account for 25% of cases and are most common in immunosuppressed patients with cancer or acquired immunodeficiency syndrome (AIDS). Malignant tumors are a rare cause of Addison's disease.

The pathologic basis of Addison's disease varies. In early stages of autoimmune adrenalitis, the cortex is infiltrated with lymphocytes and plasma cells. In later stages of the disease, the entire cortex is destroyed and may be replaced with fibrous tissue or fat cells. At autopsy it is almost impossible to identify the adrenals, which have been destroyed by granulomas and pathogen-induced necrosis. Tumoral destruction of the adrenals is marked by an overgrowth of metastatic malignant cells and a loss of adrenocortical tissue.

? **Did You Know?**

President John F. Kennedy had adrenal insufficiency (Addison's disease), most likely caused by an autoimmune disease that destroyed his adrenals. The president's disease was a well-kept secret during his lifetime.

Clinical Features

Addison's disease presents insidiously with fatigue, weight loss, and nausea. Affected patients are hypotensive and have frequent syncope. They are extremely susceptible to infections. They do not tolerate any stress and cannot work or maintain many of the usual daily routines. Numerous metabolic disturbances may be detected. The serum typically exhibits low levels of sodium and chloride, elevated potassium levels, and low glucose levels. If untreated, these mineral disorders lead to cardiac conduction problems, which can be lethal. Steroid levels in the blood are low.

The final diagnosis is made on the basis of an ACTH test. Normally, ACTH stimulates secretion of corticosteroids. In Addison's disease, such stimulation has no effect, proving that the adrenal has been destroyed and cannot respond to physiologic stimuli. Treatment with steroids results in fast recovery. However, exogenous steroids must be administered at regular intervals for the remainder of the patient's life.

The comparative features of Cushing's syndrome and Addison's disease are shown in Figure 17-14.

DISEASES OF THE ADRENAL MEDULLA

The most important diseases of the adrenal medulla are two tumors: *neuroblastoma* and *pheochromocytoma.*

NEUROBLASTOMA

Neuroblastoma is a tumor composed of neuroblasts—that is, undifferentiated precursors of neural cells that are also precursors of normal adrenal medullary cells. The adrenal medulla is derived from cells of the neural crest that migrate during fetal development and invade the primordium of the adrenal. Normally, these migrating neuroblasts differentiate into chromaffin cells of the adrenal medulla. Differentiation is recognized by the appearance of epinephrine- and norepinephrine-rich granules, visible in the cytoplasm of these cells by electron microscopy. If the migratory neuroblasts do not differentiate but instead retain their embryonic-fetal undifferentiated phenotype, they undergo malignant transformation and form a malignant tumor. Such tumors, composed of undifferentiated neuroblasts, are called *neuroblastomas.* Similar tumors can occur in the brain or at the site of extraspinal and sympathetic ganglia, which are also derived from the neural tube and neural crest. Nevertheless, the adrenal is the most common site of neuroblastomas.

Neuroblastomas are developmental malignant lesions that predominately occur in neonates and young children. These tumors grow fast, forming large abdominal masses that may be palpated by the child's mother or by an examining physician (Figure 17-15). Neuroblastomas are highly malignant tumors, evidenced by the fact that most tumors have already metastasized by the time of diagnosis. Histologically, the tumor is composed of neuroblasts, undifferentiated small cells that have very little cytoplasm (Figure 17-16). The few cells that differentiate usually evolve into neurons. Such cells release neurogenic amines, which may be detected in the urine as catecholamines or their degradation products, such as **vanillylmandelic acid** (VMA).

Neuroblastomas are rapidly growing and metastasizing tumors that previously were invariably lethal. With modern chemotherapy, however, these tumors have become more treatable; indeed, more than 90% of patients diagnosed today are cured completely with a combined regimen of surgical, medical, and radiation therapy.

PHEOCHROMOCYTOMA

Pheochromocytoma is the most common tumor involving the adrenal medulla of adults. It occurs only rarely, having an incidence of 1:10,000 per year. This tumor is important because it is a cause of surgically treatable hypertension. If the tumor is diagnosed and removed, the hypertension caused by it is cured instantaneously. Most pheochromocytomas occur sporadically, but in 10% of all cases these tumors occur in families showing an increased incidence of pheochromocytomas or are part of tumor syndromes such as MEN2, neurofibromatosis type 1, or von Hippel–Lindau syndrome.

In most instances, pheochromocytoma is a benign, solitary tumor originating from the medulla of the adrenal (Figure 17-17). Approximately 10% of all tumors originate in extra-adrenal locations and are derived from para-aortic sympathetic paraganglia. These tumors are also known as *paragangliomas*. Furthermore, 10% of all pheochromocytomas are multiple, and 10% are malignant. Histologically, the tumor is composed of polygonal cells resembling those of the normal adrenal medulla (Figure 17-18).

Clinical Features

Pheochromocytomas are, in most instances, functionally active tumors that secrete epinephrine and norepinephrine. The release of these catecholamines into the circulation causes hypertension. Patients usually have attacks of paroxysmal

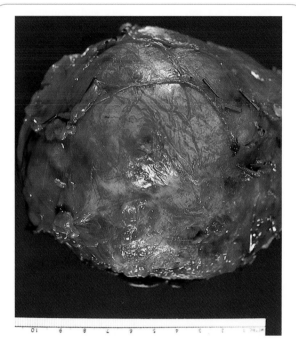

Figure 17-15 Neuroblastoma. This large tumor was removed from the abdomen of a 2-year-old boy.

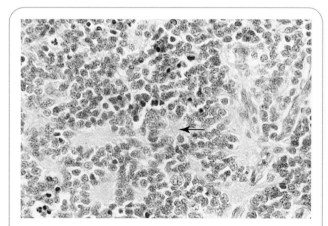

Figure 17-16 Neuroblastoma. Histologically, the tumor is composed of "small blue cells" corresponding to neuroblasts. These cells are arranged focally into "neural rosettes" (arrow) similar to those found in fetal neural tubes.

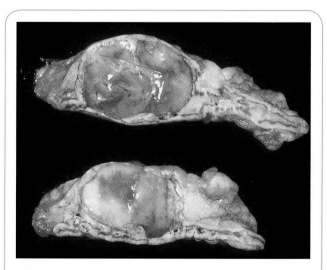

Figure 17-17 Pheochromocytoma. The adrenal contains a grayish-white nodule that is sharply demarcated from the normal tissue.

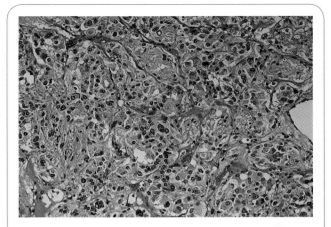

Figure 17-18 Pheochromocytoma. The tumor is composed of polygonal cells arranged into small groups surrounded by fibrous tissue containing blood vessels.

hypertension corresponding to a sudden release of catecholamines from the tumor. Prolonged exposure to epinephrine or norepinephrine may cause heart lesions *(catecholamine cardiomyopathy).*

The diagnosis of pheochromocytoma is made clinically and is confirmed biochemically by demonstrating elevated levels of epinephrine, norepinephrine, or both in blood. Levels of VMA, the primary degradation product of these biogenic amines, are elevated in urine (Figure 17-19). In complex cases it is necessary to perform functional studies that are based on the inhibition or stimulation of catecholamine release from the tumor cells.

Pheochromocytomas are treated surgically. The prognosis is excellent because most of these tumors (90%) are benign, well encapsulated, and readily removable.

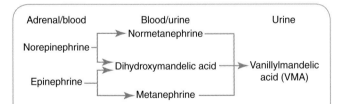

Figure 17-19 Metabolism of catecholamines leading to the formation of degradation products, which are excreted in urine. (Courtesy of Group for Research in Pathology Education [GRIPE], Oklahoma City, Oklahoma.)

REVIEW QUESTIONS

1. Which hormones are secreted by the pituitary?
2. Describe the anatomic components and cells of the thyroid, parathyroid, and adrenals and list the hormones they secrete.
3. Compare the signs of pituitary hyperfunction in children and adults.
4. What are the signs of pituitary hypofunction?
5. List the most important pituitary tumors and their clinical manifestations.
6. What are the causes of hyperthyroidism?
7. What are the clinical features of hyperthyroidism?
8. What are the causes of hypothyroidism?
9. What are the clinical features of hypothyroidism?
10. Correlate the pathologic and clinical features of nodular goiter.
11. List the most important thyroid neoplasms and discuss their prognosis.
12. What are the causes of hyperparathyroidism?
13. What are the clinical features of hyperparathyroidism?
14. What are the metabolic consequences of hyperparathyroidism?
15. Compare the clinical features of hyperparathyroidism and hypoparathyroidism.
16. What are the causes of adrenocortical hyperfunction?
17. Describe the clinical features of the three most important syndromes caused by adrenocortical hyperfunction.
18. What are the causes of adrenocortical hypofunction?
19. What are the clinical features of adrenocortical hypofunction?
20. Compare neuroblastoma and pheochromocytoma.

18

The Skin

Chapter Outline

NORMAL ANATOMY AND PHYSIOLOGY
OVERVIEW OF MAJOR DISEASES
  Pathology of Basic Skin Lesions
  Congenital Disorders
  External Injury
    Mechanical Trauma
    Thermal Injury
    Electrical Injury
    Radiation Injury
  Infectious Diseases
    Bacterial Infections
    Fungal Infections
    Viral Diseases
    Insect Infestations and Bites
    Acne

Idiopathic and Immune Disorders
  Eczema
  Seborrheic Dermatitis
  Psoriasis
Neoplasms
  Epithelial Tumors
  Pigmented Lesions
  Malignant Melanoma
  Dermal Connective Tissue Tumors
  Dermal Tumors Derived from Bloodborne Cells
Diseases of the Nails
Hair Diseases

Key Terms and Concepts

Acne
Actinic keratosis
Albinism
Alopecia
Basal cell carcinoma
Burns
Contact dermatitis
Contusion
Crust
Dermatofibroma
Dermatophytoses
Eczema
Epidermolysis bullosa
Excoriation
Fissure
Folliculitis

Freckle
Herpesvirus
Hirsutism
Ichthyosis
Impetigo
Insect bites
Kaposi's sarcoma
Keratins
Laceration
Lentigo
Macule
Malignant melanoma
Mycosis fungoides
Nevus
Nodule
Onychomycoses

Papule
Paronychia
Patch
Plaque
Pustule
Scabies
Scales
Scleroderma
Seborrheic keratosis
Squames
Squamous cell carcinoma
Sunlight injury
Tinea (capitis, corporis, cruris)
Ulcer
Urticaria pigmentosa
Vitiligo

NORMAL ANATOMY AND PHYSIOLOGY

The skin is the external covering of the body, and its primary function is to protect the body from undue outside influences. The Greek term for skin is *derma;* accordingly, the subspecialty of medicine concerned with skin diseases is called *dermatology. Dermatopathology* is the synonym for pathology of the skin.

The skin is an organ that consists of three layers: epidermis, dermis, and subcutis (Figure 18-1). The outer epidermal layer is predominantly composed of keratinocytes and scattered melanocytes (see Figure 18-1). The dermis consists of connective tissue. It also contains blood vessels, nerves, hair follicles, and skin adnexal glands. The hypodermis, or subcutis, is predominantly composed of fat tissue.

The surface of the skin is constantly abraded, and the epidermis is constantly regenerated from the proliferating cells in the basal layer. This is essential for maintaining the integrity of the skin and its primary function—protection against external injury. Intact skin represents a formidable barrier; therefore it is imperative that the body keep its "armor" intact.

The epidermis undergoes keratinization, which is the second most important protective mechanism. Epidermal cells have the capacity to produce **keratins,** which are cytoskeletal proteins that are highly resistant to mechanical and chemical injury. The keratin layer thus represents the final stage of epidermal cell differentiation. It varies in thickness from one anatomic site to another and is most prominent on the palms and soles.

The keratinized epidermis provides limited protection against sunlight by preventing the penetration of light through the skin. In this function the *keratinocytes,* the principal cells of the epidermis, are abetted by *melanocytes,* the pigment-producing cells. Melanocytes are located in the basal layer.

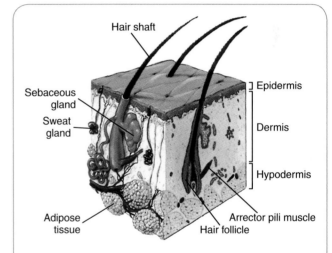

Figure 18-1 The skin consists of three layers: epidermis, dermis, and subcutaneous tissue. (Modified from Jarvis C: Physical Examination and Health Assessment, ed 5, St. Louis, 2007, Saunders.)

However, these cells have branching cytoplasmic processes that extend to several adjacent cells and link them with keratinocytes. Melanocytes produce melanin, a brown pigment, which is packaged into membrane-bound cytoplasmic bodies (melanosomes) and transferred through the cytoplasmic processes into keratinocytes. This transfer of pigment accounts for the browning of the skin on exposure to sunlight. Keratinocytes injected with melanin are more resistant to ultraviolet light and therefore protect the body against the adverse influences of sunlight more efficiently than do nonpigmented keratinocytes. Over time, the suntan fades and the skin pigmentation disappears as the pigmented keratinocytes are lost and replaced with new cells that do not contain melanin.

The epithelial components of the dermis, often referred to as *skin appendages,* are anatomically distributed in an uneven manner. *Hair follicles,* with the sebaceous glands attached to them, are prominent on the scalp but are not evident on the palms or plantar side of the foot. *Eccrine sweat glands* are present all over the body except for some sites, such as the margins of the lips and nipples. The primary function of these sweat glands is perspiration and thus, indirectly, thermoregulation. Apocrine or odoriferous sweat glands are located in some areas, such as the axilla and pubic region. Under the control of sex hormones, these glands produce a clear, sweat-like fluid that is rich in organic substances. The organic components of sweat decompose under the influence of skin bacteria, resulting in distinct odors.

The hypodermis, or subcutis, is the third layer of the skin. It is predominantly composed of fat cells and connective tissue. The thickness of this layer, which is poorly demarcated from the overlying dermis, varies. Its primary function is to provide thermal and mechanical protection to the body by its fat pad *(panniculus adiposus).* It also allows us to sit comfortably in one place and study for examinations!

OVERVIEW OF MAJOR DISEASES

The most important diseases involving the skin are as follows:

- Traumatic lesions caused by mechanical, chemical, or thermal injury
- Infectious disease
- Immune diseases and diseases of presumptive immune etiology
- Metabolic diseases and those secondary to diseases of internal organs
- Tumors

It is also important to remember that the causes of many skin diseases remain unknown. The treatment of skin diseases is still, in many cases, empirical, symptomatic, and not fully understood or scientifically justified. Thus dermatologists still have a reputation for assigning each skin disease a long Greek or Latin name and then treating them all with the same creams!

Several facts important to an understanding of skin diseases are presented here, before a discussion of specific pathologic entities.

1. *The skin protects the body primarily by maintaining its own integrity.* Intact dry skin is the best barrier against infection. Wounds caused by mechanical trauma or minor cuts provide entry sites for bacteria. Moist skin, caused by sweating (as during a hot, wet summer), also facilitates the entry of bacteria. This explains why skin infections are more common among manual laborers whose skin is easily traumatized, especially those working in tropical climates.
2. *Skin can be traumatized mechanically, thermally, or chemically or by various forms of radiation.* Various forms of mechanical skin trauma induce different lesions.

Just compare a knife wound and a penetrating bullet wound. Likewise, many of us have been burned or had frostbite, rarely stopping to consider these as forms of thermal trauma. Blisters produced by exposure to early summer sun are prime examples of radiation-induced skin trauma. Sunlight is a mixture of ultraviolet, visible light, and infrared rays, all of which can damage the skin under appropriate conditions.

3. *The effects of acute injury are distinct from those caused by chronic or repeated injuries.* For example, gradual exposure to sunlight allows gradual pigmentation of the skin. However, if the skin were exposed to the same amount of radiation in one long day on the beach, it would not tan but would burn, blister, and finally undergo acute scaling. Long-term exposure to sunlight causes chronic skin injury and accelerates aging of the skin.
4. *Skin is covered normally with bacteria that do not affect it adversely.* Our skin is not sterile; it is covered with myriad saprophytic bacteria. That is why surgeons must wash their hands before operations so that they do not infect the operating field if the gloves rupture. Saprophytic bacteria are innocuous as long as they remain on the intact skin. However, they may infect wounds and cause overwhelming infections in weak or immunosuppressed persons.

Bacteria, viruses, fungi, and parasites that are transferred onto the skin may cause diseases. Bacteria, such as staphylococci, may invade hair follicles or sebaceous glands, as occurs in *acne.* Viruses, such as *herpesvirus,* may invade the epidermis and cause vesicles. Fungi tend to grow in the keratin layer, causing dermatophytic infections, such as "athlete's foot." Lice tend to grow on hair shafts. Subcutaneous infections with worms occur often in the tropics but are not usually seen in the United States.

5. *Skin participates in an immune reaction to foreign substances.* The skin is constantly exposed to foreign substances, many of which are immunogenic and act on the immune system of the body. For example, many people are allergic to nylon underwear, cats, or house dust. Such substances may induce allergic contact dermatitis and even systemic symptoms. Childhood atopic dermatitis and eczema are the most common immune-mediated skin diseases.
6. *Skin may be affected by systemic, metabolic, and immune diseases.* The etiology of many such diseases is still unknown. For example, systemic sclerosis, a multiorgan disease of the connective tissue, produces hidebound skin known as **scleroderma.** Diabetes mellitus is a systemic disease affecting the metabolism of carbohydrates and lipids, which often manifests as skin lesions. Diabetes also predisposes individuals to bacterial infections and causes microcirculatory disturbances, which predispose them to ulcerations of the skin.
7. *Skin diseases may present with hypopigmentation or hyperpigmentation.* Albinism represents generalized genetic hypopigmentation. Localized hypopigmentation is called **vitiligo.** Hyperpigmentation may be a consequence of suntanning but also may be hormonally induced.

8. *The skin is the most common site of tumors in the human body.* This can be explained, in part, by the fact that such tumors are more easily diagnosed than small tumors of the same size in internal organs. However, one should also remember that the skin is constantly exposed to various carcinogens: chemicals, radiation, viruses, and probably many other influences of unknown carcinogenic potential. Contact with known carcinogens should be avoided. The most important skin carcinogen—the ultraviolet light in sunshine—can be avoided to some extent, but never entirely.

9. *The skin has a limited way of responding to injury.* Morphologically, identical skin lesions can be induced by different means. For example, blisters *(bullae)* can result from sunbathing; an allergic reaction to poison ivy; a systemic disease, such as porphyria; or a primary skin disease of unknown etiology, such as bullous pemphigoid.

PATHOLOGY OF BASIC SKIN LESIONS

In view of the fact that the skin has a limited reaction pattern and that many diseases produce the same symptoms, it is important to learn and understand the terms used for skin lesions in dermatologic practice. The most important of these are presented in Figure 18-2.

- **Macule**—flat lesion measuring less than 2 cm in diameter; not raised or depressed; primarily representing a change in skin color. The best example is the freckle: a brown, pigmented spot.
- **Patch**—similar to a macule but larger than 2 cm in diameter. The best example is the skin rash that occurs in measles, a childhood viral disease.
- **Papule**—slightly elevated, small induration of the skin with a diameter of less than 1 cm. Papules are the hallmark of eczema, which is usually caused by allergy.
- **Nodule**—similar to a papule but larger (1 to 5 cm in diameter). Nevi, or moles, which are pigmented, slightly raised skin lesions, are the best examples of this.

- **Tumor**—nodule with a diameter exceeding 5 cm. Such tumors may be benign or malignant.
- **Vesicle**—fluid-filled elevation of the epidermis measuring less than 1 cm in diameter. **Herpesvirus** infections produce vesicles on the border of the lips.
- **Bulla**—vesicles measuring more than 1 cm in diameter. Burns can cause bullae, some of which are confluent and may cover large surfaces of the skin.
- **Pustule**—vesicle filled with pus. *Impetigo,* a bacterial infection of the skin that usually affects children, is a typical example.
- **Ulcer**—defect of the epidermis. Syphilitic chancre, which most often appears on the skin or mucosa of the genitals, is a good example.
- **Crust**—a skin defect that is covered with coagulated plasma or blood. Healed wounds are covered with crusts.
- **Scales**—keratin layers that cover the skin in flakes or sheets and that can easily be scraped away. Pemphigus and seborrheic dermatitis are relatively common skin diseases of unknown etiology that cause scaling of the skin.
- **Squames**—large scales. **Ichthyosis,** a congenital thickening of the skin, forms numerous squames.
- **Excoriation**—superficial skin defect caused by scratching. Any chronic skin disease accompanied by an itch will ultimately result in excoriations, mostly self-induced by the patient.
- **Fissure**—sharp-edged defect of the epidermis that extends into deeper layers of the skin. Athlete's foot, a fungal disease, typically produces fissures.

CONGENITAL DISORDERS

Congenital diseases of the skin may present at birth, early in life, or later. These include minor cosmetic imperfections (so-called birthmarks) and diffuse afflictions affecting the entire body integument. The **nevus,** or birthmark, is the most common congenital skin anomaly (in Latin, *naevus* means "birthmark"). Nevi represent congenital developmental defects or hamartomas

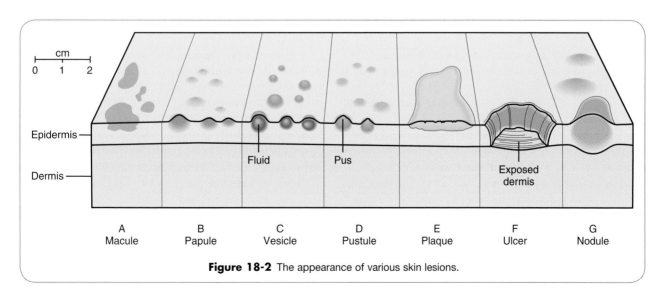

Figure 18-2 The appearance of various skin lesions.

(in Greek, *hamartion* means "body defect") whereby normal skin elements are arranged in an abnormal manner. Brown birthmarks *(melanocytic nevi)* are composed of melanocytes. *Nevus flammeus,* also known as *port-wine mark,* is a congenital aggregate of small blood vessels, usually found on the face. Congenital nevi are innocuous lesions that require no treatment.

Many skin diseases have a significant hereditary component; some are even inherited as Mendelian traits. For example, *ichthyosis congenita* is inherited as an autosomal dominant trait. In this disease the child is born covered with thick squames resembling fish skin (in Greek, *ichthys* means "fish").

Albinism (*albinus* means "white" in Latin) is a generalized hypopigmentation caused by an inborn error of metabolism. Affected persons lack one of the enzymes essential for the synthesis of melanin from the amino acids tyrosine and phenylalanine. These individuals appear strikingly pale and never tan. They have white hair and red eyes because their hair and retina also lack pigment. Albinos are at increased risk for developing sunburns and skin cancer, and they should avoid exposure to the sun altogether. There is no treatment for this pigmentary defect.

Epidermolysis bullosa is a term used to denote several congenital skin disorders, all of which are characterized by the formation of blisters on rubbing of the skin or minor trauma. The most severe form, which is fortunately rare, may present during intrauterine life. The milder forms present with blisters that form spontaneously, usually on the palms and soles. There is no effective treatment for this disease.

EXTERNAL INJURY

Skin can be injured by a variety of external means. These can be classified as follows:

- Mechanical trauma
- Thermal injury
- Electrical injury
- Radiation injury

MECHANICAL TRAUMA

Humans are exposed to mechanical trauma throughout their lives. Minor trauma does not even register. However, major trauma may have serious consequences, and because it is usually not limited to the skin alone but involves other organs as well, it may even be lethal.

It is customary to categorize mechanical trauma according to the means by which it is inflicted. *Blunt trauma* is caused by objects, such as a club or hammer. It usually results in **contusion** (*contusio* means "bruise" in Latin). Bleeding into the skin and soft tissue occurs from mechanically disrupted blood vessels. **Laceration** involves disruption of the skin and the underlying soft tissue. It usually requires surgical treatment and does not heal easily. Sharp trauma (wound) is caused by sharp objects, such as a knife or bullet.

THERMAL INJURY

Skin can be injured by relatively short exposure to very high or very low temperatures or by prolonged exposure to moderately high or low temperatures. The most important forms of injury are **burns,** caused by heat, and cold injuries, such as frostbite and immersion foot injury.

Burns

The extent of skin burns depends on the mode of exposure (e.g., sunburn, hot metal, hot air, and fumes), the duration of exposure, the temperature, and the anatomic site of injury. For example, the palms and soles have a thicker keratin layer and are more resistant to burns than the skin of the face. Thermal injury may be localized (e.g., sunburn on the face) or widespread (e.g., total body burns, as might be incurred in a house fire). The final clinical outcome of burns depends on the depth of skin injury and the extent of the body surface affected.

Burns are graded clinically by establishing the depth of skin injury. First-degree burns are the mildest form, producing only erythema and swelling. Histologically, the epidermis shows spotty, single-cell necrosis and edema. Such lesions are transitory, reversible, and heal spontaneously without any consequences.

Second-degree burns are characterized by blisters involving the epidermis. The hair follicles and skin adnexa in the dermis are spared. The epidermis heals from the edges of the blisters and from the epithelium of the hair follicles without scarring.

Third-degree burns, also known as *full-thickness burns,* cause massive necrosis of the entire epidermis and dermis, extending, to a variable degree, into the subcutaneous tissue and underlying soft tissue. Localized third-degree burns take a long time to heal, usually with prominent scarring. Large surface areas affected by third-degree burns cannot heal spontaneously and require specialized treatment, including skin transplantation. Skin may be taken for transplantation from other parts of the body (autograft) or from an unrelated donor (allograft). If properly done, skin grafting is a very efficient method for resurfacing damaged parts of the body.

To estimate the chances for survival and to determine appropriate treatment modalities, it is important to estimate the total surface of the body that has been burned. For this purpose, it is customary to apply the "rule of nines," which assigns 9% of the total body surface area to burns affecting the head and to each of the upper extremities and 9% × 2 to each lower extremity and to the frontal and posterior surface of the trunk (Figure 18-3). Any burn exceeding 9% of the total body surface is serious and must be treated intensively in a specialized burn unit. With modern treatment, most patients can be saved, even if they have extensive burns, but the scarring that follows may have crippling consequences. Mortality usually results from uncontrolled fluid loss and infection of the denuded body surfaces.

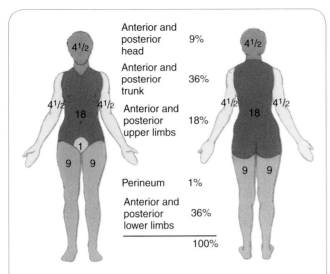

Figure 18-3 Schematic depiction of the "rule of nines," which subdivides the body into 9% areas to allow estimates of the extent of burns. (From Applegate EJ: The Anatomy and Physiology Learning System, 4th ed, St. Louis, 2011, Saunders.)

Anterior and posterior head 9%
Anterior and posterior trunk 36%
Anterior and posterior upper limbs 18%
Perineum 1%
Anterior and posterior lower limbs 36%
100%

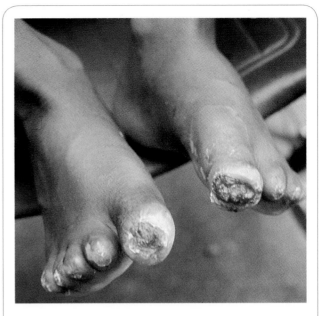

Figure 18-4 Frostbite of toes. Localized cold injury has caused necrosis of toes exposed to extreme cold on a climbing expedition in the Himalayas. (From Stevens A, Lowe J, Scott I: Core Pathology, 3rd ed, London, 2009, Elsevier.)

Cold Injuries

Cold injuries are usually less severe and less life threatening than burns, although prolonged exposure to cold can cause death by freezing. Death in snow blizzards has befallen many a mountaineer and polar explorer, but immersion foot and frostbite are more common injuries seen in daily medical practice.

Immersion foot is the term used to describe tissue injury caused by exposure to nonfreezing cold and a moist environment. It typically affects the legs and was first recognized in soldiers who had to stand for hours in trenches—hence the synonym *trench foot*. The principal damage occurs at the level of the small blood vessels, which, stunned by cold, become permanently dilated and unable to regulate local blood flow. Venous stagnation occurs, contributing to gradual cooling of tissues and accounting for the bluish color of the skin. Skin necrosis develops, with formation of blisters and ulcers.

Frostbite, or *congelation* (a Latin term meaning "freezing"), is an injury caused by exposure to subfreezing point temperature. The tissue changes resemble those induced by immersion foot injury, but they develop more rapidly and are usually more pronounced. Any part of the body may be injured. The fingers, toes, and face are most often involved. On reheating, the tissue becomes blotchy red and swollen. Recovery may occur, but necrotic tissue (gangrene) may impede healing and parts of the extremities may be lost forever (Figure 18-4). Surgical resection of nonviable tissue may be indicated, but only after spontaneous recovery is deemed impossible.

ELECTRICAL INJURY

Contact with unprotected and inadequately isolated electrical wires can cause skin wounds. Similar wounds result from lightning, which is electricity that is generated by nature. The passage of electricity through the skin generates heat, which burns the tissues, leaving linear marks along its path. At the point of entry of high-voltage electricity into the body—typically, at the site of contact with an unprotected high-voltage wire—the tissue is burned and an "electric mark" of blackened skin forms. However, electrical injury also affects the deeper tissues and possibly even internal organs, and it may cause death by interfering with the electrical conduction system of the heart. In the dermis, electricity damages the blood vessels, provoking thrombosis and subsequent infarctions in the areas to which the thrombosed blood vessels were providing blood before the injury.

RADIATION INJURY

We are constantly exposed to numerous sources of natural radiation, the most important source of which is the sun. In addition, we are exposed to various forms of artificial radiation, such as radio waves, television waves, microwaves, and ultrasound. The two most important forms of radiation injury are caused by sunshine and ionizing radiation.

Sunlight Injury

Acute exposure to the sun over a short period leads to hyperemia. Prolonged exposure causes sunburn, accompanied by blisters and peeling of the skin (Figure 18-5). Acute sunburn represents a first- or second-degree thermal injury.

Chronic exposure to the sun has cosmetically pleasing beneficial effects, but it also damages the skin. Most of the long-term consequences are related to ultraviolet light.

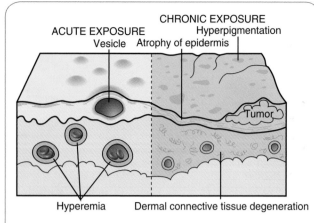

ACUTE EXPOSURE

CHRONIC EXPOSURE

Vesicle — Hyperpigmentation — Atrophy of epidermis

Tumor

Hyperemia — Dermal connective tissue degeneration

Figure 18-5 Short-term and long-term effects of sunbathing. Acute injury results in hyperemia of the dermis and blister formation. Long-term exposure may stimulate pigmentation and may also promote carcinogenesis and aging of the epidermis and dermis.

Controlled sunbathing over a relatively short period, such as 2 weeks, stimulates the transfer of melanin pigment from melanocytes to keratinocytes in the epidermis, producing a suntan. However, suntan is usually short lived, and the skin color returns to normal after the pigmented keratocytes have been shed (i.e., within about 30 days). The adverse affects of long-term exposure to sun outweigh the short-term cosmetic effects. Two major consequences of prolonged suntanning are accelerated aging of the skin and development of tumors.

Aging affects all layers of the skin. The skin becomes more brittle and less elastic, develops wrinkles, and tends to resist injury less efficiently than that of younger people. Wounds also tend to heal more slowly.

Ultraviolet light is carcinogenic for the skin. Skin tumors develop more often on sun-exposed surfaces, such as the face or arms. Furthermore, skin tumors are more common in persons who work outdoors than those who work in offices. Sailors and farmers are at increased risk, for obvious reasons. Moreover, fair-skinned persons are at a greater risk than dark-skinned persons, who are partially protected by the pigment in their skin.

? Did You Know?

For many years the cosmetic industry has been producing creams and lotions advertised as "elixirs of youth," claiming that they reduce aging of the skin. The results are usually disappointing. Recent advances in molecular biology are promising more efficient drugs. Among the drugs already on the market is Botox, the toxin isolated from the bacteria *Clostridium botulinum*. Botox injected into the skin can be used to smooth facial creases and folds.

Ionizing Radiation

Short-term exposure to x-rays or other forms of ionizing radiation (e.g., in a laboratory during handling of radioactive isotopes) is not dangerous and usually produces no obvious pathologic changes. However, prolonged or repeated exposure, or exposure to large doses of ionizing radiation, can produce significant lesions. Whereas alpha particles are large and do not penetrate the skin, beta particles can penetrate up to 1 cm and can cause epidermal changes. Gamma rays and x-rays penetrate tissues easily, causing little damage while passing through the tissue themselves. On the other hand, all these radiation particles induce secondary ionization of the molecules in tissues; thus all ionizing particles should be considered potentially damaging.

? Did You Know?

Not everybody can acquire a suntan. Indeed, dermatologists recognize six distinct groups. Those who:
1. Always burn, never tan
2. Burn readily, tan poorly
3. Burn occasionally, tan well
4. Almost never burn, tan easily
5. Are pigmented all the time (e.g., Asians)
6. Are black-skinned (e.g., blacks)

Short-term exposure to high levels of radiation may induce necrosis because radiation kills cells. Long-term exposure to small doses of radiation stimulates pigmentation and also may be carcinogenic. Thus it is no wonder that many old-time radiologists who were inadequately protected while working have developed skin cancer of the hands. Today it is unusual to see x-ray–induced cancer in health professionals.

INFECTIOUS DISEASES

Infectious diseases of the skin are common. In most instances these infections are localized and do not produce serious systemic symptoms. However, skin infections can have systemic consequences as well.

BACTERIAL INFECTIONS

Bacterial infections of the skin are classified into three major groups:
- Primary bacterial infections, which occur on apparently normal skin
- Secondary bacterial infections, which complicate preexisting skin diseases or wounds and ulcers
- Systemic bacterial infections, in which the skin involvement is only one of many manifestations of systemic, bloodborne infection

Primary bacterial infections are typically caused by pus-forming bacteria and therefore are called *pyodermas*. Most often, these infections are caused by coagulase-positive staphylococci and beta-hemolytic streptococci, which may produce either superficial or deep lesions. Bacteria that have developed resistance to antibiotics have become a major source of hospital-acquired infections. Among them the most prominent is the methicillin-resistant *Staphylococcus aureus* (MRSA), which is particularly resistant to treatment.

Impetigo (in Latin, *impeto* means "to attack") is a common superficial infection caused by streptococci or *S. aureus*. It is characterized by superficial pustules that rupture, leaving behind honey-colored scabs (Figure 18-6). Impetigo is most often found on the face of small children. Because these skin lesions are itchy, affected children often spread the infection to other sites on their body and can infect their playmates as well. Impetigo is highly contagious but responds well to systemic antibiotic therapy. It heals without any scars.

Folliculitis is a common form of infection limited to hair follicles (Figure 18-7). It is usually caused by *S. aureus*.

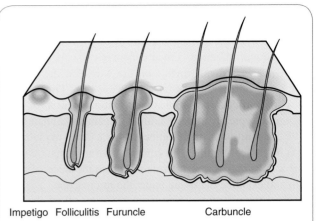

Figure 18-7 Purulent skin infections. Infections may be limited to epidermis or involve the hair follicles and dermis.

Impetigo Folliculitis Furuncle   Carbuncle

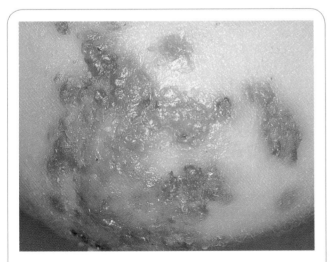

Figure 18-6 Impetigo. The skin shows typical yellow crusting blisters containing pus. (From Stevens A, Lowe J, Scott I: Core Pathology, 3rd ed, London, 2009, Elsevier.)

Typically it involves hairy areas, such as the beard. The bacteria produce a purulent exudate that fills the lumen of hair follicles. As the bacteria invade the hair shaft and the infection extends into the perifollicular tissue, a *furuncle* (boil) develops. If the infection spreads to adjacent follicles and the original abscess enlarges to include several hair follicles, a much larger boil, called a *carbuncle,* evolves. Such large abscesses are most often located on the neck and are more common in males than in females. Adequate antibiotic treatment may prevent further spread and recurrence of infection, which is otherwise common.

Secondary bacterial infections develop at the site of another disease or in wounds. Bacterial infections impede the healing of primary skin disease. The skin affected by chronic dermatitis, known clinically as *eczema,* is almost always contaminated with bacteria. Hence, the treatment of most chronic skin diseases must include some antibiotic therapy to eradicate the bacterial contamination.

Systemic infections may spread to the skin through the blood or the lymphatics or by direct extension of the infection from the underlying tissue to the skin. Such infections are more common in debilitated or immunosuppressed patients. Any case of septicemia or bacteremia—that is, entry of bacteria into the blood—may cause skin abscesses.

FUNGAL INFECTIONS

Fungal infections (**dermatophytoses**) of the skin are extremely common. Luckily, fungal pathogens—called *dermatophytes*—tend to live in "dead tissues," such as the surface keratin layer, hair, or nails, and cause almost no inflammation in the underlying skin. Nevertheless, such infections cause itching and discomfort and predispose the individual to secondary bacterial infection, which may lead to the formation of fissures and scaling.

The most common sites of superficial dermatophytoses are the feet, head, and nails and the intertriginous parts of the body, such as the axilla and groin. These lesions are called *tinea* or *ringworm. Tinea pedis,* or athlete's foot, typically begins between the toes and spreads locally. *Tinea unguium* is a chronic nail infection. **Tinea corporis** presents as circular or irregularly shaped patches on the skin that have a pale center and spreading margins (Figure 18-8). **Tinea cruris** (jock itch) affects the groin region. **Tinea capitis,** or scalp ringworm, typically affects children, causing local hair loss.

The diagnosis of fungal infections is usually made on the basis of clinical findings. To confirm the fungal nature of the disease, one may scrape the squames from the surface epithelium and examine the tissue under the microscope.

Other fungi besides dermatophytes may affect the skin. The most important of these pathogens is the ubiquitous *Candida albicans,* the cause of common thrush in children. Blastomycosis, coccidioidomycosis, and similar fungal infections are uncommon in temperate climates but are endemic in the southern United States and especially the tropics. These invasive, deep fungal infections cause large destructive lesions and tumorlike lesions called *mycetomas.* Mycetomas may produce major skin defects and deformities and are resistant to therapy.

VIRAL DISEASES

Viral infections of the skin may be acute and self-limited or chronic. Acute systemic viral diseases are common in childhood and present with either a maculopapular rash *(exanthem),* as in measles, or vesicles, as in chickenpox. Herpes labialis and herpes zoster, or shingles, are localized, blistering, viral skin diseases affecting adults.

Viral skin diseases may also have a chronic course. The best example of a chronic viral disease of the skin is the common wart *(verruca vulgaris),* which is caused by human papillomavirus (HPV). Warts are innocuous lesions that disappear spontaneously after some time, with or without treatment.

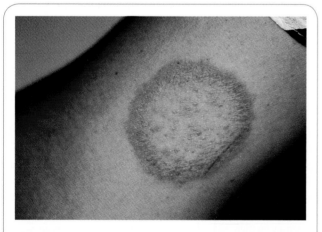

Figure 18-8 Tinea. This superficial fungal infection ("ringworm") appears as a round, scaly erythema with central clearing. (From Damjanov I, Linder J: Pathology: A Color Atlas, Mosby, 2000, St. Louis.)

INSECT INFESTATIONS AND BITES

Insect bites cause itchy, papulomacular skin lesions that usually have a red dot in the center. Blood-sucking insects that feed on human blood, such as fleas, mosquitoes, bed bugs, and lice, are the most common culprits. The skin lesions are caused by substances injected by the insect. Such substances are biologically active and cause edema, itching, or pain. These lesions are usually temporary and do not require treatment.

Many insects, such as wasps, use their sting in self-defense. The poison injected by such a sting contains vasoactive substances, which may cause edema, hemorrhage, and even systemic effects. Persons allergic to bee stings may develop a profound local reaction or a systemic anaphylactic reaction, which, if untreated, may result in death. It is important to remember that insect bites not only may cause local irritation but also may transmit serious systemic diseases, as in the case of fleas (typhus), ticks (Lyme disease), and mosquitoes (malaria). Mosquito bites have recently become an important source of West Nile virus infection.

Scabies is a contagious skin disease caused by the mite *Sarcoptes scabiei* (in Greek, meaning "flesh cutter"). This tiny organism, which is barely visible with the naked eye, burrows into the superficial layers of the epidermis. The burrows appear like irregular lines on the skin and are most prominent between the fingers and on the dorsal side of the wrist. Typical maculopapular eruptions evolve, in part induced by scratching and in part caused by a reaction to the bite, to the mites' feces, or to the ova deposited by the female. Treatment with specific antiscabies ointments is usually effective.

ACNE

Acne *vulgaris,* as the adjective in its official Latin name indicates, is a very common disease (in Latin, *vulgus* means "crowd"). Although acne is an infectious disease, it is best to consider it under a special heading, because other factors besides bacteria play an important role in the pathogenesis of typical lesions.

The pathogenesis of acne is not fully understood. Hereditary factors, hormonal factors, and general cleanliness are important. Acne typically begins at puberty, probably under the influence of sex hormones. Sex hormones, particularly androgens, stimulate the development of sebaceous glands on the face, neck, chest, and back (Figure 18-9). The secretion of sebum is increased, as evidenced by greasy skin. At the same time, the sex hormones promote hyperkeratosis at the orifice of hair follicles, which blocks the discharge of sebum. The stagnant sebum is colonized by anaerobic bacteria *(Propionibacterium acnes).* This results in formation of *comedones,* which can occur in two forms: open (blackheads) and closed (whiteheads). Through the action of bacterial lipases, the fat of the sebum is broken down to glycerin and free fatty acids, which, upon release into the tissue, cause inflammation. The entire obstructed follicle and the surrounding connective

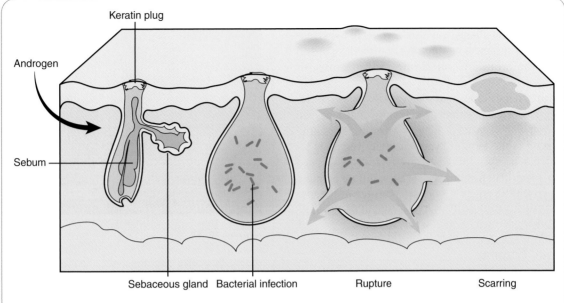

Keratin plug

Androgen

Sebum

Sebaceous gland Bacterial infection   Rupture   Scarring

Figure 18-9 Pathogenesis of acne. Hyperkeratotic epidermal plug prevents the discharge of sebum. The retained sebum is colonized by bacteria. Bacterial action expands the follicle and ultimately leads to rupture and discharge of infected purulent sebum into the adjacent dermis.

tissue are transformed into pustules or larger abscesses. These may persist, become confluent *(acne conglobata),* transform into dermal cysts, or heal with scarring *(keloid acne).* Scratching, picking, or pressing of these lesions predisposes the individual to secondary infections (Figure 18-10).

Acne is a major cosmetic problem in teenagers. Treatment is aimed at decreasing the keratinization of follicles by using retinoic acid or keratinolytic agents, such as benzoyl peroxide, and controlling infection with local or systemic antibiotics, such as clindamycin or tetracycline.

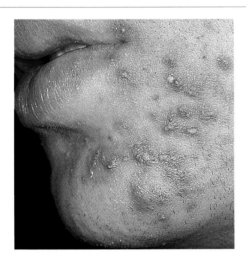

Figure 18-10 Acne. The facial skin shows a combination of comedones, papules, and pustules. (From Habif TP et al: Skin Diseases, Diagnosis and Treatment, 2nd ed, St. Louis, 2005, Mosby.)

IDIOPATHIC AND IMMUNE DISORDERS

Many skin diseases have either no identifiable cause or are presumed to be caused by immune mechanisms. Most often, such idiopathic or immune-mediated dermatoses present as eczema or chronic dermatitis or as papulosquamous or bullous disorders. Clinically, such diseases present as localized or widespread skin lesions of variable morphology. Itching is the most common symptom.

ECZEMA

Eczema (in Greek, meaning to "boil out") is a term used to denote many forms of chronic dermatitis—that is, inflammatory skin diseases with the following characteristics:

- Present with nonspecific lesions, such as localized edema, papules, and vesicles
- Are uniformly accompanied by *pruritus* (the Latin term for "itching")

Because of the itching, the primary lesions become infected, which causes secondary changes, such as scales, crusts, and oozing. Histologically, eczema is characterized by chronic inflammatory cell infiltrates in the dermis, blood vessel dilation, and edema. The epidermis shows edema and hyperkeratosis.

It is convenient to classify eczema into exogenous eczema and endogenous eczema.

Exogenous Eczema

Exogenous eczema can usually be traced to a specific cause in the environment; that is, it may be caused by irritants or allergens. Many exogenous chemicals may act as irritants. For example, detergents in soap may cause eczema in house-wives, and cement powder may cause hand lesions in construction workers. Skin allergy can also develop in hypersensitive persons. For instance, **contact dermatitis** develops in some people who are allergic to plastic, rubber gloves, or even gold rings.

Allergies to systemic drugs may also cause various skin reactions. Drug-induced skin eruptions may present as localized or systemic rash with intensive itching. In other instances drug reactions present in the form of hypersensitivity vasculitis involving small blood vessels of the dermis, typically associated with pinpoint (petechial) hemorrhages or even diffuse purpura. Chronic drug reactions are called *lichenoid eruptions* because they cause patchy thickening of the skin similar to the crustlike lichen on tree bark.

Endogenous Eczema

Endogenous eczema may occasionally have an identifiable cause, but most often its cause is unknown. Many systemic autoimmune disorders, such as systemic lupus erythematosus, present with skin lesions. Atopic dermatitis, a common disease affecting approximately 10% of all children, also is thought to have an immunologic basis. It tends to affect families with other immune disorders, such as hay fever, but its pathogenesis is still unknown.

SEBORRHEIC DERMATITIS

Seborrheic dermatitis, a widespread chronic disease that affects 10% to 20% of the U.S. population, is a multifactorial disorder. It presents with reddening, scaling, and itching of the skin, especially on the nasolabial folds and eyebrows and the upper chest. It leads to the formation of abundant dandruff. Topical steroids provide some relief, but this does not prove the allergic nature of this disease. Special shampoos and soaps containing sulfur also can be used.

PSORIASIS

Psoriasis is the most important generalized papulosquamous disease because it affects 1% to 2% of the entire world population and currently is incurable. It is more common in some families, but its mode of inheritance is not Mendelian.

The disease presents with slightly elevated papules and patches. These are covered with silvery scales, reflecting the parakeratotic surface layer (Figure 18-11). The lesions most often appear on the extensor surface of the extremities, such as the knees and elbows. The scalp and the nails are also often affected. In most patients the lesions are not itchy, although the Greek word *psora,* from which the name of the disease is derived, means "to itch."

The papules erupt in crops, symmetrically involving various parts of the body; they then slowly fade away. Exacerbations seem to be related to trauma and emotional stress. The treatment is symptomatic but not too effective. Symptoms related to internal organs may develop occasionally, most often in the form of psoriatic arthritis.

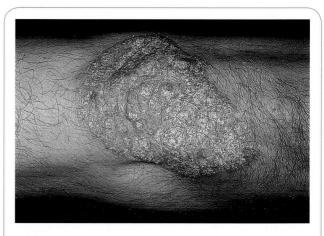

Figure 18-11 Psoriasis. A silvery, scaly psoriatic plaque is seen on the skin of the knee. (From Habif TP et al: Skin Diseases, Diagnosis and Treatment, 2nd ed, St. Louis, 2005, Mosby.)

NEOPLASMS

Neoplasms of the skin are divided into four groups:
- Tumors of epithelial cells
- Tumors of pigmentary cells
- Tumors of the dermal connective tissue
- Tumors of bloodborne "immigrant" cells

All these tumors may be benign or malignant. The most important tumors are listed in Table 18-1.

EPITHELIAL TUMORS

Epithelial skin tumors originate from the surface epidermis, hair shafts, sebaceous glands, and various eccrine and apocrine sweat glands. Most common are tumors originating from the epidermis itself. Sweat gland and sebaceous gland tumors are much less common.

Seborrheic Keratosis

Seborrheic keratosis (also called *senile warts*) is the most common benign epidermal tumor, presenting in the form of a brownish, solitary or multiple, mulberry-shaped, wartlike, exophytic, flat-topped lesion with a corrugated, furrowed surface. Histologically, the lesion consists of papillae lined with a uniform population of basaloid cells.

Seborrheic keratosis is innocuous and should not be considered premalignant. Some lesions that are very pigmented may be mistaken for malignant melanoma. In contrast to melanoma, senile warts are friable and easily removed.

Basal Cell Carcinoma

Basal cell carcinoma is the most common malignant skin tumor of epithelial origin. Fortunately, this low-grade malignant tumor does not metastasize and rarely, if ever, causes death.

TABLE 18-1 Neoplasms of the Skin

Tumor Category	Benign	Malignant	Cell of Origin
Epithelial tumors	Seborrheic keratosis Eccrine adenoma Sebaceous adenoma	Basal cell carcinoma Eccrine carcinoma Sebaceous carcinoma	Keratinocyte Sweat gland Sebaceous glands
Pigmentary cell tumors	Nevus	Malignant melanoma	Melanocyte
Connective tissue tumors	Dermatofibroma Hemangioma	Fibrosarcoma Angiosarcoma Kaposi's sarcoma	Fibroblast Endothelial cell of blood vessels
Tumors originating from bloodborne cells	Pseudolymphoma Urticaria pigmentosa	Lymphoma Malignant mastocytosis Metastatic carcinoma	Lymphocyte Mast cell Malignant disease of an internal organ

Lesions are typically located on sun-exposed skin and thus are probably related etiologically to overexposure to sunlight. The tumor presents as a slightly elevated nodule with a central depression that becomes increasingly prominent as the tumor grows (Figure 18-12). Histologically, the tumor is composed of islands and strands of invasive neoplastic cells resembling those in the basal layer of the epidermis. Treatment, whether surgical resection, cauterization, or radiotherapy, yields excellent results, although some of the flat and multifocal lesions may recur if not removed completely.

Squamous Cell Carcinoma

Squamous cell carcinoma is a truly malignant tumor of the surface epithelium. Like basal cell carcinoma, it occurs most often on sun-exposed skin. The lesion presents as a flat **plaque;** a small, persistent ulcer; or a slightly elevated, keratotic plaque (Figure 18-13). Histologically, the tumor is a

squamous cell carcinoma that is indistinguishable from squamous cell carcinoma in other organs.

On sun-exposed skin, squamous cell carcinoma is often preceded by a malignant, preinvasive stage of disease known as **actinic keratosis.** Colloquially, actinic keratosis is also known as *squamous cell carcinoma "one half,"* so named because it shows many of the cytologic characteristics of cancer but no invasion of the underlying tissue. It is also known as solar keratosis because it typically occurs on sun-exposed body surface. It appears in the form of atrophic or inducated patches that have a rough and often hyperkeratotic surface. Actinic keratosis typically progresses to an even more atypical lesion, squamous cell *carcinoma in situ (CIS).* In contrast to actinic keratosis, which is "one-half carcinoma," CIS is a full-blown carcinoma involving all layers of the epidermis. CIS is also called *preinvasive carcinoma,* to distinguish it from invasive squamous cell carcinoma, a

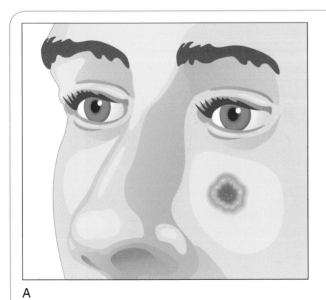

A

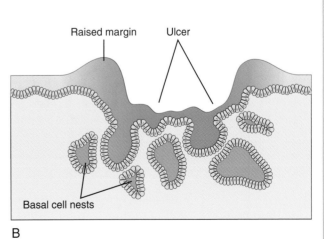

B

Figure 18-12 Basal cell carcinoma. *A,* Tumor appears as a nodule with central depression. *B,* This craterlike tumor is composed of invasive basaloid cells arranged into nests.

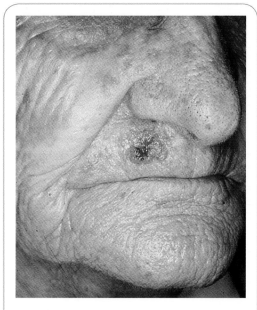

Figure 18-13 Squamous cell carcinoma.

tumor that does not respect the border between the epidermis and dermis and is a truly infiltrating malignant neoplasia.

The most important telltale signs of cancer are as follows:

- Persistent, nonhealing ulcer, containing friable, bleeding tissue
- Ulcer or nodule of irregular shape and indistinct margins
- Ulcer surrounded by atrophic and keratotic skin typical of **sunlight injury** (*actinic keratosis*)

Typical squamous cell carcinomas are locally invasive, but less than 2% of all tumors metastasize. The prognosis depends primarily on the stage of the disease; therefore it is imperative that the tumor be diagnosed early. Because none of

the clinical signs is diagnostic, it is important to perform a biopsy of all suspicious lesions for histologic examination.

PIGMENTED LESIONS

Normal skin contains numerous brownish pigmentary lesions (Figure 18-14), the most common of which are freckles, lentigo, and nevi.

- *Ephelis,* or **freckle,** is a patch of skin in which the melanocytes show a hyper-reactivity to ultraviolet stimulation. If exposed to sunlight, such spots become darker brown.
- **Lentigo** is a sharply demarcated macule occupied by an increased number of melanocytes. Lentigines do not respond to sunlight.

Nevus, or mole, as explained previously, is a developmental abnormality of the skin characterized by an accumulation of melanocytes. Nevi may be located in the dermis *(dermal nevus)* or at the dermoepidermal junction *(junctional nevus),* or they may be both junctional and dermal *(compound nevus).* Finally, there are the so-called blue nevi, which are composed of deep dermal melanocytes. Because of their deep location in the skin, such nevi have a bluish-gray color. Nevi are divided into two groups: *congenital nevi,* which are present at the time of birth, and *acquired nevi.* Congenital nevi are birthmarks with no special significance. In Japan a congenital nevus on the right earlobe portends good luck and is considered evidence that the person was born under a lucky star. Acquired nevi appear at puberty, become more prominent during adult life, and then involute. Acquired nevi are usually innocuous skin lesions and do not require treatment. The malignant potential of ordinary acquired nevi is very low. However, some nevi—so-called *dysplastic nevi*—are not so innocuous and may progress to malignant melanoma. Dysplastic nevi occur at a high rate in some cancer-prone families and, if untreated, undergo malignant transformation in more than 50% of cases.

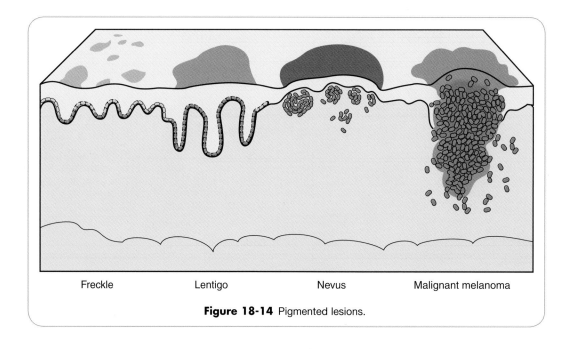

| Freckle | Lentigo | Nevus | Malignant melanoma |

Figure 18-14 Pigmented lesions.

MALIGNANT MELANOMA

Malignant melanoma is a tumor originating from melanocytes (Figure 18-15). Approximately one half of malignant melanomas originate from intact skin; the other half arise from freckles and preexisting nevi. Because melanoma is the most malignant of the skin tumors, it is important to diagnose it as early as possible. Several clinical histologic types of melanoma are recognized.

Lentigo maligna is a flat, macular lesion that typically originates in a preexisting freckle, usually in elderly persons. It remains localized for up to 10 to 15 years and, if not removed, acquires invasive properties and transforms into a superficially spreading or invasive nodular melanoma.

Superficial spreading melanoma accounts for 70% of all malignant pigmentary tumors and is the most common form of clinically recognized melanomas. These lesions present as irregularly pigmented macules with irregular edges. The lesions are pruritic and are most often located on the legs in women and the back in men. Histologically, these lesions are composed of malignant melanocytes that grow radially in the epidermis, showing, for a considerable time, no tendency for dermal invasion. As the tumor progresses, the cells tend to invade superficial layers of the epidermis and then invade the dermis, thus giving rise to nodular melanoma.

Nodular melanoma is the rapidly growing, infiltrating variant of malignant melanoma. It is marked by vertical growth and invasion of the dermis. The extent of dermal invasion is the most important prognostic sign. Pathologists estimate the depths of tumor invasion by histologic means and then use these measurements to stage the tumor. For example, if the tumor invades less than 0.75 mm and is limited to the papillary dermis, it is considered a level I lesion and is entirely curable. Tumors invading to a depth of more than 1.5 mm (i.e., those that have spread to the reticular dermis) are classified as level IV and have a 5-year survival of 40%. Invasion of the subcutaneous tissue by tumor (level V lesion) portends a poor prognosis (a 5-year survival of 25%).

Acral-lentiginous melanomas develop on the palms and plantar surfaces or underneath the nails. This is the most common variant of melanoma in blacks and Asians.

Clinical Features

Malignant melanomas are related to sun exposure and are thus more common in patients living in tropical areas than those living in northern climates. The races that have little pigment are more susceptible than pigmented races. Accordingly, melanomas are rare in blacks (except for acral-lentiginous melanomas). A familial predisposition to melanomas has been registered in individuals with multiple dysplastic nevi.

At least one third to one half of all malignant melanomas originate in preexisting lentigines or acquired and dysplastic nevi. Therefore it is important to recognize the transition of these benign or premalignant pigmentary lesions into overt malignant melanoma. Clinical experience has taught us the "A-B-C-D of diagnosis," as follows:

A—*Asymmetry of the pigmented lesion.* Any pigmented lesion that has flat and elevated parts intermixed in a haphazard manner should be considered potentially malignant and warrants careful monitoring.

B—*Borders.* Lesions that have irregular margins, with notching and leakage of brown pigment across the borders, are suspect.

C—*Color.* Marked variations in color (ranging from dark black to dark brown to red), when interspersed with areas that appear bleached, are signs of "restlessness" of the melanocytes and their potential for invasiveness. Malignant melanoma cells are not as efficient melanin producers as normal pigmentary cells. Melanomas are immunogenic and an immune reaction may destroy some cells. All these aspects of tumor biology account for the paler areas noted in the tumors.

D—*Diameter of the lesion.* Most malignant melanomas that are diagnosed clinically measure more than 6 mm in diameter. This does not mean that lesions smaller than 6 mm are not malignant. However, any lesion that

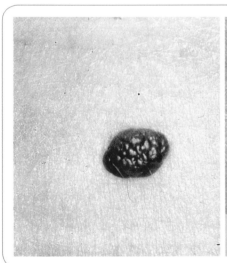
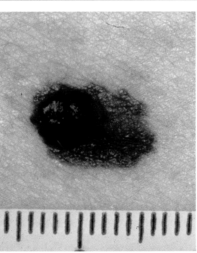

Figure 18-15 Pigmented skin lesions. *Left,* Benign pigmented nevus (mole). *Right,* Malignant melanoma. Note the differences in size and shape and the irregular borders of the melanoma. (Courtesy the National Cancer Institute, Bethesda, Maryland.)

has the previously mentioned A-B-C features and measures more than 6 mm in diameter should be removed and examined histologically.

The treatment of malignant melanomas is surgical. Tumors that have distant metastases must be treated by radiation therapy and chemotherapy. The overall 5-year survival for all forms of melanoma is 60%.

Did You Know?

Well-known children's stories can be used to raise awareness of malignant melanoma, as mentioned in some medical texts. *Ugly Duckling sign* refers to a mole that is different from others. Such moles that look "uglier" may be spotted by the patient and should be examined by the doctor. The *Little Red Riding Hood* warning reminds us that persons with fair skin and light-colored hair may develop light-colored melanomas, which might therefore escape detection.

DERMAL CONNECTIVE TISSUE TUMORS

Dermal tumors may originate from fibroblasts, blood vessels, and many other structures. These are mostly benign lesions or low-grade malignant tumors that are curable by surgical excision. Among these, the most common is the **dermatofibroma.** Dermatofibromas are benign tumors composed of fibroblasts. Surgical excision is the treatment of choice.

Did You Know?

Neurofibromas are hereditary tumors arising from the small nerves in the skin. As shown in this drawing from the nineteenth century, such tumors have been recognized for some time. Only recently, however, has neurofibromatosis been linked to a defect in a tumor suppressor gene. This defect can be transmitted from one generation to another. Approximately 100,000 Americans have some evidence of neurofibromatosis, although the tumors are rarely as numerous as those shown here.

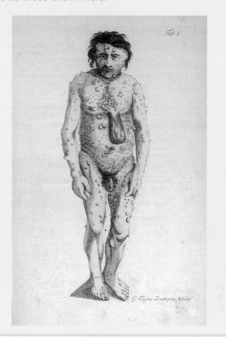

Kaposi's Sarcoma

Kaposi's sarcoma is a dermal tumor composed of blood vessels and perivascular connective tissue cells (Figure 18-16). These red tumors present as hemorrhagic nodules, which are often multiple and confluent. Previously, Kaposi's sarcoma of the skin was extremely rare. However, with the epidemic of acquired immunodeficiency syndrome (AIDS), the incidence of Kaposi's sarcoma has increased dramatically; this tumor has become the most prevalent malignant lesion in patients with AIDS. The relationship of Kaposi's sarcoma to AIDS is not fully understood, but it seems that the state of immunosuppression associated with AIDS somehow facilitates the proliferation of blood vessel–forming cells in the dermis and in other sites.

Recently, herpesvirus type 8 has been isolated from Kaposi's sarcoma cells. It has been proposed that the virus may cause tumors in immunosuppressed hosts.

Kaposi's sarcoma is a tumor of low malignant potential, which, nevertheless, tends to spread in immunosuppressed patients with AIDS. It may spread widely and cause death. No adequate treatment is available for this tumor.

DERMAL TUMORS DERIVED FROM BLOODBORNE CELLS

The skin may be affected by malignant cells that reach it from the blood circulation. It is thus fairly common to see dermal infiltrates of malignant lymphoma or other visceral malignant lesions. T-cell lymphomas have a special predilection for the skin, one form of which is called **mycosis fungoides.** Typically this disease presents as skin macules and papules that progress to nodules and ulcerating large masses.

Urticaria pigmentosa is a peculiar skin disease characterized by dermal infiltrates of mast cells. This disease, typically found in children and young adults, presents with pigmented, brownish-red macules or slightly elevated papules that flare on touching or stroking. Histologically these lesions consist

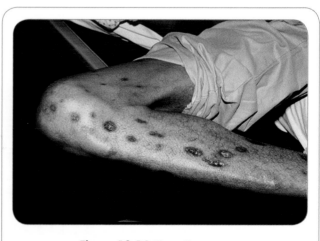

Figure 18-16 Kaposi's sarcoma.

of dermal infiltrates of mast cells. These mast cells release histamine and other vasoactive amines, causing swelling and reddened skin patches. The disease usually does not require any special treatment, and it disappears spontaneously with time, usually after puberty.

DISEASES OF THE NAILS

Nails are specialized coverings on the toes and fingers, which can be considered as modified skin. The nails are derived from the constantly dividing cells of the matrix at the base of the nail, which is partially covered with the cuticle of the nail fold (Figure 18-17).

Diseases of the nails are manifold; some of them are caused by local conditions, whereas others reflect various systemic disorders. Deformities, such as *onychogryphosis* (from the Greek *onychos,* meaning "nail," and *gryphosis,* meaning "curvature"), are usually without a known cause. Spoon-shaped nails *(koilonychia)* are usually a sign of iron-deficiency anemia, whereas nail clubbing is a sign of chronic pulmonary disease. Psoriasis is associated with nail disease in about 50% of all patients.

Nails are resistant to infection except for the base and the cuticle. Bacterial infections of the cuticle, which are common, are called **paronychia** (Figure 18-18). This is most common in individuals who work with their hands immersed in water, such as kitchen personnel. The only clinically significant nail infections are caused by fungi. These **onychomycoses** are typically chronic; resistant to treatment; and cause nail deformities, defects, and brittleness.

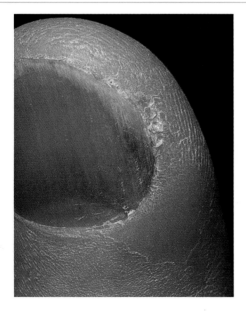

Figure 18-17 Structure of the nail. (From Habif TP et al: Skin Diseases, Diagnosis and Treatment, 2nd ed, St. Louis, Mosby, 2005.)

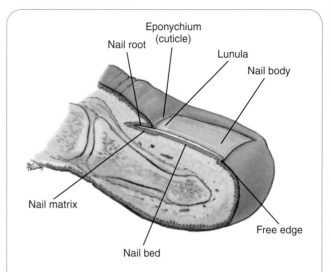

Figure 18-18 Paronychia. Swelling and redness of the cuticle on the proximal side of the nail. (Modified from Jarvis C: Physical Examination and Health Assessment, 5th ed, St. Louis, 2007, Saunders.)

HAIR DISEASES

The body is covered with several types of hair that differ with regard to their structure, growth cycle, and many other properties. Compare, for instance, the hair of the pubic skin, the scalp, and the beard. Clearly each of these forms of hair may react in a different manner to various adverse influences and will show different pathologic changes. Some of these diseases have been mentioned already, such as fungal and bacterial infections. Acne is, in essence, a disease of the hair follicle–sebaceous unit.

An excess of hair is called **hirsutism** (in Latin, *hirsutus* means "shaggy"). The hair growth on the chin and the chest is stimulated by male sex hormones; thus normal males have a beard and chest hair. Hirsutism in these areas in the females is usually a sign of hormonal disturbances, such as those caused by androgen-producing ovarian or adrenal tumors or complex hormonal disturbances caused by polycystic ovary syndrome.

Loss of hair from the scalp is called baldness, or **alopecia** (from the Greek *alopex,* meaning "fox"; thus alopecia is loss of hair, as in fox mange). Alopecia may be focal *(alopecia areata)* or diffuse. Alopecia areata may be an autoimmune disease, but in some instances it is caused by fungi *(tinea capitis)* or bacteria, such as that seen in syphilis. Hair pulling *(trichotillomania)* is usually a manifestation of nervousness and may cause focal hair loss.

Diffuse alopecia involves large portions of the scalp and typically occurs in aging males. Male-pattern baldness is marked by recession of the frontotemporal hairline with progressive loss of hair over the convexity of the head. Such baldness is considered idiopathic but has a strong hereditary component. It usually occurs after the age of 30 years and is resistant to treatment. Alopecia in women is usually a sign of hormonal disorders, such as hypothyroidism or some nutritional deficiency (e.g., iron deficiency and protein malnutrition). Alopecia may also be induced by cytotoxic drugs. Drugs used to treat cancer kill the dividing cells, including those in the hair matrix, thus preventing hair growth. Alopecia universalis caused by cytotoxic drugs involves not only the scalp but also the eyebrows and body hair. After completion of the therapy, hair growth resumes.

REVIEW QUESTIONS

1. What are the main histologic components of the epidermis, dermis, and subcutis?

2. What are the main functions of the skin?

3. Give clinical examples of a macule, patch, papule, vesicle, pustule, plaque, ulcer, and nodule.

4. What is ichthyosis?

5. What is albinism?

6. What is epidermolysis bullosa?

7. Explain the effects of mechanical trauma on the skin and subcutaneous tissues.

8. What are the differences between first-degree, second-degree, and third-degree burns?

9. Compare immersion foot and frostbite.

10. Describe an "electric mark" on the skin.

11. Compare the effects of acute and chronic sun exposure.

12. Describe and explain the pathogenesis of impetigo, folliculitis, furuncle, and carbuncle.

13. Compare superficial dermatophytosis with deep fungal infections.

14. List viruses that infect skin.

15. Describe insect bites.

16. What is scabies?

17. Describe the pathology of acne and explain its pathogenesis.

18. What is eczema?

19. What is seborrheic dermatitis?

20. Describe the pathologic and clinical features of psoriasis.

21. Classify skin neoplasms.

22. What is seborrheic keratosis?

23. Compare basal cell and squamous cell carcinoma.

24. What is actinic keratosis?

25. What are the most important telltale signs of skin cancer?

26. Compare freckle with lentigo and nevus.

27. Classify malignant melanomas.

28. List the A-B-C-D of diagnosis of malignant melanoma.

29. What is Kaposi's sarcoma, and how is it related to the AIDS epidemic?

30. Compare mycosis fungoides and urticaria pigmentosa.

31. Describe the main features of nail infections.

32. Compare hirsutism and alopecia.

Bones and Joints

Chapter Outline

NORMAL ANATOMY AND PHYSIOLOGY
OVERVIEW OF MAJOR DISEASES
  Developmental and Genetic Disorders
    Achondroplasia
    Osteogenesis Imperfecta
  Infectious Diseases
    Osteomyelitis
  Circulatory Disturbances
  Metabolic Disorders
    Osteoporosis
    Osteomalacia
    Renal Osteodystrophy
    Paget's Disease

Traumatic Injuries
  Bone Fractures
  Joint Dislocations
Bone Tumors
  Benign Bone Tumors
  Malignant Bone Tumors
Joint Diseases
  Osteoarthritis
  Rheumatoid Arthritis
  Infectious Arthritis
  Gout

Key Terms and Concepts

Achondroplasia
Ankylosing spondylitis
Aseptic bone necrosis
Bone mineral density (BMD)
Chondroma
Chondrosarcoma
Degenerative joint diseases
Ewing's sarcoma
Fracture

Giant cell tumor of bone
Gout
Hyperuricemia
Lyme disease
Osteoarthritis
Osteogenesis imperfecta
Osteoma
Osteomalacia
Osteomyelitis

Osteopenia
Osteoporosis
Osteosarcoma
Paget's disease
Renal osteodystrophy
Rheumatoid arthritis
Rickets

After reading this chapter, the student should be able to:

1. Define the portions of a typical long bone: epiphysis, metaphysis, diaphysis, and epiphyseal growth plate.
2. Define and describe the bone cells: osteocyte, osteoblast, osteoclast, and chondrocyte.
3. Describe the anatomy of joints.
4. Discuss achondroplastic dwarfism, osteogenesis imperfecta, and osteopetrosis.
5. Describe the most common forms of osteomyelitis.
6. Describe aseptic necrosis and list at least two anatomic sites affected.
7. Define osteoporosis and discuss its clinical features.
8. Explain the pathogenesis of osteomalacia and rickets and relate the bone changes to clinical symptoms.
9. Describe the healing of simple bone fractures, define callus, and explain the reasons for delayed healing of fractures.
10. List the typical age at onset and the most common anatomic sites of osteosarcoma, chondrosarcoma, and Ewing's sarcoma and describe typical features of these tumors.
11. Define osteoarthritis, explain the pathogenesis of degenerative joint disease, and describe its pathology.
12. Define rheumatoid arthritis and explain its pathogenesis and pathology.
13. List the three most important facts about ankylosing spondylitis.
14. Give two examples of infectious arthritis.
15. Define gout and describe the pathology of gout arthropathy.

The skeleton is composed of bones connected to one another by joints. The diseases affecting the skeleton are classified under the headings of orthopedic pathology and rheumatology.

NORMAL ANATOMY AND PHYSIOLOGY

The human body contains more than 200 bones, which can be classified as either long or short and flat. The long bones, also known as *tubular bones,* form the shaft of the extremities, whereas the short and flat bones form the skeleton of the trunk, the skull, and the terminal portions of the extremities (Figure 19-1).

All bones are composed of cells (osteocytes) and extracellular matrix (osteoid) that is impregnated with calcium phosphate salts in the form of hydroxyapatite. In the cortex of long bones, the cells and matrix are arranged into elementary units called *osteons,* which form the compact bone. The medullary portion of long, most short, and flat bones is composed of trabeculae, forming the cancellous or spongy bone. The inside surface of the compact bone and the trabeculae are covered with bone-forming cells (osteoblasts) and bone-resorbing cells (osteoclasts). The external surface of bones is covered with the periosteum, which also contains osteoblasts, fibroblasts, blood vessels, and nerves.

Long bones have a central part, called the *diaphysis* (Figure 19-2), and two ends, each of which is covered with a cup of articular cartilage. These terminal portions of bone are called *epiphyses* because they are above the growth plate, which is called the *physis* (in Greek, *physis* means "growth"). The growth plate and the adjacent terminal diaphysis represent the most metabolically active segment of the long bones. Because it changes dramatically during development, it is therefore called the *metaphysis.* (In Greek, the prefix *meta* denotes "changes"; thus *metaphysis* means the growth-related, changing part of the bone.)

Bone formation during fetal life and until the end of puberty occurs through two mechanisms. The longitudinal growth of long bones is based on osseous transformation of the cartilage in the growth plate, called *endochondral ossification.* Most flat bones form through intramembranous ossification, whereby bone formation results from direct transformation of fibrous matrix into osteoid, followed by mineralization (i.e., deposition of calcium phosphate salts, predominantly in the form of hydroxyapatite). Intramembranous ossification also accounts for the subperiosteal bone formation of long bones, which is the basis of the appositional growth and widening of long bones. Endochondral ossification ceases by the end of puberty and appears later only exceptionally and under pathologic conditions, as during healing of bone fractures. The intramembranous appositional growth of long bones continues, albeit at a slower rate, throughout the normal life span.

The most important functions of bone are the following:
- Mechanical support for the muscles, which makes possible the movement of limbs
- Protection of internal organs, such as the ribs forming the thorax or the skull protecting the brain
- Support of hematopoiesis, which occurs in the bone marrow
- Storage of calcium and phosphate salts

The normal structure of bones and their shape depend on two extraosseous influences: their interaction with the muscles and the hormonal regulation of calcium and phosphate metabolism. The normal structure of bones also depends on the proper balance between bone formation and bone resorption. The muscles insert onto the periosteum and, by exerting

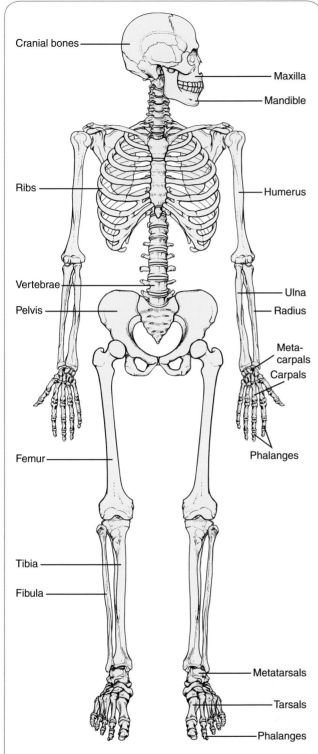

Figure 19-1 The human skeleton consists of long bones (e.g., femur and radius), short bones (e.g., tarsal bones and vertebrae), and flat bones (e.g., pelvic bone, scapula, and calvaria).

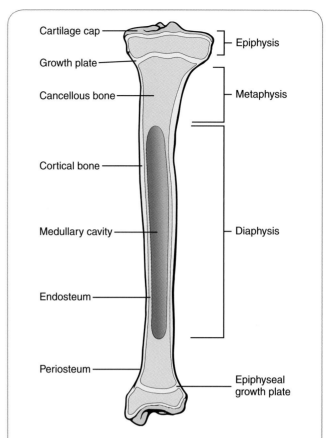

Figure 19-2 The long bone has a central part (diaphysis) and two terminal parts (epiphysis). The shaft of the bone is composed of cancellous bone on the outside and trabecular bone on the inside. The marrow contains fat tissue except in the short and flat bones of the trunk, where it is composed of hematopoietic cells. The external surface of the bone is covered with periosteum. The articular surface is covered with a cartilage cap.

tension, modulate the shape of bones according to the elementary laws of physics.

Osteoblasts form new bone, whereas osteoclasts remove and remodel old bone under the influence of hormones (e.g., parathyroid hormone [PTH]), vitamins (e.g., vitamins D and C), and various other biologically active substances (e.g., prostaglandins and interleukins). The calcium and phosphate released from the bone enter the circulation and are in balance with ionized calcium and phosphate in the serum. As discussed in greater detail in Chapter 17, this balance is tightly regulated by PTH and vitamin D.

A joint is the junction between two or more bones, designed to provide support and structural firmness and to allow movement. There are two types of joints: (1) moveable diarthrodial or synovial joints and (2) joints that allow limited or no movement at all, termed *synarthroses.* We shall limit our discussion predominantly to synovial joints, which account for most of the joints of the extremities. Synarthroses interconnect the bones of the head and trunk.

The typical synovial joint is enclosed in a connective tissue capsule composed of ligaments (Figure 19-3). On the

413

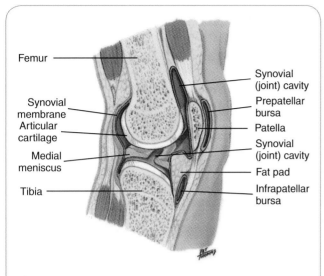

Figure 19-3 Schematic drawing of a typical diarthrodial (synovial) joint. (From Applegate EJ: The Anatomy and Physiology Learning System, 4th ed, St. Louis, 2011, Saunders.)

Labels on figure: Femur, Synovial membrane, Articular cartilage, Medial meniscus, Tibia, Synovial (joint) cavity, Prepatellar bursa, Patella, Synovial (joint) cavity, Fat pad, Infrapatellar bursa

inside, the space is lined with synovial cells secreting a viscous fluid that lubricates the joint surface. The joint surfaces are covered with cartilaginous caps covering the epiphyseal bone. Between the two adjacent cartilaginous surfaces of two adjacent bones, some joints, such as the knee, have a semilunar disk called the *meniscus;* in other joints the cartilage caps of opposing bones are in close contact with each other, separated only by a thin film of synovial fluid. Some joints, such as the knee, are reinforced by ligaments that hold the bones within the joint in close contact with one another. Joints are richly supplied with blood vessels and nerves.

OVERVIEW OF MAJOR DISEASES

The most important diseases of the bones are the following:
- Metabolic diseases affecting the growth, formation, and removal of bone
- Fractures and deformities
- Bacterial infections
- Tumors
- Inflammatory diseases
- Degenerative joint disease

Several facts important to an understanding of bone pathology are presented here, before a discussion of specific pathologic entities.

1. *Bones have two major functions: mechanical and metabolic.* Although bones are viewed only as support structures, one should not forget that bones are the major storage site of calcium and phosphate salts. Bones actively participate in the body's response to vitamin deficiency (e.g., **rickets** secondary to vitamin D deficiency). Many hormones, such as PTH, corticosteroids, and sex hormones, have an effect on bones. The joints have only a mechanical function: to stabilize the skeleton and enable movement of bones.

2. *Bones and joints are composed of living tissues that undergo constant changes.* Bones are in an active equilibrium with other parts of the body. For example, the muscles exert constant pressure and tension, influencing the shape of bones and maintaining their normal structure. Loss of muscle strength in people who are paralyzed or confined to bed because of chronic illness weakens bones. Exercise has been recommended for delaying age-related bone loss. Prolonged immobilization stiffens the joints and may cause *ankylosis* (in Greek, *ankylos* means "stiff"). Vertebrae may be affected by **ankylosing spondylitis,** a progressive disease of unknown origin that typically occurs in men with human leukocyte antigen (HLA) B27. It results in obliteration of intervertebral joints and stiffening of the vertebral column, which can be recognized on radiographs as "bamboo-spine."

3. *The extracellular matrix of bones is constantly formed, remodeled, and resorbed.* Bone consists of metabolically active cells (osteocytes) that form and maintain it. Osteoblasts form the bone, whereas osteoclasts resorb it. The structure of bones depends on a balance between osteoblastic and osteoclastic activity. Excessive resorption of minerals from the extracellular bone matrix results in softening of bones *(osteomalacia).* Excessive bone formation without commensurate resorption occurs only rarely (as in a congenital disorder called *osteopetrosis,* or "marble bone disease"). Acromegaly caused by overproduction of the pituitary growth hormone also causes excessive bone formation.

4. *The extracellular matrix of the bone consists of osteoid and minerals; cartilage, which is not mineralized, lines the joint surfaces.* Minerals such as calcium and phosphate account for 60% of the bone weight, and the osteoid, which is predominantly composed of collagen type I, accounts for the remaining 40%. Cartilage is made up of collagen type II.

   The synthesis of bone collagen and the deposition of hydroxyapatite are two distinct functions of osteoblasts that are under the control of different regulators. Either one of these functions could be deranged. In *osteogenesis imperfecta,* a genetic defect, collagen synthesis is defective. In osteomalacia, mineralization of osteoid is affected. Both conditions lead to weakening of bones, caused by a loss of bone substance **(osteopenia),** and an increased incidence of fractures.

5. *Calcium and phosphate stores in the bones are in equilibrium with ionized calcium and phosphate in the blood.* The ratio of ionized calcium and phosphate in the blood is tightly regulated and normally oscillates only within a narrow range. Calcium and phosphate can be mobilized quickly from the bones to compensate for low levels of these minerals in the blood. An excess of calcium or phosphate in blood is counterbalanced by an increased deposition of these minerals in bones or their excretion in urine or feces.

6. *Bone cells respond to stimuli by hormones, cytokines, and prostaglandins.* Bone cells respond to a variety of hormones: PTH, vitamin D, calcitonin, estrogens, androgens, growth hormone, corticosteroids, and probably many others. An excess or deficiency of these hormones adversely affects the skeleton. For example, a deficiency of vitamin D in children results in rickets and deformities of the long bones. Bone cells respond to interleukins, transforming growth factor, prostaglandins, and other bioactive substances. In response to activated oncogenes, bone cells may undergo neoplastic transformation and give rise to benign and malignant tumors. Osteoblasts, the most proliferative cells, are the most common sources of these tumors, such as benign osteomas and malignant osteosarcomas.

7. *Bone diseases are age specific.* Normal bones change considerably during the human life span. There are major differences between the growing bones of prepubertal youngsters and those of older adults. Likewise, the diseases that affect the bones in each age group are also distinct. For example, each bone tumor has a typical peak age incidence. Some bone diseases that are common in older adults, such as osteoporosis, are unusual in children. The same pathogenetic agent or mechanism can produce one set of changes in growing bones and another in nongrowing adult bones. For example, growth hormone stimulates the epiphyseal growth plate in growing bones, promoting longitudinal growth *(gigantism).* In adults, growth hormone stimulates the appositional bone growth of adult bones, resulting in acromegaly. Vitamin D deficiency in childhood causes rickets, whereas in adults it causes osteomalacia.

Growing bones need more nutrients and are therefore more vascularized and receive more blood than the bones of adults. Accordingly, the bones of adolescents are more likely to be infected by bloodborne bacteria than the bones of adults are.

8. *Joints are moving structures that may be traumatized easily.* Long-term trauma causes degenerative changes known as *osteoarthritis.* Because the joints are constantly under pressure, they can be easily injured. Such injury can cause joint dislocation *(luxation).*

9. *Unlike bones, joints may be affected by autoimmune diseases. Rheumatoid arthritis* and *systemic lupus erythematosus* are autoimmune diseases that commonly affect the joints. The inflammation typically involves the synovial membranes, the internal lining of the joint capsule.

DEVELOPMENTAL AND GENETIC DISORDERS

Developmental and genetic bone diseases are rare, occurring in the general population at a rate ranging from 1:20,000 to 1:60,000. Despite great advances in the understanding of these diseases, they remain incurable.

ACHONDROPLASIA

Achondroplasia is a genetic disorder caused by a mutation in the gene encoding fibroblast growth factor receptor 3. This mutation, which is inherited as an autosomal dominant trait, affects adversely endochondral ossification and the growth of long bones, thus causing dwarfism. Achondroplastic dwarfs can be easily recognized because they typically have short legs and arms and a body of relatively normal size. In contrast to the thwarted growth of long bone, the bones of the trunk develop normally because they are formed by intramembranous ossification. The calvaria, the domelike portion of the skull, and the bones of the hands develop normally, but the base of the head, which is of endochondral origin, is thwarted in its growth. The face appears disproportionately small in comparison to the upper part of the head; a "saddle nose" and small jaws are usually present.

OSTEOGENESIS IMPERFECTA

The term **osteogenesis imperfecta** encompasses several diseases (in Latin, it means "defective bone formation"). Recently it has been shown that the basic defects in these diseases are various mutations involving genes encoding collagen I, the principal protein of the bone matrix (osteoid). These defects, presenting in several clinical forms, are inherited as either autosomal recessive or autosomal dominant traits.

Depending on the extent and the form of the gene defect, the disease may begin *in utero*, in childhood, during puberty, or even later in life. In the most severe, lethal form of congenital osteogenesis imperfecta, the affected infant is born with numerous bone fractures, resulting in early death (Figure 19-4). Children affected by milder forms of the disease have problems

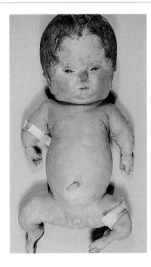

Figure 19-4 Osteogenesis imperfecta. This child, who died shortly after birth, had a large, soft head and short extremities, which on x-ray examination showed numerous fractures. (From Damjanov I, Linder J: Pathology: A Color Atlas, St. Louis, 2000, Mosby.)

with their growth, and they are often hospitalized for surgical repair of fractures and concomitant deformities. The mildest forms of osteogenesis imperfecta may become clinically apparent only in adult life and present with only minor problems, such as increased susceptibility to bone fracturing.

Collagen type I has widespread distribution in the body. Thus the symptoms of osteogenesis imperfecta are not limited solely to the bones. Many patients have thin skin, thin dental enamel *(dentinogenesis imperfecta),* and defective heart valves *(floppy mitral valve).* Defective collagen formation in the eye imparts a bluish hue to the sclera.

INFECTIOUS DISEASES

Bones are relatively resistant to infections, but once infections develop, it may be difficult to eradicate them. An infection located inside the bone is called *osteomyelitis,* whereas an infection of subperiosteal bone and periosteum is called *periostitis.*

OSTEOMYELITIS

Osteomyelitis is a bacterial infection of bones. It may present as an acute infection that progresses to chronic osteomyelitis; less commonly it takes the form of a slowly evolving, chronic disease.

Etiology

The most common causes of osteomyelitis are pyogenic cocci—most notably, *Staphylococcus aureus.* Drug addicts may develop mixed-flora hematogenous infections. Patients with sickle cell anemia are predisposed to infections caused by *Salmonella.* Mycobacterium tuberculosis bone infection is rare today but previously was a common cause of chronic osteomyelitis of the spine, known as *Pott's disease* and *hunchback deformity.*

Pathogenesis and Pathology

Staphylococcal osteomyelitis is the best prototype of bone infection. The infection, which usually originates in the metaphysis, typically occurs in growing children. It affects boys more often than girls, presumably because bone trauma is more common in boys.

The metaphysis is the most vascularized portion of the bone, receiving copious blood through one or more arteries. These vessels, known as *nutrient arteries,* penetrate the cortical bone and deliver the blood into the zone of the epiphyseal growth plate. This "direct access" facilitates the entry of bacteria into the bone during bacteremia. Once the bacteria have reached the "fertile soil" of the metaphysis, which is well supplied with nutrients and oxygen, they multiply rapidly, forming a focus of infection. Polymorphonuclear neutrophils (PMNs) are soon attracted from the blood, and these cells form pus, which spreads into the adjacent portions of the epiphysis, through the medullary cavity, and through the haversian canals of the compact bone (Figure 19-5). The pus draining from the cavity is rich in enzymes, which can lyse the bone and cartilage. The devitalized bone fragments remain in the newly formed cavities filled with pus. Pus may drain from the cavity to the surface through channels called *sinuses.* Reactive bone forms around the zone of inflammation as an attempt by the body to wall off the infection and prevent its spread. These changes result in deformities of the

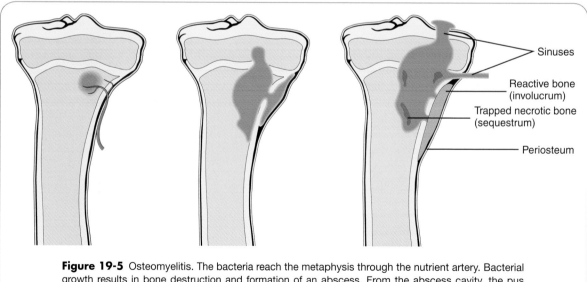

Figure 19-5 Osteomyelitis. The bacteria reach the metaphysis through the nutrient artery. Bacterial growth results in bone destruction and formation of an abscess. From the abscess cavity, the pus spreads between the trabeculae into the medulla, through the cartilage into the joint, or through the haversian canals of the compact bones to the outside. These sinuses traversing the bone persist for a long time and heal slowly. The pus destroys the bone and sequesters parts of it in the abscess cavity. Reactive new bone is formed around the focus of inflammation.

bone, predisposing the bone to fractures that heal poorly as long as there is pus in the area.

In adults, bacterial osteomyelitis occurs as a complication of bone fractures or bone surgery or because of the spread of infection to the bones from the joints and adjacent soft tissues. Gangrene of the toes that is caused by diabetes is also often complicated by osteomyelitis, often requiring amputation of the affected toes or the entire foot.

Suppurative osteomyelitis must be treated with large doses of antibiotics. However, surgical drainage of the pus and repair of the defect may be unavoidable in extensive infection associated with destruction of bone or deformities.

 Did You Know?

Spontaneous osteomyelitis that occurs without a predisposing cause has become a relatively rare disease. Most cases of osteomyelitis reported today occur after trauma or surgery on the bones. The site of open trauma, caused by severe injury or a bullet wound, typically becomes infected. Such exogenous bacteria may spread through the bone and cause osteomyelitis, which will typically delay healing of a fracture. Likewise, infectious agents may be introduced into the bone during bone surgery. Although surgery is performed under sterile conditions, 1% to 3% of orthopedic operations are associated with subsequent infection at the site of surgery. To reduce this complication, orthopedic surgeons operate in specially designed operating rooms that contain almost no bacteria in the air. The surgeons also use special dress and masks to prevent infection of their patients. Using such precautions, the best centers of orthopedic surgery have reduced the number of cases of postoperative osteomyelitis to less than 0.5%.

CIRCULATORY DISTURBANCES

A sudden onset of ischemia caused by disruption or complete interruption of blood flow results in bone infarcts. Traditionally these are called **aseptic bone necrosis.** This term, coined in the nineteenth century when most bone necroses were caused by bacteria (i.e., were septic), is still used for historic reasons. Moreover, various forms of aseptic infarcts of growing bones are still called by the names of the physicians who first described them. This list of more than 50 names provides some satisfaction and pleasure to name-droppers with a photographic memory but would cause desperation among the rest of us if we tried to memorize all these eponyms. These diseases occur mostly in children and adolescents, affecting ossification centers of various growing bones. For example, Legg-Calvé-Perthes disease involves the femoral head, Köhler's disease the lunate bone, and Scheuermann's disease the vertebrae. All these diseases represent infarcts of the ossification centers of various growing bones.

Etiology and Pathogenesis

The cause of most infarcts is unknown, but occasionally infarcts may be related to trauma, emboli, radiation, or drugs. Well-documented cases include air emboli in caisson

(decompression) disease or microthrombi and sludges of sickle cells in sickle cell anemia.

Clinical Features

Aseptic bone necrosis is a disease of growing children and adolescents, but it also occurs at a high rate in elderly persons. Certain portions of the growing skeleton are at increased risk and undergo infarction more often than others. The carpal bones are especially vulnerable because of their complex blood supply. In elderly persons the most important site of aseptic necrosis is the head of the femur. Ischemic fractures of the neck of femur, which are especially common in conjunction with osteoporosis, are often incapacitating. The hip joint, which may become afunctional, usually must be replaced because the chances of spontaneous repair are minimal.

METABOLIC DISORDERS
OSTEOPOROSIS

Osteoporosis is a multifactorial disease characterized by an absolute reduction of the total bone mass. It is probably the most prevalent bone disease worldwide. Osteoporosis, with all its complications, costs society approximately $10 billion per year. It has been estimated that one third of women older than 65 years have some minor fractures related to osteoporosis. In those older than 85 years, one third of all American women and one in every six men are temporarily or permanently confined to bed because of hip fractures, the most incapacitating complication of osteoporosis.

Etiology

It is customary to divide this disease into two basic forms: primary and secondary osteoporosis. There are no definitive clues about the etiology of primary osteoporosis, which accounts for most cases. Primary osteoporosis is a disease of elderly persons, affecting women more often than men (Figure 19-6). Secondary osteoporosis may occur at any age and is related to identifiable causes that include the following:

- Hormonal disturbances, which are marked by an excess (e.g., hyperadrenocorticism) or deficiency (e.g., hypogonadism or diabetes) of some hormones
- Dietary insufficiency caused by inadequate intake (e.g., calcium or vitamin C deficiency) or malabsorption of nutrients (e.g., intestinal disease or liver disease)
- Immobilization, as in chronic diseases or after trauma
- Drugs, such as anticonvulsants for the treatment of epilepsy or anticoagulants (e.g., heparin)
- Tumors, such as hormonally active lesions of the endocrine glands, or metastases that destroy bone directly, as in breast carcinoma

Osteoporosis often has multiple causes. For example, in a postmenopausal woman who smokes and abuses alcohol, osteoporosis results from a lack of estrogen and also from the direct and indirect effects of smoking and alcohol on bone cells. Alcoholics suffer from other nutritional deficiencies and are at risk for developing cirrhosis. Cirrhosis of the liver

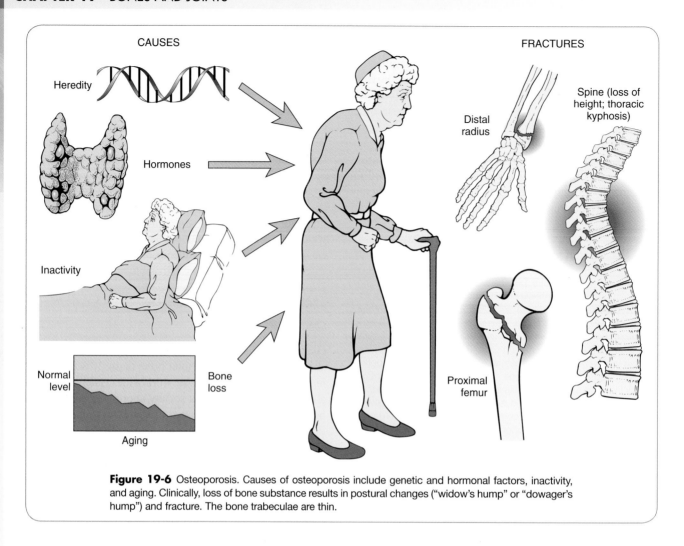

Figure 19-6 Osteoporosis. Causes of osteoporosis include genetic and hormonal factors, inactivity, and aging. Clinically, loss of bone substance results in postural changes ("widow's hump" or "dowager's hump") and fracture. The bone trabeculae are thin.

affects vitamin D metabolism, reducing intestinal absorption of calcium. Moreover, alcoholic patients often suffer from other nutritional deficiencies as well.

Pathogenesis

Osteoporosis is characterized by the simultaneous loss of the organic bone matrix (osteoid) and minerals. Although the pathogenesis of primary osteoporosis remains unknown, several determinants of bone loss have been identified. These include the following:

- Initial bone mass
- Diet and lifestyle
- Hormones
- Age-related changes in metabolism

Normal bones are remodeled during the entire life span. During the growth phase and up to approximately 30 years of age, bone formation by osteoblasts exceeds bone resorption by osteoclasts. However, after this, bone resorption outpaces bone formation, resulting in a net bone loss of 0.5% of the total bone mass per year. After menopause, the bone resorption is accelerated in women threefold to fivefold, resulting in a bone loss in the range of 1% to 3%. The reasons for this accelerated bone loss, which occurs over 8 to 10 years, are not

known, but they are believed to be related to estrogen. Estrogen replacement therapy can prevent or slow the development of postmenopausal osteoporosis. Bone loss is less prominent in men, who do not go through menopause; however, even they develop some osteoporosis with advancing age.

Osteoporosis develops more often in gracile white women of small frame, who have a smaller initial bone mass, than in women with large frames ("heavy bones"). Men have denser bones, so their bones take longer to become osteoporotic. Blacks generally have denser bones than whites. Bone density is greater in athletes and muscular persons, and the beneficial effects of exercise in maintaining the bone mass have been amply documented.

Dietary calcium and vitamin D are also important and thus are added to many items included in the typical American diet to meet the minimum daily requirements. However, if the absorption of vitamin D and calcium is impaired because of liver or intestinal disease, deficiencies may develop.

Pathology

Osteoporotic bones are thin and brittle and are prone to fracture. The bone loss involves both cortical and spongy bone. In type I osteoporosis, which occurs typically in postmenopausal women, trabecular bone loss predominates, occurring most prominently in the vertebrae and distal radius. Major complications of type I osteoporosis are therefore crush fractures of the vertebral bodies and of the distal end of the radius. Type II, or old-age, osteoporosis is characterized by a proportional loss of cortical and trabecular bone of the long bones. The most serious fractures of old age are those of the head of femur. However, none of the bones is spared. The vertebrae are common sites of microfractures, which produce wedge-shaped deformities that are most pronounced anteriorly. Multiple wedge-shaped fractures of the vertebral bodies make old people appear smaller and bent forward.

Clinical Features

The symptoms of osteoporosis are extremely variable and often nonspecific. Vertebral fractures can cause back pain or kyphosis of the spine ("dowager's hump"). Extensive osteoporosis may reduce a person's height up to 15 cm, or 10%. Fractures of the long bones, such as the femur, may be incapacitating. More than 1 million hip fractures occur each year in the United States, and at least 25% of these never heal. Other bones may be affected as well. Despite a marked loss of bone substance, patients with osteoporosis show no biochemical abnormalities. Serum calcium, phosphate, and alkaline phosphatase levels are normal.

Osteoporosis is best diagnosed by radiographic studies. Routine x-ray studies are not very sensitive and detect signs of osteoporosis only after a 30% to 50% reduction of bone mass has occurred. **Bone mineral density (BMD),** best measured by a radiologic test called dual-energy x-ray absorptiometry (DEXA scan), can provide more precise estimates of absolute bone loss caused by osteoporosis. The results are expressed as T-scores, based on the comparison of BMD of the examined person with a 30-year-old healthy adult. Normal T-score falls within 1 standard deviation (SD) of the control. A T-score in the range of -1 to - 2.5 SD indicates low bone mass (osteopenia), and values below -2.5 SD are diagnostic of osteoporosis. According to these criteria, approximately 40% of all postmenopausal Caucasian women have osteopenia, and 7% have osteoporosis.

> **? Did You Know?**
>
> The fact that osteoporosis occurs more often in postmenopausal than premenopausal women has prompted research into the role of estrogens in osteoporosis. The exact role the sex hormones play in bone maintenance is not known. Nevertheless, it has been shown that estrogens, if taken after menopause, retard the development of osteoporosis. Estrogens may increase the risk for endometrial cancer in such women.

OSTEOMALACIA

Osteomalacia (in Latin, meaning "softening of bones") is a consequence of inadequate mineralization of the organic bone matrix, caused by disturbances of either vitamin D or phosphate metabolism. Osteomalacia of growing bones is called *rickets.*

Etiology

Vitamin D and phosphates are essential nutrients. Vitamin D is derived from diet but is also synthesized in the skin under the influence of ultraviolet light. Meat and dairy products are the primary sources of dietary phosphates.

Vitamin D deficiency may result from the following (Figure 19-7):

- *Inadequate intake,* as occurs in malnourished children in underdeveloped parts of the world. In the United States, many foods are fortified with vitamin D, and the dietary deficiency occurs predominantly in vegetarians or food faddists who do not drink milk supplemented with vitamin D. Milder forms of vitamin D deficiency are found in elderly

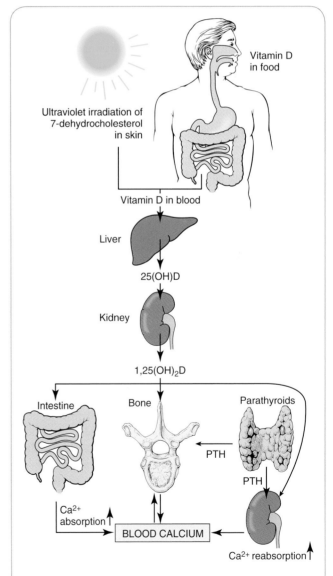

Figure 19-7 Vitamin D metabolism and the various pathologic processes that can interfere with it. PTH, parathyroid hormone.

persons with poor dietary habits (living on "tea and biscuits") or who cannot afford to buy vitamin-fortified food.

- *Inadequate exposure to sunlight,* as occurs in people living above the Arctic circle. Eskimos typically compensate for lack of endogenously synthesized vitamin D by eating fish fat.
- *Abnormal intestinal absorption,* as may occur in those with primary diseases of the small intestines in which vitamin D is not absorbed or biliary and pancreatic diseases associated with fat malabsorption.

Osteomalacia also may be caused by hypophosphatemia related to abnormal absorption or excessive loss of phosphates. Malabsorption may result from intestinal diseases and is an important complication of intestinal resection. The aluminum that is present in some antacids (e.g., Maalox) may bind to phosphorus in the intestinal lumen and prevent its absorption. PTH also prevents tubular resorption of phosphates; thus phosphate wasting in urine is a constant feature of hyperparathyroidism.

Pathogenesis

Activation of vitamin D occurs in the liver and the kidneys. Several active metabolites are formed, of which the hydroxylated $1,25(OH)_2$ vitamin D is the most important. This active form of vitamin D has three primary functions:

- Stimulation of intestinal absorption of calcium and phosphorus.
- Action on the bone, which has a dual nature and includes deposition of calcium into the osteoid and the mobilization of calcium from calcified bone. Vitamin D is essential for mineralization of osteoid. The exact mechanism of this stimulatory influence is not known. In conditions dominated by hypocalcemia, vitamin D has just the opposite effect; in concert with PTH, it mobilizes calcium from bones.
- Stimulation of the PTH-dependent resorption of calcium in the kidney.

Pathology

Vitamin D deficiency results in osteopenia, which is visible as increased bone lucency on x-ray examination. Microscopically the bone spicules are composed of broad seams of osteoid surrounding the central mineralized core. Clinically the bones are soft and pliable. Fractures and deformities are typical complications. *Rickets,* the osteomalacia of growing bones in children, affects bone formation. Endochondral ossification in the growth plates is most severely disturbed. This results in growth retardation, bone deformities, and fractures of long bones. Osteomalacia is characterized by an excess of osteoid around the calcified core of the trabeculae of spongy bone and on the endocavitary side of compact bones. Fractures are common and heal by exuberant osteoid formation. Softening of the bones may also produce deformities. These are common in children affected by rickets but are rare in adults.

Rickets causes growth retardation, softening of growing bones, and deformities. Typical *bowlegs* result from the inability of soft leg bones to carry the weight of the body. A widened junction between the rib bone and the cartilage—the costochondral junction—appears nodular and can be palpated as beads on the thorax (called *rachitic rosary*). Softening of the cranial bones is called *craniotabes.* Dentition is delayed, and the teeth may be speckled as a result of incomplete mineralization.

Clinical Features

Osteomalacia of adults is often asymptomatic, or it may cause nonspecific bone pain. Muscle weakness is common. Skeletal deformities develop slowly and are not prominent.

Rickets produces typical deformities of the legs, ribs, and head. However, many other bones are affected, and the consequences may become clinically important many years later. For example, childhood deformities of the pelvis may persist and may be severe enough to narrow the birth canal and impede normal vaginal delivery of a baby.

The diagnosis of osteomalacia is based on clinical symptoms, radiographic evidence of osteopenia, and typical laboratory findings. In vitamin D–related osteomalacia, calcium and phosphate levels are low in serum, but the PTH level is elevated because of compensatory parathyroid hyperplasia. In typical osteomalacia resulting from phosphate deficiency, the serum phosphate level is low but serum calcium and PTH levels are normal.

RENAL OSTEODYSTROPHY

Chronic renal failure is associated with complex bone changes usually grouped under the term **renal osteodystrophy.** These bone changes are directly or indirectly related to the altered homeostasis of calcium and phosphates in the body.

Pathogenesis

Because the kidneys cannot excrete phosphorus, the phosphate level in the blood rises. This is accompanied by hypocalcemia and compensatory hyperparathyroidism. PTH stimulates bone resorption and a release of calcium and phosphate into the blood, resulting in hyperphosphatemia, normalization of blood calcium levels, and occasionally even hypercalcemia. Calcium absorption in the intestines is decreased also because the damaged kidneys cannot form hydroxylated vitamin D, which is essential for intestinal calcium absorption.

Pathology

The pathologic changes in the bones are highly variable. The bone trabeculae are predominantly composed of osteoid and are poorly mineralized *(osteomalacia).* PTH stimulates osteoblasts and fibroblasts, causing medullary *osteofibrosis* and paradoxically even osteosclerosis. Increased osteoclastic activity may cause cystic changes *(osteitis cystica).* Aggregates of osteoclasts may form small nodules, which are indistinguishable from the so-called brown tumors of hyperparathyroidism. Renal osteodystrophy may improve with kidney transplantation or following dialysis.

PAGET'S DISEASE

Paget's disease, or *osteitis deformans,* is a chronic disease of unknown origin characterized by irregular restructuring of bone that leads to thickening and deformities of bone. It has been estimated that 3% of all men and women older than 60 years have radiologic signs of Paget's disease. The highest prevalence is seen among the British and their descendants in the United States and Australia; the lowest incidence of this disease is in East Asians. A familial form of Paget's disease has been linked to a gene locus on chromosome 18, but it is unknown whether these genes are important for the sporadic form of the disease as well.

Pathogenesis and Pathology

Paget's disease is most likely related to some defects in the function of osteoclasts. Cytokines stimulating the formation and activity of osteoclasts, such as interleukin-6 (IL-6) and growth factors such as RANK ligand, have been identified as the major mediators of bone restructuring, but the exact pathogenesis of the disease remains unknown. However, it is known that the disease has three phases. First, the destructive phase is marked by bone resorption. Second, in the mixed phase, bone resorption is counterbalanced by new bone formation. Third, in the osteosclerotic phase the trabeculae appear irregularly thickened and the normal compact bone is replaced by wide, sclerotic, dense bone. This bone is crisscrossed with calcified cement lines demarcating irregularly shaped osteons and the borders between the bone and incompletely calcified osteoid, giving the bones a typical histologic mosaic appearance.

Clinical Features

The course of Paget's disease is highly variable. Many patients are asymptomatic or have only minor skeletal pain. The most commonly affected sites are the cranium and the long bones of the lower extremities. The thickened cranial bones may compress the cranial nerves and cause headaches, hearing loss, or dizziness. The tibia and fibula are thickened and deformed (bowlegs) (Figure 19-8). Osteosarcoma develops as a late complication in some patients. Because osteosarcomas are rare in adults, all tumors that develop in patients older than 50 years presumably arise in bones affected by Paget's disease.

The diagnosis of Paget's disease is based on x-ray studies. The thickened bones show a "honeycomb" or "cotton-wool" appearance because of the irregular bone structure. Deformities and fractures are common.

TRAUMATIC INJURIES

Mechanical injuries may affect bones, causing fracture, or joints, causing dislocations and tearing of various ligaments.

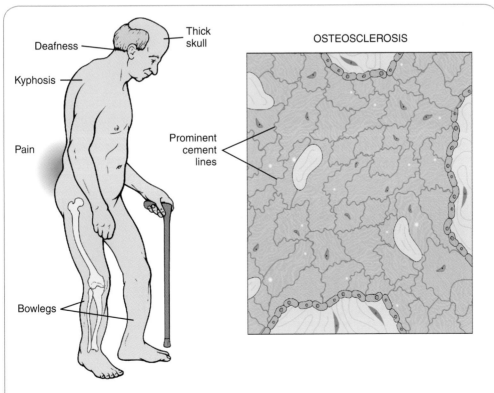

Figure 19-8 Paget's disease. Clinical features are caused by bone deformities. The mosaic pattern of dense bone is seen on histologic examination.

BONE FRACTURES

A **fracture** (in Latin, meaning "break") denotes a disruption of bone continuity caused by mechanical factors, most often by trauma. Fractures are clinically classified as *simple* if there is a single fracture line or *comminuted* if there are multiple lines and fragments (Figure 19-9). Simple fractures extending through the entire thickness of the bones are called *complete; incomplete* fractures are those that do not extend from one side to another. If the overlying skin is intact, the fracture is considered *closed,* whereas if the skin is disrupted, it is termed *open* or *compound.*

Infected fractures are also called *complicated.* Clinicians also distinguish between *traumatic* fractures, which are related to obvious mechanical injury, and *spontaneous* fractures, which occur without major external trauma. These are also called *pathologic* fractures because they occur in structurally abnormal bone that cannot withstand normal outside pressure and tension (e.g., osteoporosis) or in bone that has been destroyed by a pathologic process (e.g., bone tumor). Depending on the clinical situation, there are also other clinical terms for specific fractures characteristic of various diseases. Compression fracture of the vertebral bones is a complication of osteoporosis; linear stress fractures of the tibia are common in athletes. Greenstick fractures occur in children's bones, which tend to bend rather than break.

Healing of simple fractures occurs in a predictable manner (Figure 19-10). Cellular events in healing fractures resemble those seen in wound healing, as discussed in Chapter 2.

The initial phases of wound healing require complete immobilization of the fracture site. Any movement that could disrupt the provisional scaffolds and cause additional bleeding into the site of fracture will delay the healing. Therefore the extremity must be immobilized with casts. However, if the defect is too big, the bone must be reconstructed surgically. This usually includes the removal of necrotic tissue, which cannot be removed readily by granulation tissue, and the insertion of nails and mesh wire to hold the pieces together. Compression of two sides of the fracture promotes healing. Once the fracture heals, the final restructuring of the new bone occurs only after normal movement is reestablished. Rehabilitation exercises are occasionally needed to complete the recovery.

Healing of fractures depends also on the proper influx of nutrients. In malnourished persons, fractures heal poorly. Vitamins, especially C and D, and calcium and phosphorus are important for new bone formation. Infection and foreign bodies introduced by trauma impede fracture healing.

JOINT DISLOCATIONS

Dislocation, or luxation, of joints is a process during which the bones forming the joint lose contact and become misaligned. The trauma causing the dislocation usually tears some of the joint support structures and may also tear the ligaments that hold the bones together. Trauma may also damage the blood vessels, leading to intra-articular or periarticular hematoma (i.e., accumulation of extravasated blood inside or around the joint). The joint is also edematous and painful, and movement of such a joint becomes limited or impossible. Severe dislocation may be recognized by a deformity of the affected extremity, which may become fixated in an abnormal position.

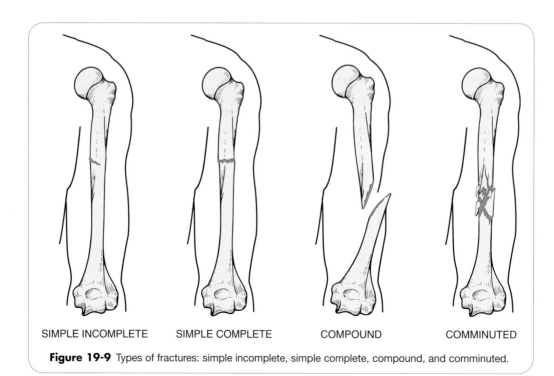

SIMPLE INCOMPLETE   SIMPLE COMPLETE   COMPOUND   COMMINUTED

Figure 19-9 Types of fractures: simple incomplete, simple complete, compound, and comminuted.

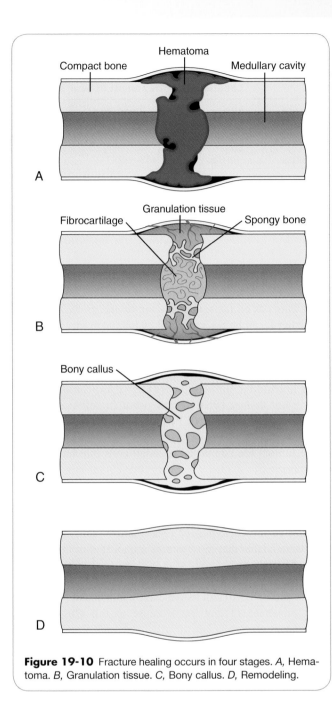

Figure 19-10 Fracture healing occurs in four stages. *A,* Hematoma. *B,* Granulation tissue. *C,* Bony callus. *D,* Remodeling.

immobilized and the patient relieved of pain with analgesics. In severe dislocations it is necessary to surgically correct the misalignment of the bones and repair possible tears in the joint capsule or the ligaments.

BONE TUMORS

Primary bone tumors are rare, accounting for less than 1% of all clinically diagnosed tumors. Approximately 50% of these are derived from blood-forming cells of the bone marrow. These neoplasms, such as multiple myeloma and leukemia, are discussed in Chapter 9. Tumors of bone-forming cells (**osteoma and osteosarcoma**), cartilage cells (**chondroma** and **chondrosarcoma**), osteoclasts (**giant cell tumor of bones),** and primitive mesenchymal bone marrow cells (**Ewing's sarcoma**) account for the other 50% and are discussed here. *Secondary tumors*—that is, metastases from other sites—outnumber primary bone tumors by a ratio of 10:1. The most common primary sites of such malignant lesions are the breast, prostate, lung, kidneys, and thyroid.

BENIGN BONE TUMORS

Benign bone tumors are composed of bone cells *(osteoma),* cartilage cells *(chondroma),* or fibroblasts *(nonossifying fibroma).* Typically these tumors appear as bumps or soft defects on the outer surface of bones or small nodules on the inside of the bone that are discovered on routine x-ray examination or because of the pain that they produce as a result of expansive growth. The growing tumors are removed only if they cause pain (e.g., those on the nose or the face). Benign bone tumors do not tend to undergo malignant transformation. The only exceptions are chondromas, which occasionally give rise to chondrosarcomas.

MALIGNANT BONE TUMORS

The essential data on the four most common malignant bone tumors are summarized in Table 19-1. It should be noted that bone tumors occur more often in males than in females and

The dislocation occurs as a result of the effects of force or abnormal movement, such as by stepping into a hole or by slipping on ice. Sports injuries are often accompanied by dislocations of the knee or shoulder joint. Slipping and falling may cause dislocation of the hand and foot or ankle joints.

Dislocation can occur at any age and affect any person. However, it occurs more often in persons who have hereditary "loose joints" and those with certain genetic and hereditary diseases affecting collagen and other connective tissue components.

If a dislocation is clinically suspected, it is of paramount importance to take an x-ray overview of the injured area to exclude fracture. If there is no fracture, the joint should be

TABLE 19-1 Malignant Bone Tumors

Tumor	Age (Years)	Gender Ratio (M:F)	Bones Commonly Involved	Location	Treatment (5-year survival)
Osteosarcoma	10–25	2:1	Long bones of extremities (knee joint), jaws	Metaphysis	S + C (60–70%)
Chondrosarcoma	35–60	2:1	Pelvis, ribs, vertebrae, long bones (proximal parts)	Diaphysis or metaphysis	S (depending on grade, 45%–90%)
Ewing's sarcoma	10–20	2:1	Long bones; may be multiple	Diaphysis	C + S (75%)
Giant cell tumor	20–40	1:1	Long bones (knee joint)	Epiphysis	S (95%)

C, chemotherapy; S, surgery.

that each of the tumors is characterized by a typical peak age incidence and anatomic location (Figure 19-11).

Osteosarcoma is the most common primary malignant tumor involving bone (Figure 19-12). The most important facts about this tumor are as follows:

- This bone-forming tumor most often involves the metaphysis of the long bones of the extremities. Approximately 50% of these tumors are located in the knee joint. The jawbone is the most common short bone involved.
- Osteosarcoma is a tumor of young persons. Osteosarcomas in adults are rare, and most develop as a result of preexisting Paget's disease.
- These malignant tumors metastasize through the blood, and most dying patients have lung metastases. Treatment is based on surgical resection combined with chemotherapy. Without chemotherapy, less than 10% of affected patients survive 5 years. However, with chemotherapy, 5-year survival has reached 60% to 70% and many patients are completely cured.

Chondrosarcoma is a malignant tumor composed of neoplastic cartilage cells (Figure 19-13). The most important facts about this tumor are as follows:

- Tumors originate in the axial skeleton (i.e., the bones of the trunk [pelvis, ribs, and vertebrae]) and the adjacent portion of long bones (e.g., the proximal femur and humerus).
- On the basis of the maturity and the level of differentiation of cells, these tumors can be classified as well differentiated, moderately differentiated, or poorly differentiated and graded on a scale from I to III. Grade I tumors usually do not metastasize and have a much better prognosis than grade II or III tumors. The 5-year survival for these three groups is as follows: grade I, 90%; grade II, 60%; and grade III, 40%.
- These tumors usually affect adults and have a peak incidence in those 35 to 60 years of age.
- Treatment is based on surgical resection, because the tumor cells are insensitive to chemotherapy. The prognosis for particular tumors varies widely in a range from 20% to 80%

and depends on the size of the tumor and its location (i.e., whether it can be resected) and histologic grade.

Ewing's sarcoma is a malignant tumor composed of undifferentiated bone marrow cells (Figure 19-14). Although rare, nevertheless it is the second most common tumor of bones in children. Similar tumors known as *primitive neuroectodermal tumors* (PNET) may occur in soft tissues. The most important facts about Ewing's sarcoma and PNET are as follows:

- The tumors are composed of small cells that have hyperchromatic bluish nuclei and very little cytoplasm. The cytoplasm may contain abundant glycogen. The nature of these cells remains poorly understood, although immunohistochemically these cells have many features in common with primitive mesenchymal or bone marrow cells. Thus it is understandable that most tumors are located in the diaphysis of long bones.
- Approximately 85% of persons with Ewing's sarcomas of bone and PNET of soft tissues have a translocation between chromosomes 11 and 22. Because of this chromosomal translocation, genes known as *FLI* and *EWS* are fused together, producing a fusion protein that plays an important role in the pathogenesis of these tumors.
- Bone tumor cells invade the cortical bone and spread into the soft tissues of the extremities. The cortical bone reacts and new bone is formed beneath the periosteum. This imparts a "sunburst" or "onion skin" appearance to the bones on x-ray examination.
- These tumors occur mostly in young persons (10 to 20 years of age) and are more common in males than in females. For unknown reasons, Ewing's sarcomas are very rare in children of African-American and Asian descent.
- The tumor may metastasize via the blood. Some multiple tumors may represent multifocal primary tumors originating in distant bones at the same time. Ewing's sarcoma is a highly malignant tumor, and without chemotherapy it is invariably lethal. With chemotherapy, up to 75% of children will survive 5 years and 50% of children with tumors become long-term survivors.

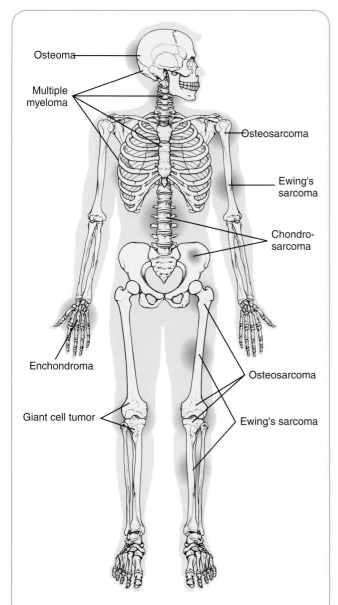

Figure 19-11 Schematic presentation of the most common sites of origin of bone tumors. Most often, osteosarcomas originate in the metaphyses of long bones, chondrosarcomas arise in the axial skeleton, Ewing's sarcomas develop in the diaphyses of long bones, and giant cell tumors originate in the epiphyses of long bones. Osteomas occur most often in the skull, and enchondromas occur most often in the small bones of the hand. Multiple myelomas involve the calvaria, vertebrae, and ribs but also other bones that contain hematopoietic bone marrow.

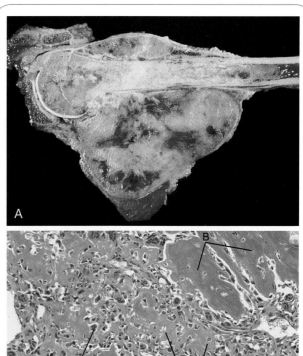

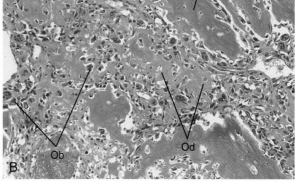

Figure 19-12 *A,* Gross appearance of osteosarcoma. *B,* Histologically, the tumor consists of osteoblasts (Ob) and osteoid (Od) or bone (B).

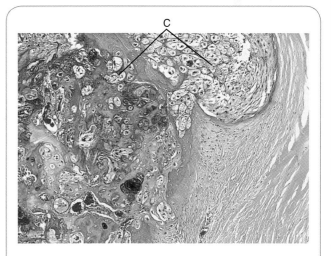

Figure 19-13 Chondrosarcoma is composed of cartilage (C) cells.

JOINT DISEASES

The most important diseases affecting the joints are *osteoarthritis,* also known as **degenerative joint disease (DJD),** and rheumatoid arthritis, which together account for more than 90% of all cases in rheumatology practice. Luxations, as mentioned before, are typically treated by orthopedic surgeons

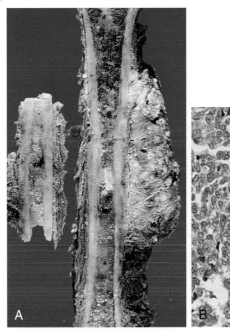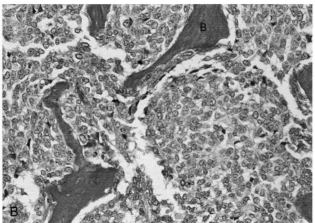

Figure 19-14 *A,* Ewing's sarcoma originates in the diaphysis of long bones. *B,* Histologically, the tumor is composed of a uniform population of small blue cells infiltrating the spaces between the bone trabeculae (B).

and are important traumatic joint lesions. Some luxations and joint deformities are congenital. For the sake of completeness, infectious arthritis and gout, an important metabolic cause of arthritis, are mentioned. Tumors of the joints are rare. The only proliferative joint disease that deserves mention is pigmented villonodular synovitis. However, it is unclear whether this is a benign tumor or a traumatic reactive lesion of the synovium. It should be noted that the tumor known as *synovial sarcoma* is actually a soft tissue sarcoma that does not involve the joints and that, despite its name, it is not derived from or related to synovial cells.

OSTEOARTHRITIS

Osteoarthritis, or DJD, is the most common joint disease. Osteoarthritis is classified as primary or secondary. The causes of primary osteoarthritis are unknown. Secondary osteoarthritis develops under conditions that stress the joint surfaces, such as repeated trauma; in congenitally abnormal joints, such as the hip or knee joints of achondroplastic dwarfs; in structurally abnormal joint structures, such as those affected by various hormonal and metabolic diseases

Pathogenesis

The pathogenesis of primary DJD is unknown, but most authorities favor a wear-and-tear explanation and consider the articular cartilage to be the primary site of injury. Empirical facts in support of the wear-and-tear hypothesis are as follows:

- DJD preferentially affects the weight-bearing joints, such as the knee, hip, and vertebral joints.

- The prevalence of the disease increases with age. Almost all persons older than 65 years have some x-ray findings suggestive of DJD.
- Mechanical instability, stress of the joint, or increased stress of the joint surface accelerates the disease.
- Abnormal connective tissue degenerates quickly, and because many of the properties of connective tissue are inherited, the disease has a tendency for familial preponderance. DJD is more common among native Americans than in other ethnic groups.

Proponents of opposing views assert that DJD either is a metabolic disorder or is caused by inflammation. Inflammation of the periarticular connective tissue is prominent in many cases, especially in the fingers, but it is impossible to state whether this inflammation is the cause or consequence of joint changes. Because finger joints are not weight bearing, the common involvement of these joints is taken as evidence against the wear-and-tear hypothesis and in support of the primary inflammatory nature of the disease. The beneficial effect of anti-inflammatory drugs is another argument in favor of this hypothesis. However, because these drugs also act as analgesics, the beneficial effect could reflect more a reduction of pain than an effect on the basic process that has caused joint pathology.

Pathology

Pathologic changes in the joints are not specific (Figure 19-15). Initial changes are seen in the articular cartilage, which shows softening, surface defects, and irregular thinning. Very early in the disease, the cartilage undergoes fibrillation, with formation

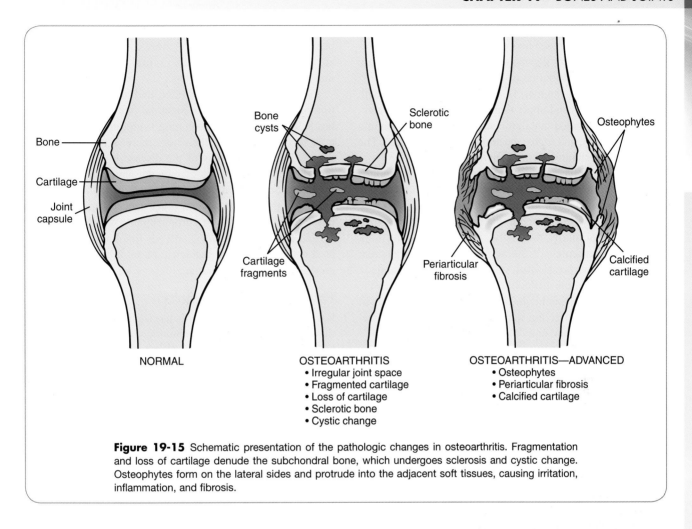

Figure 19-15 Schematic presentation of the pathologic changes in osteoarthritis. Fragmentation and loss of cartilage denude the subchondral bone, which undergoes sclerosis and cystic change. Osteophytes form on the lateral sides and protrude into the adjacent soft tissues, causing irritation, inflammation, and fibrosis.

of vertical clefts. The cartilage fragments are shed into the cavity, leaving behind the denuded surface of the subchondral bone. Continued pressure induces sclerosis of the subchondral plate, which is called *eburnation* because the bone appears dense, like ivory. Bone degeneration under stress leads to the formation of cysts, which are filled with fluid, and a bone defect that communicates with the joint cavity. At the margins of the joint, spurs of new bone *(osteophytes)* form, projecting into the adjacent connective tissue. The traumatized soft tissue undergoes swelling and inflammation.

Clinical Features

Symptoms of osteoarthritis are nonspecific, and many individuals with prominent radiographic evidence of disease and even gross deformities commonly have only minor disability. A list of common symptoms related to pathologic changes is presented in Table 19-2.

The most common symptom is pain, which is relieved by rest. Stiffness typically lasts 15 to 20 minutes and then disappears; this is in contrast to rheumatoid arthritis, in which stiffness persists an hour or more after joint immobility (e.g., during sleep or sitting). All joints show reduced mobility and tend to be deformed as a result of intra-articular changes and superimposed lesions caused by faulty movement and periarticular inflammation. Joint movement is often associated with

TABLE 19-2	Clinicopathologic Correlations in Osteoarthritis (Degenerative Joint Disease)
Symptom	**Pathologic Findings**
Pain	Osteophytes, periarticular inflammation, bone cysts, destruction, microfractures
Crepitus	Degeneration of cartilage
Swelling and warmth	Periarticular inflammation
Joint deformation	Osteophytes, periarticular fibrosis, degeneration of cartilage, reactive bone lesions
Loss of normal mobility	Degeneration of cartilage, loose intra-articular bodies, muscle spasm

crepitus, a grating of rough articular surfaces. Muscle spasm and contractures tend to develop with progression of the disease as the body attempts to reduce movement in the painful joint.

Weight-bearing joints are most often affected, including the hips, knee joints, and cervical and lumbar spine. On the hand, the disease typically involves the distal interphalangeal, proximal interphalangeal, and first carpometacarpal joints. On the foot, the first metatarsophalangeal joints are most often affected. Symptoms depend on the duration of the disease and the anatomic distribution of the joints involved.

Hip involvement, known as *coxarthrosis,* presents with pain in the buttocks and upper thigh and limited mobility, resulting in a so-called antalgic gait (from *ante,* meaning "against" in Latin, and *algos,* meaning "pain," in Greek). The patient walks hesitantly, trying to avoid pain.

Knee joint involvement may present with pain or crepitus as the joint surfaces erode and roughen. Deformities of the joint result in bowlegs or knock-knee deformities.

The spine may be affected in the cervical or lumbar area. DJD involves primarily the intervertebral apophyseal joint, which causes stiffening of the vertebral column. Radicular pain from the compression of spinal nerves is common. In many older people it is difficult to determine what caused the symptoms—DJD or spondylosis, a degenerative disease of unknown etiology affecting the intervertebral joints and resulting in exostoses and ankylosis of adjacent vertebrae.

The hands are commonly involved. The nodular deformities of the distal interphalangeal joints, the most common manifestation of DJD, are called *Heberden's nodules.*

Feet that are affected by DJD show deformities of the toes. The most common is DJD of the first metatarsophalangeal joint, which leads to the formation of a deformity called a *bunion.*

The diagnosis of osteoarthritis is based on clinical symptoms and radiologic findings. Typical x-ray findings include narrowing of the joint space, sclerosis of the subchondral bone, cystic bone changes, and osteophytes. It is important to note that DJD produces no diagnostic laboratory findings. Joint fluid analysis may occasionally be useful. Typically, it shows no signs of joint inflammation, no bacteria, and no evidence of urate crystals. This helps exclude inflammatory arthropathies and gout but does not prove that the patient has osteoarthritis.

RHEUMATOID ARTHRITIS

Rheumatoid arthritis (RA) is a very common disease, affecting 1% of the world's population. RA is most common in adults 40 to 70 years of age, but it may occasionally develop in younger persons and even in children. Clinically, it is characterized by the following features:

- Chronic, symmetric inflammation of the joints
- Significant but not diagnostic laboratory findings, usually with positive serologic data suggestive of an immune disorder
- Variable extra-articular manifestations

Etiology

The cause of RA is unknown. The disease is approximately four times more common among women than men. This could reflect the more common occurrence of autoimmune diseases in women but could also be related to sex hormones; with advancing age, the sex differences become less prominent. Lifestyle seems to have a role, because it has been shown that the disease is more common and symptoms are more severe in urban than in rural areas and in cold climates as opposed to warm ones.

Genetic factors are important, and a familial predisposition has been noted. If one identical twin has RA, the other has a 30% chance for developing symptoms as well, in contrast to fraternal twins, in whom there is only 5% concordance. The genetic basis of the disease is supported by the fact that more than 70% of patients have the same human major histocompatibility locus. HLA loci are inherited as a cluster, together with several other genes located on the immune response region of chromosome 6. Thus it is not surprising that certain HLA genotypes (haplotypes) are associated with an increased incidence of autoimmune diseases in general and RA in particular.

Pathogenesis and Pathology

RA is a systemic autoimmune disease that primarily involves the synovial joints. The inflammation begins as synovitis and leads to exudation of fluid and inflammatory cells into the joint cavity (Figure 19-16). The infiltrates consist of lymphocytes and plasma cells, but the joint fluid contains PMNs as well, albeit in variable quantities. The inflammation stimulates the ingrowth of vessels and proliferation of synovial cells. Ultimately the exuberant synovial fronds transform into granulation tissue. This is called *pannus* because it covers the articular surfaces like a sheet (in Latin, *pannus* means "cloth cover"). Like any other granulation tissue, the pannus is rich in inflammatory cells that secrete lytic enzymes and various mediators of inflammation. These biologically active substances destroy cartilage and erode the underlying bone. The joints become immobilized and the intra-articular space may even become completely obliterated as the granulation tissue transforms, in subsequent stages, into a collagenous scar, causing ankylosis. The immobilized bone on both sides of the joint undergoes osteoporosis that is readily visible on x-ray studies.

Extensive research into the pathogenesis of RA has not yet provided any definitive answers about the pathogenesis of joint inflammation. Major emphasis has been placed on elucidating the role of immunoglobulins, prostaglandins, and various interleukins, which promote inflammation and also exert metabolic influences on the adjacent bone and connective tissue. Drugs that inhibit prostaglandin synthesis, such as aspirin and indomethacin, are known to improve clinical symptoms.

Clinical Features

The onset of RA is usually insidious, although in some patients the disease presents with an acute onset of joint pain, swelling, and redness. Symmetric involvement of small joints is typical, but the symptoms may appear in any joint. The most commonly affected joints are the proximal interphalangeal joints of the fingers, the metacarpophalangeal joints, and the joints of the wrist (Figure 19-17). The elbow and the ankle are also common sites of inflammation, and the large joints of the extremities can be involved as well.

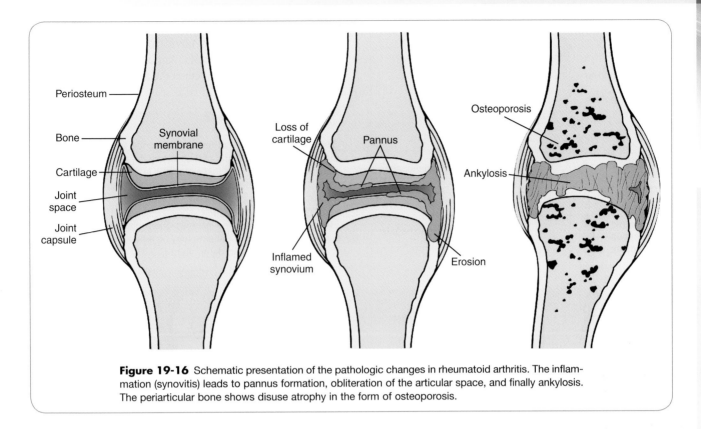

Figure 19-16 Schematic presentation of the pathologic changes in rheumatoid arthritis. The inflammation (synovitis) leads to pannus formation, obliteration of the articular space, and finally ankylosis. The periarticular bone shows disuse atrophy in the form of osteoporosis.

RA has an unpredictable course. In some patients a remission may occur spontaneously after a single episode; in most people, however, it will recur or persist. In about 10% of patients it will progress and cause severe disability. Early onset of disease carries a poor prognosis. At least 50% of patients with juvenile RA develop severe deformities and systemic complications.

The most serious complications are joint deformities and contractures, which cause a loss of full-range mobility. Ulnar deviation of the wrist, with deviation of the fingers in the opposite direction and anterior slippage of the proximal phalanges, is known as a *Z deformity*. Other terms—such as *hourglass, opera-glass, swan-neck,* and *boutonnière deformity*—are used to describe the various hand deformities.

RA is a systemic disease that can cause low-grade fever, loss of appetite, malaise, and fatigue. Anemia is common. Pathologic lesions occur in many anatomic sites besides the joints, the most common of which are subcutaneous nodules *(rheumatoid nodules)* composed of central fibrinoid necrosis surrounded by macrophages and lymphocytes. These nodules are painless, are small (less than 2 cm in diameter), and cause no symptoms. Rheumatoid nodules do not occur in other forms of arthritis and are therefore useful in the diagnosis of RA.

Internal organs often show nonspecific signs of chronic inflammation. In the lungs this presents as interstitial fibrosis or subpleural fibrosis. Rheumatoid lung disease presents with localized parenchymal lesions and is commonly associated with pleuritis and pleural effusion. The eyes show signs of inflammation *(scleritis)*. Pericarditis can develop on the surface of the

heart. Rheumatoid vasculitis, provoked by the deposition of immune complexes in the walls of arteries, can occur in all organs and can cause widespread infarcts.

RA that develops in children and adolescents is called *juvenile RA,* also known as *Still's disease.* In contrast to typical RA, juvenile RA most commonly involves the large joints. It has an acute onset and more prominent extra-articular manifestations than typical RA. It also has a worse prognosis than classic RA.

Laboratory findings include a variety of abnormalities that accompany systemic inflammation and some immune disturbances, but none of these is diagnostic of RA. Rheumatoid factor, an immune complex formed between a patient's own immunoglobulin M (IgM) and immunoglobulin G (IgG), is present in 80% of patients. Unfortunately, these immune complexes are not diagnostic of RA, because they may be found in other autoimmune disorders and even in healthy persons. Antibodies to cyclic citrullinated peptide (CCP) are present only in RA patients and are apparently more specific markers of the disease. Joint fluid analysis is helpful for demonstrating intra-articular inflammation, but it is most useful for excluding bacterial arthritis (in RA there are no bacteria) and gout (in RA there are no urate crystals). Other autoimmune diseases, such as systemic lupus erythematosus, must be excluded on clinical grounds because these diseases may produce the same symptoms and often cause arthritis.

No specific therapy exists for RA. However, treatment with anti-inflammatory drugs may provide relief and slow the progression of the disease.

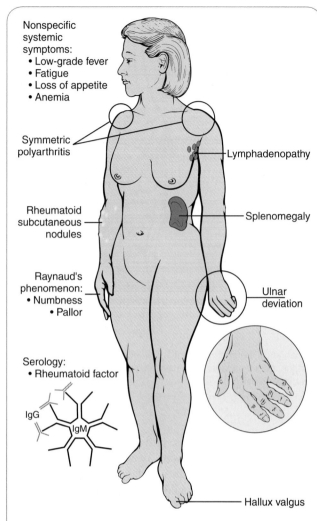

Nonspecific
systemic
symptoms:
• Low-grade fever
• Fatigue
• Loss of appetite
• Anemia

Symmetric
polyarthritis

Lymphadenopathy

Rheumatoid
subcutaneous
nodules

Splenomegaly

Raynaud's
phenomenon:
• Numbness
• Pallor

Ulnar
deviation

Serology:
• Rheumatoid factor

IgG

IgM

Hallux valgus

Figure 19-17 Signs and symptoms of rheumatoid arthritis. IgG, immunoglobulin G; IgM, immunoglobulin M.

transient exudation of fluid into the joint cavity. Histologically there is evidence of synovitis marked by infiltrates of lymphocytes and plasma cells. Antibiotic treatment usually eradicates the infection and cures the arthritis.

> **? Did You Know?**
>
> Clinicians use a variety of terms to describe hand deformities in rheumatoid arthritis. Some of these carry the names of the physicians who first described these changes (e.g., Heberden's nodes). Other terms are more colorful and less precise and serve only to help one remember that hand deformities occur often in rheumatoid arthritis. This photograph shows "opera-glass" deformities. Even people who have never used opera glasses will remember such a term, and some patients may be amused that a fancy term is used to describe their deformity.
>
>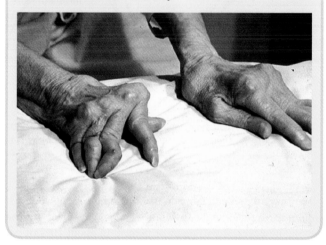

Many viral diseases cause vague pain in the muscles and joints. Such viral infections typically produce a transient, self-limited synovitis. The inflammation is usually mild, heals spontaneously, and leaves no consequences.

GOUT

Gout denotes a group of diseases characterized by *hyperuricemia* and the deposition of uric acid crystals in various tissues, primarily the joints, subcutaneous tissue, and kidneys. Hyperuricemia is a prerequisite for gout, but not all persons who have hyperuricemia will have symptoms of gout. It should be remembered that **hyperuricemia** is arbitrarily defined as blood levels exceeding 7 mg/dL (415 μmol/L). By this standard, approximately 10% of the normal population has hyperuricemia. In elderly persons and those who are hospitalized for various reasons, hyperuricemia may be found even more often. It is comforting to know that only 5% of hyperuricemic persons in any age group develop gout. Almost 95% of all patients with gout are males. A significant number of patients have a family history of gout.

Etiology and Pathogenesis

Gout may be classified as primary or secondary. Primary or idiopathic gout may be classified as metabolic (i.e., caused by hyperproduction of uric acid) or renal (i.e., caused by

INFECTIOUS ARTHRITIS

Infectious arthritis results from hematogenous spread of pathogens during sepsis, from the spread of infection from adjacent bones, from direct inoculation of bacteria by trauma or surgical procedures, or from joint fluid removal *(arthrocentesis).* Pyogenic arthritis caused by staphylococci or streptococci is rare. Tuberculous arthritis was common in the past, but it is rare today. Gonococcal arthritis, a well-known complication of this sexually transmitted disease, affects less than 5% of infected persons who have not been treated properly.

The most common bacterial arthritis is the migratory arthritis of Lyme disease. **Lyme disease** is caused by the spirochete *Borrelia burgdorferi,* transmitted by ticks *(Ixodes dammini).* Arthritis, often in a migratory form, occurs a few weeks or even months after the tick bite, in concert with fleeting skin rash *(migrating erythema)* and nonspecific systemic symptoms. The knee joint is most involved, but other weight-carrying joints, and even smaller joints, may show signs of inflammation as the bacteremia spreads the disease, causing underexcretion of uric acid). Most affected patients are over-producers, but the kidney's handling of uric acid is also important. Secondary gout is related to another disease or identifiable causes of hyperproduction of uric acid or its underexcretion in the kidneys. The main forms of gout are listed in Box 19-1.

Uric acid is the end product of purine metabolism. Surplus uric acid that is produced in the body is excreted in the urine, so that the normal concentration of uric acid in blood remains less than 7 mg/dL. However, many patients with gout show decreased clearance of urates in the proximal tubules. Renal excretion of urates includes filtration in the glomeruli, resorption in the proximal tubule, and secretion in the proximal tubules, followed by partial resorption in the loop of Henle and the collecting tubules. Although the exact mechanisms of renal malfunction in gout are not known, it is well established that the kidneys of most patients underexcrete urates in urine.

Hyperuricemia leads to deposition of uric acid crystals in tissues. Most deposits are in the form of insoluble monosodium urate. The disease typically develops after many years—usually 15 to 30 years—of asymptomatic hyperuricemia. The most common sites of uric acid deposition are the joints and periarticular connective tissue. In more than 90% of cases, the first symptoms occur in the tarsometatarsal joint of the big toe, which is clinically known as podagra (meaning "foot seizure" in Greek). Uric acid is probably released from the deposits in the joint capsule by minor trauma. It enters the joint cavity and hypersaturates the fluid. Because the feet are usually colder than the rest of the body and because the low temperature reduces uric acid solubility and promotes crystallization inside the joint, deposition of crystals occurs along the joint surfaces and the periarticular connective tissue. Uric acid crystals are chemotactic and provoke an acute inflammation within the joint (Figure 19-18). Uric acid also activates the complement system and kallikrein, which promote inflammation, cause pain, and recruit more leukocytes into the joint. Uric acid crystals are phagocytosed by the leukocytes. However, because these crystals are sharp, they pierce the

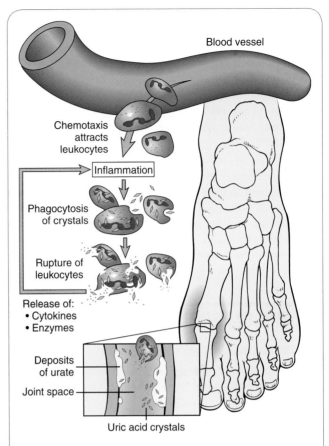

Figure 19-18 Gouty arthritis. Deposits of uric acid crystals in the connective tissue have a chemotactic effect and cause exudation of leukocytes into the joint. The inflammation most often affects the metatarsophalangeal joint of the big toe.

lysosomes, and a release of acid hydrolases ensues. Such an attack of gout not only is painful but also has all the features of acute inflammation.

Clinical Features

Gout can be classified as acute or chronic. In acute gout the joint is swollen, hyperemic, and warm, and the patient cannot walk because of the excruciating pain. Systemic symptoms include fever, leukocytosis, tachycardia, and general exhaustion. The attack may last 2 to 3 days or longer and usually subsides spontaneously. Recurrences can occur within weeks but often occur after a prolonged period. Asymptomatic periods tend to become shorter and shorter as the disease progresses. *Chronic gout* is marked by less inflammation but more pronounced bone deformities. In addition to joint involvement, gout often presents with painless subcutaneous deposits of uric acid known as *tophi*. These are most common on the ears, on the extensor sites of the arms, over the olecranon, and over the patella. Histologically, they are encapsulated; contain birefringent urate crystals; and are surrounded by macrophages, lymphocytes, and giant cells.

Deposits of urates can be found in many internal organs, but most of these are small or inconsequential. The most

BOX 19-1 Classification of Gout and Hyperuricemia

Primary metabolic
  Idiopathic overproduction
  Lesch-Nyhan syndrome
Secondary metabolic
  Hematopoietic malignant disease
  Chronic hemolysis
  Obesity
  Alcoholism
Primary renal
  Underexcretion of uric acid
Secondary renal
  Kidney disease
  Drugs (diuretics)
  Lead poisoning

significant are uric acid deposits in the kidneys, which often show signs of ischemia-, toxin-, and infection-related injury. Hypertension is common in gout, and it may also damage the kidneys. Chronic renal failure is seen in 25% of all patients with gout.

Hypersaturation of urine with uric acid may lead to the formation of uric acid stones, found in 20% of all patients. Stones may cause obstructive nephropathy or predispose these individuals to chronic pyelonephritis. Gout also predisposes patients to the formation of calcium stones.

The diagnosis of gout is based on the recognition of typical clinical symptoms and on laboratory proof of hyperuricemia. Monoarthritic joint pain involving the great toe is highly characteristic of gout. However, if there are doubts, x-ray studies may be useful in demonstrating bone erosion with tophi. Numerous leukocytes and uric acid crystals can be seen by microscopic analysis of joint fluid.

REVIEW QUESTIONS

1. What are the functions of bone cells?

2. Define epiphysis, metaphysis, and diaphysis and explain why a knowledge of these anatomic terms is important for pathology.

3. Compare endochondral and intramembranous ossification.

4. What are the main functions of bones?

5. What are the basic structure and function of joints?

6. What is achondroplasia?

7. What is osteogenesis imperfecta?

8. What are the main causes of osteomyelitis?

9. Describe the principal pathologic feature of osteomyelitis.

10. What are the possible causes of aseptic bone necrosis?

11. Describe typical clinical features of aseptic bone necrosis.

12. What are the causes of osteoporosis?

13. Discuss the pathogenesis of osteoporosis.

14. What are the complications of osteoporosis?

15. What is osteomalacia?

16. Explain the role of vitamin D in calcium homeostasis.

17. Compare rickets and osteomalacia.

18. How is osteomalacia diagnosed?

19. What are the main pathologic features of renal osteodystrophy?

20. Describe the three phases of Paget's disease.

21. Describe various forms of fracture of long bones.

22. Describe the healing of fractures.

23. What happens during joint dislocation?

24. Classify bone tumors.

25. Describe the main pathologic and clinical features of osteosarcoma.

26. Describe the main pathologic and clinical features of chondrosarcoma.

27. Describe the main pathologic and clinical features of Ewing's sarcoma.

28. What are the main pathologic and clinical features of giant cell bone tumor?

29. What is osteoarthritis?

30. Compare the facts favoring the wear-and-tear hypothesis of osteoarthritis with those favoring a metabolic or inflammatory origin for this disease.

31. Describe the pathology of osteoarthritis.

32. What are the main clinical signs and symptoms of osteoarthritis?

33. What is rheumatoid arthritis?

34. What are the roles of hormones, genes, and autoimmunity in the pathogenesis of rheumatoid arthritis?

35. What is pannus, and how does it evolve?

36. Describe the pathology of rheumatoid arthritis.

37. What are the clinical features of rheumatoid arthritis?

38. What are the main causes of infectious arthritis?

39. What is gout?

40. How common is gout in men and women?

41. Compare primary and secondary gout.

42. How does hyperuricemia lead to podagra?

43. Compare the clinical features of acute and chronic gout.

44. What are tophi?

45. What kind of urinary stones are found in persons who have gout?

Muscles and Peripheral Nerves

20

Chapter Outline

NORMAL ANATOMY AND PHYSIOLOGY
OVERVIEW OF MAJOR DISEASES
  Neurogenic Atrophy
  Myasthenia Gravis
  Muscular Dystrophies
    Duchenne's Muscular Dystrophy
    Other Dystrophies
  Congenital Myopathies

Acquired Myopathies
  Diabetic Myopathy
  Cancer Myopathy
Mechanical Injury of Muscles
Myositis
  Infectious Myositis
  Immune Myositis
Soft Tissue Tumors

Key Terms and Concepts

Acetylcholine
Angiosarcoma
Becker's dystrophy
Cerebral palsy
Creatine kinase
Crush injury
Dermatomyositis
Diabetic myopathy
Duchenne's muscular dystrophy
Dystrophin
Hemiplegia

Leiomyosarcoma
Limb-girdle dystrophy
Liposarcoma
Malignant peripheral nerve sheath
  tumor
Muscular dystrophy
Myasthenia gravis
Myositis, infectious
Myotonic dystrophy
Neurogenic atrophy
Neuromuscular junction

Paralysis
Paraplegia
Polymorphous cell sarcoma
Polymyositis
Rhabdomyolysis
Rhabdomyosarcoma
Soft tissue tumors
Synovial sarcoma
Wallerian degeneration of axons

433

NORMAL ANATOMY AND PHYSIOLOGY

Skeletal muscle is composed of striated muscle fibers. Each of the anatomically distinct muscles, which vary in size from the very large muscles (e.g., quadriceps) to exquisitely small muscles (e.g., ocular muscles), is enclosed in a connective tissue fascia called the *perimysium.* Thinner connective tissue septa branch from the epimysium, forming strands of perimysium that enclose groups of muscle fibers and separate them into fascicles. Septa within each fascicle, called *endomysium,* are composed of basement membrane–like material that envelopes each muscle fiber individually (Figure 20-1). This framework of stromal tissue provides support to muscle cells, blood vessels, and nerves.

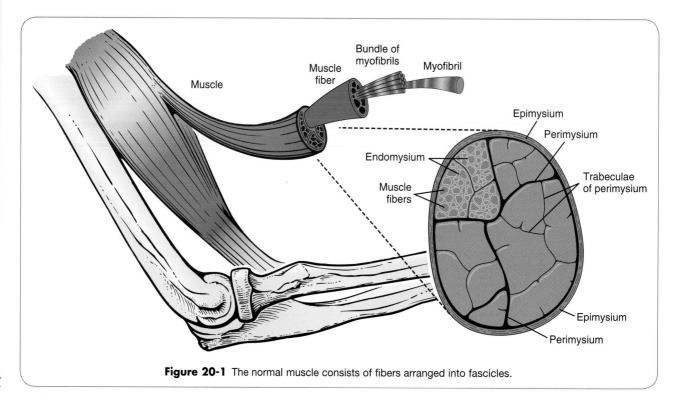

Figure 20-1 The normal muscle consists of fibers arranged into fascicles.

The muscle cells are postmitotic, terminally differentiated cells that cannot divide. The regeneration of muscle proceeds from less-differentiated reserve cells. Such regeneration is highly inefficient and limited.

Muscle cells are specialized cells that are rich in contractile proteins (actin and myosin). To perform their primary function (contractibility), these cells have a high ratio of cytoplasm to nuclei. The muscle cells are long and extensible; that is, many return to normal length after contraction. To maintain their viability, they have many nuclei, typically located beneath the cell membrane along the entire length of the fiber. The nuclei are positioned so that they do not interfere with the contraction of the fibers that occupy the rest of the cytoplasm.

Each muscle fiber is individually innervated by a branch of the motor neuron axon. The site of contact between the axon and the muscle fiber is called the **neuromuscular junction.** The nerve and muscle are separated from one another by a very narrow space. Into this space the nerve ending releases **acetylcholine** (ACh), which acts as a neurotransmitter and binds to receptors on the surface of the muscle cell, causing

membrane depolarization and thereby initiating contraction. The enzyme cholinesterase removes the neurotransmitter from the muscle receptors. This is associated with repolarization of the muscle cell membrane and relaxation. The significance of the neuromuscular junction is illustrated in the paragraph on myasthenia gravis later in this chapter.

Skeletal muscles are composed of two types of fibers: type I, or *slow fibers,* and type II, or *fast fibers*. In chickens these fibers are separated from one another. The red fibers that maintain protracted contraction are found in chicken legs, whereas the white fibers designed for rapid but short movements of the wings are found in chicken breast. In humans the red and white fibers are intermixed at random in a checkerboard pattern that is easily recognized using special histochemical techniques. Histochemistry makes it possible to distinguish between type I fibers, which are rich in oxidative enzymes, and type II fibers, which contain fewer of these enzymes (Figure 20-2).

It is important to remember that muscle fibers are not inherently fast or slow; instead, their properties depend on nerve impulses. If a fast white muscle fiber loses its original

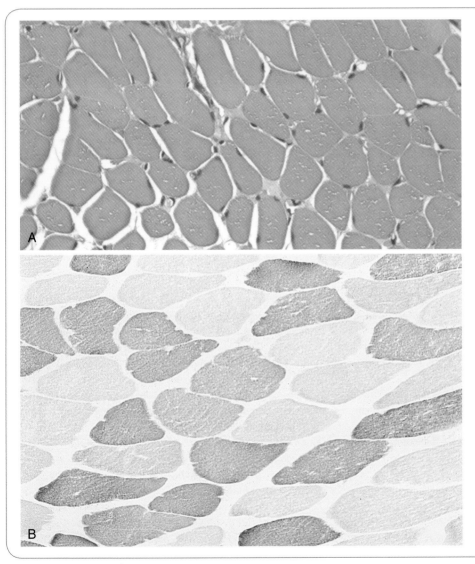

Figure 20-2 Normal skeletal muscle histology. *A,* In routine hematoxylin- and eosin-stained slides, skeletal muscle fibers have abundant pink cytoplasm and nuclei that are located peripherally underneath the cell membrane. *B,* Special stain used to distinguish type I from type II fibers shows that the muscle consists of two types of cells arranged in a checkerboard manner.

innervation and is later reinnervated by a "slow" nerve, it will change and become slow. Such changes are commonly seen in reinnervated muscle after regeneration of transected axons.

The muscles are composed of highly specialized cells whose primary function is contraction. For example, this enables the body to move, generate heat, breathe, and maintain posture. In addition, muscles are a storage site for metabolites, such as glycogen and fat. Proteins of the muscle cells can be used, under adverse conditions, as sources of energy. (Inmates of concentration camps appeared wasted because they used muscle proteins to compensate for an inadequate diet.)

OVERVIEW OF MAJOR DISEASES

The skeletal muscles have a limited capacity to respond to injury, and the range of morphologic and functional changes in diseased muscles is quite narrow. Morphologically recognizable changes include the following:

- Adaptations, such as atrophy and hypertrophy
- Cell injury, referred to in this context as degeneration
- Limited regeneration
- Inflammation
- Neoplastic proliferation

Functionally, muscle diseases are characterized by an inability to contract adequately *(weakness),* an inability to sustain action *(fatigability),* continuous spasm *(myotonus),* or irregular and uncoordinated contraction of groups of fibers *(fibrillation).* However, the most prominent symptom of muscle disease is pain *(myalgia).*

The most important muscle diseases are the following:

- Neuromuscular disorders
- Muscular dystrophies
- Mechanical trauma
- Myositis

Metabolic myopathies, inborn errors of metabolism, and muscle diseases secondary to systemic diseases are not discussed. These diseases are very rare, and it is enough to know that they exist. However, for the sake of completeness, examples of such diseases are listed in Box 20-1. Tumors of striated muscles and soft tissues that are adjacent to them are rare and are described briefly.

Several facts important to an understanding of normal muscles and muscle diseases are presented here, before a discussion of specific pathologic entities.

1. *Muscle and peripheral nerves are a single unit.* Without proper nerve stimulation, the muscle undergoes atrophy. However, the muscle can be reinnervated from the regenerative nerve. Loss of motor neurons—for example, after stroke or spinal cord injury—causes paralysis of skeletal muscles.

2. *Transmission of nerve stimuli from nerve to muscle is chemically mediated and depends on the binding of the neurotransmitter to the receptors on the muscular side of the neuromuscular junction.* Chemical destruction of ACh (the neurotransmitter) or the blockade of receptors

can impede or completely block the transmission of stimuli. Muscle paralysis in *myasthenia gravis,* an immune-mediated disease, is mediated by antibodies to the ACh receptor that impair the transmission of neural impulses.

3. *The function of muscle cells depends on the integrity of their primary cytoplasmic components.* A deficiency of normal structural components is best noted in hereditary muscle disease. A genetic defect involving the plasma membrane protein **dystrophin** causes muscle cell degeneration in Duchenne-type muscular dystrophy. Aggregation of tropomyosin in cytoplasmic bodies—so-called nemaline bodies—impairs the function of muscle cells in nemaline myopathy.

4. *Muscle cell function depends on the maintenance of transmembrane gradients in the concentration of minerals in the muscle cell and the pericellular fluids.* The hypocalcemia of hypoparathyroidism causes muscle spasms *(tetany).* A disease known as *hypokalemic periodic paralysis* is characterized by attacks of weakness caused by low serum potassium levels, which perturb the normal transmembrane mineral gradient.

BOX 20-1   Classification of Muscle Diseases*

Neuromuscular Disorders
Neurogenic muscle cell atrophy
Myasthenia gravis

Muscular Dystrophy
Duchenne's dystrophy
Limb-girdle dystrophy
Myotonic dystrophy

Congenital Myopathy
Carnitine deficiency
Nemaline myopathy
Mitochondrial myopathy

Endocrine and Metabolic Myopathy
Thyrotoxicosis
Diabetes

Paraneoplastic Myopathy
Dermatomyositis

Autoimmune and Infectious Myositis
Polymyositis and dermatomyositis
Infectious myositis
Trichinosis

Mechanical Trauma
Crush injury
Muscle sprain
Rhabdomyolysis

Tumors
Rhabdomyosarcoma

*with examples of important entities.

5. *Muscle function depends on adequate generation of energy.* Carnitine deficiency, an inborn error of lipid metabolism, and various congenital mitochondrial myopathies are characterized by muscle weakness that can be explained in terms of insufficient energy production. No machine can function without fuel, and muscles that are inadequately supplied by energy are no exception.

6. *Many hormones affect muscle function.* Hormones regulate the intermediary metabolism and influence mineral gradients in the muscle. Thyroid, adrenal, or insulin excess or deficiency may cause muscle weakness. Lack of parathyroid hormone causes spastic contractions.

7. *Many toxins and drugs may affect the muscle.* The effect may be exerted directly on the muscle cell or indirectly through the nerve. Bacterial toxins may cause paralysis or muscle spasm. Botulism, a disease caused by a toxin from *Clostridium botulinum,* is marked by muscle paralysis. Tetanus, a disease marked by muscle spasm (tetany), is caused by a toxin from *Clostridium tetani.* Curare, a natural poison used by Indians of South America on arrows, may cause muscle paralysis. Curare is also used to induce muscle relaxation during surgery.

8. *Muscle is often affected by autoimmune disorders.* Systemic lupus erythematosus, rheumatic arthritis, and dermatomyositis present with inflammatory muscle lesions. Myasthenia gravis is an autoimmune disorder affecting the neuromuscular junction.

9. *Destruction of muscle fibers is characterized by a release of muscle-specific enzymes,* such as **creatine kinase (CK).** This enzyme is released into the circulation and is a useful marker of muscle cell injury. Traumatic injury of the muscle, and even exercise-induced rhabdomyolysis (i.e., rupture of striated muscles), as occurs in most marathon runners, causes elevation of CK in blood.

10. *Muscle cells are relatively resistant to infections.* Bacterial infections of the muscles are rare in persons who have intact skin. However, infected wounds may cause the spread of bacteria into muscle. Viral infections are probably more common. Most viral infections are mild (but clinically undiagnosed) and have no residual consequences. Aches and pains of muscles during a bout of flu are the best examples of viral myositis. *Trichinella spiralis,* a worm acquired from eating inadequately cooked pork, may infest the muscle and cause chronic myositis.

11. *Muscle cells cannot regenerate properly.* Muscle cell loss cannot adequately be compensated for because the regeneration from the reserve cells is limited. Thus muscle cell loss is, for all practical purposes, irreversible. On the positive side, the nonproliferating muscle cells rarely, if ever, undergo malignant transformation. The most common malignant muscle cell tumor—*rhabdomyosarcoma*—is very rare in adults. Rhabdomyosarcoma is more common in young persons, in whom it is probably derived from fetal or growing muscle cells. Most tumors in the muscles of adults are derived from connective tissue cells. Such tumors are rare, and in medical practice they are known as *soft tissue sarcomas.*

NEUROGENIC ATROPHY

Neurogenic atrophy is a form of muscle cell atrophy caused by injury of the nerves, classified as either upper motor neuron or lower motor neuron.

The upper motor neuron is located in the central cortex. The lower motor neuron is in the anterior horn of the spinal cord. The axons of the upper neuron connect the cerebral cortical neurons with the spinal neurons. These axons run through the spinal cord. The axons of the lower motor neurons are assembled into fascicles, which form peripheral nerves extending from the spinal cord to the skeletal muscles (Figure 20-3).

The most common causes of neurogenic atrophy of muscle are listed in Box 20-2. For example, the lower motor neuron may be damaged in the spinal cord. Poliomyelitis, a viral disease that has been eradicated by successful immunization, destroys the anterior horn neurons and causes paralysis. Autoimmune diseases like Guillain-Barré syndrome may affect the motor nerves and cause weakness and paralysis. This disease is also known as postinfectious polyradiculoneuropathy because it usually develops 2 to 4 weeks after a viral disease.

The axons are extensions of motor neurons that form peripheral nerves. Nerves are long structures and can be injured easily because they are not protected adequately by

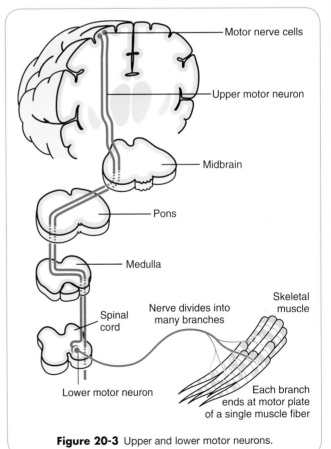

Figure 20-3 Upper and lower motor neurons.

Motor nerve cells

Upper motor neuron

Midbrain

Pons

Medulla

Spinal cord

Nerve divides into many branches

Skeletal muscle

Lower motor neuron

Each branch ends at motor plate of a single muscle fiber

Cerebral bleeding and infarcts ("strokes") that destroy cerebral neurons are the most important causes of upper motor injury. Stroke is typically associated with a massive loss of motor neurons in the cortex. Bleeding into the midbrain and the internal capsule of the basal ganglia may damage axons crossing these parts of the brain. **Paralysis** (loss of power or the ability to move voluntarily) of both legs is called **paraplegia.** **Hemiplegia** is a paralysis of the muscles on one side of the body. All these conditions are characterized by neurogenic atrophy of skeletal muscles.

Histologic signs of neurogenic atrophy vary depending on the extent of nerve loss. This condition may present as single muscle cell atrophy or fascicular atrophy. Loss of branches of axons, as is commonly seen in diabetic neuropathy or various toxic neuropathies, is accompanied by single muscle cell atrophy. Such fibers are scattered at random throughout the muscle fascicle. They appear angulated and are surrounded and compressed by adjacent normal muscle fibers, many of which actually undergo compensatory hypertrophy (Figure 20-4). Transection of the entire nerve or its parts causes atrophy of larger groups of muscle fibers or the entire fascicle *(fascicular atrophy).*

Spinal cord or cerebral injury leads to atrophy of entire muscles, as is commonly seen in paraplegic persons. Such atrophy is permanent and irreparable. Single-cell atrophy may be reversed, and each muscle can theoretically regain its size and normal shape if it is reinnervated. In practice this rarely occurs because the underlying cause of muscle disease is usually incurable.

Transection of the larger nerves also can be repaired if the proximal part of the axon is preserved (Figure 20-5). The nerve distal to the transection injury degenerates, together with its myelin sheath. This **wallerian degeneration** progresses toward the nucleus of the nerve but stops at the first node of Ranvier

surrounding soft tissues. For example, nerves can be severed in a knife stabbing. The axon can also be damaged by a toxin or by antibodies *(autoimmune neuritis).* Ischemia, most often caused by small blood vessel disease in persons with diabetes, may also damage the nerves or their axons. Diabetic neuropathy is probably the most common cause of neurogenic atrophy of the skeletal muscles.

Upper neuron injury may be related to transection of the spinal cord and the damage of descending cerebrospinal tracts. This is a common consequence of car accidents or sport injuries (e.g., football injuries).

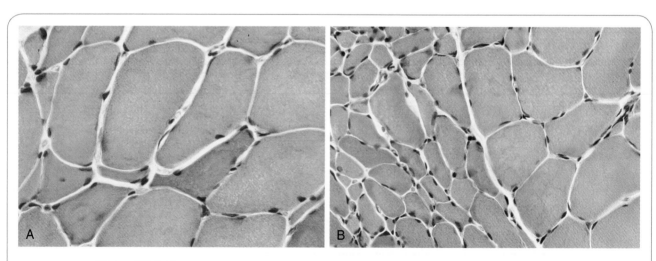

Figure 20-4 Histologic appearance of atrophic fibers. *A,* Single-cell muscle atrophy comprises individual, small, angulated fibers surrounded by fibers of normal size. This is usually a consequence of the loss of axonal branches, as in ischemia secondary to diabetes. *B,* Fascicular atrophy involves the entire muscle fascicle *(left).* It is usually related to transection of a larger nerve or injury of the motor neurons in the brain and spinal cord.

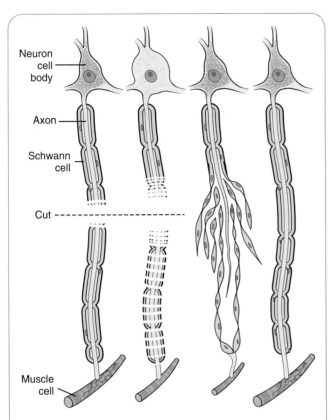

Figure 20-5 Wallerian degeneration and regeneration of peripheral nerve. The nerve degenerates distal to the transection and proximally, up to the first node of Ranvier. Schwann cells regenerate and form a new sheath through which the axon will find its way to reinnervate the muscle.

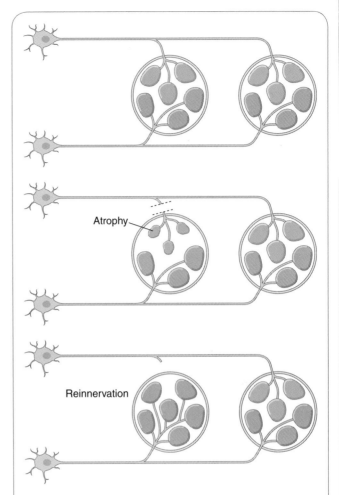

Figure 20-6 Denervation and reinnervation of the striated muscle. In the normal muscle, type I and type II fibers are intermixed in a checkerboard manner. Denervation is followed by reinnervation, during which the type of nerve determines which type the muscle will be; thus all the fibers reinnervated by one nerve will be of the same type. Hence there is grouping of type I and type II fibers.

proximal to the injury. From this area, the Schwann cells proliferate and lay down the path for axonal regrowth. Axonal growth typically progresses at a speed of 1 to 2 cm per week until the terminal branches again reach the denervated muscle. The axonal branches reinnervate the muscle, reestablishing functional neuromuscular junctions. We have all heard of "surgical miracles"—operations in which skillful surgeons have reconnected to the body a severed arm, finger, or a penis. In all these cases of reconstructive surgery, the transected nerves were sutured together and axons were allowed to regenerate.

Reinnervated muscles resume normal function and appear normal on histologic examination. The only difference from the preexisting normal state is that groups of muscle fibers are innervated by a single axon. Because the axon determines the muscle type, the fibers in the reinnervated area will all be of the same type—either type I or type II—and will not be intermixed in a checkerboard pattern as before. This is called *fiber type grouping* and is typical of reinnervated muscles (Figure 20-6).

MYASTHENIA GRAVIS

Myasthenia gravis (MG) is an autoimmune disease involving the neuromuscular junction. It is characterized by impaired neural impulse transmission. MG is a rare disease with

a prevalence of 10 to 15 per 100,000 persons. It is more common in women than in men (by a ratio of 3:2). Most affected women are 20 to 35 years of age, whereas affected men are generally older (50 to 60 years of age). In 75% of patients with MG, especially those in the younger age group, the disease is associated with enlargement of the thymus.

Etiology and Pathogenesis

The cause of MG is unknown. However, almost all patients have antibodies to ACh receptors. The reasons for the formation of such autoantibodies are not known. These antibodies bind to the receptor on the neuromuscular plate, preventing the binding of neurotransmitters and the normal transmission of nerve impulses to the muscle (Figure 20-7).

Pathology

The striated muscles examined during muscle biopsy are histologically normal or occasionally contain aggregates of lymphocytes. On electron microscopic examination, one observes

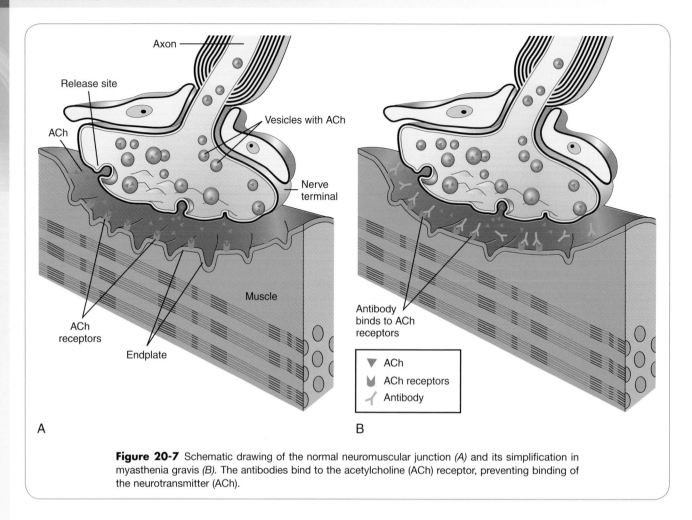

Figure 20-7 Schematic drawing of the normal neuromuscular junction *(A)* and its simplification in myasthenia gravis *(B)*. The antibodies bind to the acetylcholine (ACh) receptor, preventing binding of the neurotransmitter (ACh).

a decreased number of invaginations of the motor neural plate. How the antibodies produce these morphologic changes is unknown. The loss of invaginations correlates with biochemical and immunohistochemical data, which indicate a reduced number of surface receptor sites for ACh at the motor neural plate. Antibodies bound to the receptor can be demonstrated by immunohistochemical techniques during muscle biopsy. Antibodies are also found circulating in the blood.

Many patients with MG have enlargement of the thymus. Histologically, the enlarged thymus shows either hyperplasia or neoplasia. Tumors of the thymus are called *thymomas*. Although it appears that thymomas play a part in the development of MG, their pathogenic role has not been fully elucidated.

Clinical Symptoms

MG is characterized by easy fatigability and muscular weakness. Small extraocular muscles and facial muscles are most often involved. In approximately 15% of all patients, the disease remains limited to the eye muscles *(ocular myasthenia)*. In both generalized and ocular myasthenia the eyelids show drooping *(ptosis)* and patients typically complain of double vision *(diplopia)* and easy fatigability on reading. Facial muscle weakness produces a bland expression, and these patients often complain of an inability to chew. The disease

spreads to the upper extremities, usually involving the proximal muscles. Finally, all the muscles may become affected, and the patient is unable to move. Death occurs as a result of the paralysis of the thoracic intercostal respiratory muscles and the diaphragm.

The diagnosis of MG is made on the basis of clinical findings and is confirmed with specific tests, including an anticholinesterase test, electromyography, and serologic testing for antibodies to ACh receptors. The anticholinesterase test is performed with antagonists of cholinesterase, such as edrophonium. This drug may momentarily improve symptoms because the inhibition of the enzyme that normally destroys ACh allows the "flooding" of the neuromuscular junction with ACh to occur. Such an excess of ACh temporarily facilitates the transmission of impulses from the nerve to the muscle. Electromyographic testing, which involves inserting a needle into the muscle and connecting it with a generator of electric current, shows increased fatigability of muscles. Normal muscle fibers contract when stimulated, but as the affected muscles are stimulated with consecutive electric impulses, they respond less and less to the stimulation. Antibodies to ACh receptors, however, are the most reliable sign that the patient has an autoimmune disorder that causes the symptoms of MG. Such antibodies are easily detectable in patients' blood.

The treatment of MG is symptomatic because, for the time being, this disease is incurable. Best results are obtained with drugs that inhibit the action of acetylcholinesterase. As in the cholinesterase test, this treatment increases the concentration of ACh at the neuromuscular junction. Plasmapheresis, a procedure whereby antibodies are removed from the blood, provides temporary relief but cannot stop the progression of the disease (as reported in more than 80% of cases). Patients with thymic enlargement should undergo thymectomy, which may be beneficial, especially in young women. The prognosis is less favorable for older patients and those who cannot be helped by thymectomy; 40% of them die within the first 5 years after diagnosis.

MUSCULAR DYSTROPHIES

The term **muscular dystrophy** encompasses a group of muscle diseases, all of which show the following:
- Genetic defects inherited as Mendelian traits
- Primary muscle cell pathology
- Progressive course and symptoms related to muscle wasting

The most important diseases of this group are listed in Table 20-1.

Clinically, muscular dystrophies are a heterogeneous group. They differ with regard to the following:
- Mode of inheritance
- Age of onset
- Muscle groups that are initially affected
- Severity of the disease
- Associated findings

Muscular dystrophies may be inherited as autosomal dominant, autosomal recessive, or sex-linked traits. The diseases may have their onset in childhood, adolescence, or adulthood. Each disease initially involves different muscle groups, and some diseases are named accordingly. For example, facioscapulohumeral dystrophy involves the muscles of the face and those overlying the scapula as well as those attached to the humerus. These diseases may be severe or mild, and some are associated with lesions of other organs besides the muscles.

Because all these diseases show essentially similar pathologic changes, histologic examination of muscle biopsy specimens is of limited diagnostic value. In all patients with muscular dystrophy, the muscle cells fall apart ("degenerate"), releasing typical muscle enzymes, such as CK, into the circulation. An elevated CK level in the blood is a reliable sign of muscle injury, but it is not useful for distinguishing between the various types of muscular dystrophy. However, recent advances in molecular biology, which have already identified the genes for some muscular dystrophies, offer the most promising means for precise diagnosis.

DUCHENNE'S MUSCULAR DYSTROPHY

Duchenne's muscular dystrophy is the most common muscular dystrophy, caused by mutations of the gene encoding *dystrophin,* an integral plasma membrane protein. Dystrophin holds together other structural proteins, linking them to the cell membrane (Figure 20-8). This abnormality affects muscle fibers and many other cells in the body. Skeletal muscle cells degenerate and muscle weakness ensues.

The gene encoding dystrophin is located on the X chromosome and is very long. Larger or smaller parts of this gene may be mutated or deleted in muscular dystrophy. The symptoms of the disease vary depending on the extent of the mutation or deletion. A milder form, called **Becker's dystrophy,** is 10 times less common than Duchenne's dystrophy.

Duchenne's muscular dystrophy is a sex-linked recessive disease; thus it occurs only in boys. Mothers who are carriers of the gene are asymptomatic. In one third of cases, however, the mother is not the carrier, indicating that a new mutation occurred in the affected male.

Pathology

Skeletal muscles affected by Duchenne's dystrophy show typical alterations that are not distinct from similar changes in other dystrophies. The histologic picture varies, and as the

---

TABLE 20-1 Muscular Dystrophies

Type of Dystrophy	Inheritance/Incidence per 10,000	Age at Onset	Muscles Involved Initially	Symptoms/Course	Associated Findings
Duchenne's	XR/1:5000	3–5	Girdle	Severe (death by 25 years of age)	Mental retardation
Becker's	XR/1:50,000	5–10	Girdle	Mild but progressive (death at 40+ years of age)	—
Limb-girdle	AR/AD 1:100,000	Variable (5–10)	Shoulder, girdle	Moderate weakness	Cardiomyopathy
Myotonic	AD/1:8000	Variable (10–30)	Eyelids, face, distal limbs	Variably progressive mytonia (death at 50–60 years of age)	Mental retardation, frontal baldness, gonadal atrophy, heart disease, diabetes

AD, autosomal dominant; AR, autosomal recessive; XR, X-linked recessive.

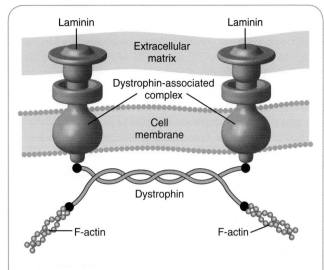

Figure 20-8 Duchenne's muscular dystrophy. The disease is caused by an abnormality in the protein dystrophin, which is responsible for the functional integrity of the muscle cells. It binds on one side with actin fibers (F-actin) and on the other side with cell membrane glycoproteins. The gene encoding dystrophin is on the X chromosome.

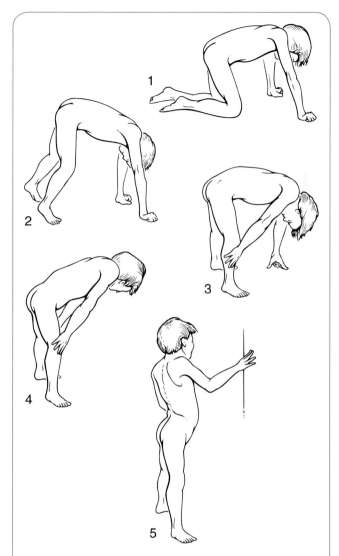

Figure 20-9 The clinical diagnosis of Duchenne's dystrophy is made on the basis of a neurologic examination. If a boy with this disease is in a squatting or "all-fours" position and is asked to rise, he will not be able to get up because of the weakness of the pelvic girdle muscles. He will use his arms to raise his body.

disease progresses, the changes become increasingly prominent. Early stages of dystrophy are marked by individual muscle cell degeneration. As the disease progresses, more and more muscle fibers are lost, resulting in progressive muscle weakness. The progressive muscle cell loss is accompanied by compensatory hypertrophy of viable fibers and an ingrowth of fibrous tissue and fat cells. With progression of the disease, the muscle fascicles are gradually lost and replaced by fibrous tissue and fat cells. Severe wasting of skeletal muscles leads to skeletal deformities.

Clinical Features

Symptoms of Duchenne's dystrophy appear in preschool boys and are caused by a weakness of the weight-carrying muscles of the pelvic girdle and lower extremities. Affected boys have difficulty getting up from a squatting position and must use their arms to lift the body (Figure 20-9). During this effort, they typically move their hands up their legs, as if climbing a tree. The gait is first waddling and soon becomes completely uncontrollable. The weakened legs become deformed and cannot be kept straight. By school age, most of these boys need braces and often cannot walk on their own. Contractures and deformities of the extremities and the trunk inevitably develop, and by the age of 10 to 12 years, these boys are confined to a wheelchair. The loss of respiratory muscles is accompanied by difficulties with breathing and recurrent pneumonias. Respiratory insufficiency is the main cause of death in affected individuals. Even with the best health care, early death cannot be prevented, and it usually occurs in the late teens or early twenties.

The diagnosis of Duchenne's dystrophy is made based on typical clinical findings, the hereditary nature of the disease,

and supporting laboratory evidence. CK is released from degenerating muscle; thus CK blood levels are elevated. The deficiency of dystrophin can be demonstrated immunohistochemically in muscle biopsies. Genetic mutations of the dystrophin gene can be demonstrated by molecular biologic techniques. This test can also be performed on fetal cells obtained by chorionic villus biopsy or amniocentesis before birth.

OTHER DYSTROPHIES

Other dystrophies are less common than Duchenne's dystrophy (see Table 20-1). Note that these dystrophies are generally milder and present later in life than Duchenne's dystrophy. *Becker's dystrophy,* a mild form of Duchenne's dystrophy, is related to the same gene and protein defect. However, these two dystrophies do not occur in the same families. The symptoms of Becker's dystrophy appear later in life and are generally milder. Nevertheless, the disease has a progressive course and all patients die in their late forties or fifties.

The term **limb-girdle dystrophy** includes several genetic disorders that can be inherited as autosomal dominant or autosomal recessive traits. The mutated genes encode cell membrane proteins, such as sarcoglycans or dystroglycans, which are linked to dystrophin in the adjacent cytoplasm of muscle cells. These diseases present clinically in adulthood and are characterized by mild to moderate muscle weakness. With appropriate physical therapy most patients are not severely incapacitated and can lead a productive life.

Myotonic dystrophy is the second most common genetic muscle disease. It is caused by the expansion of the CTG trinucleotide repeat on chromosome 19 encoding a protein kinase, appropriately called dystrophia myotonica protein kinase (DMPK). The disease is inherited as an autosomal dominant trait and affects males and females at the same rate. It is not known why the deficiency of DMPK causes muscle weakness, as well as several other pathologic changes in the body. The symptoms appear in adulthood and are dominated by muscle wasting.

In contrast to other dystrophies, which show only muscle weakness, myotonic dystrophy is characterized by myotonia. Myotonic muscles can contract, but they remain contracted for some time—that is, they cannot relax immediately. For instance, when such a patient shakes hands with somebody, the hand is held tightly in position, even after the other person has withdrawn the hand. Because of weakness of the ocular muscles in these patients, the eyelids droop. Facial muscle weakness accounts for the typical "hatchet face" appearance of those affected. Myotonic dystrophy is a multisystemic disease, and the patients usually have diabetes mellitus, testicular atrophy, and frontal baldness. Premature death (usually in the fifties) is attributable either to complications of diabetes or to heart disease.

CONGENITAL MYOPATHIES

Congenital myopathies are a group of diseases that comprise a slew of rare disorders involving not only the muscles but other organs as well. Muscle weakness caused by these disturbances of intermediary metabolism appears early in life, and they are often lethal at an early age. A few examples of such metabolic genetic disorders are listed here and include the following:

- Inborn errors of lipid metabolism (e.g., carnitine deficiency)
- Inborn errors of glycogen metabolism (e.g., glycogenosis type II, so-called Pompe's disease)

- Mitochondrial myopathies (e.g., disorders of oxidative phosphorylation in mitochondria caused by mitochondrial gene mutations)
- Chennelopathies (e.g., various forms of periodic paralysis caused by an inborn error of enzymes involved in the transport of minerals across the cell membrane)

Congenital myopathies also include diseases limited to the muscles, such as nemaline myopathy or central core myopathy. Although these are rare diseases, from time to time the practitioner may see a child who cannot move and has flaccid limbs. It is important to remember that this *floppy child syndrome* may have a genetic basis. The mother must understand that the baby's disease is not related to some mishap in pregnancy and that genetic counseling may be indicated. Furthermore, such diseases must be distinguished from cerebral palsy.

Cerebral palsy is the most common form of muscle weakness in children. Pathologically it is an upper neuron disease; it is mentioned here because in its severe form it may present as floppy child syndrome. The muscular atrophy, which varies in extent, is related to developmental defects of the motor cortex in the central nervous system. The cause of cerebral changes is unknown. It seems that they are the result of prenatal brain injury rather than birth-related cerebral trauma, as previously held. The nature of the intrauterine brain injury is poorly understood. Neurogenic atrophy of muscles impairs the ability of the child to move. Many children are confined to a wheelchair and develop secondary deformities. In the worst cases they are unable to walk at all. However, many children who are born with a milder form of disease can be rehabilitated and function almost normally.

? Did You Know?

Congenital myopathies cause generalized muscle weakness. If lifted, affected infants cannot hold up their heads. Colloquially these diseases are known as *floppy infant syndrome.*

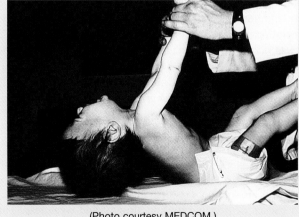

(Photo courtesy MEDCOM.)

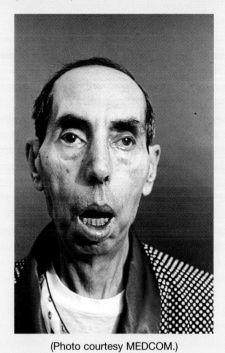
ACQUIRED MYOPATHIES

The term *acquired myopathies* is used to denote nonspecific muscle weakness secondary to some identifiable disease. The term *myopathy*—from the Greek, meaning "muscle ailment"—is in itself noncommittal. Many metabolic and hormonal diseases (e.g., diabetes or thyroid disease) and autoimmune diseases (e.g., rheumatoid arthritis) can cause muscle weakness.

The pathogenesis of acquired myopathies and their course are highly heterogeneous. In thyrotoxicosis, the high metabolic rate reduces the muscle stores of nutrients, whereas in hypothyroidism the entire metabolism, including the energy-generating metabolism of muscles, is sluggish. *Myopathia rheumatica,* a common diagnosis in persons with rheumatoid arthritis, is probably secondary to rheumatic joint disease. Muscle biopsy reveals only minor and nonspecific changes in all these diseases. Electromyography is also not diagnostic.

DIABETIC MYOPATHY

Diabetes, a disease of the small blood vessels (microangiopathy), is associated with chronic hypoperfusion of muscles with blood. Diabetes also affects the peripheral nerves and causes neurogenic muscle atrophy and weakness. The disturbances of the intermediary metabolism of carbohydrates and lipids, caused by insulin deficiency or resistance, also adversely influence muscle function. **Diabetic myopathy** has at least three causes, including a vascular, neurogenic, and metabolic component. Muscle biopsy is rarely performed because it usually contributes little to the diagnosis. Histologically the muscle may show focal atrophy. The small blood vessels have thickened walls. The nerves may show some loss of axons.

CANCER MYOPATHY

Acquired myopathy is a common paraneoplastic syndrome. Tumors may produce muscle weakness through several mechanisms. For example, antibodies to tumor antigens may incite an immune-mediated inflammation. Some tumors share common antigens with muscle and skin, and the antibodies to these antigens may cause dermatomyositis or polymyositis. Muscle weakness without any inflammation may be found in other patients. In practice, paraneoplastic myopathy is treated symptomatically with analgesics and muscle relaxants. Muscle biopsy is rarely performed in these patients, and the pathologic basis of *paraneoplastic myopathy* often remains undetermined.

MECHANICAL INJURY OF MUSCLES

Mechanical trauma may cause major injury of the skeletal muscles, the blood vessels supplying the blood to the muscles, or the nerves providing the innervation. Most often all these anatomic parts of the extremities or other body parts are injured at the same time.

Mechanical trauma may occur during car accidents but also can be related to contact sport injury (e.g., boxing, football), beating or clobbering, free fall from a high building, or compression by heavy objects. The most severe form, called **crush injury,** occurs when a person is covered with construction material during a work-related injury, by bricks in a collapsing house, or by mud and rocks in a landslide.

Mechanical impact leads to rupture of muscle fibers, causing these cells to die and release their contents into the blood. Creatine kinase is the most sensitive serologic marker of such a muscle injury, and it is invariably elevated in the blood. Other proteins released during **rhabdomyolysis** (the technical term for rupture of muscle fibers), such as myoglobin or myosin, can also be found in the blood.

The concomitant injury to the blood vessels leads to the formation of intramuscular hematomas, and the nerve injury causes paralysis. The entry of myoglobin and other proteins from the damaged muscle fibers into the circulation may promote disseminated intravascular coagulation (DIC). Myoglobin is filtered through the renal glomeruli into the urine, thus causing myoglobinuria. Myoglobin damages renal tubules, causing renal tubular necrosis and renal failure, with oliguria and finally anuria. These patients need renal dialysis, but many will actually never recover their renal function and will require renal transplantation. Unless the patient is promptly treated, the shock resulting from crush injuries is associated with high mortality. Because the skeletal muscle fibers cannot regenerate adequately, massive muscular necrosis never heals completely, resulting in deformities and loss of muscle function.

In addition to injury caused by severe mechanical trauma, muscle injury can occur even during strenuous exercise. Muscle injuries are common in weight lifters, wrestlers, cyclists, and football players. Such "pulling of muscles" usually involves rupture of muscle fibers, typically accompanied by hematoma causing local inflammation and fever. These sprained muscles usually recover with rest and physical therapy, but if the rupture is substantial, surgical intervention might be needed.

MYOSITIS

Myositis is a term used to describe inflammatory muscle diseases, which are divided into two major groups: infectious myositis and myositis caused by immune mechanisms. Inflammation usually involves more than one muscle; therefore, the disease is called **polymyositis.** The most important forms of myositis are listed in Box 20-3.

INFECTIOUS MYOSITIS

Infectious myositis may be caused by bacteria, viruses, protozoa, or worms. Isolated infectious myositis is rare except in patients with complicated wounds. Systemic diseases affect the muscles, but the symptoms of myositis are usually overshadowed by other, more serious clinical findings. Pyogenic cocci may be bloodborne and may form an abscess in the muscle. Infected emboli detached from cardiac valves in endocarditis may lodge in the muscle, also causing an *abscess.* Local extension of bacterial infection of the pharynx into the muscles of the neck causes a suppurative myositis and soft-tissue gangrene known as *Ludwig's angina.* Ludwig's angina is a very serious disease that still has a high mortality. Gas gangrene, caused by Clostridium perfringens, is an important complication of wound infections marked by necrosis of

muscles and formation of air bubbles in the tissues. Infected wounds are also a source of tetanus infection. Tetanus toxin causes spastic contractions of all muscles, even those at a distance from the site of infection. Tetanus is invariably lethal. Because there is no treatment for tetanus, it is essential that everyone be immunized against tetanus toxin early in life and receive a booster dose of vaccine every 10 to 20 years.

Viral infections are often associated with muscle pain *(myalgia).* It is not known whether myalgia is attributable to invasion of muscle cells by viruses or to inflammation in the interstitial spaces or the connective tissue. Coxsackievirus has a propensity for invading muscle cells and is the best known cause of viral myalgia. Both cardiac and skeletal muscles are affected. One can assume that the chest wall pain in patients presenting with coxsackievirus myocarditis is caused by invasion of striated muscles with the same virus.

T. spiralis is a worm that may be ingested in raw or inadequately cooked pork. The worm has a tendency to invade striated muscles and cause localized myositis (Figure 20-10).

IMMUNE MYOSITIS

Immune myositis occurs in several forms, including the following:

- *Polymyositis,* which is limited to muscles.
- *Dermatomyositis,* in which the inflammation is not limited to the muscles but may involve other organs as well. Skin changes are prominent.
- *Myositis of systemic lupus erythematosus.* This form of myositis is usually overshadowed by other, more serious symptoms of this disease, which is systemic and caused by a type III hypersensitivity reaction. The muscle disease, like the other symptoms, is caused by the deposition of immune complexes in vessel walls.
- *Sarcoidosis,* which is a systemic disease caused by a cell-mediated immunity type IV hypersensitivity reaction and characterized by granuloma formation.

BOX 20-3 Classification of Myositis*

Infectious Myositis
Pyogenic bacteria (e.g., staphylococcal sepsis)
Anaerobic bacteria (e.g., gas gangrene secondary to *Clostridium perfringens*)
Virus (e.g., coxsackievirus myopathy)
Protozoa (e.g., *Toxoplasma gondii* acquired from cats)
Worms (e.g., *Trichinella spiralis* from raw pork or game)

Immune Disorders
Polymyositis
Dermatomyositis
Systemic lupus erythematosus
Sarcoidosis

*with examples of common forms.

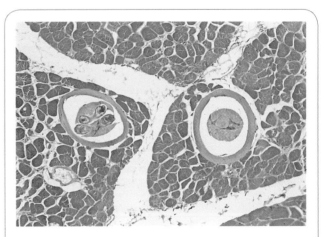

Figure 20-10 Trichinosis of the muscle. The encysted parasite is seen surrounded by normal muscle fibers.

NORMAL ANATOMY AND PHYSIOLOGY

The nervous system consists of two interrelated parts: the central nervous system (CNS), which comprises the brain and the spinal cord, and the peripheral nervous system, which includes the peripheral nerves and autonomic ganglia. The nervous system is closely interrelated to the endocrine system, with which it regulates and integrates numerous body functions. The nervous system is also closely interlinked with the skeletal muscles, the function of which depends critically on proper innervation.

The CNS consists of the brain and the spinal cord (Figure 21-1). The brain includes the cerebrum, cerebellum (the "little brain"), and brainstem, which can be further subdivided into the midbrain, pons, and medulla oblongata. The cerebrum, which represents the largest part of the brain, is organized into two hemispheres that appear morphologically identical; nevertheless, one of them is dominant over the other. The hemispheres are connected through a number of commissures, the most prominent of which is the corpus callosum.

The external surface of the brain is arranged into gyri, which are separated by invaginations called the *sulci*. On cross section, the brain forming the gyri is seen to be composed predominantly of gray matter, also known as *cortex*. The brain tissue beneath the cortex appears white and is called the *white matter*. The deep parts of the brain also contain gray areas, which form the basal ganglia, thalamus, and hypothalamus. The cortex and subcortical gray matter are composed of numerous neurons and support cells. The axons emanating from the nerve cell bodies extend into the white matter, where they become myelinated. Myelinated axons extend from the white matter into other parts of the brain and into the spinal cord.

The cerebrum has four major lobes, known as the frontal, parietal, temporal, and occipital lobes. Each of these lobes has a special function. The frontal lobe primarily controls motor functions, but it also regulates behavior, emotions, and higher intellectual functions. The parietal lobe has primarily sensory functions. The occipital lobe is the seat of the visual center. The temporal lobe has an important role in hearing and smelling. The basal ganglia supply inhibitory stimuli to skeletal muscles, coordinate skeletal muscle contractions, and block unwanted muscle contractions. The thalamus is an important center for integrating sensory stimuli and is an important determinant of consciousness. The hypothalamus serves as a crossroad that connects various parts of the brain; it also regulates many body functions. The centers for regulation of temperature, heart rate, blood pressure, thirst, appetite, and many others are located in the hypothalamus. Moreover, the hypothalamic centers are the source of the neurosecretory substances that stimulate the pituitary to produce various trophic hormones regulating the function of other endocrine glands.

The midbrain, pons, and medulla oblongata are parts of the brain that contain numerous myelinated nerve bundles connecting the brain with the spinal cord. These structures

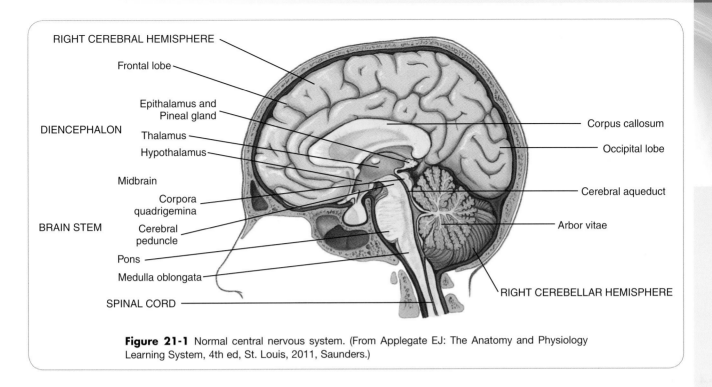

RIGHT CEREBRAL HEMISPHERE

Frontal lobe

Epithalamus and
Pineal gland

DIENCEPHALON

Thalamus

Hypothalamus

Midbrain

Corpora
quadrigemina

BRAIN STEM

Cerebral
peduncle

Pons

Medulla oblongata

SPINAL CORD

Corpus callosum

Occipital lobe

Cerebral aqueduct

Arbor vitae

RIGHT CEREBELLAR HEMISPHERE

Figure 21-1 Normal central nervous system. (From Applegate EJ: The Anatomy and Physiology Learning System, 4th ed, St. Louis, 2011, Saunders.)

also contain important centers that regulate elementary body functions. For example, the midbrain contains the visual and auditory reflex centers, whereas the medulla oblongata contains vital centers, such as the cardiac, vasomotor, and respiratory centers.

The cerebellum is the major regulator of motor activities. It controls the maintenance of balance, regulates the tone of muscles, and coordinates voluntary movement. The cerebellum receives sensory input from the spinal cord and vestibular organ of the inner ear, as well as motor impulses from the cerebral cortex. These neural signals are integrated in the cerebellum and transmitted to the skeletal muscles to coordinate their function. Damage of the cerebellum affects the coordination of limb and eye movements.

The spinal cord consists of gray matter and white matter. In contrast to the brain, the gray matter of the spinal cord is located internal to the white matter around the central canal. The gray matter has a butterfly-like shape on cross section, with anterior and posterior horns that consist of neurons and unmyelinated nerve fibers. The neurons of the anterior horn give rise to peripheral nerves, which extend to the muscles and carry motor impulses. The white matter of the spinal cord consists of myelinated nerve fibers representing the descending motor tracts or ascending sensory tracts. The motor tracts, such as the corticospinal tracts, are located in the anterior and lateral white matter. These myelinated nerves represent axonal extensions of cortical and subcortical neurons of the brain known as the *upper motor neurons.* Axons of the cerebral nerves connect with distal neurons in the anterior horn of the spinal cord called the *lower motor neurons.* The *sensory spinal tracts,* which are located predominantly in the posterior

columns, represent the axonal extension of neurons located in the spinal ganglia. Spinal ganglia are located external to the spinal cord, to which they are connected by the dorsal roots.

The peripheral nervous system consists of nerves emanating from the CNS and the autonomic nervous system. Each spinal nerve has an anterior root and a posterior root. The ventral root consists of the axons of the lower motor neuron, whereas the dorsal root is composed of spinal ganglia and their cytoplasmic extensions. The sensory and motor neurons form a circuit that is important for reflex movements.

The *autonomous nervous system* regulates involuntary (autonomic) body functions. It consists of a sympathetic and a parasympathetic part. The nerve cells of the autonomic nervous system are located in the peripheral ganglia, which may be paravertebral or located at a distance from the CNS (collateral ganglia). Like the neurons in the CNS, autonomic nerve cells have axons that innervate various internal organs. The autonomic nervous system regulates movement within the intestines, the tonus of blood vessels, urination, ejaculation, and many other automatic or reflux functions. For example, sympathetic stimulation causes vasoconstriction and hypertension, whereas parasympathetic stimuli have just the opposite effects.

The brain is enveloped by specialized connective tissue called *meninges.* The outer layer, called the *dura,* is composed of dense collagenous tissue. The middle layer, called the *arachnoid* (derived from the Greek word for spider web), is loosely structured and consists of loose connective tissue strands and blood vessels. The innermost layer, called the *pia,* is contiguous with the brain and actually represents the external surface of the brain.

The brain is separated from the arachnoid by a thin space filled with cerebrospinal fluid (CSF). CSF is produced by the choroid plexus in the third ventricles. The fluid flows (under relatively low pressure) from the lateral ventricles into the third ventricle and then into the fourth ventricle. From the fourth ventricle, the CSF may enter the central canal of the spinal cord or exit through the lateral openings (foramina of Luschka) and a median opening (foramen of Magendie) into the subarachnoid space. From the subarachnoid space, the CSF is resorbed through the arachnoid granulations of the meninges into the venous system.

The CSF serves as a cushion that protects the brain from injury. At the same time, it allows an exchange of substances between the brain and the blood. In normal adults the volume of CSF is approximately 150 mL, and it circulates at a constant rate. Children have less CSF. The circulation of CSF depends on a constant rate of production and resorption (approximately 500 mL/day).

HISTOLOGY OF THE BRAIN

The brain consists of neurons and support cells (Figure 21-2). The neurons are large, very complex cells that have highly specialized functions. Each neuron has three basic components: a cell body, also known as a *perikaryon;* one or several dendrites; and a single axon. The perikaryon contains the nucleus, which is typically surrounded by a well-developed cytoplasm full of organelles. Dendrites and axons are extensions of the cytoplasm that contain less organelles and that are specialized for the transmission of neural impulses. Axons and dendrites form the cerebral and spinal tracts and the cranial and spinal nerves.

The support cells of the CNS are called *glial cells* (neuroglia). Glial cells are classified as astrocytes, oligodendroglia, microglia, and ependymal cells. Astrocytes are star-shaped, relatively large cells with cytoplasmic processes that attach

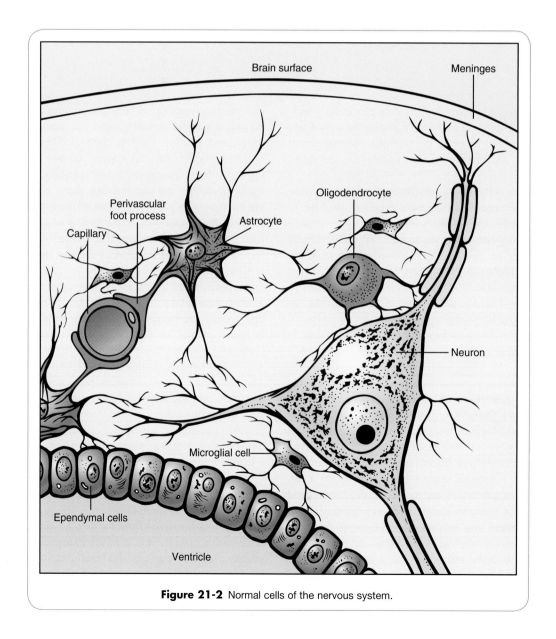

Figure 21-2 Normal cells of the nervous system.

to nerves and blood vessels. Oligodendroglial cells are small cells that form long cytoplasmic processes that wrap around the axons. Schwann cells are the peripheral nerve equivalents of oligodendroglia. They form myelin sheaths of peripheral nerves. Microglia are small cells with short cytoplasmic processes. Microglial cells are mobile and phagocytic cells that are derived from bone marrow precursors that have colonized the brain. Ependymal cells line the inside of ventricles of the brain and the central canal of the spinal cord. The cilia on the apical surface of the ependymal cells contribute to the flow of CSF.

OVERVIEW OF MAJOR DISEASES

Diseases of the nervous system are very common, and essentially all health workers must deal with them in their daily practice. The symptoms of neural diseases may be mundane, such as headache or back pain; dramatic, such as an epileptic seizure; or deep seated and unrecognized, such as depression, which may lead to suicide attempts. Common, mild neurologic diseases may be treated by family physicians, nurses, or even local pharmacists, who can often recommend a good and efficient treatment for such ailments. Long-standing headache or severe recurrent headache, known as *migraine,* may require a more detailed examination, usually performed by a neurologist. In some cases, headache is the first symptom of a brain tumor; in such instances the patient is referred to a neurosurgeon. Many headaches are psychogenic, or related to the stresses of daily life. In such cases the patient may require the assistance of a psychiatrist.

The nervous system may be affected by numerous diseases, the most important of which are the following:

- Developmental and genetic diseases
- Diseases caused by trauma
- Circulatory disorders
- Infectious diseases
- Autoimmune diseases
- Metabolic and nutritional diseases
- Neurodegenerative diseases of unknown etiology
- Brain tumors

Several facts important to an understanding of CNS pathology are presented here in summary form, before a discussion of specific pathologic entities.

1. *The nervous system consists of highly specialized functional units.* A loss of certain parts of the CNS results in typical functional defects that can be recognized on neurologic examination. The damage is typically irreversible because neurons cannot regenerate. For example, an injury of the Broca area of the frontal cortex results in a loss of speech. A loss of the visual center in the occipital lobe leads to central blindness. Lesions of the respiratory centers, which are located in the medulla oblongata, cause death.

2. *The CNS is protected from mechanical injury by the bones of the skull and vertebrae.* The skull is composed of bones that enclose the brain and shield it from external insults. The bones of the vertebrae protect the spinal cord. The joints between the bones of the skull ossify during childhood, making the entire skull a compact unit. Brain wounds occur only if the integrity of the skull is disrupted. The vertebrae, which protect the spinal cord, are linked to one another by intervertebral disks and tendons that allow them a certain degree of mobility. The spinal cord is thus more susceptible than the skull to external trauma. Any rapid body movement that is forceful enough to cause anterior, posterior, or lateral movement of the vertebrae can damage the spinal cord. If the vertebral bodies become detached from one another or severely dislocated, the spinal cord may be completely severed. This typically occurs in auto accidents.

3. *The CNS is separated from the remainder of the body by meninges and by a blood–brain barrier.* The CNS has an abundant blood supply, which ensures a constant supply of energy (i.e., oxygen and nutrients). However, the brain must remain relatively isolated from metabolic changes in the body that could adversely affect the functions of the neurons. To this end, the CNS is protected and separated from the rest of the body by the meninges and an anatomic and functional barrier known as the *blood–brain barrier.* The blood–brain barrier acts like a filter, allowing the passage of some substances from the blood into the CSF while preventing the passage of others. For example, bilirubin does not enter the CNS compartment, even in the most severe forms of jaundice. Glucose concentration in the CSF is 50 to 75 mg/dL and in general it should be less than 66% of the blood concentration. The protein concentration of normal CSF does not exceed 45 mg/dL, which is just a fraction of the concentration of proteins in serum, which is approximately 7 g/dL.

When the blood–brain barrier breaks down, the brain is affected by many substances that cross it and enter the neural tissue. The blood–brain barrier of premature infants is not fully functional and the jaundice of such infants *may be* accompanied by the passage of bilirubin into the CSF.

Jaundice in infants affected by maternal-fetal Rh incompatibility may even cause impregnation of the basal ganglia by bilirubin *(kernicterus),* which may be accompanied by irreparable brain injury.

4. *The brain and the spinal cord are surrounded by CSF.* The space between the brain and the meninges is filled with clear CSF. CSF has several functions, the most important of which are to separate the brain from the meninges and to serve as a mechanical buffer between the brain and the bones of the skull. Without the CSF, the brain would be much more vulnerable to trauma.

CSF also serves as a venue for the disposition of metabolites and waste products from the brain. Normally it has a defined biochemical composition that fluctuates very little. In patients with neurologic diseases, the CSF changes, and these changes can be detected by laboratory tests. For example, bacterial infection of the meninges **(meningitis)** is accompanied by the appearance of neutrophils in the CSF. Multiple sclerosis (MS) is associated with the appearance of gamma globulins (so-called oligoclonal bands), which are important for the diagnosis of this disease.

The rate of production, flow, and resorption of CSF remains constant under normal circumstances. Obstruction of CSF flow or blockage of CSF resorption leads to the accumulation of fluid in the brain **(hydrocephalus).** If the obstruction is at the level of the midbrain, preventing communication between the lateral ventricles and the subarachnoid space, the resulting hydrocephalus is designated as noncommunicating. In contrast, communicating hydrocephalus develops if there is an obstruction in the meninges that prevents the resorption of CSF into the venous system.

5. *Neurons, the principal cells of the CNS, are nondividing, postmitotic, permanent cells, whereas the supporting cells, such as the glial cells, are facultative, mitotic (labile) cells that are capable of dividing.* The brain contains billions of neurons, all of which are formed during prenatal, intrauterine life. Neurons are long-lived cells. Nevertheless, every hour of our lives, we lose thousands of neurons to programmed natural death. Lost neurons cannot be replaced because the remaining neurons cannot divide and the brain does not contain neuronal reserve cells. Because neural tissue cannot regenerate, every loss of brain substance results in permanent defects.

In contrast to neurons, the glial cells retain a capacity for multiplication and are capable of multiplying in response to certain forms of injury. *Gliosis* (i.e., an increased number of glial cells) is a typical sign of brain injury. Gliosis is found around tumors, brain infarcts, and foci of intracerebral hemorrhages.

The dichotomy between the neurons and glia is important for understanding the histogenesis of brain tumors. Because the adult neurons are incapable of dividing, these cells never give rise to tumors. The malignant tumors of neural cell origin are found only in children, in whom they presumably originate from undifferentiated precursors of neural cells, such as neuroblasts. The primary tumors of the brain in adults are derived from glial cells and are classified as **gliomas.** Other support structures of the brain, such as the meninges and the blood vessels, also contain cells that are capable of proliferation and malignant transformation. These tumors are known as *meningiomas* or *hemangioblastomas.*

6. *The CNS may be affected by diseases that involve other organs, as well as by diseases that are unique to the CNS.* The CNS is affected by many multisystemic diseases, especially those classified as circulatory, metabolic, or infectious. For example, atherosclerosis of the coronary arteries and aorta is often accompanied by **cerebrovascular accidents** (CVAs). End-stage kidney disease *(uremia)* or liver disease (cirrhosis) may be accompanied by metabolic disturbances that typically cause numerous neurologic symptoms. Uremia typically terminates in progressive somnolence and coma. Hepatic encephalopathy is characterized by mental confusion, flaplike movements of the hands *(asterixis),* and coma. Systemic infections caused by various bacteria or viruses may spread to the brain, usually by a hematogenous route.

Diseases restricted to the brain may be caused by neurotropic pathogens, or they may be a consequence of metabolic changes unique to neural cells. For example, neurotropic viruses, such as rabies, infect only nerve cells. *Prions*—minute infectious particles composed only of proteins, which are smaller than viruses—survive only in nerve cells and are therefore selectively harmful to the CNS. Prions cause spongiform degeneration of the brain that is typical of such diseases as kuru and **Creutzfeldt-Jakob disease.** Neurodegenerative diseases, such as Alzheimer's disease or Parkinson's disease, are characterized by neuronal degeneration and loss of neurons. The etiology and pathogenesis of these neurodegenerative diseases are unknown.

7. *The symptoms of CNS diseases result from dysfunction of or loss of function of neurons.* Overall, symptoms of diseases of the CNS can be local, such as the headaches that accompany brain tumors, or systemic, such as the generalized paralysis and coma that follow massive intracerebral bleeding.

Local symptoms of intracranial lesions result from direct compression of a nerve center by a mass (e.g., a tumor) or increased intracranial pressure caused by mass effect or cerebral edema. Intracranial tumors and all inflammations of the brain and meninges cause brain edema. Brain edema also develops in shock and in many metabolic diseases, as well as in cases of drug overdose and poisoning.

Increased intracranial pressure is a life-threatening condition. The symptoms depend on the pace at which it develops. A sudden, explosive increase in intracranial pressure, such as that caused by a bullet wound to the head, will cause death instantaneously. By contrast, a rapid but gradual increase of intracranial pressure will present as a severe headache that is usually accompanied by vomiting, blurry vision, and loss of consciousness. Such patients lapse into coma and usually die of apnea (absence of breathing) or develop pulmonary edema secondary to inhibition of the medullary vital centers. Patients with chronic elevation of intracranial pressure—for example, those with brain tumors—generally present with headaches, personality changes, intellectual decline, or emotional lability. As the pressure gradually increases, symptoms of acute intracranial hypertension supersede the nonspecific chronic symptoms.

Death caused by increased intracranial pressure usually results from the compression of vital centers in the brainstem. Most often, the centers of the medulla oblongata are compressed by the edematous tonsils of the cerebellum, which herniates through the foramen magnum (Figure 21-3). Herniation of the medial portion of the cerebral hemisphere beneath the tentorium cerebelli (uncal or transtentorial herniation) may compress the pons and can also cause death. Other forms of **herniation of the brain,** such as herniation of the cingulate gyrus of the cerebral hemisphere beneath the falx cerebri or herniation through an opening of a broken skull, are less important.

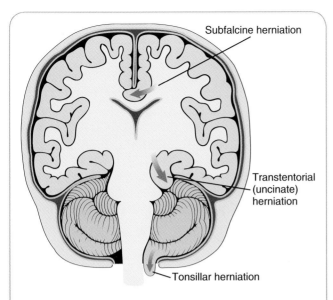

Figure 21-3 Herniations of the brain. Subfalcine herniation involves the cingulate gyrus protruding beneath the falx cerebri. Transtentorial (uncinate) herniation involves the uncus protruding below the tentorium cerebelli. Tonsillar herniation involves the cerebellar tonsils protruding into the foramen magnum.

Symptoms of CNS dysfunction may result from a loss of neurons (e.g., the loss of memory that accompanies Alzheimer's disease), from abnormal function of neurons (e.g., the rigidity of muscles in Parkinson's disease), or from abnormal excitation of neurons (such as that which can be recorded by electroencephalography [EEG] during the convulsions typical of epilepsy). Many psychiatric diseases, such as schizophrenia or bipolar psychosis, are caused by abnormal function of brain cells, but the nature of these neural cell dysfunctions remains unknown. The underlying defect of psychiatric diseases has not been defined in pathologic terms.

DEVELOPMENTAL DISORDERS

The cause of most developmental disorders is unknown. Among the identifiable well-known causes of developmental disorders, the most important are the following:
- Genetic diseases
- Chromosomal abnormalities
- Intrauterine infections

These conditions are mentioned here for the sake of completeness but are discussed in greater detail in Chapter 5.

ANENCEPHALY AND DYSRAPHIC DISORDERS

The CNS develops from the neural plate, which folds and ultimately closes into a neural tube extending along the dorsal side of the body axis (Figure 21-4). As the neural tube forms, it becomes internalized and is protected by the overlying skin.

The mesenchyme between the neural tube and the skin is induced to form bone, which gives rise to the skull and the vertebral bodies. Each of these bones originates from separate and often multiple ossification centers. The products of ossification centers must fuse to provide a continuous external envelope to the CNS.

Incomplete fusion of the neural tube gives rise to **dysraphic disorders** (derived from the Greek word *raphe,* meaning "suture"). Dysraphic malformations occur in several forms (see Figure 21-4). If the calvaria are not formed and the unprotected brain is destroyed *in utero,* the malformation is called **anencephaly** (see Figure 5-24). Milder dysraphic malformations, such as meningocele, myelomeningocele, and spina bifida, are characterized by a lack of fusion of the posterior bone coverings. If the meninges protrude through the bony defect, the malformation is called *meningocele.* In myelomeningocele, the protrusion contains not only the meninges but also a portion of the spinal cord. Spina bifida is characterized by an absence of vertebral arches, resulting in exposure of the meninges or the spinal cord to the outer world. Spina bifida may be evident at birth as a deep defect on the lower back, or it may be covered with skin and be inapparent *(spina bifida occulta).*

Anencephaly is incompatible with life. Spinal dysraphic malformations are typically associated with major neurologic deficits, such as paralysis. Although spina bifida cannot be repaired entirely and the neurologic defects are permanent, these children may be rehabilitated to a certain degree by physical therapy. *Folic acid* taken during pregnancy can reduce the occurrence of anencephaly and other dysraphic malformations.

INTRACRANIAL HEMORRHAGES

Intracranial hemorrhages can be classified into four groups, according to their location: epidural, subdural, subarachnoid, and intracerebral (Figure 21-5). These hemorrhages may be caused by trauma (as may occur in boxers) or brain contusions from a vehicular accident; rupture of blood vessels that are congenitally abnormal (as in aneurysms) or that are damaged by hypertension; or abnormalities of coagulation, as occurs in various congenital and acquired bleeding disorders.

EPIDURAL HEMATOMAS

Epidural hematomas are typically located between the skull and the dura in a space that under normal circumstances is almost nonexistent because of the close apposition of the dura to the skull bones. Epidural hematoma develops from a ruptured middle meningeal artery most often torn by a bone spicule resulting from a fracture of temporal bone. Because arterial blood fills the space, slowly separating the dura from the bone, it usually takes several hours before a large hematoma is formed. Once the hematoma reaches a volume of 50 to 60 mL, it is large enough to compress the brain and cause coma. In children, in whom the skull bones are not as firmly fixated as in adults, arterial rupture can occur because of traumatic bone

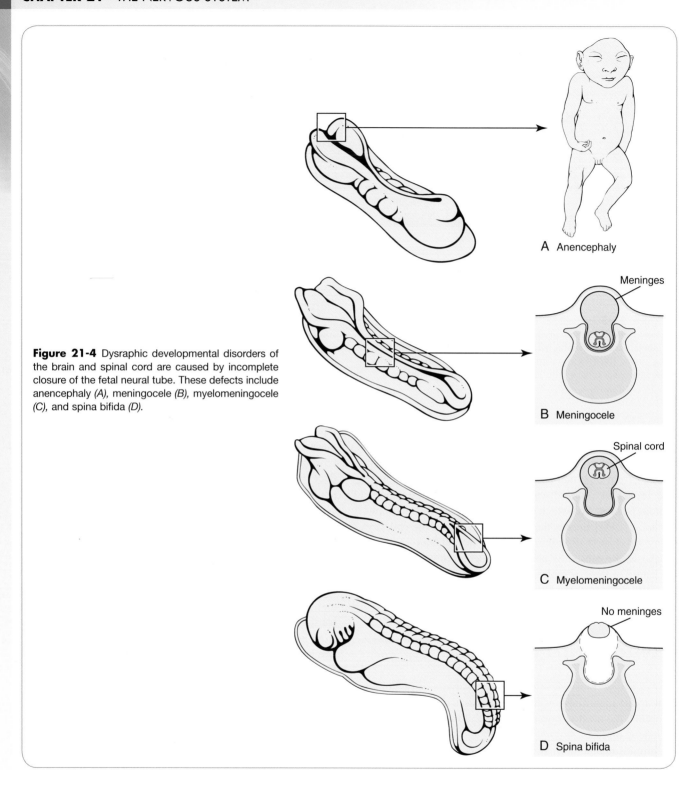

Figure 21-4 Dysraphic developmental disorders of the brain and spinal cord are caused by incomplete closure of the fetal neural tube. These defects include anencephaly *(A)*, meningocele *(B)*, myelomeningocele *(C)*, and spina bifida *(D)*.

A Anencephaly

Meninges

B Meningocele

Spinal cord

C Myelomeningocele

No meninges

D Spina bifida

displacement, even without fracture. If unrecognized, epidural hematoma is invariably lethal.

SUBDURAL HEMATOMAS

Subdural hematomas occupy the space between the dura and the arachnoid. Normally this space is bridged by thin-walled veins that can be easily torn by trauma, especially the

type of blunt trauma that causes sudden movement of the brain in one direction and the dura in another. Subdural hematomas are typically found in boxers or in unattended, bedridden elderly patients who have fallen out of bed. Repeated trauma has a cumulative effect. It is thought that the sudden movement of the brain in one direction, if unaccompanied by a similar movement of the dura, has a tearing effect on the bridging veins and can rupture them. The coagulated blood

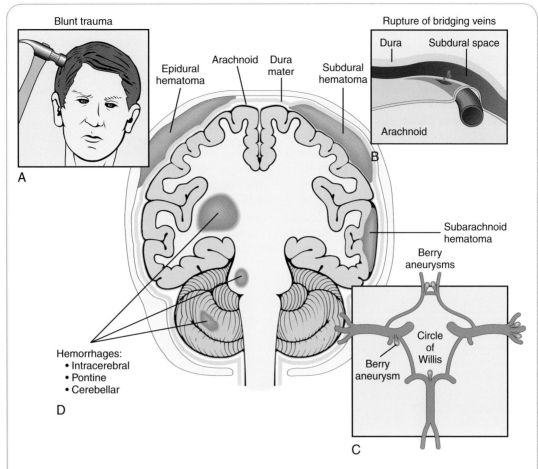

Figure 21-5 Intracranial hemorrhages. *A,* Epidural hemorrhage is caused by trauma and rupture of the middle meningeal artery. *B,* Subdural hemorrhage is caused by traumatic rupture of bridging veins. *C,* Subarachnoid hemorrhage is typical of ruptured berry aneurysm of the circle of Willis at the base of the brain. *D,* Intracerebral hemorrhage is a complication of hypertension. The most common sites of hypertensive hemorrhages are the basal ganglia, pons, and cerebellum.

typically covers the lateral hemispheres like a cap. The symptoms are initially nonspecific (e.g., headache), but as the hematoma enlarges, it may produce significant neurologic symptoms, a loss of consciousness, and even death.

SUBARACHNOID HEMORRHAGES

Subarachnoid hemorrhages are located in the space between the arachnoid and the pia (i.e., the brain surface). Most often, subarachnoid hemorrhages are caused by traumatic contusion of the brain, in which case the blood leaks into the subarachnoid space from the ruptured cerebral blood vessels at the base of the brain.

Ruptured **aneurysms of the circle of Willis** are another important cause of subarachnoid hemorrhages. These congenital saccular aneurysms, also called *berry aneurysms* because of their small size and shape, are found in 1% to 2% of the general population, although most are clinically silent. Rupture, which usually occurs between 30 and 60 years of age, can be precipitated by hypertension but

often occurs spontaneously, without any obvious cause. Bleeding into the subarachnoid space is associated with high mortality. If recognized, berry aneurysms can be treated surgically, usually by placing clips at the site of their origin, thereby preventing the entry of blood into the lumen of the aneurysm.

INTRACEREBRAL HEMORRHAGE

Intracerebral hemorrhage is a common complication of head trauma, regardless of the nature of the trauma. Blunt trauma caused by a club or open trauma, such as that caused by a metal object (e.g., a hammer), may cause contusion of the brain and bleeding from the ruptured intracerebral vessels. Gunshot wounds are also accompanied by intracerebral hemorrhage.

Among the nontraumatic forms of intracerebral hemorrhages, the most important are various forms of stroke. Intracerebral hemorrhage is also common in leukemia and other hematologic diseases associated with abnormal coagulation.

CEREBROVASCULAR DISEASES

Cerebrovascular disease (CVD) is the third most common cause of death and the most common crippling disease in the United States. The most important clinical manifestation of CVD is **stroke,** also known as *brain attack* to indicate that it represents a medical emergency similar to a heart attack. Strokes can be divided into two categories: *ischemic* (85%), related to atherosclerosis of the cerebral arteries or thromboembolic occlusion of cerebral arteries, and hemorrhagic (15%), which is most often a complication of arterial hypertension.

Atherosclerosis of the cerebral vessels has the same morphologic features as atherosclerosis in other sites. The lesions may involve the major blood arteries or their intracerebral branches (Figure 21-6). Narrowing of the arteries may be gradual, as a result of progressive atherosclerotic fibrosis and calcification, or it may occur suddenly, as when an atherosclerotic plaque ruptures, provoking intravascular thrombosis and complete occlusion of the arterial lumen. Depending on the type of vascular lesions, CVD causes either widespread or localized lesions.

GLOBAL ISCHEMIA

Patients who have widespread atherosclerotic narrowing of the entire cerebrovascular system develop multiple foci of ischemic necrosis. Such lacunar infarcts cause minor neurologic deficits but, over time, result in slowly progressive mental deterioration *(multi-infarct dementia).*

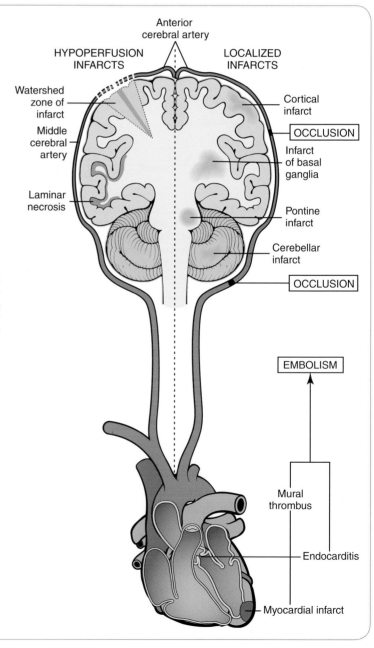

Figure 21-6 Cerebral infarcts. Localized infarcts are caused by an occlusion of the internal or basilar artery or their major branches. Diffuse infarcts, caused by hypoperfusion of the brain, occur in watershed areas and in the form of laminar necrosis in the innermost layers of the cortex. Occlusion may be caused by thrombosis or emboli.

Cardiac failure or any other form of vascular collapse (e.g., hypotensive shock secondary to hemorrhage into the intestines of patients whose cerebral blood flow is marginal) results in widespread infarcts. Such hypoperfusion infarcts are typically located in the parasagittal cortex, in the areas representing the marginal zones of arterial supply by the branches of the carotid artery on one side and the basilar artery on the other. Systemic hypotension lowers the perfusion from both sides, and the area in the border zone becomes hypoxic, resulting in so-called **watershed infarcts.** Hypoperfusion also leads to laminar necrosis of the deeper zones of the gray matter. These zones receive blood from the short penetrator arteries entering the cortex from the surface. Because of hypotension, the blood entering the cortex does not reach the deep cortex, and necrosis ensues. If heart function is restored, patients recover with only minor neurologic deficits. Nevertheless, these minor CVAs have a cumulative effect and ultimately cause mental deterioration.

CEREBRAL INFARCT

An infarct or ischemic necrosis of a distinct anatomic part of the brain caused by CVD clinically presents as a stroke. **Cerebral infarcts** are most often caused by thrombotic occlusion of an atherosclerotic artery. Thromboemboli originating in the heart chambers (e.g., after a myocardial infarction) or on the cardiac valves (e.g., resulting from endocarditis) are the second most common causes. Other diseases, such as arteritis, are rarely associated with stroke.

The pathologic changes in the brain vary depending on the time that has elapsed since the onset of occlusion. Ischemic brain liquefies, and the ischemic area undergoes necrosis, transforming into a puttylike mush. This focus of **encephalomalacia** ("softening of the brain") may remain pale (pale or bland infarct), or it may be perfused with blood from the collateral circulation and transform into a hemorrhagic infarct. White matter infarcts usually remain pale, whereas those in the gray matter tend to transform into red infarcts. Red infarcts are common after cerebral embolization with arterial thromboemboli because such infarcts are more readily perfused by arterial blood from adjacent, unoccluded blood vessels.

The brain tissue surrounding the infarcts, regardless of their color, is edematous. During this phase of maximal cerebral swelling, patients experience the most profound neurologic deficits and are at the greatest risk of dying. Within a few days after infarction, the cerebral edema subsides, and the condition of patients surviving this critical period improves in most instances. The margins of the viable tissue surrounding the infarct become vascularized. The necrotic material is removed from the infarct by scavenger cells that invade the area from the newly formed blood vessels. Ultimately the infarct transforms into a fluid-filled cavity *(pseudocyst)*. Brain infarcts cannot heal, and the neurologic deficits caused by them are permanent.

The clinical presentation of cerebral infarction depends on the site of arterial occlusion. For example, occlusion of the middle cerebral artery, which is the most common cause of cerebral infarction, results in contralateral *hemiplegia* (loss of the capacity to move the extremities), sensory loss on the same side of the body, and bilateral symmetric loss of vision in half the visual fields, with the eyes deviating to the side of the lesion. *Global aphasia* (an inability to speak or write) develops if the infarct occurs in the dominant hemisphere.

After a stroke, the treatment of unconscious patients includes intensive life-supporting measures. Brain edema, which is the most important life-threatening feature of an acute stroke, must be treated vigorously with corticosteroids and dehydrating hyperosmolar agents that drain the water fluid from the brain tissue into the circulation.

Physical therapy is important in the long-term rehabilitation of these patients, and occupational therapy may improve their general well-being and quality of life. Approximately 80% of patients survive the initial stroke, and 60% are alive 3 years thereafter. Patients recovering from stroke have a 25% chance of another stroke.

INTRACEREBRAL HEMORRHAGE

In patients who have no vascular anomalies, such as aneurysms, arteriovenous malformations, or hemangiomas, intracerebral hemorrhage or apoplexy is most often caused by arterial hypertension. Hemorrhage results from the rupture of small blood vessels that have been damaged mechanically by hypertension. The most common sites of hemorrhage are the basal ganglia, which are affected in about two thirds of cases. Cerebellar and pontine hemorrhage account for most of the remaining cases, whereas other sites are rarely involved. With recent improvements in the treatment of hypertension, intracerebral hemorrhages have become less common.

Intracerebral hemorrhage typically results in a well-circumscribed hematoma (Figure 21-7) that is clearly visible on CT scans of the brain. Like infarcts, such hematomas are surrounded by edematous brain tissue. Cerebral edema subsides in patients who survive the apoplexy, with resorption of the extravasated blood and the destruction of necrotic tissue by the hemorrhage. Ultimately the infarct transforms into a pseudocyst, which usually contains yellow fluid. The wall of the pseudocyst typically contains hemosiderin-laden macrophages.

The clinical features of intracerebral hemorrhage may resemble those of cerebral infarction. However, in most cases the clinical picture is more dramatic, with about 30% of patients

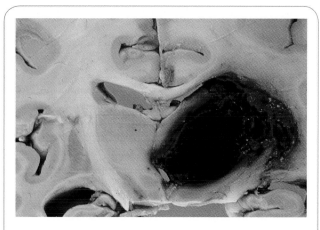

Figure 21-7 Hypertensive hemorrhage.

losing consciousness and appearing stricken. Other patients may complain of severe headache or may experience an urge to vomit. Hemorrhage into the basal ganglia is accompanied by a rapid onset of hemiplegia and hemiparesis, which are fully developed in most patients admitted to the hospital. Cerebellar hemorrhage typically presents with nausea and vomiting, loss of balance, and severe headache. Patients rapidly lapse into coma, and most die within 48 hours. Pontine hemorrhages are almost invariably lethal, with most patients dying within hours of the onset of the first, usually nonspecific, symptoms.

Treatment of patients with hypertensive hemorrhages includes supportive measures. Recovery depends on the site and extent of the brain lesion.

TRAUMA

Injuries of the head, neck, and spinal cord are major causes of disability and mortality worldwide. In the United States, head injuries occur at an estimated yearly rate of 200 per 100,000, neck injuries at a rate of 5 per 100,000, and spinal cord injuries at a rate of 3 per 100,000.

BRAIN INJURY

Brain injuries vary in severity and are classified as concussion, contusion, or laceration. In addition, head trauma is often accompanied by hematomas, as discussed earlier in this chapter.

Brain **concussion** presents as a transient loss of consciousness, usually after blunt head trauma. Loss of consciousness is based on functional disturbances affecting the temporal lobes and the reticular activating system of the brainstem. There are no significant macroscopic or microscopic changes in the brain.

Brain **contusion** (bruise) is characterized by a disruption of cerebral or meningeal blood vessels by severe blunt trauma. The lesions are hemorrhagic and are typically located at the site of impact *(coup lesion)* and its diametrically

opposite pole *(countercoup lesion)* (Figure 21-8). A coup lesion is caused by direct force, whereas a countercoup lesion is a result of the deceleration of the moving brain caused by the skull bones that serve as shock absorbers. Rotation of the head on impact causes even more damage. Contusions of the brain are serious injuries associated with considerable mortality. Survivors may have severe neurologic deficits, some of which may be permanent.

Laceration of the brain is typically caused by open trauma that disrupts the integrity of the brain. Gunshot wounds also produce laceration of the brain tissue. Such wounds have high mortality. Death is related to acute expansion of the intracranial volume and the consequent compression of the vital centers in the brainstem. Patients who survive gunshot wounds of the brain usually have major neurologic deficits, and some of them may develop epilepsy (seizures).

NECK AND SPINAL CORD INJURIES

Spinal cord injuries may occur anywhere along the spinal cord. The mobility of the neck accounts for the greatest vulnerability of the cervical spine, which is especially susceptible to injury during traffic accidents. *"Backlash injury"* of the neck is the most common. However, none of the segments of the spinal cord is immune to injury.

Injuries of the cervical spine have traditionally been classified as either hyperextension or hyperflexion injuries. In **hyperextension injury,** an impact on the forehead causes hyperextension and rupture of the anterior spinal ligaments,

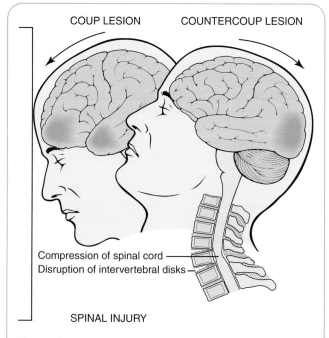

Figure 21-8 Spinal cord trauma. A coup lesion of the brain occurs at the site of impact, whereas a countercoup lesion is diametrically opposite to the coup lesion. The spinal cord lesion depicted here is caused by hyperextension.

with subsequent compression of the posterior side of the spinal cord. In **hyperflexion injury,** the impact on the occiput causes extensive anterior flexion of the spinal cord and compression of the anterior portion of the spinal cord. Both hyperextension and hyperflexion injuries may cause complete transection of the spinal cord, resulting in a loss of both motor and sensory functions below the site of injury. Typically, the injured person experiences flaccid paralysis accompanied by a loss of sensation below the site of injury. Urination and defecation reflexes are also lost. With time, the reflex functions return and the paraplegia or quadriplegia becomes spastic. The reflexes governing the bladder and bowel functions may also be partially restored.

INFECTIONS

Infections of the CNS are common. Any infectious pathogen can cause CNS disease, although in clinical practice, bacterial, viral, protozoal, and fungal infections are the primary culprits.

Etiology and Pathogenesis

Infections of the CNS can be acquired through several routes: by direct extension, hematogenously, or via the nerves.

Bacterial infections of the brain typically develop hematogenously during sepsis and bacteremia or from septic emboli (Figure 21-9), as in infectious endocarditis. Open wounds of the brain are usually infected by bacteria that have gained direct entrance into the brain parenchyma. Bacterial infections of the paranasal sinuses or the middle ear also may spread into the cranium and cause CNS infection.

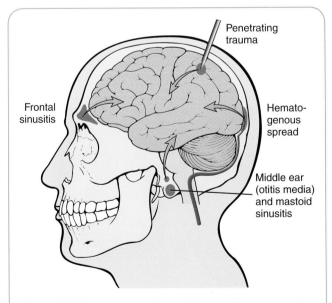

Figure 21-9 Bacterial infections of the central nervous system. Infectious organisms may reach the brain through several routes: hematogenously, by direct entry secondary to penetrating trauma, or by direct spread from adjacent structures such as the inner ear or the nasal sinuses.

Streptococcus pneumoniae accounts for most cases of bacterial meningitis in adults. Group B streptococci, which often colonize the female genital tract, can infect babies during birth and are the most important cause of bacterial meningitis in neonates. In that age group, meningitis also can be caused by *Escherichia coli* and *Listeria monocytogenes*. The most important bacterial pathogens in older infants, children, and adolescents are *Neisseria meningitidis* (meningococcus) and *S. pneumoniae*. Previously, meningococcal infections tended to present as mini-epidemics occurring in closely related clusters, such as military recruits living in common barracks. Modern immunization has reduced such outbreaks. Tuberculosis of the brain was important in the past but is rare today. Neurosyphilis is a feature of tertiary syphilis, an infection with the sexually transmitted spirochete *Treponema pallidum*.

Viral infections are usually spread to the brain by a hematogenous route. Viral pathogens include common childhood viruses, such as the measles virus, rubella, or adenovirus. The ubiquitous viruses, such as herpesvirus or cytomegalovirus, may infect the brain of children or adults and cause either meningitis or encephalitis. Neurotropic viruses (i.e., viruses that exclusively infect neural tissue), which are known for their geographic provenance (e.g., St. Louis encephalitis), are transmitted by insects, such as mosquitoes and ticks. These viruses often cause seasonal epidemics.

? Did You Know?

Even before prions, the causative agents of spongiform encephalopathies (e.g., Creutzfeldt-Jakob disease), were discovered, it was known that the brain tissue of patients affected with this form of dementia was infectious. This was best documented for kuru, a prion-induced disease affecting the natives of New Guinea. The aborigines of that area were cannibals who ate the brains of other people. The disease was transmitted by the infected brain tissue. At highest risk were the women and children who ate human brain as a delicacy.

Herpesvirus is the most common viral cause of localized encephalitis in the United States. *Japanese B encephalitis,* caused by an arthropod-borne virus, is the most common neurotropic virus associated with epidemic forms of encephalitis. *West Nile virus,* a mosquito bite–related viral infection that has become quite common in the United States, is associated with encephalitis in about 10% to 20% of cases. In elderly persons or in those otherwise sick and debilitated, this infection may be lethal.

Among the neurotropic viruses, rabies virus should also be mentioned. The rabies virus usually enters the human body through wounds inflicted by rabid dogs, foxes, or various other animals, such as raccoons and bats. In contrast to other viruses, the rabies virus reaches the CNS by traveling along the peripheral nerves from the site of inoculation through the spinal cord and specific neural pathways. Intracytoplasmic viral inclusions, or so-called Negri bodies, are found most prominently in the neurons of the brainstem. Symptoms typically appear 1 to 3 months after infection.

Prions are small infectious particles composed of protein. Previously classified as "slow viruses," prions seem to be distinct from viruses in that they do not contain DNA or RNA. Prions infect the nervous system selectively and are transmitted by direct exposure to infected material. For example, Creutzfeldt-Jakob disease has been transmitted by corneal transplants. Even human brains that are removed at autopsy are infectious.

Protozoal infections of the CNS are usually acquired hematogenously. The most important protozoal pathogen is *Toxoplasma gondii,* an important cause of encephalitis in neonates. Toxoplasmosis is also an important infection in patients with acquired immunodeficiency syndrome (AIDS). Clinical symptoms of toxoplasmosis evolve over a period of 1 to 2 weeks and may be both focal and diffuse. Brain lesions may be seen by computed tomography as ring-enhancing lesions resembling those caused by lymphoma or fungal infections.

Fungal infections reach the brain hematogenously. Fungal encephalitis or meningitis is usually found in immunosuppressed patients and is especially common in those with AIDS. The most important pathogens are *Candida albicans, Aspergillus flavus,* and *Cryptococcus neoformans.*

Pathology

Infections of the CNS may involve the brain and the spinal cord or the meninges. Such infections may present in several pathologic forms.

ENCEPHALITIS

Encephalitis presents as localized or diffuse inflammation of the brain parenchyma. Typically, it is caused by viruses that invade neural or glial cells. Herpes simplex encephalitis usually affects the temporal lobe, causing foci of necrosis and hemorrhage. Viral particles can be recognized in the nuclei of infected cells. Epidemic, arthropod-borne viral encephalitides usually present with widespread lymphocytic infiltrates that typically fill the perivascular Virchow-Robin spaces (Figure 21-10).

MYELITIS

Myelitis is a diffuse infection of the spinal cord. Like encephalitis, it is usually caused by viruses. Poliomyelitis, a viral infection most prominently affecting the anterior horns of the spinal cord, was previously a major crippling disease, but it has been eradicated by immunization.

CEREBRAL ABSCESS

A **cerebral abscess** is a localized suppurative infection of the brain. It presents as a mass lesion and may be mistaken for a tumor. The abscess consists of a cavity filled with pus and a capsule composed of glial cells and fibroblasts. Most abscesses are caused by pyogenic bacteria, but in immunosuppressed patients, some abscesses may be of fungal origin or may contain mixed flora.

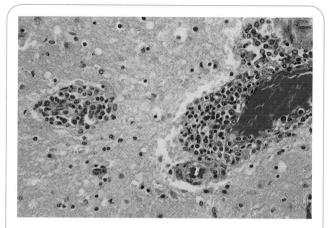

Figure 21-10 Viral encephalitis. The perivascular spaces contain prominent infiltrates of lymphocytes.

MENINGITIS

Meningitis is an inflammation of the meninges. Viral meningitis, probably the most common and the most underdiagnosed infectious disease of the CNS, occurs in many viral diseases, such as the common flu. It is characterized by a lymphocytic exudate in the subarachnoid space. Viral encephalitis may also extend into the meninges. In such cases, CSF analysis reveals lymphocytosis. Bacterial meningitis caused by pyogenic bacteria, such as *S. pneumoniae* or *N. meningitidis,* is characterized by an exudation of neutrophils. In severe cases the entire surface of the brain is covered with pus that fills the subarachnoid spaces (Figure 21-11). The CSF typically contains numerous neutrophils, a finding that is important in establishing the diagnosis.

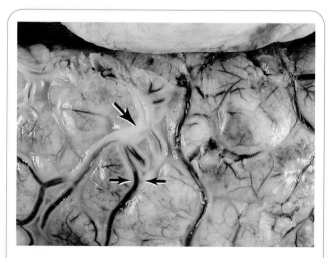

Figure 21-11 Bacterial meningitis. The surface of the brain is covered with pus *(arrows).* (From Damjanov I, Linder J: Pathology: A Color Atlas, St. Louis, 2000, Mosby.)

NEUROSYPHILIS

Neurosyphilis usually presents as chronic meningitis. The meninges are infiltrated with lymphocytes and plasma cells, which are typically centered on small blood vessels. In the healing stages of syphilitic infection, meningeal fibrosis predominates. Fibrosis of the spinal meninges may compress the dorsal roots, resulting in atrophy of afferent, sensory axons entering the spinal cord. This causes the best-known complication of neurosyphilis: *tabes dorsalis.* Tabes dorsalis is pathologically recognized on cross sections of the spinal cord by the atrophy of the dorsal (sensory) columns. Syphilitic perivascular inflammation of the brain impairs the blood flow, causing ischemic necrosis of the cortical centers. The loss of neurons correlates clinically with motor and mental deterioration, collectively known as the *syphilitic general paresis of the insane.*

AIDS-RELATED INFECTIONS

Various pathologic forms of AIDS-related CNS lesions are sometimes combined and found in the same patient. This is best illustrated by the so-called **AIDS-related encephalopathy,** a rather common finding in terminally ill patients infected with the human immunodeficiency virus (HIV). HIV infects macrophages and T lymphocytes, and these cells "import" the virus into the CNS. The infected "newcomers" secrete various cytokines, some of which appear to be toxic to brain cells. AIDS dementia seems to be a consequence of these adverse influences. In addition, the HIV-infected brain is less resistant to invasion by a variety of bacterial, viral, parasitic, and fungal pathogens that rarely enter the normal brain. Among these pathogens, the most prominent are Toxoplasma and Cryptococcus. Meningitis, encephalitis, or brain abscesses may develop. Most of these infections are resistant to treatment, and many patients die of CNS infection.

Did You Know?

Many famous personalities of the past died of neurosyphilis. Because neurosyphilis causes both neurologic and psychiatric symptoms, many of these individuals were confined to asylums for the insane before they died. The blood-thirsty Russian czar Ivan the Terrible was thought to have gone mad from syphilis.

AUTOIMMUNE DISEASES

Autoimmune diseases of the CNS are poorly understood. Although it has been known for some time that such diseases exist, and despite the fact that there are several good animal models for studying such diseases, neuroimmunology is still a rather obscure field. An immune form of encephalitis has been described in patients immunized against various infectious diseases. Some late forms of postinfectious encephalitis may represent an immune disease. However, the most important of all immunologic disorders is multiple sclerosis.

MULTIPLE SCLEROSIS

Multiple sclerosis (MS) is a demyelinating disease that is presumed to be of autoimmune origin. It is the most common immunologic CNS disease, affecting approximately 250,000 Americans, most of whom are 20 to 45 years of age. It has a prevalence of 1 in 1000 and is thus the leading neurologic disease in young adults. Women are affected twice as often as men. Symptoms may appear at any age but rarely occur before puberty or after the age of 50 years.

Etiology and Pathogenesis

The cause of MS is unknown. However, the search for possible causes has revealed many interesting epidemiologic, genetic, and immunologic facts. One day these leads may help us better understand the disease, uncover its etiology, and find a cure.

Epidemiologic data indicate that MS occurs more often in whites of Western and Northern European origin who live in temperate climate zones above the 40th parallel than in people living in the tropics. However, if persons at risk live for the first 15 years of life in a moderate climate and move to the tropics, they have the same high risk that they would have in their original climate.

Genetic studies have shown that MS affects certain families more often than others. The first-degree relatives of an affected person have a 15 times higher risk of developing the disease than the general population living under the same conditions. If one monozygotic twin develops symptoms, the second twin will also become ill in 25% of cases. Genetic linkage studies have disclosed a high prevalence of certain human major histocompatibility antigens among the affected individuals, further supporting the theory of genetic predisposition.

Immunologic studies have shown that MS resembles experimental allergic encephalomyelitis (EAE), which can be induced in animals by immunizing them with CNS myelin. T-helper and T-suppressor lymphocytes and macrophages have been demonstrated in early lesions in the human brain. T cells in the MS lesions belong to a few clones that have been immunized to some local antigen in the brain. In contrast to such oligoclonal T-cell populations in the brain, the peripheral T lymphocytes in the blood do not show any evidence of clonal expansion. This has led scientists to conclude that the T cells attracted to the brain play an important pathogenetic role and that most likely these cells have been sensitized to some component of myelin. The nature of this hypothetical antigen has not been elucidated. It is also not known whether the macrophages in the brain lesion are only secondary bystanders whose function is to remove the debris from damaged cells or whether the macrophages are essential for the initial presentation of antigen to the T cells. In addition, the role of B lymphocytes and plasma cells is enigmatic. These antibody-producing cells and their precursors are usually found around the cerebral blood vessels near the lesion. Immunoglobulin G (IgG), secreted by these cells, is found in the CSF. By immunoelectrophoresis, it may be shown that the

463

IgG in the CSF is composed of oligoclonal bands, suggesting that the B cells in the brain also represent selected clones responding to some unidentified antigen. Although the significance of all these immunologic findings remains uncertain, oligoclonal IgG bands in the CSF are useful in the diagnosis of MS.

Pathology

MS is a demyelinating disease that typically involves the white matter. Demyelination of the axons leads to the formation of typical plaques (Figure 21-12) that are usually found in the white matter of the brain, optic nerves, or spinal cord. Periventricular plaques in the lateral hemispheres of the brain are typical. Histologically, the early lesions are infiltrated with lymphocytes and macrophages. The older lesions consist of demyelinated axons surrounded by reactive astrocytes. Oligodendroglial cells—the cells responsible for the myelination of axons—are remarkably absent, because they were most likely destroyed in the acute stages of the disease.

Clinical Features

MS is a chronic disease characterized by episodes of exacerbation and remission of neurologic symptoms. Symptoms include both sensory and motor abnormalities. Among the sensory defects, the most common is loss of sensation of

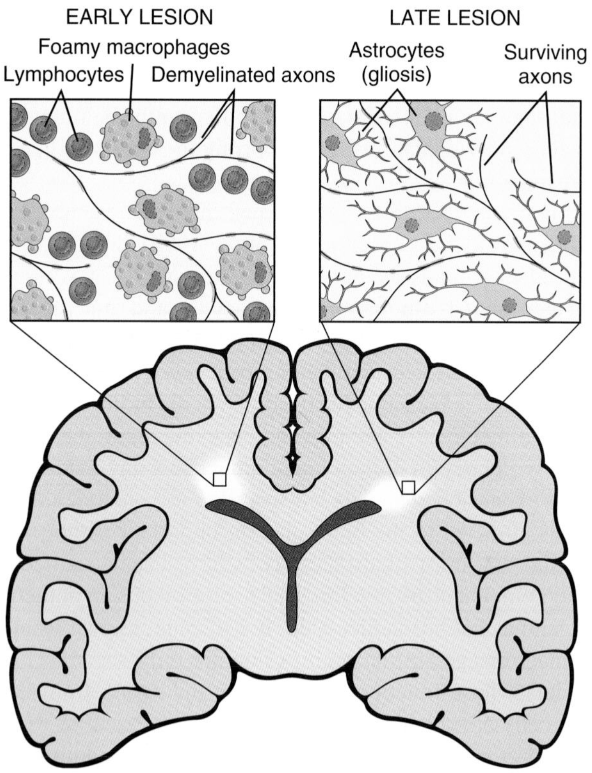

Figure 21-12 Multiple sclerosis. Early lesions contain demyelinated axons surrounded by lymphocytes and foamy macrophages. Late lesions—that is, fully formed demyelinated plaques—consist of demyelinated axons and astrocytes.

touch, accompanied by tingling. Blurred vision is a common early symptom. Motor symptoms include muscle weakness, unsteady gait, incoordination of movements, and sphincter abnormalities such as urinary incontinence. These symptoms usually appear to be unrelated to one another, and the diagnosis of MS may therefore be rather difficult.

The diagnosis of MS is made on clinical grounds. Current criteria require documentation of two separate sets of CNS symptoms that occur in at least two episodes, separated by a period of 1 month or more. Magnetic resonance imaging (MRI) is a useful diagnostic technique. With this specialized x-ray technique, a brain lesion is evident in 80% of patients. Oligoclonal IgG bands are typically found in the CSF, and although this abnormality is not pathognomonic of MS, it strongly supports the diagnosis.

MS has an unpredictable course. Most patients become physically incapacitated over a period of 20 to 30 years. Patients who develop MS after the age of 40 years and those with marked motor disability early in the course of disease have a poor prognosis.

METABOLIC AND NUTRITIONAL DISEASES

INBORN ERRORS OF METABOLISM

Metabolic injury of the brain is a common feature of many inborn errors of metabolism. Diseases involving the enzymes essential for maintenance of myelin and cell membranes of neurons are accompanied by extensive lesions of the CNS. The best known among these incurable diseases are the following:

- *Tay-Sachs disease,* a deficiency of the enzyme hexosaminidase A that leads to accumulation of gangliosides in neurons. The disease presents early in life and is characterized by progressive mental and motor deterioration and blindness.
- *Niemann-Pick disease,* a deficiency of sphingomyelinase that leads to an accumulation of sphingomyelin. This disease also begins in childhood and is characterized by progressive mental deterioration. The accumulation of sphingomyelin in the cytoplasm damages the cells. Neuronal loss leads to profound atrophy of the brain.

NUTRITIONAL DISEASES

Among the nutritional deficiencies affecting the brain, the most important are those related to an inadequate intake of vitamins. Some vitamin deficiencies occur because of gastrointestinal disorders that prevent normal absorption (e.g., pernicious anemia, which is marked by an inability to absorb vitamin B_{12}). The most important vitamin deficiencies that affect the brain are deficiencies of thiamine (vitamin B_1), vitamin B_{12}, and nicotinic acid.

Thiamine deficiency presents clinically as Wernicke's encephalopathy or Korsakoff's syndrome. Wernicke's syndrome includes disturbances in ocular function, gait, and mental function. Korsakoff's syndrome presents with mental deterioration whereby patients lose memory (amnesia) and make up incredible stories (confabulation). Degenerative neuronal changes are typically found in the hypothalamus, the periaqueductal region of the midbrain, and mamillary bodies. These two syndromes are often combined and can be referred to as **Wernicke-Korsakoff syndrome.**

Vitamin B_{12} deficiency presents with uncoordinated movements and a sensorimotor peripheral neuropathy with signs of spinal cord disease. Typically, affected patients have an abnormal gait. Psychiatric symptoms are also present but are highly variable. Some patients are demented, others delirious or depressed, and still others mentally slow. Pathologically, vitamin B_{12} deficiency leads to subacute combined degeneration of the spinal cord, which is characterized by degeneration of ascending tracts of the posterior columns and descending pyramidal tracts.

Nicotinic acid deficiency results in pellagra, a clinical syndrome characterized by dermatitis, diarrhea, and delirium (the "three Ds"). The neurologic and psychiatric symptoms of pellagra are usually present but are highly variable.

ALCOHOLISM

Alcohol has profound effects on the brain. In small amounts it stimulates the brain, causing euphoria and lack of inhibition. In larger amounts, alcohol induces sleep and depresses brain functions. Alcohol, when ingested in excessive amounts, may even act as a neurotoxin and cause death.

Chronic **alcoholism** affects the nervous system directly and indirectly. In addition to its direct neurotoxic effects, alcohol damages the liver and alters intermediary metabolism. These general metabolic changes are often combined with nutritional deficiencies, such as deficiencies of thiamine, folic acid, or nicotinic acid, all of which can affect the brain.

The neuropathologic changes related to chronic alcoholism usually reflect the complex nutritional and metabolic disturbances in these patients. Thiamine deficiency probably accounts for Wernicke-Korsakoff syndrome and the variety of psychiatric and neurologic deficiencies encountered under these conditions. The pathologic lesions are located in the same regions of the midbrain as in thiamine deficiency (Figure 21-13). Cerebellar atrophy accounts for uncoordinated movements during walking and work. General cortical atrophy of the brain, probably related to a loss of neurons exposed to the neurotoxic effects of alcohol, results in progressive mental deterioration, loss of memory, an inability to concentrate, irritability, and many other symptoms. Myelopathy and sensory-motor neuropathy account for sensory deficiencies and the tremor and fatigability of muscles. Alcohol also has a direct adverse effect on the striated muscle cells.

Some of the pathologic changes encountered in chronic alcoholics are only indirectly related to alcohol abuse. For example, subdural hematoma, which is often found in such patients, may be related to repeated head trauma sustained in falling when inebriated. *Pontine myelinolysis* is a peculiar lesion in the pons that is related to vigorous correction of sodium imbalance in chronic alcoholics with cirrhosis.

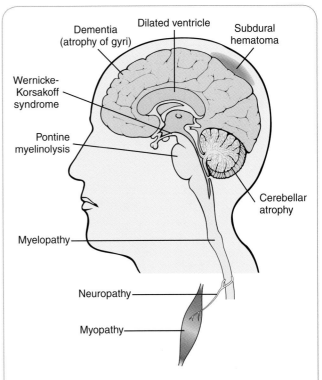

Figure 21-13 Pathologic changes in the nervous system caused by chronic alcoholism.

Withdrawal of alcohol, as in chronic alcoholics who are hospitalized, may induce an acute confusional state, known as *delirium tremens* (DT). DT develops suddenly and is characterized by agitation, confusion, and hallucinations. The patient cannot concentrate, pays no attention to others, and may hear strange voices or see objects that do not exist (e.g., white mice or devils on the wall).

NEURODEGENERATIVE DISEASES

The term **neurodegenerative disorders** is used (for lack of a better one) to describe a group of diseases of unknown etiology that are limited to the CNS. These diseases, which are unrelated to one another, present with a variety of neurologic and psychiatric symptoms. For example, Parkinson's disease presents with movement disorders, Huntington's disease is characterized by abnormal body movements and progressive mental deterioration, and Alzheimer's disease presents with only a loss of mental capacities but no motor deficits.

The diagnosis of neurodegenerative disorders can readily be made in typical cases. However, many patients do not have all the typical clinical features, and the diagnosis may be made only by excluding all other brain diseases that could cause the same set of symptoms. Because these neurodegenerative diseases are incurable, one must be certain that the patient does not have a curable disease before establishing a diagnosis of neurodegenerative disease (Figure 21-14).

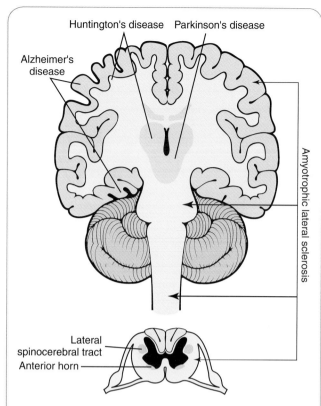

Figure 21-14 Degenerative diseases of the brain preferentially involve various parts of the brain. Alzheimer's disease causes atrophy of the frontal and occipital cortical gyri. Huntington's disease affects the frontal cortex and basal ganglia. Parkinson's disease is marked by changes in the substantia nigra. Amyotrophic lateral sclerosis affects the motor neurons in the anterior horn of the spinal cord, brainstem, and frontal cortex of the brain.

ALZHEIMER'S DISEASE

Alzheimer's disease is a form of dementia (loss of mental capacities) of unknown etiology. It is characterized pathologically by atrophy of the frontal and temporal cortex of the brain and shows typical histologic features. It affects older people, particularly those 70 years and older. The symptoms of Alzheimer's disease are seen only rarely in people younger than age 60. The number of clinical cases increases progressively with age, from 1% in those 60 to 64 years old to 40% in those who are over 85 years old. At present, approximately 7 million people in the United States are affected by Alzheimer's disease, and a new case of Alzheimer's disease is diagnosed every 70 seconds.

Etiology and Pathogenesis

The causes of Alzheimer's disease and the pathogenesis of cerebral lesions are not known. Investigations have centered on possible genetic factors and the elucidation of the reasons for the degeneration of neurons that leads to atrophy of the cortex and mental deterioration.

Genetic factors play a role in the pathogenesis of the familial form of Alzheimer's disease, which accounts for 5% to 10% of all cases. Familial Alzheimer's disease has been linked to genetic changes on chromosomes 21 and 19. In this context, it is of interest to mention that trisomy 21 is typical of Down's syndrome, which shows identical neuropathologic changes to those of Alzheimer's disease. In both conditions the brain contains deposits of a special form of amyloid, composed of beta-amyloid (Aβ) peptide, which is derived from amyloid precursor protein (APP). Chromosome 19 carries the gene for apolipoprotein E4 (apoE4), a plasma protein that is deposited in the brain lesions characteristic of Alzheimer's disease. It has been shown that the deposited apoE4 is actually a variant of normal plasma protein. The abnormal protein is produced by a mutated *APOE4* gene. This mutated *APOE4* gene is found in 3% of the normal population. The carriers of this abnormal gene develop Alzheimer's disease at an astounding rate (90%), which suggests that this gene may play an important pathogenetic role.

Neuronal loss in the brain of patients with Alzheimer's disease has been studied extensively. Existing evidence points to possible neurotoxic effects of beta-amyloid, a fibrillar extracellular substance that is deposited in the brain lesions. Intracellular defects such as hyperphosphorylation of tau protein, an axonal microtubule binding protein in neural cells, and abnormal phosphorylation of neurofilaments have also been implicated. Neuronal loss may be related to decreased levels of nerve growth factor, which is essential for maintenance of normal nerve cells. However, none of these findings fully explains the pathogenesis of brain lesions in Alzheimer's disease, and so the search for its causes goes on.

Pathology

The pathologic diagnosis of Alzheimer's disease is based on gross and microscopic neuropathologic findings. On gross examination, the brain appears atrophic and shows narrowing of the gyri and a widening of the sulci. Atrophy affects the frontal and temporal lobes most prominently. Histologic changes are most prominent in the cortex. Typical histologic features are neuritic (senile) plaques, neurofibrillary tangles, granulovacuolar degeneration, and deposition of amyloid in the neuritic plaques and the wall of the cerebral vessels. Some of these changes can be recognized on routine hematoxylin-eosin–stained slides, but they are more easily identified on slides prepared by special procedures. For example, neuritic plaques and neurofibrillary tangles are best seen after silver impregnation of tissue sections, whereas amyloid is best demonstrated by the Congo red stain or immunohistochemically with specific antibodies.

Clinical Features

Alzheimer's disease presents clinically as a dementia. **Dementia** is defined as a progressive loss of cognitive functions and a functional decline that typically interferes with work and social activities. The loss of memory predominates; this loss is usually insidious but tends to progress until the patient becomes completely dysfunctional and cannot perform any mental operations. As clinical function deteriorates, most patients also develop speech problems, must limit their daily activities, and finally become bedridden and completely dependent on nursing care. With adequate care, most patients with Alzheimer's disease live long lives. Death is not related to Alzheimer's disease itself but rather usually reflects the decreased resistance to infection that normally occurs with advancing age.

The clinical diagnosis of Alzheimer's disease is based on the demonstration of progressive dementia. It should be remembered that dementia can result from a variety of cardiovascular, endocrine, and metabolic diseases and that it may be induced by certain drugs. Brain tumors and infections also can cause dementia. The diagnosis of Alzheimer's disease should be made only after all these other possible causes of dementia have been excluded.

Specialized x-ray studies, such as computed tomography (CT) scans and MRIs, are useful for documenting atrophy of the cortex, but similar atrophy may be found in nondemented elderly people and in those with multi-infarct dementia. Thus the x-ray findings are not diagnostic. Laboratory findings are nonspecific and do not provide any direct support to the clinical diagnosis. Nevertheless, such studies may be useful in excluding other "organic" forms of dementia.

 Did You Know?

The term *sundowning* is used for evening or late afternoon changes in the behavior of patients with Alzheimer's disease. As the day comes to a close, some of these patients become more confused, restless, and insecure or more demanding, upset, and suspicious. The reasons for sundowning are not known, but most likely this change in behavior is related to fatigue and a loss of neural energy.

PARKINSON'S DISEASE

Parkinson's disease (PD) is a subcortical neurodegenerative disorder characterized by movement disorders and pathologic changes of the extrapyramidal (involuntary) motor system nuclei of the midbrain. PD is relatively common, and it typically affects elderly patients.

Etiology and Pathogenesis

The cause of PD is unknown. The disease is characterized by a decreased number of dopaminergic neurons in the substantia nigra. These neurons release dopamine, a neurotransmitter, which is transported into another nucleus called *striatum*. The striatum and the substantia nigra form a functional unit. The substantia nigra of patients with PD is not dark (as is normal) but rather is depigmented because of the loss of pigmented neurons. The amount of dopamine in the striatum is also reduced, which correlates with the retarded transmission of neuronal impulses between these nuclei. The loss of neurotransmitters correlates with the clinical appearance of

movement disorders. The midbrain centers regulate and coordinate these movements and the impulses essential for the performance of such movements. L-Dopa, a precursor of dopamine, and other drugs that increase the levels of dopamine in the brain may temporarily improve the symptoms in some patients. However, in most cases PD is progressive and incurable.

Most patients with PD have the idiopathic form of the disease. In addition to this form, clinicians also recognize a secondary form, which is also called *parkinsonism*. The symptoms of parkinsonism are indistinguishable from those of PD except that in the former group the onset of symptoms can be traced to another pathologic event, such as encephalitis. Many drugs, especially those used in the treatment of psychiatric disease, can cause parkinsonism.

Clinical Features

PD presents with disturbances of movement, primarily tremor, rigidity, bradykinesia, and postural instability (Figure 21-15). Tremor or twitching of the muscles is most prominent in the

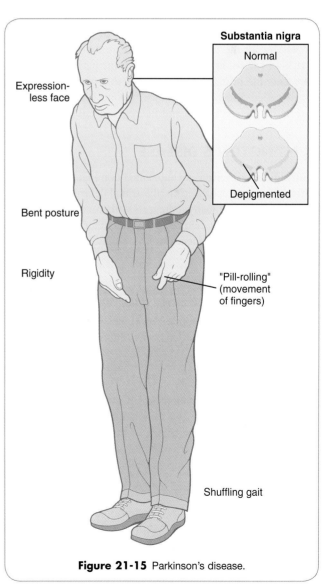

Figure 21-15 Parkinson's disease.

hands or face and is typically enhanced by emotional stress. It is less prominent during voluntary movements. Rigidity and resistance to passive movements are increased. For example, if an affected patient is asked to move the arms against slight pressure exerted by the examiner, the movement has a staggering, cogwheel-like character. *Bradykinesia* refers to slowing of movements. Affected patients exhibit instability while walking. They walk bent forward, as if "chasing their point of gravity." A significant number of patients with PD become depressed, and dementia develops in about 10%. The treatment of PD is symptomatic, because no cure is available.

Pathology

PD presents with rather consistent pathologic changes involving the striatonigral part of the brainstem. On gross examination, the substantia nigra appears pale. Histologically, this change is related to a loss of melanin-rich neurons in this subcortical nucleus. The remaining neurons contain typical round eosinophilic inclusions, known as *Lewy's bodies*. These bodies are composed of beta-synuclein, a protein linked pathogenetically to the familial of PD, but also contain neurofilaments, ubiquitin, and a protein called *parkin*. In a minority of cases, Lewy's bodies can be seen in cortical neurons, accounting for the development of depression and dementia in 10% to 15% of all PD patients. In some patients, dementia represents the primary manifestation, in which case the disease is called *dementia with Lewy's bodies* (DLB). The exact relationship between DLB and PD remains unknown.

HUNTINGTON'S DISEASE

Huntington's disease is an autosomal dominant neurodegenerative disease affecting primarily striatal neurons but also the cerebral cortex. Clinically it presents with motor disturbances, progressive dementia, and abnormal behavior. The disease is familial and has an incidence of 1 in 20,000 people.

Pathogenesis

The gene for the disease, *HTT,* known as *Huntingtin,* has been localized to chromosome 4. The coding region of *Huntingtin* contains a CAG trinucleotide repeat, accounting for the fact that the disease appears at an earlier age and is more severe with each generation.

Pathology

Huntington's disease is characterized by atrophy and loss of nerve cells in the caudate and the putamen, accompanied by a variable atrophy of motor cortex of the frontal lobe. Histologic changes are nonspecific and include atrophy, degeneration, and loss of neurons, accompanied by reactive gliosis.

Clinical Features

Symptoms usually begin by the age of 40 years but may appear even earlier, and 10% of cases are diagnosed in childhood. In adults, symptoms include involuntary, gyrating movements of the trunk and limbs (choreiform movements); postural instability; rigidity; and progressive

dementia. Bradykinesia and rigidity dominate in children. Once the symptoms appear, however, the patient's condition rapidly deteriorates. Most affected patients become completely mentally incapacitated and die within 20 years of onset.

AMYOTROPHIC LATERAL SCLEROSIS

Amyotrophic lateral sclerosis (ALS) is a neurodegenerative disease characterized by motor weakness and progressive wasting of muscles in the extremities, leading ultimately to generalized muscle loss and death. It is also known as *Lou Gehrig's disease,* named after the famous baseball player who was afflicted by it. Although ALS is a rare disease, affecting 2 in 100,000 people, it has been of interest to scientists because of its unique features, which could provide new insight into the pathogenesis of other, more common neurodegenerative diseases.

Etiology and Pathogenesis

The cause of ALS is unknown. A familial form of ALS, accounting for 10% of all patients, has been linked to the mutation of the copper-zinc superoxide dismutase *(SOD1)* gene on chromosome 21. Speculations are that this mutation deprives the neurons of the protection against superoxide and that this oxygen radical therefore kills the cells at an increased rate. However, this hypothesis does not account for the loss of motor neurons in sporadic cases. Furthermore, there are no acceptable explanations for the selective loss of motor neurons and the sparing of other nerve cells.

Pathology

The disease is characterized by a loss of motor neurons in the spinal cord, midbrain, and finally cerebral cortex. Most prominent is the loss of the lateral cerebrospinal pathways in the spinal cord (which prompted the name of the disease), as the lateral parts of the white matter are replaced by sclerosis. This change is related to the loss of motor axons and the skeletal muscle atrophy that is readily visible on muscle biopsy.

Clinical Features

ALS usually affects older men and women, but it can be seen in younger and middle-aged persons as well. For example, Lou Gehrig was only 37 years old when he died, 2 years after he was diagnosed with ALS. ALS presents with weakness and wasting of the small hand muscles. Fasciculation (involuntary twitching) of muscles is typical. Such movements occur as fast, involuntary contractions that do not move the limbs. Speech becomes slurred in advanced cases, but the intellect is not affected. Most patients become immobile and ultimately die as a result of paralysis of the respiratory muscles.

The diagnosis of ALS is made clinically. Electromyography shows typical denervation and muscular atrophy. Muscle biopsy can confirm this finding but is rarely necessary. ALS is an incurable, progressive disease that inevitably leads to death over a period of a few years.

EPILEPSY

Epilepsy is a group of diseases that present with recurrent seizures. Seizures are typically characterized by convulsions (i.e., uncoordinated twitching of muscles and spastic contractions). Epileptic attacks may also include short periods of altered consciousness, abnormal motor activity, altered sensory phenomena, or inappropriate behavior. All these manifestations of epilepsy are thought to result from abnormal synchronized electrical activity of the brain.

Etiology and Pathogenesis

Seizures may result from focal or generalized dysfunction of the neurons in the cerebral cortex as a result of neurologic or systemic diseases. In most cases the cause of epileptic seizures is not known; such epilepsy is classified as idiopathic. Typically these forms of epilepsy begin in childhood between the ages of 2 and 15 years and have presumptively genetic causes. Seizures that develop as a result of identifiable disorders are called *secondary seizures*. Common causes of secondary epilepsy are listed in Table 21-1.

Clinical Features

There are several types of epilepsy. Only the two most important ones are discussed here: generalized epilepsy and focal epilepsy.

GENERALIZED EPILEPSY

Generalized epilepsy is in most instances idiopathic and begins in childhood. The overall risk of developing epilepsy up to the age of 20 years is 1%. The cause of generalized epilepsy is not known, and the disease is not related to defined pathologic lesions that can be identified on gross or microscopic examination of the brain. Clinically it presents with generalized seizures, resulting from bilateral diffuse electric discharges involving the entire cerebral cortex. The convulsions are tonic-clonic and the person usually loses consciousness. The attack may be preceded by sensory or psychic premonitions called *auras*. After the attack the patient is in a postictal state characterized by deep sleep, confusion, headaches, and muscle soreness.

FOCAL EPILEPSY

In focal epilepsy the electric discharges originate from a well-defined cortical area. The discharges may remain localized to their site of origin, or they may spread to adjacent parts of the brain. Focal epilepsy may occur in any age group, and in most instances one can identify its causes or at least link it to a defined event, such as viral infection of the meninges. In children the causes include developmental abnormalities of the brain and infections. In adults focal epilepsy may be a consequence of trauma or infections. In many instances it is the first sign of a brain tumor.

The diagnosis of epilepsy is based on clinical data, which must be further documented with appropriate neurologic examinations, including electroencephalographic (EEG) recordings of the electric activity of the brain. Most importantly, one must distinguish idiopathic from secondary epilepsy, which usually has a less favorable prognosis. In patients with secondary epilepsy, one must identify the cause of the disease and if possible remove the epileptogenic focus. Drug therapy eliminates seizures in one third of all patients and greatly reduces the frequency of seizures in another third. In most of these patients the drugs can be discontinued after proper control of seizures. Most patients treated for idiopathic epilepsy do not have loss of function and lead a normal life.

NEOPLASMS

Neoplasms of the CNS are relatively rare, accounting for only 2% of all cancer deaths. Nevertheless, these tumors are important clinically for several reasons:

- Brain tumors have a very high mortality. This high mortality is partially related to the malignant nature of brain tumors and partially to their location. Any enlarging mass inside the cranial cavity can eventually cause death by compressing the vital centers.
- Brain tumors occur at any age but are relatively prominent in younger age groups. In childhood, brain tumors account for 20% of all malignant diseases. In the 20- to 40-year age group they are still among the most common cancers, accounting for 10% of cancer deaths. The occurrence of brain tumors does not decrease with age, but in the older age groups, tumors of the CNS do not stand out as such because they are overshadowed by the more common neoplasms.

Approximately 50% of brain tumors are primary neoplasms, whereas the other 50% represent metastases from other sites. Because there is a 50% chance that a tumor could be a metastasis, it is important to determine whether the patient has a malignant lesion elsewhere before establishing a

TABLE 21-1 Causes of Secondary Epilepsy

Condition	Examples
Drugs and toxins	Alcohol, psychotropic drugs, lead poisoning
CNS infections	Meningitis, encephalitis, brain abscess
Brain trauma	Accident, intracranial surgery, birth trauma
Intracranial bleeding	Subdural hematoma
CNS tumors	Glioma, metastatic tumors
Metabolic disorders	Hypoglycemia, hyperglycemia, hypocalcemia
Fever (especially in children)	Infection, heatstroke, sunstroke

CNS, central nervous system.

diagnosis of a primary malignant brain lesion. This approach also avoids unnecessary brain surgery.

Intracranial tumors can be histologically classified as benign or malignant. Malignant tumors have a tendency for infiltrative growth; therefore it is almost impossible to remove them completely by surgery. Benign tumors are curable but may also cause death because of their inaccessibility or their location close to a vital center. Although histologically benign, such tumors could clinically be considered malignant.

Malignant tumors of the CNS differ from malignant diseases in other parts of the body in that they do not metastasize. Death occurs as a result of intracranial mass effects and the compression of vital centers. This can occur from the direct impingement of the tumor on vital centers or because of increased intracranial pressure and the compression of the brainstem by the herniated cerebellar tonsils or the uncal gyri of the hippocampus (see Figure 21-3).

Classification

Tumors of the CNS can be classified, according to their derivation, into several groups, the most important of which are the following:

- Tumors of glial cells (75%)
- Tumors of neural cell precursors (2%)
- Tumors of the meninges (15%)
- Tumors of the cranial and spinal nerves (5%)

Other tumors, such as hemangiomas and hemangioblastomas originating from cerebral blood vessels, primary cerebral lymphomas, or pinealomas (tumors of the pineal gland), are generally rare. An increased incidence of primary brain lymphoma has been noted in immunosuppressed patients with AIDS.

Tumors can occur in any part of the CNS. Various histologic tumor forms differ in their predilection for certain anatomic sites (Figure 21-16). For example, medulloblastoma is always located in the cerebellum. Cystic astrocytomas of childhood are most often found in the cerebellum, whereas solid astrocytomas and glioblastoma multiforme occur most often in the cerebrum. Meningiomas arise from the meninges, most often along the falx cerebri, the midsagittal line between the two cerebral hemispheres.

Etiology and Pathogenesis

The causes of brain tumors are not known. No definitive risk factors have been identified for most CNS tumors. Nevertheless, there are several promising leads for future research that have been derived from the study of some less common forms of CNS tumors. For example, nerve sheath tumors involving cranial nerve VIII (acoustic neuromas) are familial and are a feature of the hereditary neurofibromatosis type II syndrome. These tumors have been linked to changes in a tumor suppressor gene typically found in affected families. An increased incidence of meningiomas has been noted in patients with familial neoplastic syndromes, such as neurofibromatosis type I and multiple endocrine adenomatosis type II, a syndrome characterized by the appearance of medullary carcinoma of the thyroid and adrenal medullary tumors (pheochromocytomas). Approximately 75% of meningiomas show a peculiar chromosomal change: deletion of the long arm of chromosome 22. This chromosomal segment carries the neurofibromatosis tumor suppressor gene. These findings link meningiomas to neurofibromatosis and provide evidence for the possible genetic etiology of these tumors. Cerebellar **hemangioblastomas** are also familial. These tumors are

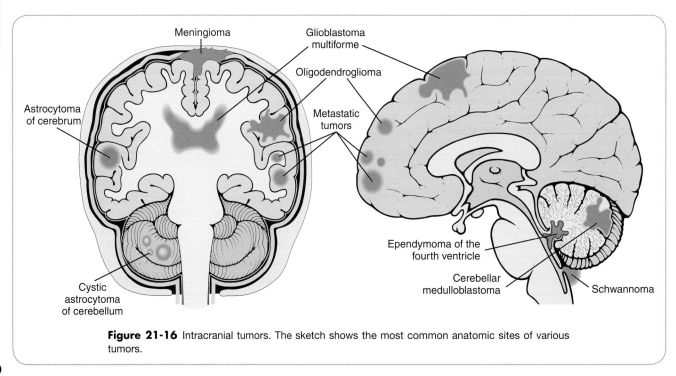

Figure 21-16 Intracranial tumors. The sketch shows the most common anatomic sites of various tumors.

found in families affected by von Hippel–Lindau disease, a hereditary condition characterized by blood vessel tumors in the brain and retina; cysts in the kidney, liver, and pancreas; and a strong tendency for renal cell carcinoma. These patients carry a mutated suppressor gene *(VHL)* that has been localized to chromosome 3.

The molecular biologic and chromosomal changes in glial cell tumors, the most common CNS neoplasms, are more complex. Like colon cancer and several other malignant diseases, most glioblastomas show mutation of the *P53* suppressor gene. A loss of alleles from chromosomes 17 and 19 is found at a high rate, but the significance of these genetic and chromosomal changes remains enigmatic. No genetic markers unique to brain tumors have yet been identified.

GLIOMAS

Tumors arising from glial cells can be classified as astrocytic, oligodendroglial, or ependymal. Tumors previously considered to be of microglial origin have been reclassified as cerebral lymphomas.

Astrocytic tumors, known as **astrocytomas** and *glioblastoma multiforme,* account for about 80% of these tumors. Oligodendrogliomas and ependymomas are less common, each accounting for 10% of all gliomas. All gliomas are malignant.

Astrocytic gliomas can be subdivided into two groups: infiltrating and noninfiltrating tumors. *Noninfiltrating astrocytomas,* also known as *pilocytic astrocytomas,* are relatively well circumscribed tumors that occur most often in the cerebellum of children and young adults. Less often they are located in the floor of the third ventricle and even in the cerebral hemispheres. These tumors are most often cystic but may be also solid. Histologically, astrocytomas are composed of relatively well differentiated hairlike *(pilocytic)* astrocytes. These astrocytomas grow slowly and can be resected, although many of them recur.

Infiltrating astrocytomas are the most common brain tumors, accounting for 80% of all intracerebral tumors. They are classified into three groups: diffuse astrocytoma, anaplastic astrocytoma, and glioblastoma. These tumors infiltrate and distort or destroy the normal brain, often causing secondary changes such as hemorrhage or necrosis.

Glioblastoma is the most common CNS tumor. Its peak incidence is at age 65, but it may occur in younger persons as well. Most of these tumors are found in the lateral hemispheres of the brain (Figure 21-17). As its name implies, the tumor has a highly variegated gross appearance. Parts of the tumor are necrotic and yellow, parts are hemorrhagic red, and parts are white, like normal brain. Typically the lesion is irregularly shaped and poorly demarcated from normal brain parenchyma, often extending through the corpus callosum from one cerebral hemisphere into the other. On cross-sectional examination of the brain at autopsy, or by CT scanning and MRI in living patients, such bilateral lesions have a butterfly-like appearance.

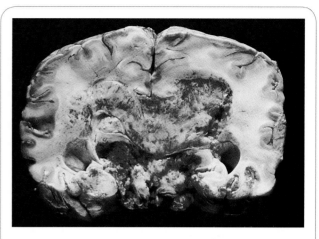

Figure 21-17 Glioblastoma. Gross appearance of a bilateral "butterfly" tumor. (From Okazaki H, Scheithauer BW: Atlas of Neuropathology, New York and London, Gower Medical Publishing, 1988, acquired by Elsevier, Ltd, Oxford, UK.)

Histologic studies reveal that glioblastomas are composed of highly anaplastic astrocytic cells. These cells may retain a fetal appearance, in which case they have small blue nuclei and no cytoplasm. Alternatively, they may become enlarged, take on a bizarre shape, or be multinucleated with well-developed cytoplasm. Mitotic figures are numerous. Typically, the blood vessels in the tumor show marked proliferative changes. Invasive, rapid growth of cells and the vascular changes account for the common occurrence of necrosis and hemorrhage in the tumor.

? Did You Know?

George Gershwin, the famous American composer, died at the age of 38 of a brain tumor. Initially he only had headaches and was diagnosed as having neurosis. He developed olfactory hallucinations and had the feeling that somebody was trying to suffocate him by burning rubber. He collapsed while conducting an orchestra and was taken to a hospital, where an inoperable glioblastoma was diagnosed.

Oligodendrogliomas are rare gliomas that usually involve the cerebral hemisphere of middle-aged adults. These tumors are usually well circumscribed, often partially cystic, and calcified. Histologically, these tumors are composed of well-differentiated oligodendroglial cells. The tumors can be classified histologically as low-grade or high-grade malignant lesions, but the correlation between histologic findings and survival is not perfect. The poor correlation between histology and prognosis is related to the fact that 50% of all oligodendrogliomas contain astrocytes, which may not be evident in a brain biopsy. Because astrocytes proliferate at a higher rate than do oligodendroglial cells, mixed tumors (occasionally called *oligoastrocytomas*) grow faster than pure oligodendrogliomas. Such tumors may progress to glioblastoma multiforme. Pure, well-differentiated oligodendrogliomas have a more indolent course.

Ependymomas are derived from ependymal cells lining the ventricles and central canal of the spinal cord. Ventricular ependymomas are typically found in children. In adults, ependymomas are usually located in the terminal part of the spinal cord, called the filum terminale and cauda equina. On histologic examination, ependymoma cells have round or elongated nuclei and are enmeshed in a fibrillar background. Tumor cells line the papillary structures or form rosettes (i.e., structures reminiscent of ependymal canals and fetal neural tubes). Ependymomas of the terminal part of the spinal cord are often composed of papillae in loose myxomatous connective tissue (myxopapillary ependymoma).

The prognosis for gliomas depends on their location and their histologic composition. Noninfiltrating astrocytomas of the cerebellum have the best prognosis and can be even cured by complete resection. Glioblastoma is almost invariably fatal, regardless of its location; most patients die within 12 to 18 months of diagnosis. With modern surgical and radiation therapy, patients with astrocytomas usually survive 5 years after diagnosis, but most die because the tumors cannot be removed in their entirety. Cerebral oligodendrogliomas and ependymomas have a somewhat more favorable prognosis, with a survival of 5 to 10 years. Ependymomas of the filum terminale can be removed surgically and have a good prognosis.

TUMORS OF NEURAL CELL PRECURSORS AND UNDIFFERENTIATED CELLS

Terminally differentiated neurons cannot proliferate and are thus incapable of malignant transformation. Hence it is thought that neuroectodermal tumors probably arise from undifferentiated, fetal precursors retained in the brain of infants and children. It has also been proposed that the neural cells may undergo reverse development, or "dedifferentiation," regressing to a fetal stage, becoming mitotic, and giving rise to neoplasms. There is no support for any of these theories; thus the source of neuroectodermal tumors remains obscure.

Approximately 10% to 15% of all brain tumors are composed of primitive neuroectodermal cells resembling those found in the fetal neural tube. The most important tumor in this group is *medulloblastoma,* a cerebellar childhood tumor of uncertain origin. It is generally assumed that medulloblastomas originate from fetal neural cell precursors, although it is unclear why such fetal cells would remain in the cerebellum. An alternative explanation, involving dedifferentiation of neurons or proliferation of the outer granular layer of cerebellum, is speculative and is not supported by solid evidence.

Medulloblastomas are composed of fetal-like neuroectodermal cells (i.e., cells that are reminiscent of those in fetal medulla spinalis). These tumors are limited to the cerebellum and are found only in children. The tumors grow quickly, and although they are sensitive to radiation therapy and chemotherapy, they have a poor prognosis. Medulloblastoma cells

can enter the CSF and be carried by CSF. These cells may travel through the central canal of the spinal cord and form implantation metastases in the spinal cord. With modern surgery and chemotherapy, 50% of children harboring these tumors survive 10 years.

MENINGIOMA

Meningiomas arise from the meninges (Figure 21-18). Most meningiomas are benign, and only about 4% are malignant. Most tumors are located in the midline, impinging from outside the cerebral hemispheres. However, meningiomas can also arise from the meninges at the base of the brain and along the spinal cord. For unknown reasons, spinal meningiomas are 10 times more common in women than in men. Compression of the brain may cause epileptic seizures or motor deficits. Meningiomas are surgically curable and have an excellent prognosis except the few that are malignant or located in an unreachable location.

TUMORS OF THE CRANIAL AND SPINAL NERVES

Tumors originating from the nerves, collectively called neuromas, are composed of cells enveloping the axons. Those composed of Schwann cells are called **schwannomas** or *neurilemomas,* whereas those composed of neurofibroblasts are termed **neurofibromas.**

Schwannomas can originate anywhere along the length of the cranial or spinal nerves. Because Schwann cells envelop not only the peripheral portion of the nerves but also the initial intradural parts, some schwannomas are intradural (i.e., located inside the vertebral canal or the cranial cavity). Intracranial schwannomas arise most often from the cranial nerve VIII and are called acoustic neuromas.

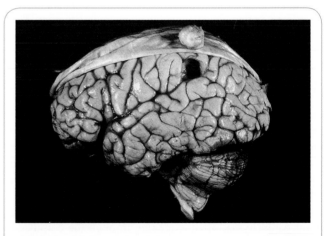

Figure 21-18 Meningioma. The round tumor has been shelled out from the hole that it has produced in the brain. (From Okazaki H, Scheithauer BW: Atlas of Neuropathology, New York and London, Gower Medical Publishing, 1988, acquired by Elsevier, Ltd, Oxford, UK.)

Neuromas may be solitary or multiple. Multiple tumors of the peripheral nerves are a feature of neurofibromatosis type I, an autosomal dominant disease that affects approximately 100,000 Americans. Acoustic neuromas are typical of neurofibromatosis type II. These neuromas may cause hearing loss and vertigo. Because of their location in the cerebellopontine angle, these benign tumors may compress the cerebellum and pons and even cause death.

METASTASES TO THE BRAIN

Approximately 50% of all brain tumors represent metastases from a malignant tumor involving some other site. Metastases may be solitary or multiple. Although any malignant tumor may metastasize to the brain, certain malignant tumors have a special predilection for spread to the brain, including lung cancer, breast cancer, and melanoma. Any part of the brain may be involved.

REVIEW QUESTIONS

1. List the main components of the central and peripheral nervous systems.
2. Describe the functions of the four major lobes of the brain.
3. Compare the functions of the midbrain, pons, and medulla oblongata with that of the cerebellum.
4. Describe the function of the spinal cord.
5. Describe the circulation of the cerebrospinal fluid.
6. List the main cells of the nervous system.
7. What are the most important diseases of the nervous system?
8. What are the sites of brain herniation caused by intracranial hypertension?
9. List the main dysraphic disorders of the central nervous system and describe their pathogenesis.
10. List the most important intracranial hemorrhages and describe their causes.
11. What is stroke?
12. What is global cerebral ischemia, and what are its consequences?
13. What is the pathogenesis of "watershed infarcts" and laminar necrosis of the brain?
14. Describe the pathology of cerebral infarcts.
15. Correlate the pathology of intracerebral hemorrhage with the clinical features of this disease.

16. What are the main pathologic findings after brain injury?
17. Compare hyperextension and hyperflexion injuries of the cervical spine.
18. Compare bacterial and viral infections of the central nervous system.
19. What are prions?
20. List the most important protozoal and fungal causes of opportunistic diseases of the central nervous system.
21. Compare the pathology of encephalitis and meningitis.
22. Describe the features of neurosyphilis.
23. What are the most important AIDS-related central nervous system lesions?
24. What is multiple sclerosis?
25. Correlate the pathologic features of multiple sclerosis with the clinical signs and symptoms of this disease.
26. How do inborn errors of metabolism affect the central nervous system?
27. What is the cause and what are the signs of Wernicke-Korsakoff syndrome?
28. How does alcohol affect the brain?
29. What are the most important neurodegenerative diseases?
30. What is Alzheimer's disease, and how is it diagnosed?
31. Describe the macroscopic and microscopic pathologic findings in Alzheimer's disease.
32. What is Parkinson's disease?
33. Correlate the pathology of Parkinson's disease with the clinical features of this disease.
34. What is amyotrophic lateral sclerosis?
35. Correlate the pathology of amyotrophic lateral sclerosis with the clinical features of this disease.
36. Classify brain tumors.
37. List the most common brain tumors and their predominant location.
38. Compare glioblastoma with other gliomas.
39. Which brain tumors occur most often in children?
40. Why do medulloblastomas metastasize?
41. What are meningiomas?
42. Which tumors originate from the peripheral nerves?

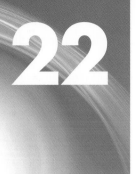

22 The Eye

Chapter Outline

NORMAL ANATOMY AND PHYSIOLOGY
OVERVIEW OF MAJOR DISEASES
    Developmental Disorders
    Trauma
    Infections
    Immunologic Disease
    Circulatory Disorders
        Hypertensive Retinopathy
        Diabetic Retinopathy

Glaucoma
Cataract
Neoplasms
    Retinoblastoma
    Malignant Melanoma

Key Terms and Concepts

Age-related macular degeneration (ARMD)
Astigmatism
Blepharitis
Cataracts
Conjunctivitis
Corneal abrasion
Dacryocystitis
Diabetic retinopathy

Endophthalmitis
Glaucoma
Hordeolum
Hyperopia
Hypertensive retinopathy
Iridocyclitis
Keratitis
Malignant melanoma
Microphthalmia

Myopia
Panophthalmitis
Papilledema
Presbyopia
Retinitis pigmentosa
Retinoblastoma
Stye
Trachoma
Uveitis

Learning Objectives

After reading this chapter, the student should be able to:

1. Describe the normal anatomy and physiology of the eye and its appendages.
2. Describe two developmental disorders affecting the eyes.
3. Discuss the adverse effects of ocular trauma.
4. Describe the various forms of infection of the eye and define conjunctivitis, keratitis, and endophthalmitis.
5. Describe the adverse effects of arterial hypertension and diabetes on the eye.
6. Describe the pathogenesis of glaucoma and its effect on vision.
7. Discuss the significance of cataracts.
8. Discuss eye tumors, with special emphasis on retinoblastoma and melanoma.

The visual system consists of the eye, the optic nerve, the optic nerve pathways, and the visual centers in the occipital lobe of the brain.

NORMAL ANATOMY AND PHYSIOLOGY

The eyes are the primary organs of vision (Figure 22-1). Each eyeball (the *globe* or *bulbus*) is located within the bony orbit of the skull, which provides protection and support from the posterior side. On the anterior side, the eyes are protected by the eyelids. The lacrimal glands, which are also located in the bony orbit, secrete tears, which keep the anterior surface of the eye, the cornea, and the sclera moist. Tears also contain antibacterial substances and protect the eye from infections. The extraocular muscles attached to the posterior and lateral sides of the globe make eye movement possible.

The globes are composed of three layers: (1) the fibrous layer, called the *sclera;* (2) the vascular layers, which are composed of three distinct parts: *choroid, ciliary body,* and *iris;* and (3) the inner layer called the *retina,* which is composed of pigmented and neural cells. On the anterior side, the sclera extends into the *cornea,* a translucent layer that allows the passage of light into the inside of the globe. The external surface of the cornea and sclera are covered with a thin, translucent layer called the *conjunctiva,* which covers the inside of the eyelids. The space behind the cornea is called the *anterior eye chamber.* Posteriorly this space is delimited by the lens and the iris. The lens is attached laterally by ligaments to the smooth muscles of the ciliary body. The space behind the lens, called the *vitreous cavity,* is filled with a gelatinous, clear, vitreous body. The posterior wall of the globe is multilayered. The innermost layer is the retina, lying on the uvea, which in turn is attached to the sclera. The neural part of the retina is composed of photoreceptor, bipolar, and ganglionic neurons. The axons of the ganglionic neurons form the optic nerve, which exits the eye posteriorly.

All these components of the eye are important directly or indirectly in sustaining the sensory function of the eye—that is, the ability of the eye to receive visual stimuli. The light entering the eye through the anterior side of the globe is refracted through the cornea and the lens. Passing through the vitreous, it reaches the rods and cones of the retina. There are approximately 3 million cones and 100 million rods in the retina. Cones are especially prominent in the central uvea in the center of the retina, which is called the *macula lutea* (in Latin, "yellow spot") because of its yellow color. The fovea is the area of sharpest vision. All parts of the retina can receive light signals except the site at which the optic nerve leaves the globe, called the *blind spot,* or optic disk.

Vision depends on the proper function of all parts of the eye. The cornea, lens, aqueous humor, and vitreous body must be translucent to allow the passage of light. The cornea and the lens must also have a normal shape and be able to accommodate so that rays of light are refracted properly. The lens is kept in place by connective tissue ligaments, which must be firm and resilient to keep the lens in place. The shape of the lens is modified by the contraction of the smooth muscles in the ciliary body. The ciliary body also secretes the aqueous humor, the fluid that fills the anterior eye chamber. The iris contains pigment cells that prevent side entry of light into the globe. The iris can dilate *(mydriasis)* or constrict *(myosis)* under the influence of sympathetic or parasympathetic stimuli, respectively.

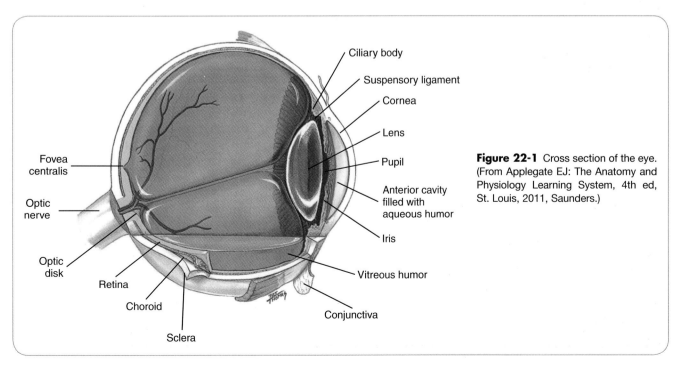

Figure 22-1 Cross section of the eye. (From Applegate EJ: The Anatomy and Physiology Learning System, 4th ed, St. Louis, 2011, Saunders.)

TABLE 22-1 Functions of the Major Parts of the Eye

Structure	Function
Sclera	External protection
Cornea	Light refraction
Choroid	Blood supply
Iris	Light absorption and regulation of pupillary width
Ciliary body	Secretion of vitreous fluid; its smooth muscles change the shape of the lens
Lens	Light refraction
Retinal layer	Light receptor that transforms optic signals into nerve impulses
Rods	Means of distinguishing light from dark and perceiving shape and movement
Cones	Color vision
Central fovea	Area of sharpest vision
Macula lutea	Blind spot
External ocular muscles	Movement of the globe
Optic nerve (cranial nerve II)	Transmission of visual information to the brain
Lacrimal glands	Secretion of tears
Eyelid	Eye protection

The most important functions of the various anatomic parts of the eye are listed in Table 22-1.

OVERVIEW OF MAJOR DISEASES

Diseases of the eye are very common. Minor visual problems, such as shortsightedness, are not even considered "true" diseases but rather represent cosmetic defects. Eyeglasses to correct for farsightedness can be bought in drugstores without a prescription. These functional disturbances are not caused by specific pathologic changes in the eye.

Functional eye problems—that is, problems of *refraction*—are treated by optometrists. *Ophthalmologists* (from the Greek *ophthalmos,* meaning "eye") are the medical specialists who treat pathologically altered eyes using sophisticated surgical instruments, laser beams, and medications.

The most important diseases of the eye and its appendages are the following:

- Infections
- Immunologic diseases
- Traumatic lesions
- Circulatory disturbances, including disorders of blood circulation or flow of aqueous humor
- Degenerative diseases, such as cataract
- Neoplasms

Several facts important to an understanding of eye pathology are presented here, before a discussion of specific pathologic entities.

1. *Most functional visual problems do not have a defined pathology.* The most common reason people visit an eye doctor is to get corrective lenses (eyeglasses). One third of the population in the United States wears eyeglasses or contact lenses. Eyeglasses are an efficient means of correcting nearsightedness **(myopia)** or farsightedness **(hyperopia).** An irregular surface of the cornea or the lens may result in uneven refraction of light, leading to **astigmatism,** which can also be corrected with eyeglasses or contact lenses. Farsightedness of old age, or *presbyopia (presbys* meaning "old" in Greek), is thought to be related to the loss of elasticity of the lens in elderly people. The reasons for the high prevalence of refractory abnormalities in younger people are not known. The eyes of affected individuals do not show any pathologic changes.

2. *Eye problems occur at any age, but overall their prevalence increases with advancing age.* **Presbyopia,** the physiologic loss of the capacity for visual accommodation that develops with advancing age, occurs predictably, and essentially all people older than age 60 require glasses for reading. The prevalence of other eye diseases also increases proportionally with age. The most prominent among these diseases are various circulatory disturbances related to atherosclerosis, diabetes mellitus, and hypertension. *Glaucoma,* a disease related to impeded circulation of vitreous fluid, is also very common in elderly people. *Cataracts* (i.e., opacification and blurring of the lens) are another common cause of impaired vision in elderly people. **Age-related macular degeneration (ARMD),** a disease of unknown pathogenesis, leads to a loss of vision as a result of a loss of retinal pigmentary epithelium. Predisposition to ARMD is inherited in about 70% of patients, but external factors, such as smoking, may contribute to its pathogenesis. The diagnosis can be made with an ophthalmoscope, which helps ophthalmologists to identify two forms of the disease: atrophic (nonneovascular) and exudative (neovascular). The proliferation of retinal blood vessels is experimentally treated with inhibitors of vasculogenesis, but in most instances the disease is progressive and incurable, ultimately leading to blindness.

3. *Infections of the eyes and eye appendages are common because the eyes are exposed to the external world.* Eyes are prone to infections with bacteria, viruses, and many other pathogens that reach the eye in droplets by dirt on fingers or dust. Because the lacrimal canals drain into the upper respiratory tract, flulike infections of the nose, mouth, and pharynx often extend into the eye.

4. *Eyes are often affected by allergies.* Various antigens from the external world, such as pollen or organic components of house dust, are readily deposited on the conjunctiva; such substances may evoke an immunoglobulin E (IgE)–mediated type I hypersensitivity reaction. Conjunctivitis is therefore a common feature of hay fever and similar hypersensitivity reactions. Type I hypersensitivity reaction is primarily mediated by histamine released from IgE-stimulated mast cells; accordingly, good results can be obtained by treating these allergic eye diseases with topical antihistaminics in the form of eye droplets. Corticosteroids are used in recalcitrant cases.

5. *Nutritional deficiencies and metabolic disturbances may affect a person's sight.* The best known among the nutritional deficiencies is avitaminosis A, which results in night blindness. In addition, diabetic retinopathy is an important cause of blindness, as mentioned in Chapter 12 (see Figure 12-11).

6. *Blindness, or complete loss of vision, may be caused by many diseases involving the eye, the optic nerve, or the brain.* Blindness is an important health problem. In the United States, 4 of every 1000 persons are blind, but in other parts of the world, blindness is even more common. The most important causes of blindness in the United States are metabolic and developmental anomalies, *eye trauma,* diabetes, glaucoma, and cataracts. ARMD, a poorly understood disease that is diagnosed in 8% of all persons over the age of 80 years, is an important cause of blindness in elderly persons. In parts of Africa, infections with *Mycoplasma trachomatis* and the parasite *Onchocerca volvulus* still cause blindness in millions of people.

7. *Tumors of the inner layers of the eye originate most often from the melanocytes and retinal cells.* Overall, tumors of the eye globe are rare. However, these tumors have unique features because of their location and because they originate from highly specialized cells: the retinal melanocytes and specialized neural cells. Tumors of the cornea are squamous cell carcinomas.

? Did You Know?

Reading in dim light does not damage the eyesight! It is a common misconception that bookish people, especially those who read in inadequately lighted rooms, are at risk of damaging their eyesight. The cause of nearsightedness is not known, nor is the structural basis of shortsightedness understood.

Skin tumors of the lids are 100 times more common than intraocular tumors. These neoplasms, which are usually diagnosed histologically as basal or squamous cell carcinomas, have all the features of histologically identical skin tumors and are not included here. Similarly, tumors of the lacrimal glands are histologically identical to those in the salivary glands and are not discussed here.

? Did You Know?

This congenitally deformed child has only one eye. Because the child resembles a Cyclops, the one-eyed monster of Greek mythology, the disease is called *cyclopia*. Fortunately, such severe malformations are rare.

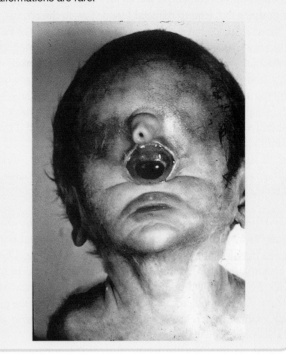

DEVELOPMENTAL DISORDERS

Developmental disorders of the eye may occur in an isolated form and without an obvious cause, or they may be associated with other congenital defects and are part of complex developmental syndromes.

Structural congenital abnormalities of the eyes are common consequences of intrauterine infections with the pathogens that cause the *TORCH* syndrome (*t*oxoplasmosis, *o*ther agents, *r*ubella, *c*ytomegalovirus, and *h*erpesvirus), illustrated in Chapter 5 (see Figure 5-4). Maternal infection during pregnancy with any of these pathogens may result in one-sided or bilateral blindness, *congenital cataracts* (clouding of the lens), or **microphthalmia** (underdeveloped, small bulbus).

Many chromosomal abnormalities are associated with congenital eye abnormalities. The best known are the eye changes in Down's syndrome, which include pigmentary abnormalities of the iris (so-called Brushfield's spots). The eyes are tilted laterally and have a medial palpebral rim known as *epicanthus* (see Figure 5-7). Epicanthus is also seen in fetal alcohol syndrome, discussed in Chapter 5 (see Figure 5-3).

Not all congenital eye defects are as obvious as those described previously. Some are minor cosmetic defects, such as *coloboma,* a slitlike defect in the iris. A *pigmented nevus* of the iris is nothing more than a beauty mark, similar to nevi of the skin.

Retinitis pigmentosa is a generic name for a group of hereditary degenerative diseases affecting the retina. Despite the name retinitis, there is no inflammation of the retina. Instead these diseases are characterized by a progressive loss of retinal photoreceptors, with subsequent accumulation of pigment released from rods and cones within the retina, as well as vascular changes that lead to reduced blood flow to the retina.

Several genes have been identified accounting for retinal degeneration, and thus the disease can be transmitted as an autosomal dominant, autosomal recessive, or sex-linked trait. Although diseases that cause retinal degeneration are inherited, the symptoms, such as night blindness and partial loss of the visual field, typically begin in adulthood. The loss of peripheral vision leads to narrowing of the visual field ("tunnel vision") and even total blindness.

TRAUMA

Eye trauma may be induced mechanically by various objects or chemically by acids, alkali, or metals. Mechanical trauma can be classified as blunt, superficial, or penetrating. Chemical trauma may be classified as irritating or mordant. In some cases the mechanical injury is combined with chemical aftereffects. For example, a small sliver of iron lodged in the globe may oxidize and release potentially dangerous ferric ions, which could propagate the injury.

Blunt trauma usually leads to intraocular hemorrhages. Such hemorrhages typically originate from disrupted small blood vessels. The bleeding from the conjunctiva usually leads to hematoma of the cornea, which is clearly visible on the white background on which it has occurred. Intraocular hematomas that are not readily recognized on external examination are typically reported by the patient as reddish blurring of the vision. Such hematomas can be documented by ophthalmoscopy.

Hemorrhages behind the retina, called retroretinal hemorrhages, are especially dangerous because they typically cause blindness. Retroretinal hemorrhages are characteristically found in battered children. In such cases the bleeding occurs when the child's head is forcefully shaken by an adult. Histologic confirmation of retroretinal hemorrhage is important for legal documentation of battered child syndrome.

Superficial trauma causes minor defects on the eye surface, such as **corneal abrasion.** Typically, the trauma is caused by a sharp object (knife, needle), by scratching, or by a foreign body (speck of dust). The lesion presents with pain, redness of the cornea, and tearing. Healing occurs in most cases, but occasionally scarring may be an important late complication.

Penetrating trauma of the eye, usually inflicted with a sharp object such as a knife or screwdriver, punctures the globe. Because of the loss of intraocular fluid, the bulbus collapses and the eye may be irreparably damaged. Infections are important late complications.

Chemical trauma usually damages the cornea and sclera. Superficial ulcerations are prone to infection but may heal without consequence. Scarring is an important complication of severe chemical burns of the cornea. Such injury may necessitate corneal transplantation.

INFECTIONS

Infections of the eye are common and are designated according to the anatomic structure involved (Figure 22-2). Fortunately, most infections are superficial and limited to the conjunctiva and eyelids. Endophthalmitis, an infection of the inside of the eye that is usually a complication of trauma, is rare.

Conjunctivitis (*"pinkeye"*), an infection of the conjunctiva lining the anterior side of the globe and the inside of the palpebrae, is a very common disease. It is usually caused by viruses, most often adenoviruses, which also cause upper

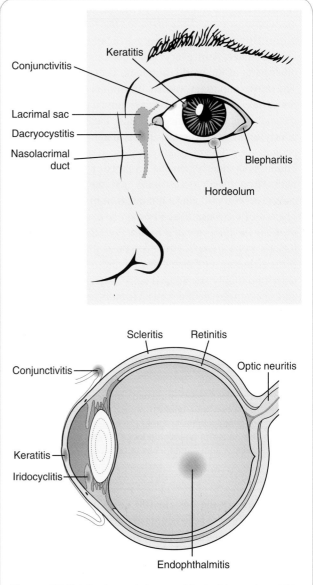

Figure 22-2 Infections of the eye: blepharitis, conjunctivitis, keratitis, dacryocystitis, iridocyclitis, and endophthalmitis.

respiratory tract infections. The inflamed eye shows marked redness as a result of active hyperemia, often accompanied by watery discharge. Viral conjunctivitis is highly contagious and may spread by hand to eye inoculation or close contact. The disease heals spontaneously, or it may respond to local antibiotic treatment. Bacterial infections may be superimposed on viral conjunctivitis, or they may occur on their own. Bacteria causing such infection usually include *Staphylococcus aureus* and *Streptococcus pneumoniae,* but conjunctivitis may be caused by any other pathogen. Bacterial conjunctivitis is characterized by redness of the eye and a purulent discharge, which may cause the eyelids to stick together. Purulent discharge should always be cultured and the infection then treated with appropriate antibiotics to prevent serious complications resulting from extensive ulceration of the cornea or the entry of infection into the bulbus.

Conjunctival inflammation may spread to adjacent structures. For example, it may involve the lacrimal glands **(dacryocystitis). Stye,** or **hordeolum,** is a suppurative inflammation involving the glands of the eyelids. Inflammation of the eyelids **(blepharitis)** results in edema and redness of the eyelids and may be so severe that the patient cannot open the eyes.

Keratitis develops when an infection extends into the cornea or when conjunctivitis presents as an ulcerating disease. In the United States this is usually a feature of herpesvirus infection. Herpesvirus initially causes corneal vesicles, which ulcerate and then are covered with crusts. These lesions heal but may cause permanent defects in the form of scars.

Trachoma is a conjunctivitis caused by *Chlamydia trachomatis;* it is prevalent in underdeveloped countries of Africa and Asia. Worldwide it is the leading infectious cause of blindness, affecting more than 80 million people. The infection is typically associated with corneal ulcers and scarring. Blindness is an important late complication in such cases.

Keratitis, uveitis, and retinitis are uncommon complications of superficial eye infections that have extended into the deeper layers of the eye. Nevertheless, they are a component of some chronic infectious diseases, such as syphilis. The infection may involve the entire eye **(panophthalmitis),** or it may be localized to the inside of the eye **(endophthalmitis).** In many cases, only part of the globe inside is involved. For example, inflammation of the uveal tract can involve the entire structure **(uveitis)** or only one part and thus may be limited to the iris and ciliary body **(iridocyclitis).**

All eye infections require prompt treatment because they may cause loss of eyesight. Superficial infections have a good prognosis; however, ulcerating infections and those involving the deeper layers of the eye may result in blindness.

 Did You Know?

Pinkeye can be treated efficiently with nonprescription eye drops. Treatment should not be indiscriminate, however. Indeed, no treatment is usually the best treatment because pinkeye is most often caused by viruses, which do not respond to antibiotics. Bacterial infections, which can be treated with antibiotics, are less common. Allergy is a common but treatable cause of pinkeye.

IMMUNOLOGIC DISEASE

Infectious diseases of the eye must be distinguished from allergies, which often present with the same clinical symptoms:

- *Type I hypersensitivity reaction* is the cause of allergic conjunctivitis, an itchy superficial inflammation that responds well to antihistamines and steroid treatment.
- *Type III hypersensitivity reactions* involving the ciliary body or the choroid are occasionally found in patients with systemic lupus erythematosus.
- *Type IV hypersensitivity reactions* (i.e., granulomas of the eye bulbus) are rare. The prototypical disease of this type is sarcoidosis, a systemic disease of unknown etiology. In the eye it usually presents with granulomas of the lacrimal glands.

CIRCULATORY DISORDERS

The delicate, thin-walled blood vessels of the eye are susceptible to damage caused by circulatory disorders associated with several systemic diseases. Most notable among these are hypertension and diabetes.

HYPERTENSIVE RETINOPATHY

Sustained arterial hypertension or sudden bouts of arterial hypertension may damage retinal and choroidal blood vessels and cause damage on the eye background. Such arteriolar changes are readily diagnosed as **hypertensive retinopathy** by fundoscopy using an ophthalmoscope (Figure 22-3). The extent of the changes can be graded on a scale from I to IV as mild, moderate, advanced, or severe, respectively. Prolonged hypertension, which is typically associated with arteriosclerosis, leads to reactive narrowing of the retinal arterioles. On ophthalmoscopic examination, such arterioles appear like copper wires. As the blood flow diminishes because of increasing arteriolar constriction, the arterioles become whitish, like silver wires. Elevated blood pressure leads to formation of microaneurysms and hemorrhages into the retinal nerve fiber layer, known as *dot and flame-shaped hemorrhages.* Exudates, known as hard exudates, soft exudates, macular star, and cotton-wool spots, are also found. In severe hypertensive retinopathy there is edema of the optic disk **(papilledema).** Because these changes are irreversible, it is clearly advisable to prevent them by treating the underlying hypertension rather than to wait passively until the retina has been damaged irreparably.

DIABETIC RETINOPATHY

Diabetes mellitus is one of the major causes of blindness in the United States. Diabetes affects the eye in several ways, most notably by promoting the formation of cataracts and by causing diabetic retinopathy.

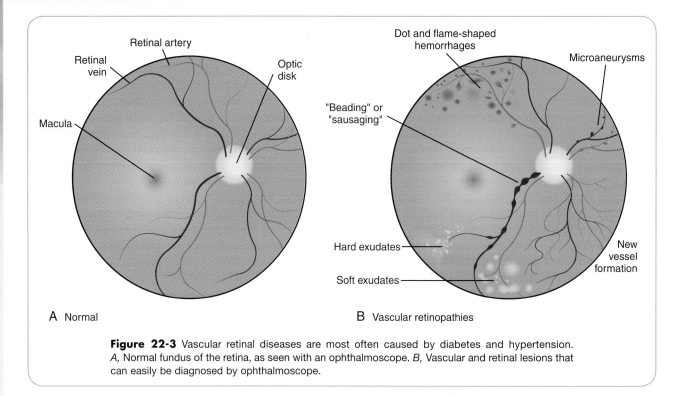

Figure 22-3 Vascular retinal diseases are most often caused by diabetes and hypertension. *A,* Normal fundus of the retina, as seen with an ophthalmoscope. *B,* Vascular and retinal lesions that can easily be diagnosed by ophthalmoscope.

Pathology

Diabetic retinopathy occurs in two forms: background and proliferative retinopathy. Both forms of diabetic retinopathy can be explained in terms of changes in the basement membrane of the arterioles and capillaries of the choroid and retina. Diabetic microangiopathy manifests either as a narrowing of the vascular lumina or as focal dilation and formation of microaneurysms (Figure 22-4). The diabetic blood vessels are more permeable than normal vessels, which leads to edema and hemorrhages into the eye *(background retinopathy)*. Such serous exudates are recognized on fundoscopy as cotton-wool spots. Ischemia secondary to vascular changes results in degenerative changes and fibrous streaks. Reperfusion of ischemic areas is accomplished by neovascularization *(proliferative retinopathy)*. In severe forms of the disease, there is retroretinal fibrosis and retinal detachment, typically associated with blindness.

GLAUCOMA

Glaucoma is a term used to describe several eye diseases characterized by increased intraocular pressure and leading to atrophy of the optic nerve and retinal ganglion cells with consequent loss of peripheral and central visual fields. It is very common, affecting 1% to 3% of all people older than 40 years. Early diagnosis and treatment can prevent progression of ocular changes and blindness.

Pathophysiology

Glaucoma is related to disturbances in the formation and circulation of the intraocular fluid. Under normal circumstances the aqueous humor is secreted by the ciliary body into the posterior chamber. From there it moves into the anterior chamber, passing through a narrow space delimited anteriorly by the iris and posteriorly by the lens and the zonular ligaments that hold the lens in place. From the anterior chamber, the fluid is resorbed into the small veins at the anterolateral margin of the iris. In glaucoma the flow of fluid is disrupted, with the result that it accumulates inside the globe, causing intraocular hypertension.

Pathology

Glaucoma is considered primary when it occurs without any obvious cause. It is classified as secondary when it is related to a preexisting eye disease, such as iridocyclitis, intraocular hemorrhage, trauma, or tumors. Primary glaucoma is more common than the secondary form of this disease.

Primary glaucoma may be pathogenetically classified into two subtypes: open-angle and closed-angle glaucoma (Figure 22-5). The etiology of primary open-angle glaucoma, the most common form of disease, is unknown. As implied by its name, the angle of the anterior chamber through which the aqueous humor is resorbed is open. The disease develops insidiously and is characterized by a progressive, slowly evolving elevation of intraocular pressure. This can be measured using an ophthalmic tonometer

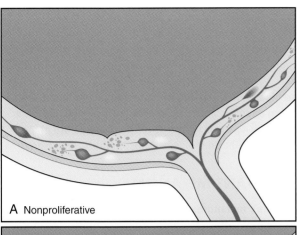

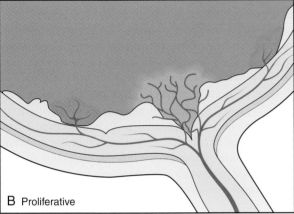

Figure 22-4 Diabetic retinopathy. *A,* Nonproliferative retinopathy shows edema, microaneurysm, and exudates. *B,* Proliferative retinopathy shows new blood vessel formation.

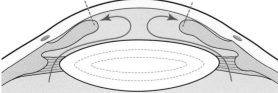

Figure 22-5 Glaucoma. *A,* In open-angle glaucoma the obstruction occurs in the trabecular meshwork. *B,* In closed-angle glaucoma the trabecular meshwork is covered by the root of the iris or adhesions between the iris and the cornea.

applied to the anterior side of the eye globe. There are no obvious histologic abnormalities, and the reasons for impeded resorption of aqueous humor are not known. If left untreated, the disease leads to optic nerve and retinal atrophy and blindness. Although the disease is bilateral, one eye is usually affected to a greater degree than the other.

 Did You Know?

Sharp pain that is typical of acute closed-angle glaucoma most often occurs in dim light. As the pupil dilates in response to dim light, the iris folds, closing the lateral angle of the anterior chamber and impeding the outflow of aqueous humor from the eye. The sharp rise in intraocular pressure may cause sudden blindness and pain.

Primary closed-angle glaucoma is characterized by a visible obstruction of the angle, typically produced by the iris during contraction. This form of glaucoma often presents with an acute onset of intraocular pain and loss of vision and redness of the eye. The intraocular pressure is elevated but only during the attacks.

Glaucoma is, in most cases, a slowly progressive disease. It causes loss of peripheral sight, which often remains unnoticed by the patient. The diagnosis is made by measuring the intraocular pressure. Early diagnosis and treatment are essential for preventing irreversible eye lesions. Glaucoma can be medically treated with drugs that decrease the production of aqueous humor or reduce intraocular pressure. If left untreated, glaucoma leads to blindness.

CATARACT

Cataract, an opacification or clouding of the crystalline lens of the eye, is the most common cause of decreased vision in the United States. However, cataracts also represent one of the most successfully treated chronic eye ailments. More than 1 million cataracts are removed surgically every year.

On the basis of etiology, cataracts can be classified as either senile or secondary:

- *Senile cataracts* are the most common form. Approximately 60% of all people older than age 70 have some evidence of clouding of the lens. It is considered a disease of aging that has no obvious causes except for wear-and-tear of the material that makes up the lens.
- *Secondary cataracts* are the result of lens opacification that is a consequence of trauma, inflammation, or radiation injury. Metabolic diseases, such as diabetes, also predispose individuals to cataracts. Some secondary cataracts are congenital and are found in infants.

Cataracts usually develop slowly over years. Patients typically complain of blurry vision. As the disease progresses, the visual acuity diminishes and eventually the vision may be lost

481

entirely. The symptoms depend on the extent of changes and their location in the lens. Axial opacities—that is, those affecting the nucleus of the lens or the central subscapular area—are more troublesome than peripheral opacities.

Early cataracts are readily diagnosed only on the basis of an ophthalmoscopic examination. As the cataract "matures," the lens becomes progressively more cloudy and the cataract becomes visible by naked eye inspection. Surgical removal of the cataract usually improves the patient's vision, but the patient will require glasses or contact lenses.

NEOPLASMS

Except for skin tumors of the eyelids, all other neoplasms of the eye are rare. The most common intraocular tumors are retinoblastoma and malignant melanoma. The incidence of retinoblastoma is 1:20,000 children, whereas the incidence of intraocular melanoma is 4:100,000 adults. Lymphomas are the most common retrobulbar neoplasms.

RETINOBLASTOMA

Retinoblastoma is a rare tumor, but still it is the most common malignant eye tumor of infancy and childhood, accounting for approximately 3% of all malignant childhood tumors. Nevertheless, it has generated considerable interest among researchers for several reasons. In approximately 5% of cases, the tumor is hereditary. In approximately 25% of sporadic cases and almost all hereditary forms, the retinoblastoma is bilateral. All these facts were instrumental in the discovery of

the retinoblastoma suppressor gene *(RB),* the first tumor suppressor gene that was fully characterized.

Retinoblastomas grow as intraocular masses that ultimately fill the entire globe and extend into the optic nerve (Figure 22-6). Clinically the tumor is recognized as a white pupil. Vision progressively deteriorates until it is lost. If untreated, retinoblastoma is almost always lethal, but with modern therapy, more than 90% of affected children survive. Long-term survivors of retinoblastoma are at a risk for developing other neoplasms, most notably, osteosarcoma.

MALIGNANT MELANOMA

Malignant melanomas are the most common primary intraocular tumors affecting adults. Tumors originate from the pigmentary cells of the uveal tract (i.e., the iris, ciliary body, or choroid). The tumors grow as pigmented masses and ultimately fill the entire globe. If diagnosed early and treated adequately, they have a good prognosis, especially if the tumor is composed of spindle cells. Tumors composed of nonspindle cells with areas of necrosis and high mitotic activity have a less favorable outcome. Spindle cell melanomas of the iris tend to grow slowly and are amenable to local resection. Because the eye has no lymphatics, metastases of ocular melanomas are hematogenous. For unknown reasons, the liver is one of the most common metastatic sites. Malignant melanomas of the choroid usually require removal of the entire globe (enucleation). Approximately 80% of patients undergoing enucleation of an eye involved by malignant melanoma survive 5 years. The cumulative mortality at 10 years is 40%, increasing 1% every year thereafter.

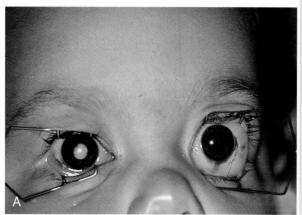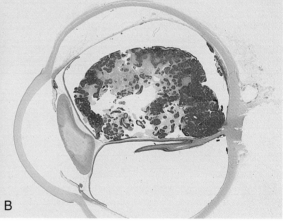

Figure 22-6 Retinoblastoma. *A,* The tumor occupies a large portion of the inside of the eye bulbus. *B,* Histologically, the tumor is composed of cells resembling fetal retinal cells ("retinoblasts"). (From Damjanov I, Linder J: Pathology: A Color Atlas, St. Louis, 2000, Mosby.)

REVIEW QUESTIONS

1. What is the function of the sclera, cornea, choroid, iris, ciliary body, lens, and retina?

2. Compare myopia with hyperopia.

3. What is presbyopia?

4. How do metabolic and circulatory disorders affect the eyes?

5. What causes microphthalmia?

6. What is retinitis pigmentosa?

7. Describe the effects of trauma on the eyes.

8. What are the causes of pinkeye?

9. Compare conjunctivitis, keratitis, and iridocyclitis.

10. Describe the pathology of hypertensive and diabetic retinopathy.

11. What is glaucoma, and what are its causes?

12. Compare open-angle and closed-angle glaucoma.

13. What are cataracts?

14. Compare senile and secondary cataracts.

15. List two of the most important eye neoplasms.

16. What is retinoblastoma?

17. What is ocular malignant melanoma?

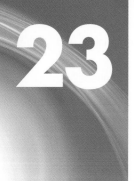

23 The Ear

Chapter Outline

NORMAL ANATOMY AND PHYSIOLOGY
OVERVIEW OF MAJOR DISEASES
   Diseases of the External Ear
   Diseases of the Middle Ear
      Otitis Media
      Otosclerosis

Diseases of the Inner Ear
   Ménière's Disease
Deafness
   Classification

Key Terms and Concepts

Ceruminous plug
Cholesteatoma
Deafness
Ménière's disease
Otitis externa

Otitis media
Otosclerosis
Perforation of the tympanic
   membrane

Presbycusis
Vertigo

Learning Objectives

After reading this chapter, the student should be able to:

1. Describe the normal anatomy and physiology of the ear.
2. List the most common diseases involving the external ear.
3. Discuss the causes and the symptoms of otitis media.
4. Discuss the causes and pathogenesis of vertigo.
5. Discuss the causes of deafness.

NORMAL ANATOMY AND PHYSIOLOGY

The ears are the primary auditory organs. Each ear consists of three major anatomic parts: the external ear, the middle ear, and the inner ear (Figure 23-1).

The external ear consists of the cartilaginous auricle or *pina* and the external auditory canal. The auricle is attached to the lateral side of the head. It is composed of elastic cartilage covered by skin. Its main function is to collect the sound waves and direct them toward the eardrum, which is located on the internal side of the auditory canal. The auditory canal is an extension of the auricle that forms as an S-shaped tube inside the temporal bone of the skull. The auditory tube ends blindly at the tympanic membrane, which separates it from the middle ear.

The middle ear consists primarily of the air-filled tympanic cavity, which is laterally delimited by the tympanic membrane and medially delimited by the partially fenestrated petrous bone. The openings on the petrous bone are known as the *oval window* and the *round window*. The oval window separates the middle ear from the semicircular canals. Three middle ear ossicles (malleus, incus, and stapes) represent a link between the tympanic membrane and the semicircular canals. These ossicles are essential for the transmission of sound impulses.

The inner ear comprises the osseus and the membranous labyrinth. The membranous labyrinth, which is filled with endolymph, is enclosed by the bone that forms the chambers of the osseous labyrinth. The inner ear has three parts: the vestibule; the semicircular canals, which are organs of equilibrium; and the *cochlea*, which is the primary auditory organ. The inner ear is linked to cranial nerve VIII, which transmits the signals from the cochlea, vestibule, and semicircular canals to the auditory centers in the temporal lobes of the brain.

OVERVIEW OF MAJOR DISEASES

Diseases of the ear are very important because they impair hearing and can cause deafness. Hearing is essential for many social activities, and loss of hearing can impair the normal social interaction of affected persons and their function in society. Loss of the sense of equilibrium may also be incapacitating.

Diseases of the ear are treated by specialists known as *ear-nose-throat (ENT) surgeons* or *otorhinolaryngologists*.

The most important diseases affecting the ear are the following:
- Diseases of the auditory canal
- Otitis media
- Disturbances of the sense of equilibrium
- Deafness

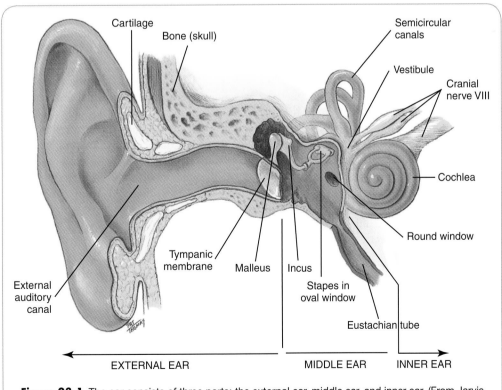

Figure 23-1 The ear consists of three parts: the external ear, middle ear, and inner ear. (From Jarvis C: Physical Examination and Health Assessment, 5th ed, Philadelphia, 2008, Saunders.)

Several facts important to an understanding of ear pathology are presented here, before a discussion of specific pathologic entities:

1. *The external ear is covered with skin and thus is affected by the same diseases that occur on the skin.* External ear allergies, infections, and tumors are indistinguishable from those on other parts of the face. In other words, the skin covering the outer ear has no unique features. Infection of the cartilage of the ear lobes is rare.

2. *The shape of the external ear varies in human populations.* Some people have small ears, whereas others have disproportionately large ears. Ear dimensions and shapes may be of importance to cosmetic surgeons, but they have no significance in terms of auditory functions of the ear.

3. *The external auditory canal contains ceruminous glands that secrete cerumen, a greasy substance also known as earwax.* **Ceruminous plug** may occlude the auditory canal, causing temporary deafness. Impacted earwax can easily be removed by nurses or physicians. If patients attempt removal themselves, using forceps or some other instrument, the eardrum could be perforated or unnecessary irritation of the ear could result.

4. *The tympanic membrane serves as a resonator for sound while also protecting the middle ear.* Rupture of the tympanic membrane can be caused by ear picking with a sharp instrument or barotrauma from increased pressure or an explosion or can occur after a purulent inflammation. Such holes will impair hearing. The defect in the tympanic membrane also facilitates the entry of bacteria into the middle ear, predisposing the individual to recurrent infections.

5. *The ear is connected to the nasopharynx by the eustachian tube.* The function of this tube is to equalize the pressure in the middle ear cavity with the pressure of the outer world. At the same time, this anatomic passageway may serve as a conduit for the spread of infections from the nasopharynx into the middle ear. Otitis media, an infection of the middle ear, is therefore a common complication of upper respiratory tract infections.

6. *The auditory ossicles in the middle ear function properly only if mobile.* The malleus, incus, and stapes are tiny ossicles that transmit the sound vibrations of the tympanic membrane to the oval window of the semicircular canals. If one or all of the ossicles become immobile (sclerotic), as in **otosclerosis,** their function is lost, resulting in deafness.

7. *The function of the semicircular canals is to process stimuli that are essential for the maintenance of equilibrium.* Diseases involving this part of the inner ear result in **vertigo** (i.e., a sensation of whirling motion or rotation and dizziness).

8. *Diseases of the ear, cranial nerve VIII, or the auditory centers in the brain may cause deafness.* There are several forms of deafness, and it is up to the ENT physician or an audiologist to determine the site of injury.

9. *Tumors of the middle ear and inner ear are rare.* Although neoplasms may arise in the middle and inner ear, or cranial nerve VIII, these lesions are uncommon. Nevertheless, acoustic neuromas of cranial nerve VIII account for most tumor-related hearing losses.

DISEASES OF THE EXTERNAL EAR

Diseases of the external ear can be caused by trauma, infection, or allergies. Tumors also occur in the external ear.

Trauma of the ear may result in rupture, hematoma, or complete loss *(avulsion)* of the earlobe. Major laceration of the ear or repeated hematoma caused by boxing can result in a deformity known as a *cauliflower ear.*

Infection of the outer ear is called **otitis externa** (Figure 23-2). It may be caused by bacteria, viruses (e.g., herpesvirus), or fungi. Infection of the external auditory canal, called *swimmer's ear,* is a well-known disease affecting athletes who spend long hours in water.

Allergic otitis externa is most often found in children suffering from atopic dermatitis (eczema). Contact dermatitis in the external ear canal may develop as a result of hypersensitivity to hearing aids. Contact dermatitis of the earlobe may be caused by earrings.

Tumors are usually found on the auricles of elderly persons. Histologically, such tumors are typically squamous cell or basal cell carcinomas, resembling those from other sun-exposed dermal sites.

DISEASES OF THE MIDDLE EAR

Like the diseases of the external ear, diseases of the middle ear may be related to trauma or infection. Allergies and tumors are less important. Some middle ear diseases, such as otosclerosis, are considered idiopathic because their cause is unknown.

Perforation of the tympanic membrane is the most important consequence of middle ear trauma. The tympanic membrane may rupture as a result of direct injury with a sharp object (e.g., a toothpick used to remove impacted cerumen), high-pitch acoustic trauma, barotrauma secondary to high air pressure caused by an explosion, or infections. Small defects usually heal spontaneously. Infection prevents healing and may result in deafness. In many cases the defects can be repaired by microsurgery.

OTITIS MEDIA

Otitis media, inflammation of the middle ear, occurs in two forms: acute or chronic infection. *Acute otitis media* typically results from viral upper respiratory tract infection involving the nasopharynx (Figure 23-2). The disease most often involves children in daycare settings, especially those who suffer from allergies. Such infection causes edema of the eustachian tube with subsequent obstruction of the tube and accumulation of fluid in the inner ear, termed *serous otitis media.* Bacterial superinfection may transform it into purulent otitis media.

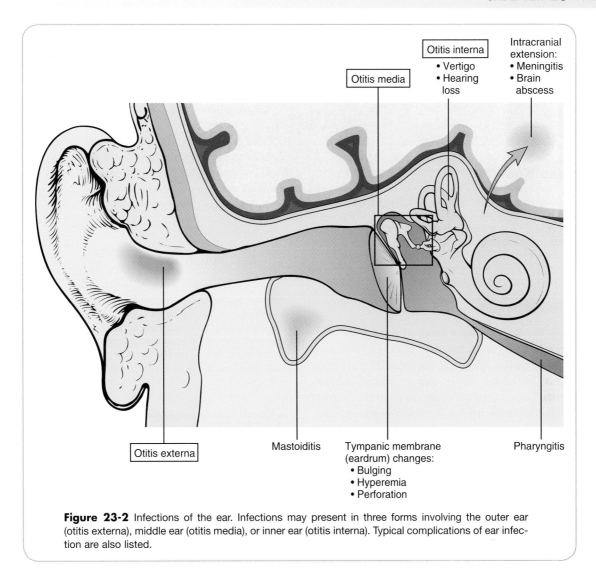

Figure 23-2 Infections of the ear. Infections may present in three forms involving the outer ear (otitis externa), middle ear (otitis media), or inner ear (otitis interna). Typical complications of ear infection are also listed.

The patient often complains of ear pain and hearing loss. The ear is typically sensitive to touch. On otoscopic examination the tympanic membrane appears red and bulging; if left untreated, it may perforate. In such cases, pus pours out of the ear canal. Bacterial otitis media usually responds well to antibiotic treatment. *Tympanocentesis*—that is, puncture of the tympanic membrane with a needle to drain the exudate—may occasionally be indicated in resistant cases. Insertion of plastic tubes into the narrow eustachian tubes is used to surgically prevent recurrent bouts of otitis media.

Complications of acute purulent otitis media include chronic otitis media and extension of the infection into the mastoid (mastoiditis), the inner ear, or the brain.

Chronic otitis media is usually a consequence of recurrent acute infections, but it also may follow traumatic rupture of the tympanic membrane. Clinically, the hallmark of the disease is a chronic purulent ear discharge. The disease is accompanied by chronic pain and loss of hearing. The tympanic membrane is usually ruptured or entirely missing. Treatment is directed at eradicating the bacterial infection.

After resolution of the infection, the eardrum and the middle ear structures can be reconstructed surgically.

Cholesteatoma, an epidermal inclusion cyst, is a common complication of chronic otitis media. This tumorlike growth results from invagination of the squamous epidermis, which grows from the auditory canal through the defect of the tympanic membrane into the middle ear and the mastoid bone. The epidermis forms keratin layers, which accumulate in the lumen of the cyst and resemble pearly white material. Cholesteatoma is treated surgically.

 Did You Know?

At least 50% of all children ages 1 to 3 years have a middle ear effusion once a year. In most cases the effusion regresses on its own, and few children develop serious ear infections.

Glue ear is a special form of nonbacterial chronic otitis media. A consequence of acute otitis in children, it is characterized by a persistent viscous effusion in the middle ear cavity. At least 5 of every 1000 children younger than 5 years are treated surgically for this condition. The treatment often includes insertion of grommets or plastic tubes into the eustachian tubes or adenoidectomy to improve the drainage of fluids from the middle ear.

 Did You Know?

Vertigo is a common complaint, and one should not immediately consider it to be a sign of inner ear disease. Vertigo may be induced by alcohol and is a typical feature of motion sickness, height sickness, or seasickness.

OTOSCLEROSIS

Otosclerosis is the most common cause of conductive hearing loss in middle-aged Americans. This disease of unknown etiology is inherited as an autosomal dominant trait, affecting approximately 10% of all whites and 1% of all African Americans in the United States. The incidence of otosclerosis is two times more common among women than among men.

The disease affects both ears, although one ear usually incurs more damage than the other. Pathologically it is characterized by the deposition of newly formed bone on both sides of the oval window. The sclerotic bone first encases the foot of the stapes, impeding its movements. As the otosclerosis progresses, the entire stapes is replaced by new bone. Treatment involves stapedectomy, or removal of the sclerotic stapes, and replacement of the sclerotic stapes by a plastic prosthesis.

DISEASES OF THE INNER EAR

MÉNIÈRE'S DISEASE

Ménière's disease is a condition of unknown etiology that affects adults. Its peak incidence is in those who are 30 to 60 years of age. The overall prevalence of this disease is not known, but estimates indicate that it affects up to 5% of all adults.

The disease is associated with hydrops of the endolymphatic system of the cochlea. Clinically it presents with the following triad:
1. Episodic vertigo that lasts 1 hour to several hours, typically subsiding but then recurring after a few hours or days
2. Sensorineural hearing loss for low-frequency sound
3. Tinnitus, or ringing in the ears

The cause of increased endolymphatic pressure is not known, but a low-salt diet and diuretic therapy, aimed at lowering endolymphatic pressure, may yield good results.

The diagnosis of Ménière's disease requires that other causes of vertigo be excluded. The differential diagnosis includes the following:
- Viral labyrinthitis, which usually follows upper respiratory tract infections
- Post-traumatic vertigo, which is typically a consequence of head trauma
- Vertigo related to migraine and other functional diseases that are not associated with inner ear pathology
- Central vertigo related to diseases of brain such as brain tumors, multiple sclerosis, or strokes

 Did You Know?

Noise monitoring in the workplace has been instituted by governmental regulatory agencies to prevent hearing loss secondary to noise trauma. All sounds exceeding 85 dB are potentially harmful to the cochlea. As an example, at takeoff, jet engines have a loudness of 150 dB. Thus earplugs and protective gear should be worn while working on the tarmac.

DEAFNESS

Deafness, or hearing loss, is a very common disease with multiple causes (Figure 23-3). Approximately 12% to 14% of people older than 65 years suffer from hearing loss, but many younger adults have a hearing loss for high-pitched tones. Approximately 2 to 3 per 1000 newborns are born deaf, indicating that hearing loss is not restricted to old age.

CLASSIFICATION

Conductive Hearing Loss

Conductive hearing loss is caused by external or middle ear lesions. In the auditory canal the cause of hearing loss may be obstruction, such as with impacted cerumen *(ceruminous plug)*. Additionally, loss of the tympanic membrane or its perforation by trauma or infection also causes conductive hearing loss. Effusion in the middle ear, cholesteatoma, or hemorrhage into the middle ear cavity can all lead to hearing loss. Otosclerosis causes deafness by impeding the transmission of signals from the tympanic membrane to the oval window.

Sensory Hearing Loss

Sensory hearing loss results from cochlear abnormalities. Noise trauma at the workplace is an important cause of sensory hearing loss. Ototoxic drugs, such as streptomycin, antimalarial drugs, and certain diuretics, may also cause deafness. **Presbycusis,** hearing loss of unknown etiology that affects elderly people, is also classified as a sensory defect.

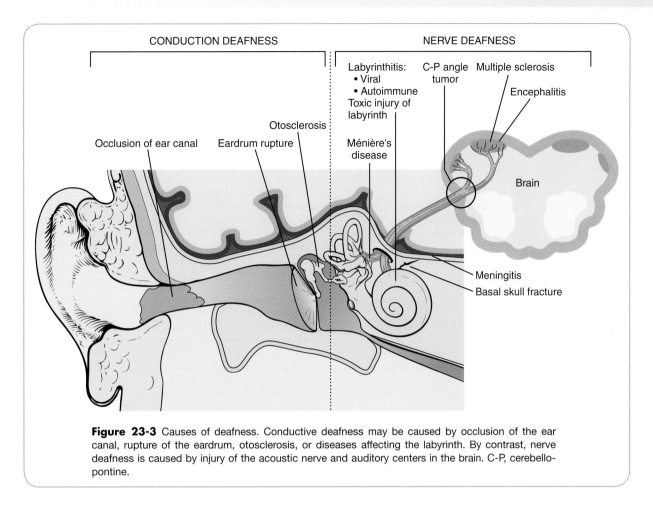

Figure 23-3 Causes of deafness. Conductive deafness may be caused by occlusion of the ear canal, rupture of the eardrum, otosclerosis, or diseases affecting the labyrinth. By contrast, nerve deafness is caused by injury of the acoustic nerve and auditory centers in the brain. C-P, cerebellopontine.

Neural Hearing Loss

Neural hearing loss results from lesions of cranial nerve VIII or of the central nervous system. This is the least common form of hearing loss. Typical causes include neuromas of cranial nerve VIII, multiple sclerosis, and cerebrovascular accidents.

The diagnosis of deafness is based on clinical data but must be documented by audiologic techniques. Some causes of hearing loss can be treated surgically, whereas others require the use of permanent hearing aids.

REVIEW QUESTIONS

1. Describe the principal anatomic components of the external, middle, and inner ear.

2. What are the main functions of the ear?

3. List the most important diseases of the external ear.

4. List the most important diseases of the middle ear.

5. Compare the clinical features of acute and chronic otitis media.

6. What is cholesteatoma?

7. What is otosclerosis?

8. What is Ménière's disease?

9. Compare the clinical findings of conductive, sensory, and neural deafness.

Glossary

abortion Interruption of pregnancy; may be spontaneous or induced.

abscess A localized collection of pus.

acetylcholine A direct-acting cholinergic neurotransmitter found at nerve endings and also at the neuromuscular junction.

achalasia Failure of the lower esophageal sphincter to relax leading to proximal dilation of the entire esophagus.

achondroplasia Genetic dwarfism caused by a mutation of fibroblast growth factor receptor 3; characterized by abnormal endochondral ossification and thwarted growth of long bones.

acne An inflammatory skin disease involving the hair follicles and sebaceous glands.

acquired immunodeficiency syndrome (AIDS) A systemic disease caused by the human immunodeficiency virus (HIV)

acromegaly Abnormal enlargement of the terminal parts of the extremities, jaws, and nose caused by an excess of growth hormone.

actinic keratosis A thickening and scaling of the skin as a result of prolonged sun exposure can affect neonates or adults and is also known as *adrenal virilism.*

acute respiratory distress syndrome (ARDS) A form of respiratory failure caused by severe pulmonary alveolar-capillary membrane injury accompanied by pulmonary edema and hyaline membrane formation.

adaptations A change in response to stress or chronic injury.

Addison's disease Adrenocortical insufficiency secondary to destruction of the adrenal glands.

adenocarcinoma A malignant tumor composed of glandular or ductal epithelium.

adenoma A benign tumor composed of glandular or ductal epithelium.

adrenaline A hormone secreted from the adrenal glands in times of stress.

adrenocortical tumor A neoplasm of the cortical part of the adrenal gland.

adrenogenital syndrome A disease caused by hypersecretion of the adrenal sex steroids.

agenesis Developmental disorder in which an organ or structure is not formed.

age-related macular degeneration (ARMD) A group of eye diseases causing irreversible changes in the retina, thus leading to progressive loss of vision in the elderly.

AIDS-related encephalopathy An abnormal condition of the structure or function of brain tissues related to AIDS.

alanine aminotransferase (ALT) An enzyme normally present in the serum and tissues of the body. Its serum concentration is elevated after liver cell injury.

albinism Congenital absence of skin pigmentation.

alcoholic hepatitis An acute toxic liver injury that is brought on by excess alcohol consumption.

alcoholism An extreme dependence on alcohol associated with a pattern of deviant behavior.

aldosterone Adrenal steroid hormone that acts on the renal tubules to retain sodium.

alkaline phosphatase An enzyme that is found in the cell membrane of many cells and is released into serum and body fluids. Its serum concentration is elevated in obstructive jaundice but also in disorders characterized by new bone formation.

allergic rhinitis An immunologically mediated inflammation of nose and nasal passages associated with watery naval discharge and itchiness of eyes and nose.

allografts Transplants between individuals of the same species who are not genetically identical are called homografts or allografts.

alopecia Baldness or loss of hair; may be diffuse or focal.

alpha$_1$-antitrypsin deficiency An autosomal recessive disorder that is related to the presence of the Piz allele of the gene that encodes for α_1-AT. Clinically it presents with emphysema and liver disease.

alpha-fetoprotein (AFP) A protein normally synthesized by the fetal liver and yolk sac. Its serum concentration is elevated in the sera of adults with hepatocellular carcinoma and nonseminomatous germ cell tumors of the testis and in those with yolk sacs containing mixed germ cell tumors of ovaries and extragonadal sites.

Alzheimer's disease A progressive neurologic disease characterized by mental deterioration, including confusion, memory failure, disorientation, restlessness, agnosia, speech disturbances, inability to carry out purposeful movement, and hallucinations.

amenorrhea The absence of menstruation.

amylase An enzyme produced by the pancreas and salivary glands that catalyzes the hydrolysis of starch into simpler compounds. Its serum concentration is elevated in acute pancreatitis and, to a lesser extent, in salivary gland inflammation.

amyloidosis A disease caused by the deposition of amyloid, an aggregate of insoluble fibrillar proteins.

amyotrophic lateral sclerosis (ALS) A degenerative disease of the motor neurons, characterized by weakness and atrophy of the muscles of the hands, forearms, and legs, spreading to involve most of the face and body.

anaphylactic shock A severe and sometimes fatal allergic reaction to a sensitizing substance.

anaphylatoxins Polypeptides derived from complement that mediate the vascular changes in inflammation or anaphylactic shock.

anaphylaxis A form of hypersensitivity (allergic) reaction that is usually mediated by histamine.

anaplasia Abnormal differentiation of cells found in malignant tumors.

anasarca Generalized edema marked by the accumulation of fluid in organs and body cavities.

anastomosis A communication between blood vessels or tubular organs (e.g., the intestines).

androgens A group of male steroid hormones.

anemia A decrease in the number of circulating red blood cells or hemoglobin to below normal levels.

anencephaly A congenital defect characterized by incomplete formation of the cranium and destruction or loss of the brain.

aneurysm A localized dilation of an artery.

aneurysms of the circle of Willis A dilation of the cell wall of a blood vessel in the circle of Willis.

angina pectoris Thoracic pain caused most often by myocardial anorexia as a result of atherosclerosis or spasm of the coronary arteries.

angioblast A blood vessel–forming cell typically found in granulation tissue.

angiodysplasia of the intestines A localized vascular lesion of the colon that may cause unexplained bleeding in elderly persons.

angiogenesis New blood vessel formation as in granulation tissue or in response to tumors.

angiography A radiographic technique for visualizing blood vessels after an injection of contrast medium.

angiosarcoma A malignant tumor of endothelial cells forming blood vessels.

angiotensin A polypeptide in the blood that causes vasoconstriction, increased blood pressure, and the release of aldosterone from the adrenal cortex.

ankylosing spondylitis A chronic inflammatory disease of unknown origin, first affecting the spine and adjacent structures and commonly progressing to eventual fusion of the involved joints.

ankylosis A stiffening and reduced mobility of a joint that has been obliterated by fibrous tissue.

anomaly Marked deviation from the normal; may be congenital or acquired.

anovulatory cycle A menstrual cycle during which the ovaries fail to produce, mature, or release eggs.

anoxia Oxygen deficiency.

anthracosis An accumulation of inhaled coal particle in the lungs.

antibodies Immunoglobulins produced by lymphocytes in response to bacteria, viruses, or other antigenic substances.

antigen Any substance that can induce an immune response of the body; also called *allergen* or *immunogen*.

antigen-presenting cells (APCs) Macrophages and related cells that can break down protein antigens into peptides and present the peptides on the cells of the immune system.

aphtha A superficial mucosal ulceration covered with a thin inflammatory exudate. Aphthae are typical features of aphthous stomatitis.

aplastic anemia A deficiency of all the formed elements of blood.

apoplexy Stroke caused by cerebral hemorrhage or ischemic infarction.

apoptosis Programmed cell death that occurs normally in developing and adult tissues but that can also be induced pathologically by various drugs, toxins, immune cells, or viruses.

appendicitis Inflammation of the appendix.

arachidonic acid A long-chain fatty acid that serves as a precursor of prostaglandins and leukotrienes.

arachnodactyly Spider-like, long, slender fingers and toes (typically found in Marfan's syndrome).

arrhythmia Abnormal heart rhythm.

arteriosclerosis Hardening or calcification of arterial walls, most often representing a complication of atherosclerosis.

arthritis An inflammation of one or more joints; may be infectious or immunologic (as in rheumatoid arthritis).

Arthus phenomenon A type III hypersensitivity reaction to the injection of a foreign substance, typically involving blood vessels.

asbestosis A lung disease caused by the inhalation of asbestos fibers.

ascites An abnormal accumulation of serous fluid in the abdomen, as may occur in end-stage liver disease.

ascorbic acid Vitamin C.

aseptic necrosis of bone (aseptic bone necrosis) A localized death of bone tissue in the absence of an infection.

aspartate aminotransferase (AST) An enzyme normally present in body serum and in certain body tissues. Its serum concentration is elevated after liver cell injury.

aspiration Entry of foreign material into the larynx, trachea, or lungs.

asthma Recurrent allergic pulmonary disease marked by bronchospasm, wheezing, and excessive mucus formation, often but not always caused by hypersensitivity to inhalation antigens.

astigmatism A light refraction disorder of the eye caused by deformity or an irregular surface of the cornea.

astrocytoma A malignant brain, cerebellar, or spinal cord tumor composed of astrocytes.

asymptomatic Devoid of symptoms.

atelectasis Collapse of all or part of a lung; characterized by an absence of air in the pulmonary alveoli.

atheroma The basic lesion of atherosclerosis, characterized by excessive accumulation of lipids in the wall of the aorta and major arteries.

atherosclerosis A systemic arterial disease characterized by an accumulation of lipids, fibrosis, and calcification of the arterial wall.

atopic dermatitis An intensely pruritic, often excoriated inflammation commonly found on the face and antecubital and popliteal areas of allergy-prone individuals.

atresia A congenital absence of a lumen in a tubular organ, such as the intestines or trachea.

atrial myxoma A benign, pedunculated, gelatinous heart tumor that most often occurs in the left atrium.

atrial septal defect A congenital cardiac anomaly characterized by an abnormal opening between the atria.

atrophy A decrease in the size of cells, tissues, or organs.

auscultation A physical examination technique based on listening to the sounds of the heart or the lung with a stethoscope.

autoantibodies An immunoglobulin produced by a person that recognizes an antigen on that person's own tissues.

autoantigen An endogenous body that stimulates the production of autoantibodies and an autoimmune reaction.

autocrine stimulation A stimulation of the effect of a hormone on cells that produce it.

autograft A surgical transplantation of any tissue from one part of the body to another location in the same individual.

autoimmune diseases A large group of diseases characterized by altered function of the immune system of the body.

autoimmune hepatitis A form of chronic immunologically mediated hepatitis.

autolysis Postmortem dissolution and disintegration of cells or tissues by the enzymes present in those tissues.

autophagosome An intracytoplasmic vacuole containing elements of a cell's own cytoplasm.

autosomal dominant inheritance A pattern of inheritance in which the transmission of a dominant allele on an autosome causes a trait to be expressed.

autosomal recessive inheritance A pattern of inheritance resulting from the transmission of a recessive allele on an autosome.

B cells A type of lymphocyte that may differentiate into antibody-producing plasma cells.

bacteremia The presence of bacteria in the blood; also known as *septicemia*.

balanitis An inflammation of the glans penis.

Barrett's esophagus A disorder of the lower esophagus marked by a benign ulcerlike lesion covered with metaplastic, intestine-like columnar epithelium.

basal cell carcinoma A low-grade malignant epithelial tumor of the skin that invades locally but usually does not metastasize.

basophil A white blood cell containing bluish (basophilic) granules filled with histamine; it is a precursor of tissue mast cells.

Becker's dystrophy An X-linked hereditary progressive muscle disease causing progressive muscle cell loss and progressive generalized muscle weakness in adult males carrying a mutation of the dystrophin gene.

benign prostatic hyperplasia (BPH) An enlargement of the prostate of elderly men involving the proliferation of glandular and stromal components of the prostate.

benign tumor A slow-growing tumor composed of well-differentiated cells that does not invade or metastasize, and generally has a good clinical prognosis.

bile duct carcinoma A malignant tumor originating from intrahepatic and extrahepatic bile ducts.

biopsy The removal of a small piece of living tissue from an organ or other part of the body for microscopic examination to confirm or establish a diagnosis, estimate prognosis, or follow the course of a disease.

birth injury Trauma suffered by a baby while being born.

bleeding disorders Pathologic alterations of bleeding; also called *hemorrhagic disorders*.

bleeding tendency Decreased synthesis of coagulation proteins results in a bleeding tendency.

blepharitis Inflammation of the eyelids.

blindness The absence of sight, which may be congenital or, more often, acquired in adult life.

bone marrow A part of the bone composed of fat cells, hematopoietic cells, and fibrous tissue filling the spaces in cancellous bone.

bone mineral density (BMD) test A noninvasive test based on dual-energy x-ray absorptiometry (DEXA scan) used to estimate absolute bone loss caused by osteoporosis.

bradykinin A vasoactive peptide formed during inflammation by the enzyme kallikrein.

BRCA1* and *BRCA2 Symbols for two breast cancer susceptibility genes.

breast carcinoma A group of malignant epithelial tumors of the breast, most of which are classified as invasive ductal or lobular carcinomas.

breast self-examination A procedure in which a woman examines her breasts and their accessory structures for evidence of change that could indicate a malignant process.

bronchiectasis Dilation of bronchi secondary to chronic inflammation.

bronchiolitis An acute viral infection of the small bronchi and bronchioles that occurs primarily in infants younger than 18 months old.

bronchitis An acute or chronic inflammation of the mucous membranes of the bronchi.

bronchopneumonia A form of patchy pneumonia involving the alveoli around the smaller bronchi and bronchioles.

bulla A blister or large skin vesicle.

Burkitt's lymphoma A rapidly growing Epstein-Barr virus–related B-cell lymphoma often involving the jaws and abdominal organs. The endemic form is typically found in children in sub-Saharan Africa, whereas the sporadic form may occur in other parts of the world as well.

cachexia A state of general ill health and poor nutrition that typically occurs in chronic diseases (e.g., cancer).

calcification Deposition of calcium salts in tissue.

calculus A stone or abnormal accumulation of mineral salts that usually forms in the lumen of the gallbladder or urinary tract.

callus New bone formation that occurs during healing of a fracture.

cancer A malignant neoplasm characterized by the uncontrolled growth of anaplastic cells that tend to invade surrounding tissue and to metastasize to distant body sites.

carcinoembryonic antigen (CEA) A glycolipid or glycoprotein antigen released from adenocarcinoma cells into the blood. It is used as a serologic marker in the follow-up of patients treated for adenocarcinoma of the large intestine and other anatomic sites.

carcinogen A substance or agent that causes the development of or increases the incidence of cancer.

carcinoid A low-grade malignant tumor of neuroendocrine cells found mostly in the gastrointestinal and respiratory systems.

carcinoma A malignant tumor composed of epithelial cells.

carcinoma *in situ* A preinvasive form of carcinoma limited to the epithelial layer; most often seen in the skin, cervix of the uterus, or the mouth and upper respiratory tract.

cardiac tamponade Compression of the heart by blood in the pericardial cavity, usually presenting as a complication of a ruptured myocardial infarct or a dissection of the aorta at its root.

cardiac transplantation A surgical transplant procedure performed on patients with end-stage heart failure.

cataract An opacity of the ocular lens compromising the eyesight.

celiac sprue A disease caused by hypersensitivity to gluten gliadin, resulting in pathologic changes of the small intestine and a malabsorption syndrome.

cerebral abscess Localized purulent bacterial infection of the brain accompanied by liquefactive necrosis and formation of a pus-filled cavity.

cerebral infarct An ischemic brain injury resulting in localized liquefactive necrosis of brain tissue, presenting with motor or sensory defects.

cerebral palsy Congenital weakness or paralysis of muscles resulting from intrauterine brain damage.

cerebrovascular accident (CVA) An ischemic brain injury related to vascular occlusion by an embolus, thrombus, or cerebrovascular hemorrhage; also known as *stroke*.

cerumen Earwax.

ceruminous plug A mass of earwax occluding the auditory canal, causing temporary deafness.

cervicitis An acute or chronic inflammation of the uterine cervix.

chancre A genital mucosal or skin ulceration lesion found in primary syphilis.

chemotaxis Movement of inflammatory cells toward a chemical attractant.

chemotherapy Treatment of disease with chemical agents.

Chlamydia trachomatis A small bacterium that may cause pneumonia, genital infections, and chronic eye infection known as trachoma.

cholangiocarcinoma An epithelial malignant tumor of the intrahepatic and extrahepatic biliary ducts.

cholecystitis An inflammation of the gallbladder that may be acute or chronic.

cholelithiasis A presence of stones in the gallbladder.

cholesteatoma A keratin-filled cystic mass formed in the middle ear as a complication of chronic or recurrent inflammation.

chondroma A benign cartilaginous tumor, most often found in bones.

chondrosarcoma A malignant cartilaginous tumor, most often found in bones.

choriocarcinoma A malignant tumor composed of trophoblastic cells resembling the chorionic epithelium of the placenta. These tumors may originate from the placenta in the uterus or within gonads and gonadal mixed germ cell tumors.

chorionic gonadotropin A hormone produced by the placental chorionic cells and excreted in the urine of pregnant women. Its detection in urine may serve as a pregnancy test.

chorionic villus biopsy The removal of a piece of living tissue from the vascular fibrils on the surface of the chorion, usually used for prenatal genetic diagnosis.

chromatin The condensed material within a cell nucleus, composed of DNA, RNA, and histones.

chromosomal abnormalities, numerical and structural Numerical chromosomal abnormalities involve a loss or a gain of chromosomes. Structural chromosomal abnormalities are caused by deletion of a portion of the chromosomal arms and translocation of a portion of one chromosome to another chromosome.

chronic disease Any disease that is of long duration.

chronic obstructive pulmonary disease (COPD) A progressive and irreversible condition characterized by diminished respiratory capacity of the lungs. Pathologically it may present as chronic bronchitis or emphysema.

cicatrization Formation of a cicatric (scar), usually after wound healing, healing of infarction, or other tissue injuries.

cirrhosis Chronic disease of the liver characterized by liver cell damage, nodular regeneration, and fibrosis that results in a loss of normal liver architecture; clinically synonymous with *end-stage liver failure.*

cleft lip A congenital anomaly consisting of one or more clefts in the upper lip as a result of the failure of the maxillary and median nasal processes to close.

clonal expansion Identical cells ("clones") derived from a single precursor. It is a feature of neoplastic growth.

coagulation Another name for clotting, a physiologic process that leads to formation of blood clots.

coagulation factors A group of 13 plasma proteins that are responsible for blood clotting.

coal-workers' lung disease (CWLD) A chronic occupational lung disease caused by dust particles inhaled in mines.

colitis An inflammation of the large intestine.

collagen A collective term for a group of mostly fibrous structural proteins found in connective tissues. Type I collagen is the most abundant structural protein in the body.

colposcopy A transvaginal examination of the cervix with an optical magnifying instrument.

complement A group of serum proteins that mediate inflammation and coagulation and amplify immune reactions.

concussion Damage to the brain caused by a blow or violent shaking.

condyloma acuminatum A genital wart caused by human papillomavirus infection.

condyloma latum A broad-based plaque that appears in secondary syphilis, usually in the anogenital region and in moist areas such as the thighs and axillae.

congenital Present at birth; a term used to describe a trait or anomaly with which one is born.

congestion An engorgement of vessels with blood.

congestive heart disease A circulatory disturbance caused by cardiac pump failure.

conjunctivitis An inflammation of the conjunctiva, caused by bacterial or viral infection, allergy, or environmental factors.

contact dermatitis An immunologically mediated skin rash resulting from reexposure to a sensitizing antigen.

contact inhibition Cessation of replication of *in vitro* dividing cells that come into contact with the edge of the plastic dish in which they are grown.

contracture An abnormal, usually permanent deformity of a joint, characterized by fixation in a flexed or semiflexed position.

contusion Mechanical injury resulting in extravasation of blood into tissue; a bruise.

cor pulmonale Acute or chronic right-sided heart failure caused by lung disease or left ventricular failure. In the chronic form it is associated with dilation and hypertrophy of the right ventricle, chronic passive congestion of internal organs and lower extremities, and edema formation.

corneal abrasion A loss of the outer layers of the cornea, usually as a result of mechanical trauma or surgery.

creatine kinase An enzyme found in the blood and in several organs. Its concentration is typically elevated in serum after skeletal muscle or cardiac muscle injury.

Creutzfeldt-Jakob disease A form of infectious dementia caused by prions. Pathologically it presents as spongiform encephalopathy.

Crohn's disease Regional enteritis; an ulcerative disease of unknown etiology characterized by inflammation of the terminal ileum or colon.

croup A spastic infectious laryngitis characterized by a barklike cough.

crush injury A form of traumatic injury of the skeletal muscles of the extremities in people covered with rubble or earth during earthquakes or squeezed by metal sheets or vehicular debris during traffic accidents.

crust Also known as a scab, it represents a solidified outer layer of wounds or oozing ulcers. It is formed from coagulated blood and cell debris.

cryptorchidism A congenital absence of a testis from the scrotum.

curettage The scraping or cleaning of a diseased surface or the internal surface of an organ for diagnosis or treatment, as in uterine curettage.

Cushing's syndrome A disease caused by an excess of corticosteroids secondary to tumors of the adrenal cortex or exogenously injected synthetic hormones.

cyanosis A bluish discoloration of the skin indicating a lack of oxygen.

cyclooxygenase An enzyme that is responsible for the formation of prostaglandins and thromboxane from arachidonic acid. It may be inhibited by aspirin and related compounds.

cyst A closed, usually fluid-filled sac lined by epithelium.

cystadenocarcinoma A malignant tumor composed of cysts lined internally by adenocarcinoma cells, which produce mucus or serous fluid. Most often such tumors are found in ovaries.

cystadenoma A benign tumor composed of one or several cysts that are lined by benign mucus or serous fluid-producing glandular cells. Like its malignant equivalent (cystadenocarcinoma), these tumors are most often found in ovaries.

cystic fibrosis An autosomal recessive genetic disorder caused by the mutation of the cystic fibrosis transmembrane conductance regulator (CFTR). It is characterized by abnormal secretion by sweat and mucous glands and complicated by pancreatic and pulmonary insufficiency.

cystitis An inflammation of the urinary bladder that may be acute and short lived or chronic.

cystitis, acute Inflammation of the bladder that is only a problem at the moment.

cytogenetics The study of chromosomes performed to detect congenital genetic disorders or genetic changes in cancer cells.

cytokines One of a large group of low-molecular-weight proteins secreted most prominently by leukocytes and macrophages during inflammation and immune reactions. They may be secreted by other cells as well and mediate cell-to-cell communication and signaling.

cytology The study of cells.

cytoplasmic organelles Cytoplasmic membrane-bound structures visible by electron microscopy in essentially all cells except mature erythrocytes.

cytoskeleton The filamentous part of the cytoplasm comprising microfilaments, microtubules, and intermediate filaments.

dacryocystitis An infection of the lacrimal glands.

deafness A condition characterized by a loss of hearing.

death The cessation of life as indicated by the absence of all vital functions, most notably loss of brain activity *(brain death)*.

degeneration A historic term for the deterioration of cell function after nonlethal cellular injury.

degenerative joint diseases (DJD) A form of arthritis, also known as osteoarthritis, characterized by erosion of articular cartilage, reactive changes in the periarticular bones, and consequent joint deformities, resulting in pain and decreased mobility of joints.

dehydration A loss of water from the body or from body tissue.

dementia A progressive, incapacitating mental deterioration marked by a loss of intellectual and cognitive functions.

demineralization Excessive elimination or loss of minerals (calcium and phosphates) from the bones.

dental caries A destructive tooth disease characterized by a loss of enamel and the decay of the underlying dental tissue.

dermatitis Skin inflammation, which may be caused by infection, immune reaction to allergens, or exposure to irritants or may occur as part of a systemic disease.

dermatofibroma A benign skin tumor composed of fibroblasts, usually presenting in the form of small, painless nodules.

dermatomyositis An immunologically mediated disease involving the skin and skeletal muscles.

dermatophytoses A group of superficial fungal infections of the skin.

dermoid cyst Also known as *cystic teratoma of the ovary*, it is a benign tumor of germ cell origin, presenting as a cyst lined by skin and various other somatic tissues. It may contain, among other substances, hair, teeth, bits of bone, and cartilage.

desmoid tumor A benign soft tissue tumor composed of fibroblasts and dense collagenous extracellular matrix.

desmoplasia A proliferation of connective tissue forming the stroma of a carcinoma.

diabetes insipidus A metabolic disorder caused by injury of the neurohypophyseal system, clinically presenting with uncontrollable polyuria and polydipsia (drinking of water because of incessant thirst).

diabetes mellitus A metabolic disease caused by a lack of insulin or by tissue resistance to insulin that adversely affects the metabolism of glucose and results in hyperglycemia.

diabetic microangiopathy Damage to small blood vessels and capillary circulation brought on by diabetes mellitus.

diabetic myopathy A muscular disease caused by diabetes mellitus, presenting as progressive muscle weakness.

diabetic nephropathy A kidney disease caused by diabetes, typically involving diabetic glomerulosclerosis, hyalinization of arterioles, nephroangiosclerosis, recurrent pyelonephritis, and occasional bouts of renal papillary necrosis. It is a common cause of end-stage kidney disease in diabetics.

diabetic retinopathy A form of chronic loss of visual acuity as a result of damage to the retinal blood vessels in diabetes mellitus.

diapedesis Exit of blood cells from a blood vessel into the tissue (as occurs in inflammation).

diarrhea The frequent passage of loose, watery stools because of intestinal or pancreatic and hepatobiliary disturbances.

diastole The resting phase of the heart contraction cycle; characterized by the dilation of ventricles.

differentiation The process by which cells acquire specialized functions and tissue- or organ-specific features.

diffuse Widespread; not limited or localized.

diffuse large B-cell lymphoma An aggressive form of non-Hodgkin's lymphoma that previously was invariably fatal but today responds favorably to chemotherapy in more than 60% of cases and can be cured.

DiGeorge syndrome A congenital disorder involving the thymus and parathyroid glands characterized by severe immunodeficiency and hypoparathyroidism in infancy and early childhood.

dilation A widening of a hollow organ or orifice, such as heart chambers, intestines, or excretory ducts of exocrine glands.

disseminated intravascular coagulation (DIC) A systemic coagulopathy characterized by formation of microthrombi in small blood vessels and subsequent uncontrollable bleeding as a result of the consumption of blood coagulation factors. It is found in many patients who suffer from shock, systemic infection, or neoplasia.

diverticulosis The presence of pouchlike herniations through the muscular layer of the colon.

diverticulum Saccular outpouching of the wall of a hollow organ, such as the large intestine.

Down's syndrome A congenital disease caused by trisomy of chromosome 21, presenting with typical facial features, mental retardation, short stature, and many developmental disorders involving the internal organs.

drowning Suffocation caused by immersion in water or other liquids.

Duchenne's muscular dystrophy An X-linked recessive muscle disease caused by mutations of the dystrophin gene, resulting in generalized muscle weakness and death in early adulthood.

ductal carcinoma in situ of the breast A form of preinvasive malignant tumor limited to the inside of the ducts. It is readily curable by timely resection, but if untreated it may progress to invasive ductal adenocarcinoma.

dwarfism Abnormally short stature caused by a lack of pituitary growth hormone or genetic mutations that prevent normal bone growth.

dysgerminoma A rare germ cell malignant tumor of the ovary, equivalent to seminoma of the testis.

dysphagia Difficulty in swallowing.

dysplasia Abnormal differentiation or maturation of tissue; refers also to preneoplastic changes in the epithelium (e.g., cervical dysplasia).

dysraphic anomaly Incomplete fusion of the midline structures covering the brain, the meninges, the bones of the calvarium, and the overlying skin of the convexity of the head.

dystrophin A protein attached normally to the sarcolemma of the skeletal muscle, missing from muscle cells of patients who have Duchenne's muscular dystrophy.

dysuria Painful urination (as occurs in cystitis).

ecchymoses Hemorrhagic spots on the skin and mucosae that are larger than petechiae; that is, they measure more than 5 mm in diameter.

eclampsia The gravest form of toxemia of pregnancy, characterized by hypertension, renal dysfunction, and seizures.

ectopia Congenital displacement of an organ or structure.

eczema Chronic skin inflammation (dermatitis) caused by various mechanisms; often caused by allergy.

edema An abnormal accumulation of fluid in tissues of body cavities.

embolism An abnormal condition in which an embolus travels through the bloodstream and becomes lodged in a blood vessel.

embolus Blood clot or foreign matter in the circulation that may obstruct blood flow.

embryonal carcinoma A malignant nonseminomatous germ cell tumor composed of undifferentiated stem cells resembling embryonic cells from the developing embryo. Embryonal carcinoma cells are also the stem cells of teratocarcinoma, in which they can differentiate into various somatic and extraembryonic tissues.

emphysema A chronic lung disease characterized by a loss of pulmonary parenchyma, resulting in widening of the terminal respiratory spaces and consequent shortness of breath and reduced ventilatory capacity.

empyema A collection of pus in a body cavity, as in the pleural cavity.

encephalitis Inflammation of the brain, most often caused by viruses.

encephalomalacia A localized softening of the brain, typically at the site of an infarct.

endocardial mural thrombus A clot attached to the wall of the vessels of the innermost layer of the heart's chambers.

endocarditis An inflammation of the inner heart lining and cardiac valves, usually caused by bacteria.

endocrinology The study of the endocrine system and hormonal disturbances.

endometrial biopsy A procedure for surgically obtaining a sample of endometrial tissue for microscopic examination. It is used in evaluating the causes of uterine bleeding in women suspected of having endometrial carcinoma or in women who are treated for infertility.

endometrial hyperplasia An abnormal condition characterized by overgrowth of the endometrium resulting from sustained stimulation by estrogen.

endometrioid Any tissue microscopically resembling the endometrial tissue.

endometriosis A condition in which foci of endometrium are located outside the uterine cavity.

endometritis An inflammation of the endometrium, often as part of pelvic inflammatory disease or after delivery and criminal abortion.

endophthalmitis An inflammation of the internal eye, usually resulting in blindness.

enteritis An inflammation of the small intestines.

eosinophil A white blood cell, usually binucleated, that contains red (eosinophilic) cytoplasmic granules.

eosinophilia An increase in the number of eosinophils in the blood, usually accompanying parasitic infections or allergic reactions.

ependymoma A tumor arising from the ependymal cells lining the ventricles and central canal of the spinal cord.

epidermal growth factor receptor A cell surface receptor binding soluble epidermal growth factor. It is expressed on many normal and neoplastic cells. On some neoplastic cells it is amplified and probably plays a role in the propagation of tumor cells.

epidermolysis bullosa A group of rare hereditary skin diseases in which vesicles and bullae develop, usually at sites of trauma.

epididymitis An acute or chronic inflammation of the epididymis.

epididymo-orchitis An acute or chronic inflammation of the epididymis and testis.

epidural hematoma A blood clot in the space between the dura mater and the bone of the skull, usually caused by arterial bleeding.

epilepsy A neurologic disease characterized by convulsions.

epiphysis A part of the bone forming the most proximal or distal ends of long bones.

epistaxis A nosebleed.

epithelial cell One of the basic cells forming (1) all solid internal organs except the heart and brain, (2) the epidermis of the skin, and (3) the internal lining of the hollow organs.

Epstein-Barr virus (EBV) The herpesvirus that causes infectious mononucleosis and probably plays a role in the formation of some malignant tumors, such as nasopharyngeal carcinoma and Burkitt's lymphoma.

erosion A destruction of tissue surface; ulceration.

erythrocyte A red blood cell.

erythroplasia A red mucosal lesion representing an intraepithelial neoplasia on the glans or corona of the penis.

erythropoietin A hormone produced by the kidneys that promotes red blood cell production (erythropoiesis).

esophageal atresia A congenital developmental disorder of the esophagus, which ends in a blind pouch or narrows to a thin cord and thus does not provide a continuous passage to the stomach.

esophageal varices A complex of longitudinal tortuous dilated veins at the lower end of the esophagus that are congested as a result of portal hypertension.

esophagitis Inflammation of the esophagus.

estrogen A female sex hormone produced by the ovaries and adrenals, and peripherally in fat cells, which generate it by conversion of testosterone.

etiology A study of the origin of disease; also used as a synonym for the cause of disease.

Ewing's sarcoma A malignant bone tumor involving the shaft of the long bones; composed of small, undifferentiated cells, the origin of which is unknown.

exacerbation An increase in the severity of a disease.

excoriation An injury to a surface of the body marked by a loss of epidermis, usually caused by trauma.

exophthalmos Abnormal protrusion (bulging) of the eyeball.

extranodal lymphoma Lymphomas originating outside the lymph nodes in solid organs, gastrointestinal system, brain, eyes, or skin.

extrauterine pregnancy A pregnancy occurring outside the uterus, most often in the fallopian tubes.

exudate Protein-rich fluid in the interstitial spaces or body cavities that contains leukocytes and is usually caused by inflammation.

familial adenomatous polyposis coli An inherited disorder related to the mutation of the tumor suppressor gene *FAP* and characterized by the development of myriad polyps in the colon, which can transform into colonic adenocarcinoma.

fatty liver An accumulation of fats, mostly in the form of triglycerides, in the liver.

fetal alcohol syndrome (FAS) A set of congenital psychologic, behavioral, and physical abnormalities in infants whose mothers consumed large amounts of alcohol during pregnancy.

fever An elevation of body temperature above the normal (37° C).

fibrin An insoluble fibrillar protein found in clots formed from fibrinogen in the plasma during blood coagulation.

fibrinous inflammation An exudative inflammation in which there is an usually large amount of fibrin in the exudate. If the exudate also contains neutrophils transforming into pus, it is called *fibrinopurulent inflammation.*

fibroadenoma A benign tumor composed of glandular epithelium and fibroblastic stroma; typically found in the breast.

fibroblast A connective tissue cell that synthesizes collagen.

fibrocystic changes Changes in the breast that occur in many women as part of the normal aging process.

fibroma A benign connective tissue tumor composed of fibroblasts.

fibronectin An adhesive glycoprotein normally found in the blood and interstitial spaces, but especially abundant at the site of inflammation and in the granulation tissue.

fibrosis A hardening of tissues secondary to deposition of collagen; excessive fibrosis may cause scarring.

fissure A groove or slitlike tissue defect, especially in the skin, anus, and mouth.

fistula An abnormal channel, caused by inflammation or tumor, that connects two hollow organs (e.g., loops of intestines or rectum and vagina).

flow cytometry A technique for sorting and counting normal or tumor cells for further characterization. The cells are marked by fluorescein-ated antibodies and counted by a special machine, which allows one to determine how many cells of a specified profile are present in the specimen. For example, blood lymphocytes may be separated and counted as T and B lymphocytes, and the T cells can then be separated into CD4+ helper cells and CD8+ suppressor/cytotoxic cells.

focal segmental glomerulosclerosis (FSG) A form of chronic glomerular disease representing the most common cause of nephrotic syndrome in adults. It is characterized by sclerosis of segments of some glomeruli.

folliculitis An inflammation of hair follicles, usually caused by bacteria.

fracture A traumatic injury to a bone in which the continuity of the bone tissue is broken.

fragile X syndrome A form of mental disorder affecting males, characterized by testicular enlargement and typical cytogenetic changes including a nearly broken X chromosome, which has a tip hanging by a flimsy thread.

freckle A brown or tan macule on the skin that results from exposure to sunlight.

fungal infection An inflammatory condition caused by a fungus.

furuncle A localized suppurative skin infection originating in hair follicles infected with staphylococci.

gallbladder carcinoma An adenocarcinoma originating in and involving the gallbladder.

gallstone A stone formed in the biliary tract, consisting of cholesterol or bile pigments and calcium salts.

gangrene A form of death of tissue, usually caused by loss of blood supply, bacterial invasion, and subsequent putrefaction.

gastrin A polypeptide hormone, produced by neuroendocrine cells of the stomach, that stimulates gastric acid secretion.

gastrinoma A neuroendocrine tumor producing gastrin and causing the Zollinger-Ellison syndrome with multiple peptic ulcers. It is most often found in the pancreas and in the duodenum.

gastritis An inflammation of the mucosa of the stomach.

genital herpes A sexually transmitted infection caused by type 2 herpes simplex virus.

germ cell tumors A group of benign and malignant tumors originating in the ovary or testis and less often in extragonadal sites, such as retroperitoneum and mediastinum.

gestational trophoblastic disease A group of rare uterine tumors and tumorlike conditions, including hydatidiform mole and choriocarcinoma, which typically develop from the placenta during or after pregnancy.

giant cell arteritis A group of progressive, immunologically mediated inflammatory disorders involving the temporal artery or aorta.

giant cell tumor of bone A benign epiphyseal long bone tumor composed of multinucleated giant cells that resembles osteoclasts scattered in a matrix of spindle cells. Some giant cell tumors may recur; rarely, some may be even malignant and metastasize.

Gilbert's disease A benign hereditary liver disease characterized by periodic hyperbilirubinemia and jaundice.

glaucoma An eye disease characterized by elevated intraocular pressure caused by obstruction of the outflow of aqueous humor or its production and circulation.

glioma A malignant brain tumor composed of glial cells.

glomerulonephritis A kidney disease characterized by inflammation of the glomeruli.

glomerulosclerosis A descriptive term for the hyalinization of capillary loops of the glomeruli, which may be affected segmentally or globally. Typically it is seen in end-stage kidney disease, but also in hypertensive renal disease, diabetic renal disease, and focal segmental glomerulosclerosis.

glucosuria Excretion of glucose in urine.

glue ear A painless condition in which a thick, sticky fluid collects behind the eardrum.

goiter An enlargement of the thyroid, usually caused by hyperplasia of follicles filled with colloid.

Golgi apparatus One of several cytoplasmic organelles involved in the cellular secretory functions.

gonorrhea Sexually transmitted disease caused by *Neisseria gonorrhoeae.*

Goodpasture's syndrome A form of rapidly progressive glomerulonephritis (RPGN) caused by the antiglomerular basement membrane antibodies, resulting in glomerular capillary destruction and extracapillary crescent formation in the urinary space between the capillary loops and the Bowman capsule.

gout A hereditary form of arthritis related to hyperuricemia and deposition of uric acid crystals in joints.

grading of tumors Histologic evaluation of tumor to determine whether the tumor cells are well differentiated, resembling the normal cells in the particular organ of their origin, or poorly differentiated.

graft-versus-host reaction An immune reaction initiated and perpetuated by the T cells from the host's bone marrow transplanted into the recipient. The transplanted T lymphocytes attack the host's tissues and typically cause damage of the skin, gastrointestinal tract, and liver.

granulation tissue Newly formed tissue, composed of blood vessels, macrophages, and fibroblasts, that typically forms during healing of wounds and fractures and the healing stages of inflammation.

granuloma An inflammatory lesion that is composed of macrophages, lymphocytes, and/or giant cells and that forms microscopic aggregates or nodules.

granulosa cell tumor A hormonally active ovarian tumor composed of granulosa cells. It is usually benign but may be malignant.

Graves' disease A form of immunologically mediated hyperthyroidism caused by antibodies to the thyroid-stimulating hormone receptor.

gynecologic Pertaining to the study of the female genital tract.

gynecomastia Enlargement of the male breast.

Hageman factor A coagulation factor, also known as factor XII, present in normal plasma that triggers the formation of bradykinin and associated enzymatic reactions.

hamartoma A nodule composed of an abnormal accumulation or overgrowth of mature cells and tissues that are normally present in the affected organ; results from abnormal development and is, in most instances, congenital, although not necessarily diagnosed at birth or in infancy.

haptens A nonproteinaceous substance that acts as an antigen by combining with particular bonding sites on an antibody.

Hashimoto's thyroiditis An autoimmune form of thyroiditis presenting with lymphocytic infiltration of the thyroid gland and hypothyroidism.

hay fever An acute, seasonal, allergic rhinitis stimulated by tree, grass, or weed pollen. It is mediated by mast cells and histamine and represents a type I hypersensitivity reaction.

hemangioblastoma A benign tumor consisting of a mass of blood vessels, most often found in the brain.

hemangioma A benign vascular tumor.

hematemesis Vomiting of blood.

hematochezia The passage of bright red blood in the stool.

hematocrit Relative volume of red blood cells in whole blood, expressed as a percentage.

hematogenous Disseminated by or derived from blood.

hematology The study of blood and blood-forming tissues.

hematoma A mass formed by coagulated blood located outside a blood vessel.

hematuria A condition characterized by spilling of blood in the urine. It may be macroscopic, which is grossly visible, or microscopic, which can be detected only by microscopic examination of urine sediment.

hemiparesis A form of muscle paralysis involving one side of the body, usually related to a stroke.

hemiplegia A paralysis of the muscles on one side of the body.

hemochromatosis May be genetic (hereditary hemochromatosis) or secondary due to excessive iron uptake or blood transfusions.

hemoglobin A complex, protein–iron compound in the blood that carries oxygen from the cells to the lungs and carbon dioxide away from the cells to the lungs.

hemolysis The destruction of red blood cells.

hemolytic anemia A disorder characterized by chronic premature destruction of red blood cells because of abnormalities of red blood cells or immunologic factors.

hemophilia An X-linked hereditary bleeding disorder caused by a deficiency of factor VIII or IX.

hemopoietic Related to the process of formation and development of the various types of blood cells.

hemorrhage An escape of blood from a ruptured blood vessel.

hemorrhoids A varicosity in the lower rectum or anus caused by congestion in the veins of the hemorrhoidal plexus.

hemosiderin An iron-rich pigment that is a product of red cell hemolysis.

hemostasis The termination of bleeding by mechanical or chemical means or by the complex coagulation process of the body.

hemothorax A collection of blood in the thoracic cavity.

hepatic encephalopathy A potentially lethal neuropsychiatric manifestation of extensive liver damage caused by chronic or acute liver disease.

hepatitis An inflammation of the liver, which may be acute or chronic, that is caused by viruses, immune mechanisms, or drugs.

hepatitis viruses A group of hepatotropic viruses that affect the liver, causing acute or chronic hepatitis or both.

hepatocellular carcinoma Liver cell carcinoma.

hepatomegaly An enlargement of the liver.

hepatorenal syndrome A type of kidney failure found in persons with liver cirrhosis; it is characterized by a gradual loss of urine production without signs of renal tissue damage.

hereditary spherocytosis A genetic form of anemia inherited as an autosomal dominant trait and characterized by hemolytic anemia caused by the presence of red blood cells that are spheric rather than round and biconcave.

hermaphroditism A rare condition in which both testicular and ovarian tissue exist in the same person.

hernia A protrusion of a part of an organ or the entire organ through an abnormal opening in the structure normally containing it, such as the abdominal wall.

herniation of the brain A protrusion of parts of the brain through a cranial opening or from one to another intracranial compartment, usually caused by brain edema and increased intracranial pressure.

herpes virus Any one of several DNA viruses, the most common of which are herpes simplex virus 1, the cause of labial herpes, and herpes simplex virus 2, the cause of genital herpes.

heterophagosome A cell vacuole formed from lysosomes and involved in phagocytosis of particulate material.

hiatal hernia A protrusion of a portion of the stomach upward through the diaphragm.

Hirschsprung's disease A form of congenital megacolon (widening of the large intestine) caused by incomplete development of colonic ganglia in the rectum.

hirsutism An excess of hair on the face or the body.

histamine A biogenic amine, released from mast cells, that mediates inflammation in type I hypersensitivity reactions.

histoplasmosis An infection caused by inhalation of spores of the fungus *Histoplasma capsulatum*.

Hodgkin's lymphoma A malignant neoplastic disease involving the lymph nodes; previously known as Hodgkin's disease.

homeostasis A state of stability or equilibrium between cells and fluids in the human body.

homografts A graft of tissue between two genetically dissimilar individuals of the same species who are not identical twins.

hordeolum A suppurative inflammation of the sebaceous glands of the eyelid.

human immunodeficiency virus (HIV) An RNA retrovirus that is the cause of acquired immunodeficiency syndrome (AIDS).

human papillomaviruses (HPVs) A group of DNA viruses that cause a variety of lesions, including common warts of the hands and feet; genital warts; and carcinoma of the oral, anal, and genital mucosa.

human T-cell lymphoma/leukemia virus (HTLV-1) A type C oncovirus of worldwide distribution but most common in Japan, Africa, and the Caribbean basin, having an affinity for helper/inducer T lymphocytes, that causes chronic infection and is associated with adult T-cell leukemia/lymphoma.

Huntington's disease An autosomal dominant hereditary condition caused by trinucleotide expansion in the huntingtin gene area. It presents with early onset of dementia and uncontrollable choreoathetotic movements.

hyaloplasm The semiliquid portion of the cytoplasm that surrounds the cell organelles.

hydatidiform mole A placental developmental abnormality characterized by trophoblastic proliferation and hydropic degeneration of chorionic villi. It occurs in complete and incomplete forms.

hydrocephalus An accumulation of cerebrospinal fluid in the ventricles of the brain.

hydronephrosis A distention of the renal pelvis with urine.

hydropic change An enlargement of the cell cytoplasm caused by an influx of water after reversible cell injury.

hydrops fetalis Massive edema of the fetus or newborn, usually in association with severe erythroblastosis fetalis and Rh incompatibility between the mother and the fetus.

hydrothorax A collection of clear fluid (transudate) in the thoracic cavity

hyperaldosteronism A condition characterized by an excess of aldosterone, usually produced by adrenocortical tumors originating from the zona glomerulosa.

hyperbilirubinemia A condition characterized by greater than normal amounts of the bile pigment bilirubin in the blood.

hypercalcemia A condition characterized by greater than normal amounts of calcium in the blood, most often resulting from excessive bone resorption and release of calcium.

hyperemia An excess of blood in part of the body caused by increased blood flow.

hyperestrinism A condition characterized by the presence of excess estrins in the body and often accompanied by functional bleeding from the uterus.

hyperextension injury of spinal cord A form of spinal cord injury caused by a straightening movement that goes beyond the normal, healthy boundaries of the spinal cord.

hyperflexion injury of spinal cord A form of spinal cord injury caused by flexion of the spinal cord beyond its normal limit.

hyperlipidemia An excess of lipids, including glycolipids, lipoproteins, and phospholipids, in the plasma.

hyperopia Farsightedness.

hyperparathyroidism An excess of parathyroid hormones caused by parathyroid adenoma or hyperplasia.

hyperplasia Enlargement of an organ as a result of an increased number of cells.

hypersensitivity pneumonitis An inflammatory form of interstitial pneumonia that results from an immunologic reaction in a hypersensitive person.

hypersensitivity reactions An inappropriate and excessive response of the immune system to a sensitizing antigen, also called an *allergen.*

hypertension Elevation of arterial blood pressure.

hypertensive retinopathy A retinal disease caused by poorly controlled arterial hypertension.

hypertensive stroke A form of stroke caused by intracerebral hemorrhage in hypertensive persons, usually related to a sudden rupture of damaged brain arteries.

hyperthyroidism A condition characterized by an excess of thyroid hormones caused by hyperactivity of the thyroid gland and, less often, by hyperfunctioning thyroid tumors.

hypertrophy An enlargement in an organ or body part caused by an increase in cell size; usually pertains to skeletal muscles or the heart.

hyperuricemia A condition characterized by an excess of uric acid in the blood.

hypoalbuminemia A condition characterized by abnormally low levels of albumin in the blood.

hypocalcemia A condition characterized by low concentration of serum calcium; typically found in hypoparathyroidism.

hypogonadism A condition characterized by an inadequate development and function of the ovary or testis.

hypoparathyroidism A condition characterized by insufficient secretion of parathyroid hormone.

hypoplasia Underdevelopment of an organ or structure.

hypotension A condition characterized by low arterial blood pressure.

hypothyroidism A condition characterized by decreased activity of the thyroid gland.

hypovolemia A condition characterized by an abnormally low circulating blood volume.

hypoxia A reduction in oxygen supply to the tissues.

hysterectomy Surgical removal of the uterus.

iatrogenic Resulting from intervention by physicians.

ichthyosis Any of several inherited dermatologic conditions in which the skin is dry, resembling fish scales.

icterus Jaundice caused by an elevation of bilirubin in blood.

idiopathic Of unknown cause.

idiopathic thrombocytopenic purpura A deficiency of platelets that results in bleeding into the skin and other organs.

IgA deficiency A genetic disorder characterized by a lack of immunoglobulin A (IgA) in serum, which may present with immune disorders and increased susceptibility to infections but is often asymptomatic.

ileus An obstruction or paralysis of the intestines.

immunity The body's defense mechanism against infection or foreign substances; may be antibody or cell mediated.

immunodeficiency, congenital Any of a group of diseases caused by a defect in the immune system.

immunoglobulin A protein that is produced by the plasma cells and that is capable of reacting with antigens and acting as an antibody.

immunohistochemistry A technique in which labeled antibodies are used to analyze tissues for the presence of specific tumor cells.

impetigo A superficial bacterial skin infection.

incidence The number of newly diagnosed cases of a disease in a given time period, usually a year.

infarct A localized area of tissue necrosis resulting from anoxia.

infection An invasion of the body by pathogenic microorganisms that reproduce and multiply, causing disease by local cellular injury, secretion of a toxin, or antigen-antibody reaction in the host.

infertility An inability to conceive or have children.

inflammation The body's reaction to injury, characterized by typical cellular, humoral, and circulatory changes.

inflammatory bowel disease (IBD) A chronic, episodic, inflammatory disease of the large intestine and rectum, which usually presents as either Crohn's disease or ulcerative colitis.

injury Tissue damage caused by external or internal adverse influences, such as trauma, infection, or metabolic disturbances.

insect bites The bite of any parasitic or venomous arthropod such as a louse, flea, mite, tick, or spider.

insulin A hormone secreted by the beta cells of the pancreatic islets of Langerhans that mediates uptake and utilization of glucose in cells.

insulinoma An endocrine tumor of the pancreas composed of neoplastic beta cells that secrete insulin.

interleukin A biologically active substance secreted by activated cells (most notably, leukocytes and macrophages).

intermediate filament proteins A family of related proteins that form intermediate filament and share common structural and sequence features. The best known proteins of this group are keratins, found in epithelial cells, and vimentin, found in connective tissue cells.

interstitial pneumonia A lung disease involving the alveolar septa and producing no intra-alveolar exudates. It is typically caused by viruses or *Mycoplasma* and clinically presents as atypical pneumonia.

intracerebral hemorrhage A type of hemorrhagic stroke in which bleeding directly into the brain occurs, usually as a complication of hypertension or ruptured berry aneurysms.

intratubular germ cell neoplasia (ITGCN) Malignant transformation of germ cells results in an intratubular tumor; also known as *carcinoma in situ.*

intussusception A prolapse of one segment of bowel into the lumen of another segment.

invasion The spreading of cancer into normal tissues.

invasive ductal carcinoma of the breast The most common type of breast cancer, which starts in the milk ducts and spreads to the nearby breast tissue.

invasive lobular carcinoma of the breast A malignant tumor composed of small cells arranged into single cell files without cell to cell attachment.

iridocyclitis An inflammation of the uvea of the eye.

497

iron deficiency anemia A microcytic hypochromic anemia caused by inadequate supplies of iron needed to synthesize hemoglobin.

ischemic A change caused by a decreased supply of oxygenated blood to a body part, marked by pain and organ dysfunction.

ischemic bowel disease A group of several disorders that compromise blood flow through segments of the intestine.

islet cell tumor Any of several tumors originating from the islands of Langerhans, including, among others, insulinoma, gastrinoma, glucagonoma, and somatostatinoma.

jaundice A yellowish discoloration of the skin or mucous membranes resulting from hyperbilirubinemia; synonymous with *icterus*.

juvenile hyperplasia An abnormal local tissue response rather than an excess of hormones.

Kaposi's sarcoma A malignant tumor composed of blood vessels; caused by human herpesvirus 8 infection and most often seen in persons with AIDS.

keloid A nodular, hyperplastic scar.

keratin A fibrillar protein forming the intermediate filaments in the cytoplasm of epithelial cells.

keratitis An inflammation of the cornea.

Klinefelter's syndrome A congenital form of male hypogonadism and infertility characterized by a 47,XXY karyotype.

Krukenberg tumors A bilateral neoplasm of the ovary resulting from metastases of gastrointestinal adenocarcinomas, most often located in the stomach.

laceration The tearing or slashing of tissues, organs, or other parts of the body.

lactate dehydrogenase An enzyme found in the cytoplasm of almost all body tissues. Its serum concentration is elevated in any condition that involves major cell breakdown, such as after chemotherapy of tumors.

leiomyoma A benign tumor of smooth muscle, most often found in the uterus.

lentigo A tan or brown macule on the skin not brought on by sun exposure.

lesion An abnormal structural change in tissues or organs resulting from injury or disease.

leukemia Any of several malignancies of the blood-forming organs characterized by the appearance of malignant white blood cells in circulation.

leukocytes White blood cells.

leukocytosis An increased number of circulating white blood cells.

leukopenia A reduction of white blood cells in the blood that can increase the risk of infection in an individual (in Greek, *penia* means "lack of").

leukoplakia A white plaque on the mucous membrane of the mouth, which may be due to hyperkeratosis or preinvasive malignancy of the squamous epithelium.

leukotrienes A class of biologically active proinflammatory compounds derived from arachidonic acid through the action of the enzyme lipoxygenase.

Leydig cell tumor Testicular tumor composed of hormone-secreting interstitial (Leydig) cells. It is usually benign and may be hormonally active, secreting testosterone or estrogens.

limb-girdle dystrophy A group of muscular dystrophies involving the skeletal muscle of the limbs and girdle. It is not a single disease but rather a clinical manifestation of numerous mutations involving genes that code muscle proteins.

lipase A fat-splitting enzyme secreted by the pancreas. Its concentration in blood is increased in acute pancreatitis.

lipid Fat.

lipofuscin A brown pigment composed of oxidized fats that accumulate in the autophagosomes of aging and chronically damaged cells.

lipoid nephrosis A form of nephrotic syndrome that occurs mostly in childhood. It is associated with no pathologic changes in the glomeruli and a good response to steroid treatment. Also known as *minimal change disease.*

lipoma A benign tumor composed of fat cells.

liposarcoma A malignant tumor composed of fat cells.

liquefaction A form of necrosis characterized by the transformation of solid tissue into fluid.

lithiasis Formation of calculi (stones), as may occur in the gallbladder (cholelithiasis) or urinary tract (urolithiasis).

lithotripsy A procedure for eliminating a calculus in the kidney, pelvis, ureter, bladder, or gallbladder.

liver transplantation A surgical treatment for end-stage hepatic dysfunction in which a donor liver is used to replace the cirrhotic liver of the recipient.

lobar pneumonia A severe infection of one or more of the five major lobes of the lungs characterized by intralobular exudation of neutrophils. It is caused by bacteria; if untreated, it may be lethal or eventually result in consolidation of lung tissue.

lumpectomy A surgical removal of the breast tumor and a thin rim of surrounding normal tissue so that the remaining normal breast is preserved.

lung abscess A localized suppurative form of pneumonia associated with cavitation as a result of the destruction of the inflamed lung parenchyma.

lung cancer A group of malignant tumors originating from the bronchial mucosa or the lung parenchymal cells, most often related to chronic cigarette smoking.

Lyme disease An infection caused by the spirochete *Borrelia burgdorferi*, transmitted by the bite of an infected tick.

lymph nodes Small oval structures that filter the lymph and fight infection and in which lymphocytes, monocytes, and plasma cells are formed.

lymphadenopathy An enlargement of lymph nodes that is caused by inflammation or neoplasia.

lymphangitis An inflammation of lymphatic vessels, usually resulting from an acute streptococcal infection of one of the extremities.

lymphocytes Mononuclear small white blood cells involved in the immune response of the body. They can be found in blood, lymph nodes and related lymphoid tissue, thymus, and spleen and are classified as B cells, T cells, and NK cells.

lymphomas A group of malignant neoplasms composed of lymphocytes.

lymphopenia A condition characterized by a decreased number of lymphocytes in the peripheral circulation, occurring as a primary hematologic disorder or in association with systemic diseases, cancer, immunodeficiency, and various forms of treatment.

lysis Destruction or decomposition. Derivative words include *lysosomes* (cytoplasmic digestive organelles), and *autolysis* (decomposition of tissues after death).

lysosomal storage diseases A group of genetic disorders resulting in an accumulation of metabolites or metabolic degradation products in lysosomes.

lysosome A cytoplasmic, membrane-bound particle that contains hydrolytic enzymes that function in intracellular digestive processes.

macrophage A mononuclear phagocytic cell normally found in tissues but also participating in chronic inflammation. It gives rise to epithelioid and multinucleated giant cells in granulomas.

macule A small, flat blemish or discoloration that is level with the skin surface.

malabsorption Impaired intestinal absorption of nutrients, usually as a result of intestinal or hepatobiliary diseases.

malignant hypertension A form of arterial hypertension of sudden onset, characterized by high elevation of systolic and diastolic blood pressure and high mortality.

malignant melanoma A pigmented malignant tumor, composed of melanocytes, most often arising in the skin or eyes.

malignant peripheral nerve sheath tumor A sarcoma (i.e., malignant tumor) of the connective tissue surrounding the nerves.

malignant tumor A neoplasm that has a poor outcome because of its invasive growth and tendency to metastasize and kill the host.

malnutrition Any disorder caused by inadequate nutrition.

MALT An acronym for mucosa-associated lymphoid tissue; found in the gastrointestinal and respiratory tract.

MALToma A low-grade lymphoma originating from the mucosa-associated lymphoid tissue, most often in the gastrointestinal tract.

mammography An x-ray examination of the breast for the detection of tumors.

Marfan's syndrome A hereditary disorder of the connective tissue caused by a mutation of the fibrillin gene and characterized by structural weakness of connective tissue, tendons, and blood vessels.

mast cell A tissue cell derived from circulating basophils.

mastectomy A surgical procedure to remove a cancerous breast.

mastitis Inflammation of the breast, most often caused by bacteria during lactation.

measles A contagious viral disease of childhood; also called *rubeola.*

Meckel's diverticulum An anomalous protrusion of the small intestine 30 and 90 cm from the ileocecal sphincter.

medulloblastoma A brain tumor affecting the cerebellum of children.

megacolon A congenital or functional dilation of the colon that results from the defective inervation of the rectum. Congenital megacolon is also known as *Hirschsprung's disease.*

megaloblastic anemia A hematologic disorder characterized by abnormal maturation of red blood cell precursors, which assume megaloblastic morphology. Most often it is caused by folic acid and vitamin B_{12} deficiency (pernicious anemia).

megaloureter Congenital ureteral dilation without obvious cause.

melena Abnormally black, tarry stool resulting from upper gastrointestinal bleeding in which the hemoglobin from blood is partially digested by hydrochloric acid into a black pigment.

membrane attack complex (MAC) The end product of the activation of the complement cascade during inflammation, formed from aggregated complement proteins. MAC perforates cell membranes and contributes to the cytotoxic action of complement.

membranous nephropathy An immunologically mediated glomerulopathy in which the glomerular basement membranes are studded with immune complexes. Clinically it presents with nephrotic syndrome that is unresponsive to treatment.

Mendelian genetics A part of genetics dealing with the inheritance of autosomal dominant and recessive disorders according to the basic principles of inheritance discovered by Gregor Mendel.

Ménière's disease A chronic disease of the inner ear, characterized by recurrent episodes of vertigo.

meningioma A benign tumor of the meninges.

meningitis Inflammation of the meninges of the brain and spinal cord.

menopause The period of a woman's life characterized by the cessation of menses.

menorrhagia An abnormally heavy or long menstrual period.

mesothelioma A rare malignant tumor of the mesothelium of the pleura or peritoneum, pathogenically linked to asbestos exposure.

metaphysis The growing part of the long bones between the diaphysis and epiphysis.

metaplasia A change from one cell type to another.

metastasis The transfer or spread of cancer cells from one site to another.

metrorrhagia A form of uterine bleeding unrelated to menstruation.

microfilaments The thinnest of the cytoskeletal fibers, composed of actin and myosin.

microphthalmia A developmental anomaly characterized by abnormal smallness of one or both eyes.

microtubules The thickest of the cytoskeletal filaments, composed of proteins called *tubulins.*

micturition The act of passing urine.

mitochondrion A rodlike, threadlike, or granular organelle that functions in aerobic respiration and occurs in varying numbers in all eukaryotic cells except mature erythrocytes.

mitosis A type of cell division that occurs in somatic cells and results in the formation of two genetically identical daughter cells containing the diploid number of chromosomes characteristic of the species.

mixed tumors A neoplasm composed of epithelial and mesenchymal neoplastic cells, most often found in salivary glands and the uterus.

monoclonal gammopathy A condition marked by the appearance of a spike of monoclonal immunoglobulins in serum, usually as a result of neoplastic proliferation of plasma cells (multiple myeloma).

morbidity The frequency of disability from a disease within a population.

mortality The condition of being subject to death.

multicystic renal dysplasia A congenital maldevelopment of the kidneys in which the normal kidney is replaced by cysts and abnormal renal tissue composed of immature tubules and glomeruli and heterologous tissues such as cartilage.

multifactorial inheritance The tendency to develop a physical appearance, disease, or condition, such as stature and blood pressure, that is the result of many genetic and environmental factors.

multinucleated giant cells Inflammatory cells with multiple nuclei and abundant cytoplasm. They are formed by the fusion of macrophages and are typically found in granulomas.

multiple endocrine neoplasia (MEN) One of two hereditary syndromes (MEN1 and MEN2) presenting with multiple endocrine tumors.

multiple myelomas A malignant neoplasm composed of neoplastic plasma cells, most often located in the bone marrow.

multiple sclerosis (MS) An incurable immunologic disease of the central nervous system, characterized by focal demyelination of axons in the white matter of the brain, leading to numerous neurologic defects, including progressive muscle weakness.

muscular dystrophy A group of genetically transmitted diseases characterized by progressive loss of muscle cells and muscle weakness.

myalgia A condition characterized by diffuse muscle pain, usually accompanied by malaise.

myasthenia gravis An autoimmune disease mediated by antibodies to acetylcholine receptor on the neuromuscular junction and presenting as muscle weakness.

Mycoplasma A genus of ultramicroscopic organisms lacking rigid cell walls and considered to be the smallest free-living organisms.

mycosis An infectious disease caused by a fungus.

mycosis fungoides A rare, slowly evolving T-cell lymphoma primarily localized in the skin.

myeloproliferative disorders A group of conditions characterized by neoplastic proliferation of myeloid cells in the bone marrow.

myocardial infarct Ischemic necrosis of the heart muscle presenting clinically as chest pain, heart failure, or sudden death.

myocarditis An inflammation of the myocardium, usually caused by viruses.

myofibroblasts A connective tissue cell that has hybrid features of fibroblasts and smooth muscle cells and thus can synthesize collagen and contract at the same time. It is found typically in granulation tissue and in desmoplastic tumors.

myopathy A term for muscle diseases of various etiologies, which may be congenital or acquired.

myopia Shortsightedness.

myositis An inflammation of muscle tissue, usually of voluntary muscle, caused by an infection or autoimmune mechanisms.

myotonic dystrophy An autosomal dominant hereditary muscle disease characterized by myotonia (muscle spasms) and progressive muscle wasting, as well as mental deterioration and diabetes.

myxedema Generalized doughy edema of the subcutaneous tissue, most prominent on the face, a typical feature of hypothyroidism.

natural killer (NK) cell A lymphocyte that is capable of binding to and killing virus-infected cells and some tumor cells.

necrosis The morphologic changes in tissue caused by cell death.

neoadjuvant chemotherapy An approach to cancer treatment that includes chemotherapy before surgical teatment.

neonatal respiratory distress syndrome A clinical presentation of neonatal hyaline membrane disease of premature infants, resulting from postnatal injury of immature lungs lacking alveolar surfactant. It presents with shortness of breath and severe hypoxia, which can be treated with instillation of artificial surfactant into the lungs.

neoplasm Any abnormal and uncontrolled growth of cells, benign or malignant; a synonym for *tumor*.

nephritis Inflammation of the kidney; most often immunologically mediated.

nephroangiosclerosis A consequence of hypertension, atherosclerosis, and/or diabetes resulting in narrowing of small renal arteries and arterioles, with consequent hyalinization of glomeruli and loss and atrophy of renal tubules. It is a common cause of renal insufficiency in the elderly.

nephrolithiasis Formation of renal calculi.

neuroblastoma A malignant tumor composed of neuroblasts (i.e., immature neural cell precursors) most often found in the adrenal medulla in children and adolescents.

neurodegenerative disorders Any of several diseases of unknown etiology resulting in a loss of the neurons in the brain and subsequent loss of mental capacity or motor and sensory functions of the brain.

neurofibroma A benign tumor of peripheral nerves composed of neoplastic perineural fibroblasts.

neurofibromatosis A hereditary tumor condition transmitted as an autosomal dominant trait, characterized by numerous neurofibromas of peripheral nerves, skin, and even internal organs.

neurogenic muscle atrophy A form of muscle wasting related to muscle denervation. It is a consequence of injury involving peripheral nerves, lower motor neurons in the spinal cord, motor pathways of the spinal cord, or the upper motor neurons in the brain.

neuromuscular junction The area of contact between the ends of a large myelinated nerve fiber and a fiber of skeletal muscle.

neurosyphilis A set of neurologic symptoms of tertiary syphilis involving the central nervous system.

nevus A mole or localized, benign, pigmented skin lesion.

nodule A small nodelike structure composed of neoplastic or inflammatory cells in the skin or internal organs.

nonseminomatous germ cell tumor (NSGCT) A group of malignant germ cell tumors of the testis comprising embryonal carcinoma, teratocarcinoma, choriocarcinoma, and yolk sac carcinoma When admixed to seminoma it is called *malignant mixed germ cell tumor.*

norovirus A virus causing acute viral gastroenteritis in children and adults; previously known as *Norwalk virus.*

nucleus The central part of most living cells (except mature red blood cells) containing the genetic material and thus controlling the major functions of each cell.

obstruction A blockage of a tubelike organ, such as the intestines.

occlusion A blockage of vessels.

occult Hidden or inapparent.

oligodendroglioma A malignant brain tumor composed of oligodendroglial cells.

oliguria A condition characterized by excretion of a reduced amount of urine.

oncogenes Genes that normally encode cellular proteins but that, if altered or mutated, can cause or contribute to the development of cancer.

oncogenic viruses Any one of more than 100 viruses able to cause the development of a malignant neoplastic disease.

oncology The branch of medicine concerned with the study of malignancy.

onychomycoses A disease caused by fungal infection of the nails.

oocyte The female germ cell capable of maturing into an ovum.

opportunistic infection An infection caused by normally nonpathogenic organisms in a hospitalized person or a host whose resistance has been decreased by disorders such as diabetes mellitus, human immunodeficiency virus infection, or cancer.

opsonin An antibody or complement split product that, on attaching to foreign material, microorganisms, or other antigens, enhances phagocytosis of that substance by leukocytes and other macrophages.

opsonization The coating of bacteria with opsonins, such as C3 fragments of complement or immunoglobulin g (IgG), that facilitate phagocytosis.

oral cancer Any one of several malignant neoplasms of the lips or the mouth, usually originating from the squamous mucosa or, less often, from other intraoral structures such as salivary glands.

orchitis An inflammation of one or both of the testes, most often caused by viruses, and characterized by swelling and pain and a damage of seminiferous tubules.

osteoarthritis A multifactorial degenerative disease predominantly affecting the weight-bearing joints and small joints of fingers and toes; also known as *degenerative joint disease.*

osteogenesis imperfecta A hereditary bone disease caused by mutations of genes encoding collagens and resulting in bone weakness and fractures.

osteoid The soft, organic part of the bony matrix composed predominantly of collagen type 1.

osteolytic Relating to osteolysis or dissolution of bone.

osteoma A benign bone tumor composed of well-differentiated osteocytes and mature bone.

osteomalacia A condition marked by softening of the bones caused by hormones or vitamin D deficiency.

osteomyelitis An infection of bone, usually caused by bacteria.

osteopenia A condition recognized radiologically as a reduced amount of mineralized bone, usually as a result of osteomalacia or osteoporosis.

osteopetrosis A hereditary disorder resulting in abnormally dense bone ("marble-bone disease") that is more friable than normal bone and tends to encroach on the hematopoietic bone marrow, causing anemia.

osteoporosis A condition characterized by excessive thinning and fragility of bones as a result of atrophy and loss of bone substance.

osteosarcoma A malignant bone-forming tumor composed of neoplastic osteoblasts.

otitis externa An inflammation of the outer ear, usually caused by bacteria.

otitis media An inflammation of the middle ear, usually caused by bacteria.

otosclerosis A disease of the inner ear characterized by conductive deafness as a result of the deposition of newly formed bone on both sides of the oval window.

ovarian cyst A globular sac filled with fluid or semisolid material that develops in or on the ovary. It may evolve from ovarian follicles and corpora lutea or from inclusions of the surface epithelium of the ovary, or may represent serous and mucinous neoplasms.

ovarian neoplasms A group of benign or malignant tumors that may originate from the ovarian surface epithelium, germ cells, sex cord cells, or nonspecific stromal cells.

oxygen radicals A group of oxygen-rich compounds, such as superoxide, hydrogen peroxide, or hydroxyl radical, that are formed in tissues and body fluids under normal or pathologic conditions. If formed in excessive amounts and if not neutralized by antioxidants, oxygen radicals can cause cell injury. They are thought to play a key role in the pathogenesis of many pathologic processes, including cancer and atherosclerosis.

Paget's disease (osteitis deformans) A bone disease marked by bone densities and deformities.

pancreatic pseudocyst A cystic cavity not lined by epithelium but by necrotic pancreatic tissue or fibrous scar tissue containing fluid rich in pancreatic enzymes admixed to cell debris. It is a complication of acute pancreatitis resulting from enzymatic lysis of the pancreas and adjacent fat tissue.

pancreatitis Inflammation of the pancreas, either acute or chronic, most often caused by alcohol abuse or obstruction of the pancreatic duct by biliary stones.

pancytopenia A marked reduction in the number of circulating red blood cells, white blood cells, and platelets.

panhypopituitarism A generalized pituitary insufficiency characterized by a deficiency of all pituitary hormones. It may be a consequence of an injury of the hypothalamus, pituitary stalk, or anterior pituitary itself.

pannus A layer of granulation tissue covering the free articular surface of a joint, typically found in rheumatoid arthritis.

panophthalmitis An inflammation of the entire eye, usually caused by virulent pyogenic bacteria.

pap smear The common name for the cytologic screening test used in gynecology to detect premalignant and malignant processes in the cervix.

papilledema A swelling of the optic disc, usually caused by increased intracranial pressure.

papilloma A wartlike benign epithelial tumor protruding from the mucosa or skin.

papillomatosis An abnormal condition characterized by widespread development of multiple papillomas, typically caused by human papillomavirus infection.

papule A small, raised, solid skin lesion less than 0.5 to 1 cm in diameter, such as the common wart.

paralysis A loss or impairment of motor function of a body part.

paraneoplastic syndrome A clinical condition caused by distant effects of a tumor on various organs that are not involved physically by the tumor itself or its metastases. The symptoms most often result from the hormonal or immunologic effects of the tumor on one or several organ systems, including the central nervous system, endocrine organs, musculoskeletal system, skin, and others.

paraplegia Paralysis of the lower extremities.

parathyroid glands Four small endocrine glands that secrete parathyroid hormone and thus regulate the homeostasis and metabolism of calcium and phosphate in the body.

parathyroid hyperplasia An enlargement of all four parathyroid glands. It may have no obvious cause (primary) or may occur in response to renal or other metabolic disorders (secondary).

Parkinson's disease A neurologic disease characterized by movement disorders.

paronychia An infection of the fold of the skin at the base of a nail.

pathogenesis The sequence of events playing a role in the development of a disease.

pathophysiology A study of functional changes in abnormal conditions or disease states.

pelvic inflammatory disease (PID) A bacterial infection of the internal female genital organs, such as the uterus, fallopian tube, and ovary.

peptic ulcer A defect in the mucosa of the stomach or duodenum that is caused by unregulated action of pepsin and hydrochloric acid on the gastroduodenal mucosa.

perforation A hole in the wall of a hollow organ, such as the intestine.

perforation of the tympanic membrane A hole or opening made through the entire thickness of the tympanic membrane at the border between the middle ear and the external ear canal.

pericarditis Inflammation of the pericardium, usually accompanied by formation of a serous, fibrinous, or purulent exudate on its internal surface and an accumulation of fluid in the pericardial cavity.

periodontal Pertaining to the gums or the soft tissues surrounding the teeth.

periodontal disease A set of pathologic changes involving the tissues that support the teeth, such as the periodontal membrane or periodontal ligament.

peritonitis An inflammation of the peritoneum, usually caused by bacteria that have gained access to the abdominal cavity.

pernicious anemia A form of anemia related to the body's inability to absorb vitamin B_{12}.

petechia A pinpoint intradermal or subcutaneous skin hemorrhage, smaller than ecchymoses or purpura.

phagocytosis The ingestion of microorganisms by leukocytes or macrophages.

phenylketonuria A genetic disease caused by a deficiency of phenylalanine hydroxylase, characterized by the presence of phenylketone and other metabolites of phenylalanine in the urine.

pheochromocytoma A tumor of the adrenal medulla that usually secretes epinephrine and norepinephrine, causing hypertension. It is usually solitary and benign, but in 10% of cases it is multiple and malignant.

phyllodes tumor A rare breast tumor composed of epithelial and stromal cells, thus resembling fibroadenomas, from which it differs in its larger size and a propensity to grow. It may be benign or malignant, in which case it may grow exceptionally large.

pituitary adenoma Any of several benign tumors of the anterior lobe of the pituitary gland. Some pituitary adenomas produce polypeptide pituitary hormones, whereas others are nonfunctional and only compress the normal gland, causing pituitary insufficiency.

placenta accreta An abnormally implanted placenta that invades the uterine muscle, making its separation from the muscle difficult.

placenta previa An abnormally placed placenta implanted over the internal end of the cervical canal.

plaque A slightly raised patch on the skin, as typically seen in psoriasis.

plasma The watery, straw-colored, protein-rich fluid forming the noncellular (fluid) part of blood and lymph.

plasma cell A cell derived from B-cell lymphocytes that secretes immunoglobulins.

plasma membrane The outer covering of a cell. It is important for the preservation of cell integrity, homeostasis with the intercellular fluid, and the contact and communication of the cell with other cells and the extracellular matrix.

plasmacytoma Malignant tumor of plasma cells, usually located in the bone marrow but also found in many internal organs (extramedullary plasmacytoma). Plasmacytomas may be solitary or multiple, in which case they are typically the defining features of multiple myeloma.

platelet A very small blood cell derived from the fragmented cytoplasm of megakaryocytes in the bone marrow. Platelets participate in coagulation, wound healing, and inflammation.

pleomorphic adenoma The most common benign tumor of the salivary glands. It is composed of epithelial, myoepithelial, and connective tissue tumor cells and is thus also known as *mixed tumor of the salivary glands*.

pleomorphism Variation in size, shape, and staining properties of tumor cell nuclei.

pleuritis An inflammation of the pleura, often associated with formation of an exudate and fluid filling the pleural cavity.

pneumoconiosis A pulmonary disease characterized by the accumulation of dust and particulate matter in the lungs.

pneumonia A bacterial, viral, or fungal infection of the lungs.

pneumothorax Air in the thoracic cavity.

poliomyelitis An acute viral disease that attacks the central nervous system; it has been almost completely eradicated by vaccination.

polyarteritis nodosa An immunologic inflammatory disease involving the arteries.

polycyclic aromatic hydrocarbons A group of chemical compounds that consist of fused aromatic rings, typically found in the tar and smoke of cigarettes.

polycystic kidney disease A hereditary kidney disease inherited as an autosomal dominant trait linked to the mutation of the gene for polycystin. The disease is characterized by the appearance of multiple renal cysts in adulthood, leading to a progressive loss of renal function and uremia.

polycystic ovary syndrome (POS) A hormonal disorder characterized by formation of multiple cysts in both ovaries; clinically it presents with hormonal disturbances, menstrual irregularities, infertility, hirsutism, and obesity.

polycythemia An increase in the total red cell mass in the blood, which may be classified as primary if the cause is unknown or secondary if related to excessive stimulation with erythropoietin.

polymorphonuclear leukocyte A white blood cell containing a segmented lobular nucleus surrounded with cytoplasm rich in granules that stain with both acidic and basic dyes. Thus it is also called a *neutrophil*.

polymorphous cell sarcoma A malignant soft tissue tumor previously known as *malignant fibrous histiocytoma*.

polymyositis An autoimmune inflammatory muscle disease affecting several muscle groups and causing muscle pain and weakness.

polyp A mass protruding from the mucosal surface or the skin. Large intestinal polyps may be either neoplastic (tubular and villous adenomas) or non-neoplastic (usually hyperplastic).

polyuria A condition characterized by the excretion of a large amount of urine.

portal hypertension A condition characterized by increased pressure in the portal vein, usually caused by cirrhosis.

postmenopausal After menopause; that is, after the cessation of regular menstruation.

poststreptococcal glomerulonephritis An immunologic renal disease that occurs in children after throat infection with certain (nephritogenic) strains of *Streptococcus*.

preeclampsia A form of toxemia of pregnancy resulting from abnormal maternoplacental interaction and presenting with edema, hypertension, and proteinuria.

prematurity When a baby is born before the expected time, usually less than 37 weeks of pregnancy.

prenatal diagnosis Any of various diagnostic techniques to determine whether a developing fetus in the uterus is affected with a genetic disorder or other abnormality.

presbycusis Hearing loss associated with aging.

presbyopia A hyperopic shift to farsightedness in the elderly resulting from a loss of elasticity of the lens of the eye.

prevalence The total number of cases of a disease at any one place and time.

primary biliary cirrhosis An autoimmune liver disease characterized by destruction of the bile duct in the portal tracts of the liver. It affects middle-aged women and is characterized by jaundice and gradual loss of hepatic function as a result of bridging fibrosis, progressing to cirrhosis. Diagnostic antimitochondrial antibodies can be found in the serum of most persons with this condition.

primary sclerosing cholangitis A chronic liver disease of possible autoimmune origin that often occurs as a complication of ulcerative colitis. It is characterized by periductal fibrosis surrounding intrahepatic and extrahepatic bile ducts, thus causing biliary obstruction and progressing to cirrhosis.

prion One of several kinds of infectious proteinaceous particles causing transmissible neurodegenerative diseases, including Creutzfeldt-Jakob disease and mad cow disease.

procarcinogen A chemical substance that becomes carcinogenic after metabolic conversion in the liver or other tissues.

prognosis The predicted outcome of a disease.

prolactinoma A benign pituitary tumor that produces prolactin, causing amenorrhea-galactorrhea syndrome in women and impotence or a lack of libido in men.

proliferative breast disease A group of noncancerous conditions that may increase the risk of developing breast cancer.

prostaglandins (PGs) A group of substances, derived from arachidonic acid through the cyclooxygenase pathway, that mediate inflammation, smooth muscle cell contraction or relaxation, and vascular permeability.

prostate-specific antigen (PSA) A protein secreted by the prostate gland into the semen but also produced by prostate cancer cells, which discharge it into the serum. PSA is thus used as a serologic marker for prostatic adenocarcinoma.

prostatitis Acute or chronic inflammation of the prostate gland, usually caused by bacterial infection.

proteinuria Excretion of increased amounts of protein in the urine.

protozoal infections Any disease caused by single-celled organisms of the subkingdom Protozoa.

pseudocyst A space or cavity containing gas or liquid but without a lining membrane.

pseudomembranous colitis. A diarrheal disease caused by ulceration of the colonic mucosa, which is partially covered with pseudomembranes composed of fibrin, mucus, and cell debris. It is often found in hospitalized patients who have received antibiotics allowing overgrowth of the anaerobic, spore-forming, toxin-producing bacteria *Clostridium difficile.*

pseudomembranous inflammation An acute inflammatory response to a powerful necrotizing toxin, such as diphtheria toxin, with formation, on a mucosal surface, of a false membrane composed of precipitated fibrin, necrotic epithelium, and inflammatory white cells.

purpura Any of several bleeding disorders characterized by hemorrhage into the tissues, particularly beneath the skin or mucous membranes.

purulent Associated with pus formation.

pus A yellow inflammatory discharge (exudate) composed of viable as well as dead and dying neutrophils.

pustule A small, circumscribed elevation of the skin containing pus.

pyelonephritis Infection of the kidney and renal pelvis, usually caused by bacteria, which may be acute or chronic and unilateral or bilateral. Bilateral chronic pyelonephritis may cause end-stage kidney disease and uremia slowly after bacterial infection of the kidney and may progress to renal failure.

pyothorax A collection of pus in the thoracic cavity.

pyrogens Substances that cause fever.

radicular dental cyst A cyst with a wall of fibrous connective tissue and a lining of stratified squamous epithelium that is attached to the root apex of a tooth with dead pulp or a defective root canal filling.

rapidly progressive glomerulonephritis (RPGN) An immune-mediated kidney disease that, if untreated, leads to end-stage renal failure within several weeks. Pathologically it presents as a crescentic glomerulonephritis and may occur as part of renal-pulmonary syndromes such as Goodpasture's syndrome or Wegener's granulomatosis.

Raynaud's disease A disease of unknown etiology characterized by intermittent attacks of ischemia of the extremities, including fingers, toes, ears, and nose, presumably as a result of vascular spasm. Similar symptoms found in persons with systemic lupus erythematosus and systemic sclerosis of cryoglobulinemia are called *Raynaud's phenomenon.*

regeneration The preferred method of body repair by which the original function of the cell is restored.

renal cell carcinoma (RCC) A malignant epithelial neoplasm of the kidney.

renal failure An inability of the kidneys to excrete wastes, concentrate urine, conserve electrolytes, and participate in the maintenance of acid-base equilibrium.

renal osteodystrophy A condition resulting from chronic renal failure and characterized by uneven bone growth and demineralization.

renal tubular necrosis Acute death of renal tubular cells as a result of ischemia or toxins, resulting in acute loss of renal excretory functions and elevation of blood urea nitrogen (BUN) and creatinine in serum.

renin An enzyme, produced by the juxta glomerular apparatus cells in the kidneys, that increases blood pressure by acting on angiotensinogen.

retinitis pigmentosa A group of progressive genetic forms of blindness presenting as gradual loss of peripheral vision.

retinoblastoma A malignant eye tumor of infancy and childhood.

Rh incompatibility A lack of compatibility between two groups of blood cells that are antigenically different because of the presence of the Rh factor in one group and its absence in the other.

rhabdomyolysis A paroxysmal, potentially fatal destruction of skeletal muscle as a result of physical or chemical causes, such as trauma, toxins, or drugs. It is characterized by the appearance of myoglobin in blood and urine. The filtration of myoglobin through the glomeruli into the tubules may cause extensive renal tubular necrosis.

rhabdomyoma A benign tumor of striated muscle that may occur in many places, such as the pharynx, tongue, or heart.

rhabdomyosarcoma A malignant tumor of skeletal muscle.

rheumatic fever An immunologic reaction to streptococci that affects the joints and the heart.

rheumatoid arthritis An immune-mediated, chronic, systemic disease producing inflammatory changes in the joints.

rhinitis An inflammation of the mucous membranes of the nose that results in a nasal discharge.

rickets A disease caused by a deficiency of vitamin D that results in softening and deformity of bones in children.

rotavirus A double-stranded ribonucleic acid virus that may cause diarrhea, especially in neonates and small children.

rough endoplasmic reticulum (RER) A cytoplasmic organelle composed of ribosome-covered laminar membranes (cisterns). These cisterns are the site for synthesis of proteins destined for export and secretion from the cell.

rupture Forcible tearing of tissue or organs.

salpingitis An inflammation or infection of the fallopian tube, usually as part of pelvic inflammatory disease.

sarcoidosis An immune-mediated disease characterized by the formation of noncaseating granulomas.

sarcoma A malignant tumor of connective tissue cells.

scabies A contagious disease caused by *Sarcoptes scabiei,* the human itch mite, characterized by intense itching of the skin and excoriation from scratching.

scales Aggregates of thin flakes of keratinized epithelium found on the surface of the skin in many chronic diseases.

scar The formation of fibrous tissue after healing of inflammation or injury of certain organs, such as the skin or intestines.

scirrhous carcinoma A hard, invasive tumor composed of tumor cells surrounded by dense fibrous tissue. This fibrous tissue reaction is called *desmoplasia,* and such scirrhous tumors are thus called *desmoplastic.* Breast and prostate carcinomas are scirrhous; the firm consistency of these tumors can be felt by palpation during physical examination

scleroderma See *systemic sclerosis.*

sclerosing adenosis A non-neoplastic breast lesion composed of proliferating glands surrounded by dense fibrous tissue.

scoliosis A lateral curvature of the spine, causing a deformity of the body.

scurvy A disease caused by a deficiency of vitamin C.

seborrheic keratosis A benign skin tumor, commonly known as a senile wart.

sella turcica A transverse depression crossing the midline on the superior surface of the body of the sphenoid bone and containing the pituitary gland.

seminoma A malignant germ cell tumor of the testis composed of clear cells resembling spermatogonia; equivalent to dysgerminoma of the ovary.

senile Pertaining to old age.

sepsis A systemic infection in which bacteria gain access to the blood, where they grow and secrete their toxins; also known as *bacteremia* or *septicemia.*

septal defect A congenital heart abnormality, presenting as a hole in the atrial or ventricular septum, that may occur as an isolated anomaly or as a part of a more complex congenital heart disease, such as tetralogy of Fallot.

septic embolus A type of emboli that is infected with bacteria. Infarcts caused by septic emboli tend to transform into abscesses because the bacteria enter the necrotic tissue from the embolus that has carried them.

septicemia Bacteremia; the presence of bacteria in the blood.

serous inflammation A form of inflammation characterized by the copious effusion of nonviscous serous and clear fluid, resembling serum obtained by centrifugation of the blood.

Sertoli cell tumor A testicular sex cord cell tumor composed of Sertoli cells, usually benign.

Sertoli-Leydig cell ovarian tumor An ovarian sex cord cell tumor usually secreting androgenic hormones that cause virilization.

serum The clear, straw-colored, liquid part of plasma that contains no cells or coagulation factors.

serum sickness An immunologic disorder characterized by the formation of circulating immune complexes that develop 2 to 3 weeks after the administration of an antiserum.

severe combined immunodeficiency An abnormal condition characterized by the complete absence or marked deficiency of B cells and T cells, with the consequent lack of humoral and cell-mediated immunity.

sex cord cell tumors of the ovary A group of tumors originating from granulosa cells, theca cells, and related sex cord cells of the ovary (e.g., thecoma, granulosa cell tumor).

sexually transmitted diseases (STDs) A group of diseases acquired by sexual intercourse (e.g., syphilis and gonorrhea).

Sheehan's syndrome A postpartum condition of pituitary necrosis and hypopituitarism after circulatory collapse resulting from uterine hemorrhaging.

shock A systemic circulatory collapse resulting in hypoperfusion of tissues and generalized hypoxia, usually after massive bleeding, sepsis, or a systemic anaphylactic reaction.

sialadenitis An inflammation of one or more of the salivary glands.

sickle cell anemia A severe, chronic, incurable genetic hemoglobinopathic anemia that occurs in people homozygous for hemoglobin S. It is caused by a mutation of the gene encoding the beta chain of hemoglobin.

silicosis A fibrotic lung disease caused by the inhalation of silica particles.

sinus A cavity or channel permitting the escape of pus.

smooth endoplasmic reticulum (SER) A cytoplasmic organelle composed of smooth vesicles that contains microsomal enzymes involved in the metabolism of toxins, drugs, and enzymes.

soft tissue tumors A group of sarcomas originating from fibroblasts, fat cells, smooth muscle cells, endothelial cells, and perivascular and perineural cells; that is, cells that are normally found in the soft tissue of the subcutis, around the skeletal muscles, and in parts of the body such as retroperitoneum or mediastinum. Microscopically similar malignant tumors may occur in the internal organs and bones.

spasm An involuntary, usually painful, muscle contraction.

spina bifida A congenital defect in the posterior part of the vertebrae that exposes the spinal cord to injury.

splenomegaly Enlargement of the spleen.

squames Layers of flattened, keratinized scales covering the surface of the epidermis.

squamous cell carcinoma A malignant epithelial tumor composed of epidermoid (squamous) cells.

staging of tumors Classification of tumors according to the extent of their spread in the body. Most often the staging is performed using the TNM (tumor, node, metastasis) system.

steatohepatitis A type of liver disease characterized by inflammation of the liver with concurrent fat accumulation in liver cells, which are surrounded by fibrous strands.

steatorrhea The passing of fatty stools resulting from intestinal malabsorption of fats.

stomatitis An inflammation of the mouth.

stroke A neurologic disease, also known as apoplexy, caused by intracerebral bleeding or infarction and characterized by a loss of sensory, motor, or mental functions performed by the damaged part of the brain.

stye A purulent infection of a meibomian or sebaceous gland of the eyelid, often caused by staphylococci.

subdural hematoma A blood clot between the dura and arachnoid.

sudden infant death syndrome (SIDS) A form of unexpected and sudden death of an apparently normal and healthy infant that occurs during sleep and with no physical or autopsic evidence of disease.

sunlight injury (sunburn, sunscald) Injuries an individual gets from sun exposure.

syndactyly A developmental anomaly characterized by the fusion of the fingers or toes.

synovial sarcoma A malignant tumor, composed of undifferentiated spindle cells, usually affecting the soft tissue of extremities in young adults.

syphilis A contagious venereal disease caused by *Treponema pallidum.*

systemic lupus erythematosus (SLE) A systemic autoimmune disease caused by circulating immune complexes and most often affecting the facial skin, joints, and kidneys.

systemic sclerosis An autoimmune disease, also known as *scleroderma,* characterized by formation of thickened collagenous fibrous tissue and thickening of the skin and internal organs, such as the esophagus or lungs.

T cells A subset of lymphocytes that play a central role in cell-mediated immunity.

tachycardia Excessively rapid heartbeat.

Tay-Sachs disease A genetic neurodegenerative disorder of lipid metabolism caused by a deficiency of the enzyme hexosaminidase.

teratocarcinoma A malignant testicular or ovarian germ cell tumor composed of malignant embryonal carcinoma cells and somatic tissues derived from all three embryonic germ layers, as well as trophoblastic and yolk sac cells. In the testis it is classified as a nonseminomatous germ cell tumor.

teratogens Agents that cause fetal abnormalities (malformations).

teratomas A benign germ cell tumor usually found in the ovary, composed of haphazardly arranged tissues derived from three embryonic germ layers and not normally found at the site of origin of the tumor.

tetralogy of Fallot A congenital heart disease characterized by four specific defects, including interventricular septal defect, dextroposition of the aorta overriding the septal defect, stenosis of pulmonary arteries, and right ventricular hypertrophy.

thalassemia A group of genetic hemolytic hemoglobinopathic anemias characterized by microcytic, hyperchromic, and short-lived red blood cells. The diseases are caused by deficient synthesis of hemoglobin polypeptide chains and are classified according to the chain involved, with alpha-thalassemia and beta-thalassemia being the two major categories.

theca cell tumor A benign ovarian sex cord tumor, also known as *thecoma*, composed of estrogen-secreting spindle cells resembling ovarian theca cells.

thrombocytopenia A reduction in the number of platelets below the normal values.

thrombophlebitis An inflammation of thrombosed veins, usually in the lower extremities.

thrombosis An abnormal condition in which a clot develops within a blood vessel.

thrombotic thrombocytopenic purpura A bleeding disorder characterized by thrombocytopenia, hemolytic anemia, and neurologic abnormalities.

thrombus A blood clot or mass of clotted blood; usually found within a blood vessel or cardiac chamber.

thymoma A usually benign tumor of the thymus gland found in the anterior mediastinum. It may be associated with myasthenia gravis or an immune deficiency disorder.

thymus A single unpaired lymphoid organ that is located in the mediastinum. It is important for the maturation of T lymphocytes, and its absence results in T-cell immunodeficiency.

thyroid tumors A group of benign and, less often, malignant tumors originating from the follicular or C cells of the thyroid gland.

thyroiditis Inflammation of the thyroid gland.

tinea (capitis, corporis, cruris, pedis) A group of fungal skin diseases involving the body (t. corporis), head (t. capitis), groin (t. cruris), or feet (t. pedis).

tophus A nodular urate deposit occurring in gout; usually found in the joints or subcutaneous tissues.

TORCH syndrome A syndrome comprising several developmental anomalies caused by infection of a fetus by one of the TORCH agents (toxoplasm, rubella, cytomegalovirus, herpesvirus, and others).

toxemia of pregnancy A group of disorders, such as preeclampsia and eclampsia, presenting during pregnancy with hypertension, proteinuria, edema, and, in the most severe form, convulsions.

trachoma A chronic infectious disease of the eye caused by the bacterium *Chlamydia trachomatis*.

transplant rejection An immunologic reaction to the transplant that can lead to its rejection.

transudate A serous fluid passed through a membrane or squeezed through a tissue or into the space between the cells of tissue.

trauma An injury caused by an external force.

trophic hormone One of several hormones secreted by the adenohypophysis that stimulate target organs.

troponins A group of proteins, normally found in cardiac myocytes, that are released from damaged heart cells in infarction. Its serum concentration is elevated soon after the onset of myocardial infarction and therefore a troponin test is used for the diagnosis of myocardial infarction.

tuberculosis An infectious, inflammatory disease caused by *Mycobacterium tuberculosis*, usually involving the lungs.

tubo-ovarian abscess An abscess involving the ovary and fallopian tube, as typically seen in pelvic inflammatory disease (PID).

tubular necrosis See *renal tubular necrosis*.

tumor A mass resulting from the abnormal growth of cells; also called *neoplasm*.

tumor antigens An immunogenic substance found on the surface of tumor cells or produced by tumor cells. It may trigger an immune response in the host or enter the serum, where it may be detected by laboratory techniques.

tumor marker A substance in the body that may be associated with the presence of a cancer.

tumor suppressor genes A group of genes that do not permit the development of neoplasia. Mutation or loss of tumor suppressor genes may lead to tumor formation.

Turner's syndrome A developmental syndrome related to monosomy of X chromosome (45,X). It is characterized by streak gonads and infertility, low stature and webbed neck, as well as other anomalies of internal organs.

typhoid fever A bacterial infection usually caused by *Salmonella typhi*, transmitted by contaminated milk, water, or food.

ubiquitin A small polypeptide that is involved in removal of effete or abnormally folded proteins from the cell cytoplasm.

ulcer A superficial defect in the mucosa of a hollow organ (e.g., stomach) or the skin.

ulceration The process of ulcer formation.

ulcerative colitis A disease of unknown origin affecting the large intestine and causing widespread confluent ulceration.

upper respiratory tract infections (URIs) A group of infectious illnesses caused by viruses and involving the nose, nasal sinuses, and upper respiratory passages.

uremia End-stage kidney disease characterized by azotemia and numerous other disturbances caused by the inability of the kidneys to excrete metabolic waste products.

urethritis Inflammation of the urethra.

urinary tract infection (UTI) A group of infectious diseases usually involving the urethra and the urinary bladder, but sometimes spreading to the upper parts of the urinary system as well.

urolithiasis Stone formation in the urinary tract.

urothelial carcinoma An epithelial malignant tumor of the urothelial epithelium lining the urinary bladder, ureters, renal calices, and pelvis and the posterior part of the urethra.

urticaria pigmentosa An uncommon form of mastocytosis, usually appearing in infancy, characterized by pigmented skin lesions that become urticarial on mechanical or chemical irritation.

UV light A form of light beyond the range of human vision at the short end of the spectrum, normally present in the sunlight; artificially it can be produced by sun-tanning machines.

uveitis An inflammation of the entire uveal tract of the eye, including the iris, ciliary body, and choroid.

vaginitis An inflammation of the vagina typically caused by *Trichomonas vaginalis, Candida albicans,* or *Gardnerella vaginalis*.

vanillylmandelic acid (VMA) A urinary metabolite of epinephrine and norepinephrine useful for the laboratory diagnosis of tumors of the adrenal medulla, such as pheochromocytoma or neuroblastoma.

varicella A viral childhood disease characterized by a vesicular skin eruption; also known as *chickenpox*.

varices Dilated veins, also known as *varicose veins*. They are most often found on lower extremities, but may be found in the lower esophagus in cirrhosis of the liver and in the form of hemorrhoids in the anus.

ventilatory failure A condition that occurs when the lungs cannot inhale enough oxygen nor remove all the carbon dioxide the body produces.

ventricular aneurysm A localized dilation or saccular protrusion in the wall of the left ventricle, usually caused by scarring of a healed myocardial infarct.

ventricular rupture A tear in the muscle wall of the left ventricle as a result of myocardial necrosis in an infarct. It may cause bleeding into the pericardial cavity, cardiac tamponade, and sudden cardiac death.

ventricular septal defect The most common cardiac anomaly, characterized by one or more abnormal openings in the septum separating the left from the right ventricle.

vertigo A sense of spinning or rotation, but often used for the sense of dizziness in general; usually caused by changes in the body position but may be related to diseases of the inner ear or the nervous system.

virilization A process in which secondary male sexual characteristics are acquired by a female, usually as a result of an excess of androgens produced by ovarian or adrenal tumors. In infants it is most often caused by congenital adrenal cortical hyperplasia, but it can be induced by exogenous male hormones as well.

vitiligo An acquired skin disease of unknown cause, consisting of irregular white patches of depigmentation.

volvulus A twisting of one part of the bowel on itself.

von Willebrand disease An inherited disorder characterized by abnormally slow coagulation of the blood and spontaneous epistaxis and gingival bleeding caused by a deficiency of a component of factor VIII.

vulvitis An inflammation of the vulva, often caused by *Candida albicans,* especially in women with diabetes mellitus.

wallerian degeneration of axons The fragmentation and necrosis of the axon distal to the site of transection.

Waterhouse-Friderichsen syndrome A syndrome caused by *Neisseria meningitidis* infection that presents with sudden onset of fever, purulent meningitis, petechial skin bleeding or purpura, and massive, bilateral adrenal hemorrhage.

watershed (brain) infarct An area of necrosis in the brain caused by hypotension in shock or acute heart failure. It results from hypoperfusion of borderline areas of the brain that are supplied in an overlapping manner by two major arteries.

Wegener's granulomatosis An immunologic disease of unknown etiology that typically affects the upper respiratory tract, lungs, and kidneys; usually associated with diagnostic antineutrophil cytoplasmic antibodies (ANCA) in serum.

Wernicke-Korsakoff syndrome A neuropsychiatric disorder caused by thiamine deficiency; most often associated with chronic alcoholism.

Whipple's disease A rare, systemic disease caused by *Tropheryma whippelii,* affecting predominantly the small intestine. It is characterized by severe intestinal malabsorption, steatorrhea, anemia, weight loss, arthritis, and arthralgia.

Wilms' tumor A malignant renal tumor of infancy and childhood; also known as *nephroblastoma.*

Wilson's disease A rare genetic disorder of copper metabolism. It is characterized by low serum ceruloplasmin and accumulation of copper in the liver and its deposition in the brain and eyes. Liver injury leads to cirrhosis, and the excess of iron in the eyes and brain causes damage of these organs.

wound dehiscence The premature "bursting" open of a wound along a surgical suture.

xanthoma A benign yellowish plaque, nodule, or tumor that develops in the skin as a result of the accumulation of lipid-laden macrophages in the subcutis and often around tendons.

xenograft A transplant of tissues or organs from one species to another (e.g., pig heart valves to humans).

xeroderma pigmentosum A rare, genetic skin disease involving mutation of the DNA repair genes. It is characterized by extreme sensitivity to ultraviolet light, which may produce pigmentation of the skin in the form of freckles, telangiectases, keratoses, papillomas, and skin cancer.

xerostomia Dry mouth caused by reduced salivation that accompanies salivary gland diseases.

yolk sac carcinoma A malignant tumor composed of cells and tissues that resemble those in the fetal yolk sac. It can be a component of testicular nonseminomatous germ cell tumors, but pure yolk sac carcinoma may also occur as an ovarian tumor or extragonadal tumor. Yolk sac carcinoma cells secrete alpha-fetoprotein into the blood, which thus can serve as a serologic tumor marker and is useful for the diagnosis and follow-up of these tumors.

yolk sac tumor A potentially malignant tumor of the testes in neonates and infants. It is composed of cells and tissue that resemble those in the fetal yolk sac. The tumor secretes alpha-fetoprotein.

zoonoses A group of diseases that affect both humans and animals.

Index

Page numbers followed by b indicate boxes; f, figures; t, tables.

A

AA amyloid, 65
ABL, 213
ABO blood groups, 55, 56f, 210f
Abortion, 361
Abscess
  brain, 32f
  cerebral, 462
  definition of, 31, 32f
  lung, 173
  pneumonia-related, 170
  pylephlebitic, 280
  tubo-ovarian, 346
Acetaminophen, 276
Acetylcholine, 51, 435-436
Acetylcholine receptors, 439-440
Achalasia, 235, 236f
Achondroplasia, 415
Acid hydrolases, 4
Acid–base balance, 164
Acid-fast bacillus, 171
Acinus, 161
Acne, 402-403, 403f
Acoustic neuromas, 472
Acquired immunity, 42
Acquired immunodeficiency syndrome, 61-64
  clinical features of, 62-63
  diagnosis of, 63
  encephalopathy associated with, 463
  epidemiology of, 61
  etiology of, 61
  global distribution of, 61
  infections secondary to, 63, 463
  Kaposi's sarcoma associated with, 62, 63-64, 408, 408f
  lymphomas associated with, 63
  maternal transmission, 109
  misconceptions about, 61b
  opportunistic infections, 61, 63
  pathogenesis of, 61-62
  pathology of, 63-64, 64f
  during pregnancy, 109
  respiratory infections, 63
  skin lesions associated with, 63
  treatment of, 64
Acral-lentiginous melanoma, 407
Acromegaly, 381f, 382
Actinic keratosis, 405-406
Activated partial thromboplastin time, 221-222
Active hyperemia, 117
Acute appendicitis, 248, 249f
Acute edematous pancreatitis, 290
Acute glomerulonephritis, 308-309, 309f
Acute inflammation, 22, 30, 34
Acute lymphoblastic leukemia, 213-214, 215f

Acute myelogenous leukemia, 213-214, 215f
Acute pancreatitis, 290-293
  alcohol abuse as cause of, 290
  chronic pancreatitis secondary to, 292
  clinical features of, 292-293
  complications of, 292, 293f
  etiology of, 290-291, 291b
  gallstones, 290
  mortality rate for, 292-293
  pathogenesis of, 290-291, 291f
  pathology of, 291, 292f
  tissue damage caused by, 291
Acute renal failure, 308
Acute respiratory distress syndrome, 126, 184-186, 185b, 185f, 186f
Acute transplant rejection, 55
Acute tubular necrosis, 315-316
Acute viral hepatitis, 267-271. *See also* Hepatitis
Addison's disease, 390f, 391
Adenocarcinoma. *See also* Cancer; Carcinoma; Neoplasms; Tumor(s)
  definition of, 72, 188
  endometrioid, 352
  gastric, 240-241
  histopathology of, 74f
  intestinal, 255-257, 256f
  microscopic features of, 70f
  pancreatic. *See* Pancreatic cancer
Adenomas
  carcinomas vs., 389
  cystadenomas, 72, 357t, 358f
  description of, 72, 74f, 351
  fibroadenomas, 369, 370f
  follicular, 385
  gastrointestinal, 72
  hepatocellular, 282-283
  macroadenomas, 382
  microadenomas, 381-382
  parathyroid, 380-381, 387
  pituitary, 381, 382f
  pleomorphic, 235
  thyroid, 384
  tubular, 72, 254-255
  tubulovillous, 255
  villous, 72
Adenomatous polyposis coli, 254
Adenosine triphosphate, 4
Adrenal cortex
  anatomy of, 379-380
  diseases of, 388-391, 389f, 390f
  hyperfunction of, 388-391, 388f, 389f, 390f
  hypofunction of, 390f, 391
Adrenal glands, 379
Adrenal insufficiency, 390f, 391

Adrenal medulla
  anatomy of, 380
  diseases of, 391-393, 392f
Adrenaline, 148
Adrenocortical tumors, 388-389, 390f
Adrenocorticotropic hormone, 191, 380
Adrenocorticotropic hormone test, 391
Adrenogenital syndrome, 388, 390-391
Aflatoxin B_1, 79, 80f, 81
Age-related macular degeneration, 476
Agglutination, 47
Aging
  of cells, 15-16, 16f
  hypotheses of, 16
AIDS. *See* Acquired immunodeficiency syndrome
Air pollutants, 181t
AL amyloid, 65
Alanine aminotransferase, 10, 265
Albinism, 396, 398
Albumin, 267
Alcohol
  abuse of, 95
  fetal alcohol syndrome caused by maternal ingestion of, 95, 95f, 135
Alcoholic cirrhosis, 271, 273f, 276-277. *See also* Cirrhosis
Alcoholic fatty liver, 15, 16f
Alcoholic hepatitis, 276
Alcoholic liver disease, 276-277, 277f
Alcoholism, 465, 465f
Aldosterone, 149, 304-305
Allergic rhinitis, 175. *See also* Hay fever
Alloantigens, 210, 211f
Allografts, 54
Alopecia, 409-410
Alpha$_1$-antitrypsin deficiency, 174, 272, 278, 278f
Alpha-fetoprotein, 76, 76f, 94, 109, 283, 331-332
Alveolar macrophages, 163
Alveolar pneumonia, 167, 168f, 169
Alveoli, 161, 163f
Alzheimer's disease, 466-467
Amastia, 366
Amebiasis, 248
Amenorrhea, 340
Amniocentesis, 98
Amniotic fluid analysis, 109
Amniotic fluid embolism, 224-225
Amniotic membrane rupture, 110
Amylase, 288
Amyloid, 64-65
Amyloid precursor protein, 466
Amyloidosis, 64-66, 65f
Amyotrophic lateral sclerosis, 468

Anaphylactic shock, 26, 49-50
Anaphylatoxins, 25-26
Anaplasia, 69, 75-76
Anaplastic carcinoma, 70f, 386, 386f
Anasarca, 115, 126-127
Anastomoses, 263, 264f, 275
Anchorage-dependent growth, 76
Androgenesis, 361
Androgens, 323
Anemia, 200-211
    aplastic, 201, 203
    classification of, 200-201
    definition of, 200
    etiology of, 201, 201b
    hemolytic. *See* Hemolytic anemia
    hypochromic, microcytic, 204
    hypoxia associated with, 200
    iron deficiency, 198, 203-204, 204f
    macrocytic, normochromic, 202
    megaloblastic, 201, 204-206, 205f
    microcytic, hypochromic, 202
    morphology of, 202-203, 202f
    normocytic, normochromic, 202
    pathogenesis of, 201
    pernicious, 205
    sickle cell, 198, 202-203, 206-208, 207f, 208f
Anencephaly, 108, 108f, 455, 456f
Aneuploid, 70, 96-97
Aneurysms
    aortic, 101, 117
    definition of, 138
    dissecting, 140, 141f
    fusiform, 140, 141f
    saccular, 140, 141f
Angina pectoris, 134, 146
Angioblasts, 36
Angiogenesis, tumor-induced, 72, 72f
Angiosarcoma, 447, 447t
Angiotensin I, 149
Angiotensin II, 149
Aniline derivatives, 80f
Anisocytosis, 209-210
Ankylosing spondylitis, 414
Ankylosis, 428
Anorchia, 325
Anovulatory cycle, 346-347
Anoxia, 8, 10, 10t, 11f, 126
Anterior pituitary gland, 379
Anthracosis, 15
Antibodies, 45-47
    antinuclear, 58
    definition of, 45
    major histocompatibility complex, 46
    production of, 46
    to red blood cells, 47, 47f
    in systemic lupus erythematosus, 58
Antibody-dependent cellular cytotoxic reaction, 50
Antibody-producing cells, 86
Anticoagulants, 225
Antidiuretic hormone, 191, 297, 304-305, 379
Antigen(s)
    cluster differentiation, 44
    definition of, 42
    human leukocyte, 46, 54
    tumor, 86
Antigen-antibody complexes, 51-52
Antigen-antibody reaction, 46-47

Antigenic drift, 165
Antigen-presenting cells, 46
Antineutrophil cytoplasmic antigens, 310
Antinuclear antibodies, 58, 446
Anuria, 305-306
Aortic aneurysm, 101, 117
Aortic atherosclerosis, 137, 137f, 140, 140f
Aortic dissection, 140
Aortic hemorrhage, 117
Aortic stenosis, 151
Aortic valve, calcified, 18f
APC, 84t
Aphonia, 163
Aphthous stomatitis, 234
Aphthous ulcers, 244-245
Aplastic anemia, 201, 203
Apocrine sweat glands, 396
Apoptosis
    description of, 17, 18-20
    importance of, 18, 19f
    lack of, 20
    in liver, 19f
    necrosis vs., 19f, 20t
    pathologic, 20
    physiologic, 20
Appendicitis, acute, 34, 248, 249f
Arachidonic acid
    cyclooxygenase pathway of metabolism, 26
    derivatives of
        in inflammation, 26-27, 26f
        slow-reacting substances of anaphylaxis as, 48
    drugs that inhibit, 27
    lipoxygenase pathway of metabolism, 26
    metabolism of, 26, 26f
    source of, 26
Arachnoid, 451
Aromatic amines, 79t
Arterial embolism, 122, 124
Arterial hemorrhage, 118
Arterial pressure, 147, 148f. *See also* Blood pressure
Arterial thrombi, 120
Arteries
    anatomy of, 131-132, 132f
    diseases of, 156-157, 157f
Arterioles, 132, 149
Arthritis
    gouty, 431f
    infectious, 430
    osteoarthritis, 415, 426-428, 427f, 427t
    rheumatoid, 415, 428-429, 429f, 430b, 430f
Arthus phenomenon, 51-52, 52f
Asbestos, 165, 181t, 182
Asbestosis, 182-183
Ascending cholangitis, 280
Aschoff bodies, 151
Ascites, 115, 116-117, 274-275, 274f, 275f
Ascorbic acid, 36
Aseptic bone necrosis, 417
Asherman's syndrome, 360
Aspartate aminotransferase, 10, 265
Aspirin
    ancient use of, 27
    cyclooxygenase inhibition by, 27
Asthma, 49, 164, 176-178, 176b, 177f, 178f
Astigmatism, 476

Astrocytes, 452-453
Astrocytomas, 470-471
Atelectasis, 186-187, 187f
Atheromas, 137-138, 138f
Atherosclerosis, 137-147
    aortic, 137, 137f, 140, 140f
    cerebral, 137, 137f
    complications of, 138
    coronary, 137, 137f
    coronary heart disease. *See* Coronary heart disease
    definition of, 137
    description of, 133, 458
    etiology of, 137-138
    forms of, 137, 137f
    gender predilection, 139
    hypertension and, 134, 139
    intestinal arteries, 141
    pathogenesis of, 137-138, 138f
    peripheral, 137, 137f, 141-142
    renal arteries, 141
    risk factors for, 138-140, 139t
    smoking and, 140
"Athlete's foot," 396
Atomic bomb, 81
Atopic dermatitis, 49, 404
ATP7B, 277
Atresia
    definition of, 20
    esophageal, 230
    intestinal, 241
Atrial myxoma, 155
Atrial natriuretic hormone, 304-305
Atrial septal defect, 135
Atrioventricular valves, 130
Atypical pneumonia, 171
Auditory ossicles, 486
Aura, 469
Autoantigens, 210, 211f
Autocrine stimulation, 6, 76-77
Autograft, 54
Autoimmune diseases, 30, 58-59. *See also specific disorder*
    diagnosis of, 58
    genetic factors, 58
    muscle affected by, 437
    nervous system, 463-464
    types of, 58b
Autoimmune hemolytic anemia, 210-211, 210f, 211f
Autoimmune hepatitis, 278, 278t
Autoimmune neuritis, 437-438
Autolysis, 17
Autonomous nervous system, 451
Autophagosomes, 4-5, 12-13
Autosomal dominant disorders, 100-102, 100t
    familial hypercholesterolemia, 101-102, 101f, 102f
    inheritance pattern for, 100f
    Marfan's syndrome, 100-101, 101f
    polycystic kidney disease, 306, 306f
Autosomal recessive disorders, 102-105
    cystic fibrosis, 102-104, 103f
    inheritance pattern for, 102f
    lysosomal storage diseases, 104, 104f
    phenylketonuria, 104-105, 105f
    Tay-Sachs disease, 104, 105f

Autosplenectomy, 207
Avitaminosis A, 294, 477
Azoospermia, 359

B

B lymphocytes, 44
    definition of, 44
    origins of, 43-44
    T lymphocytes vs., 44
Bacille Calmette-Guérin, 86, 173
Bacteremia, 134
Bacteria
    phagocytosis of, 27-28, 28f
    toxin production by, 11
Bacterial conjunctivitis, 478-479
Bacterial diarrhea, 247, 247f
Bacterial endocarditis, 152-153, 152f, 153f
Bacterial meningitis, 462, 462f
Bacterial pericarditis, 31, 31f
Balanitis, 325-326
Barrel chest, 175
Barrett's esophagus, 235-236
Basal cell carcinoma, 404-405, 405f
Basal ganglia, 450
Basophils
    functions of, 199-200
    in inflammation, 29, 29f
BCL2, 20
BCR, 213
Becker's muscular dystrophy, 106-107, 441,
        441t, 442-443
Bence Jones protein, 220
Benign prostatic hyperplasia, 332-335, 333f,
        334f
Benign tumors
    breast, 369-370
    description of, 69-71, 69f, 71t
3,4-Benzyprene, 79, 80f
Berger's disease, 311-312
Beta-amyloid, 466
Bile, 262
Bile ducts
    anatomy of, 263-265
    cancer of, 283
Biliary cirrhosis, 272-273, 278-279, 279f
Biliary tract diseases
    neoplasms, 282-285, 282t, 284f, 285f
    overview of, 263-286
Bilirubin
    albumin binding of, 267
    binding of, 267
    heme conversion to, 199, 199f
    liver's role, 264
Biopsy
    breast, 374, 375f
    chorionic villus, 98, 109, 110f
    cone, 351t
    endometrial, 353
    needle, 374-375, 375f
    punch, 351t
Birth injuries, 111-112
Birthmark, 397-398
Bitemporal hemianopsia, 380-381, 382-383
Bites, insect, 402
Bladder cancer, 318-320, 319f
Bladder tumors, 316
Blastomas, 73

Bleeding disorders, 221-225
Blepharitis, 478f, 479
Blind spot, 475
Blindness, 477
Blood. See also Hematologic diseases
    anatomy of, 195-198
    hypercoagulability of, 88, 120
    peripheral, 197-198, 197b
Blood groups, 55, 56f, 210f
Blood pressure
    definition of, 147
    determinants of, 147-149
    regulation of, 148f
Blood samples, 198, 198f
Blood transfusion, 55-58, 210
Blood urea nitrogen, 306
Blood vessels. See also Arteries; Arterioles;
        Capillaries; Veins; Venules
    inflammation-related changes in, 24, 24f
    mechanical trauma to, 222
    wall weakness of, 222
Blood–brain barrier, 453
Bloom's syndrome, 85
"Blue bloaters," 175, 176f, 176t
Body fluids
    compartments for, 114f
    description of, 114
    edema. See Edema
Bone(s). See also Skeleton
    anatomy of, 412-414, 413f
    calcium stores in, 414
    extracellular matrix of, 414
    extraosseous influences on, 412-413
    formation of, 412
    fracture of, 422-423, 422f, 423f
    functions of, 412, 414
    long, 412, 413f
    phosphate stores in, 414
    remodeling of, 418
    traumatic injuries to, 421-423, 423f
Bone cells, 415
Bone diseases
    achondroplasia, 415
    age-specific nature of, 415
    circulatory disturbances, 417
    developmental, 415-416, 415f
    genetic, 415-416, 415f
    infectious, 416-417, 416f
    metabolic, 417-420, 421
    osteogenesis imperfecta, 100, 414,
        415-416, 415f
    osteomalacia, 419-420
    osteomyelitis, 416-417, 416f
    osteoporosis, 417-419, 418f
    overview of, 414-432
    Paget's disease, 421, 421f
    renal osteodystrophy, 420
Bone infarcts, 417
Bone marrow
    neutrophil production by, 200
    transplantation of, 55, 214
Bone marrow stem cells, 43
Bone mineral density, 419
Bone tumors, 423-424. See also specific tumor
    benign, 423
    malignant, 423-424, 424t, 425f
Borrelia burgdorferi, 430
Botox, 400

Botulism, 437
Bowman's capsule, 309
Brachial plexus palsy, 111
Bradykinesia, 467-468
Bradykinin, 24-25, 25f
Brain. See also specific part of brain
    abscess of, 32f
    anatomy of, 450, 451f
    bacterial infections of, 461, 461f
    concussion of, 460
    contusion of, 460, 460f
    herniation of, 454, 455f
    histology of, 452-453
    laceration of, 460
    metabolic injury of, 464
    metastases to, 473
    traumatic injuries to, 460, 460f
Brain death, 16
Brain tumors, 469-473
    astrocytomas, 470-471
    ependymomas, 471-472
    etiology of, 470-471
    glioblastoma, 471
    gliomas, 471-472, 471f
    medulloblastoma, 472
    meningiomas, 472, 472f
    metastases, 469-470
    oligodendrogliomas, 471-472
    pathogenesis of, 470-471
    types of, 470, 470f
BRCA1, 84t, 370
BRCA2, 84t, 370
Breast
    anatomy of, 365-366, 365f
    inflammation of, 366-367, 367f
    juvenile hyperplasia of, 367
    lymphatic system of, 365
    male
        gynecomastia, 367-368
        lesions of, 376
    physiology of, 365-366, 365f
    pubertal changes in, 367
    size of, 365
    terminal duct lobular units of, 365
Breast biopsy, 374, 375f
Breast cancer, 370-376
    chemotherapy for, 375
    clinical features of, 372-376
    clinical presentation of, 372, 373f, 373t,
        376, 376f
    distribution of, 373f
    epidermal growth factor receptor
        expression by, 376
    etiology of, 370-371
    incidence of, 370, 370f
    in males, 376
    mammography of, 368, 373-374, 375f
    metastasis of, 372
    mortality of, 366
    pathogenesis of, 370-371
    pathology of, 372, 372f
    prevalence of, 366
    prevention of, 88
    prognosis of, 375-376, 375f
    race and, 371
    risk factors for, 371, 371t
    staging of, 375-376
    statistics about, 370

Breast cancer *(Continued)*
    subtypes of, 372
    surgical procedures for, 375
    survival rates for, 375f
    treatment of, 375
Breast diseases
    age-related incidence of, 366f
    cancer. *See* Breast cancer
    developmental anomalies, 366
    fibrocystic, 368-369, 369f
    gynecomastia, 99, 367-368
    hormonally induced changes, 367-369
    mastitis, 366-367, 367f
    overview of, 366-376
    proliferative, 369
Breast self-examination, 372, 374f
Breast tumors
    benign, 369-370, 370f
    malignant. *See* Breast cancer
Bronchi
    definition of, 161
    histology of, 163f
Bronchiectasis, 174, 174f
Bronchiolitis, 167
Bronchioloalveolar carcinomas, 189
Bronchitis, chronic, 173-174
Bronchopneumonia, 167, 168f, 169f
Brushfield's spots, 477
"Bubble children," 61
Budd-Chiari syndrome, 283
Buffy coat, 198
Bulla, 397
Bunion, 428
Burkitt's lymphoma, 83-84, 218
Burns, 398, 399f
Butterfly rash, 59, 59f

C

C cells, 379, 386
Cachexia, 88
Café au lait spots, 100
Calcification, 18
Calcitonin, 386
Calcium
    in bone, 414
    dietary intake of, 418
Calcium stones, 313
Cancer. *See also* Adenocarcinoma;
        Carcinoma; Neoplasms; Tumor(s)
    bladder, 318-320, 319f
    breast. *See* Breast cancer
    case reports of, 78
    causes of, 77-85
        carcinogens. *See* Carcinogens
        DNA viruses, 83
        heredity, 84-85
        tumor suppressor genes, 84, 84t, 85f
    clinical studies of, 78, 78f
    colorectal. *See* Colorectal cancer
    definition of, 68
    epidemiology of, 78, 88-90
    experimental studies of, 78
    hereditary, 84-85
    hypercoagulability associated with, 88
    incidence of, 89
    lip, 234, 234f
    lung. *See* Lung cancer

Cancer *(Continued)*
    mortality of, 90
    oral, 88, 234, 234f
    ovarian, 355
    pancreatic. *See* Pancreatic cancer
    prevalence of, 89-90
    prostate. *See* Prostate cancer
    risk factors for, 88t
    sites of, 89, 89f
    skin, 88, 89-90
    spontaneous healing of, 86
    symptoms of, 87-88, 87f
    testicular, 328f
Cancer cells, 75-77, 76f
Cancer epidemiologists, 68
Cancer myopathy, 444
Candida albicans, 230, 345, 402
Capillaries, 132-133, 132f
Capillary hemorrhage, 118
Carbon monoxide, 181t
Carbon tetrachloride, 10-11, 271-272
Carbuncle, 401
Carcinoembryonic antigen, 75-76, 76f, 86,
        231, 257
Carcinogenesis, 79-80, 80f
Carcinogens
    chemical, 79-80, 79t, 80f, 370-371
    description of, 77
    drugs as, 79
    gastrointestinal tract exposure to, 232
    identification of, 78-79
    industrial, 78-79
    natural biologic, 81
    physical, 80-81
    types of, 77f
    viral, 81-83
Carcinoid
    definition of, 190, 257
    gastrointestinal, 257, 258f
Carcinoid syndrome, 257
Carcinoid tumors, 231
Carcinoma. *See also* Adenocarcinoma;
        Cancer; Neoplasms; Tumor(s)
    adenoma vs., 389
    anaplastic, 386, 386f
    basal cell, 404-405, 405f
    bladder, 318-320, 319f
    cecal, 256f
    cervical. *See* Cervical carcinoma
    cholangiocellular, 282t, 283, 284f
    definition of, 72
    embryonal, 328-329, 330
    endometrial. *See* Endometrial carcinoma
    esophageal, 236-237, 237f
    follicular, 385-386, 386f
    gallbladder, 282t, 283-285, 284f
    hepatocellular, 265, 269, 282t, 283
    histopathology of, 72, 74f
    keratin expression by, 5
    laryngeal, 187-188, 187f
    medullary, 386, 386f
    microscopic features of, 70f
    papillary, 385, 386f
    penile, 337, 337f
    renal cell, 317, 317f
    squamous cell. *See* Squamous cell
        carcinoma
    stomach, 240-241, 240f

Carcinoma *(Continued)*
    thyroid, 385, 386f
    urothelial, 318
    vaginal, 348
Carcinoma in situ, 405-406
Carcinosarcomas, 75
Cardiac failure, 459
Cardiac hemorrhage, 117
Cardiac output, 148
Cardiac tamponade, 143, 144f
Cardiac transplantation, 155-156
Cardiac tumors, 155
Cardiogenic shock, 125, 146
Cardiomegaly, 149
Cardiomyopathy, 154-155, 155f
Cardiovascular diseases. *See also* Heart
        diseases
    arterial diseases, 156-157
    atherosclerosis, 133
    cardiomyopathy, 154-155, 155f
    congenital heart disease. *See* Congenital
        heart disease
    coronary heart disease. *See* Coronary
        heart disease
    hypertension. *See* Hypertension
    incidence of, 133f
    lymphatic diseases, 158
    overview of, 133-159
Cardiovascular system
    anatomy of, 130-133, 131f
    arteries. *See* Arteries
    blood vessels, 131-133, 132f
    diabetes mellitus complications of, 299
    heart. *See* Heart
    lymphatics of, 133
    physiology of, 130-133
    veins. *See* Veins
Caries, dental, 232-233, 233f
Carnitine deficiency, 437
Case reports, 78
Caseous necrosis, 17, 33
Catalase, 10
Cataracts, 476, 481-482
Catecholamines, 393f
Cavernous hemangioma, 282
CD3, 44
CD4, 44
CD8, 44
Cecal carcinoma, 256f
Celiac sprue, 252
Cell(s). *See also specific cell*
    aging of, 15-16, 16f
    atrophy of, 12-13, 13f
    cytoplasm of, 2f, 3-5
    death of, 17-20
    endoplasmic reticulum of, 4
    endothelial, 119-120, 139f
    function of, 2-5, 6-12
    Golgi apparatus of, 2f, 4
    homeostasis, 7
    hormonal signals, 7
    hydropic change in, 8
    hyperplasia of, 13-14, 13f
    hypertrophy of, 13-14, 13f
    immune system, 43-44
        embryology of, 43
        lymphocytes, 43-44
        plasma cells, 44, 45f

Cell(s) *(Continued)*
  inflammation, 24f
  integration of function in, 6-8
  lysosomes of, 4-5, 5f
  metaplasia of, 14
  mitochondria of, 2f, 4
  neoplastic, 68
  nucleus of, 2-3, 2f
  plasma membrane of, 6, 6f, 8f
  ribosomes of, 4
  in steady state, 7-8, 7f
  structure of, 2-5, 6
  swelling of, 8, 8f
  tumor, 75-77, 76f
  in wound healing, 35-36
Cell adaptations, 12-16
Cell death, 6
Cell injury
  causes of, 10-12
    anoxia, 8, 10, 10t
    genetic and metabolic disorders, 10t, 12
    hypoxia, 8, 10, 10t
    inflammation and immune reactions, 10t, 12
    microbial pathogens, 10t, 11
    toxins, 10-11, 10t
    viruses, 11, 12f
  irreversible, 9-10, 9f, 10t
  reversible, 8-9, 8f, 9f
Cellular oncogenes, 83, 83f
Celsus, 22
Central fovea, 476t
Central nervous system
  anatomy of, 450, 451f
  brain. *See* Brain
  infections of, 461-463
  protozoal infections of, 462
  spinal cord. *See* Spinal cord
Central nervous system tumors, 469-473
  brain. *See* Brain tumors
  classification of, 470
  neural cell precursors, 472
Centrifugation, 114
Centrilobular emphysema, 174, 175f
Cerebellum, 451
Cerebral palsy, 443
Cerebrospinal fluid, 452
Cerebrovascular accidents, 454
Cerebrovascular diseases, 458-460
  cerebral infarct, 459
  global ischemia, 458-459
  intracerebral hemorrhage, 459-460
  stroke associated with, 458
Cerebrum
  abscess of, 462
  anatomy of, 450
  edema of, 459
  hemorrhage of, 106
  infarcts of, 458f, 459
  ischemia of, 149-150
Ceruloplasmin, 277
Ceruminous plug, 486, 488
Cervical carcinoma, 348-351
  clinical features of, 350-351
  description of, 341
  diagnostic tests, 351t
  etiology of, 348
  pathogenesis of, 348-349, 349f

Cervical carcinoma *(Continued)*
  pathology of, 349-350
  prevention of, 88
  screening for, 341-343
  staging of, 349-350, 350f
  therapeutic procedures for, 351t
Cervical intraepithelial neoplasia, 349
Cervicitis, 344f
Chagas' disease, 154
Chancre, 327
Channelopathies, 443
Chemical carcinogens, 79-80, 79t, 80f, 370-371
Chemical esophagitis, 236
Chemical teratogens, 95, 95f
Chemotaxis, 25-26, 27
Chemotherapy, 375
  leukemia treated with, 214
  malignancies secondary to, 79
Chest wall lesions, 184
Chief cells, 7
Chlamydia trachomatis, 327, 479
Chlamydial infections, 327, 345-346
Chloride, 8
Chlorpromazine, 276
Cholangiocellular carcinoma, 279, 282t, 283, 284f
Cholecystoenteric fistula, 281
Cholecystokinin, 229-230, 288-289
Cholelithiasis. *See* Gallstone(s)
Cholera, 230
Cholesteatoma, 487
Cholesterol stones, 280
Chondroma, 72, 423
Chondrosarcoma, 72, 423-424, 424t, 425f
Choriocarcinoma, 330, 358t, 362
Chorionic villus biopsy, 98, 109, 110f
Chorioretinitis, 96
Choroid, 476t
Chromatin, 2
Chromosomal abnormalities, 96-99
  numerical, 96-98, 97f
  sex chromosomes, 98-99, 99f
  structural, 96, 97f
Chromosomal fragility syndromes, 85
Chromosomes
  definition of, 2
  translocation of, 96, 97f
Chronic hepatitis, 269, 270-271, 271f
Chronic inflammation, 22, 30, 33
Chronic lung disease, 33, 170
Chronic lymphocytic leukemia, 213, 215f, 216
Chronic myelogenous leukemia, 213, 214-216, 215f
Chronic obstructive pulmonary disease, 173-175
  bronchiectasis, 174, 174f
  bronchitis, 173-174
  definition of, 173
  emphysema, 174-175, 175f
Chronic pancreatitis, 292, 293-294, 294f
Chronic proliferative glomerulonephritis, 311-312
Chronic transplant rejection, 55
Chymotrypsin, 294
Ciliary body, 476t

Circle of Willis aneurysms, 457
Circulation
  bone diseases, 417
  enterohepatic, 262
  esophageal diseases, 236
  eye diseases, 479-480, 480f, 481f
  inflammation-related changes, 23-27, 23f
  kidneys, 315-316
Cirrhosis, 271-276
  alcoholic, 271, 273f
  ascites in, 274-275, 274f, 275f
  biliary, 272-273, 278-279, 279f
  clinical features of, 273-276, 273f
  definition of, 271
  description of, 263
  etiology of, 271, 271b
  histology of, 273, 273f
  pathogenesis of, 271-273, 272f
  pigmentary, 277
  portal, 271-272
  primary biliary, 278-279, 279f
  splenomegaly associated with, 275
  vitamin D metabolism affected by, 417-418
Cleft lip, 94, 230, 232, 232f
Cleft palate, 230
Clinical oncologists, 68
Clinical studies, 78, 78f
Clitoromegaly, 390-391
Clonal expansion, 79-80, 80f
Clonorchis sinensis, 281
Closed-angle glaucoma, 480-481, 481f
Clostridium spp.
  C. difficile, 32, 230, 247
  C. perfringens, 445
  C. tetani, 437
Clot formation, 221-222, 221f
Clotting factors. *See also* Coagulation factors
  deficiencies of, 223-225
  description of, 119, 140, 221-222, 222f, 222t
Cluster differentiation antigens, 44
c-myc, 84
Coagulation factors. *See also* Clotting factors
  deficiencies of, 223-225
  description of, 221-222, 222f, 222t
Coagulation proteins, 119, 119f
Coagulative necrosis, 17, 17f
Coal-workers' lung disease, 164-165, 181, 182f
Cobalamin, 205
Cochlea, 485
Cold injuries, 399, 399f
Colic, urinary, 305
Collagen, 36
Colloid osmotic pressure, 115
Coloboma, 477
Colony-stimulating factors, 197
Colorectal cancer
  description of, 232
  incidence of, 255
  prevention of, 88
  sites of, 256f
Colposcopy, 349-350, 351t
Comedones, 402-403
Comminuted fracture, 422, 422f

Common cold, 165
Compensated shock, 127
Complement system
    activation of, 25f
    in inflammation, 25-26, 25f
Complete abortion, 361
Compound fracture, 422, 422f
Compound nevus, 406
Compression fracture, 422
Concussion, 460
Conductive hearing loss, 488, 489f
Condyloma acuminatum, 344f, 345
Condyloma latum, 327, 327f
Cone biopsy, 351t
Cones, 476t
Congenital adrenal hyperplasia, 343
Congenital heart disease, 134-137
    atrial septal defect, 135
    description of, 134
    etiology of, 135
    incidence of, 134
    pathogenesis of, 135
    pathology of, 135
    septal defects, 135-136, 136f
    tetralogy of Fallot, 136-137, 136f
    ventricular septal defect, 135-136, 136f
Congenital myopathies, 443-444, 443b, 443f
Congenital rubella syndrome, 96f, 135
Congestive heart failure, 144-146
    definition of, 142
    edema of, 116, 116f
    left-sided, 145f
    myocardial infarction as cause of, 146
Congo red, 65
Conjugated hyperbilirubinemia, 266
Conjunctiva, 475, 475f
Conjunctivitis
    definition of, 478-479
    description of, 49, 477
    gonococcal, 346
    treatment of, 479
Conn's syndrome, 388
Constrictive pericarditis, 33, 154
Contact dermatitis, 53, 53f, 403-404
Contact inhibition, 76
Contractures, 37
Contrecoup lesion, 460, 460f
Contusion, 398, 460, 460f
Cor pulmonale, 149, 165
Cornea, 475, 475f, 476t
Corneal abrasion, 478
Coronary artery bypass grafting, 148
Coronary heart disease, 142-147
    clinical features of, 144-147, 145f
    complications of, 143-144, 144f
    description of, 134
    myocardial infarction secondary to, 142
    pathology of, 142-143, 143f
Coup lesion, 460, 460f
Courvoisier's sign, 295
Coxarthrosis, 428
Coxsackievirus myocarditis, 445
Cranial nerve tumors, 472-473
Crater, 234
Creatine kinase, 437, 442, 444
Crepitus, 427
Crescentic glomerulonephritis, 309-310, 310f
Cretinism, 384

Creutzfeldt-Jakob disease, 454
Crohn's disease, 244-246, 244f, 246t
Crossmatching, 56
Croup, 166-167, 167f
Crush injury, 444
Crust, 397
Cryptorchidism, 324-325, 325f, 328
CT scanning, 13
Cuboidal epithelium, 162, 163f
Curare, 437
Curling's ulcers, 238
Cushing's disease, 382, 388-389
Cushing's syndrome, 381, 388-389, 390, 390f
Cushing's ulcers, 238
Cyanide, 10, 11b
Cyanosis, 135-136
Cyclic citrullinated peptide, 429
Cyclopia, 477, 477f
Cyclosporine, 55
Cystadenocarcinoma, 357, 358f
Cystadenoma, 72, 357, 357t, 358f
Cystic fibrosis, 102-104, 103f
Cystic fibrosis conductance regulator, 102-103
Cystitis, 314-315, 315f
Cytogenetic analysis, 217
Cytogenetics, 97
Cytokines
    adhesion molecule activation by, 23-24
    polymorphonuclear neutrophil production of, 28
    T lymphocyte secretion of, 6
Cytoplasm, 2f, 3-5
Cytoplasmic organelles, 2f, 3-4
Cytoskeleton, 3-4, 5, 5t
Cytotoxic T cells, 44

D

Dacryocystitis, 478f, 479
Dane particle, 268
Deafness, 485, 488-489, 489f
Death, 16-20
    brain, 16
    cell, 17-20
Decompensated shock, 127
Defecation, 229
Degenerative joint diseases, 425-426
Deglutition, 229
Delayed puberty, 324
Delirium tremens, 465
Dementia, 466-467
    with Lewy's bodies, 468
Dental caries, 232-233, 233f
Dentinogenesis imperfecta, 416
Dermal connective tissue tumors, 408, 408f
Dermal nevus, 406
Dermatofibroma, 408
Dermatology, 395
Dermatomyositis, 444-445, 446
Dermatopathology, 395
Dermatophytes, 401
Dermatophytoses, 401-402
Dermis, 395f
Dermoid cysts, 357
Developmental abnormalities. See also
        specific disorder
    bone, 415-416, 415f
    breast, 366

Developmental abnormalities (Continued)
    esophagus, 235
    eyes, 477-478
    female reproductive system, 343
    neonatal respiratory distress syndrome,
        110-111, 111f
    nervous system, 455
    oral cavity, 232
    small intestine, 241
    stomach, 237
    urinary tract, 306-307
Diabetes insipidus, 297, 382
Diabetes mellitus, 12, 108-109, 297-300
    classification of, 297, 297b
    clinical features of, 300
    complications of, 299-300, 300f
    definition of, 297
    description of, 289
    genetics of, 108-109, 298-299
    kidneys affected by, 313
    pathogenesis of, 297-299, 298f
    pathology of, 299, 299f
    skin manifestations of, 396
    treatment of, 300
    type 1, 297, 298t
    type 2, 297, 298t
Diabetic microangiopathy, 12, 37, 134,
        300, 308
Diabetic myopathy, 444
Diabetic nephropathy, 313
Diabetic retinopathy, 477, 479-480, 481f
Diapedesis, 27
Diaphragmatic hernia, 250
Diarrhea
    bacterial, 247, 247f
    small vs. large intestine, 246t
    traveler's, 247
Diarthrodial joint, 414f
Diastole, 130-131
Differentiated cells, 2-3
Differentiation, 68
Diffuse alveolar damage, 185-186
Diffuse large B-cell lymphoma, 218
DiGeorge syndrome, 61
Digestion, 229
Dilated cardiomyopathy, 154-155, 155f
Dilation and curettage, 353
Diphyllobothrium latum, 205
Dislocation of joint, 422-423
Dissecting aneurysms, 140, 141f
Disseminated intravascular coagulation,
        120, 126, 223, 223f, 224-225, 308,
        444-445
Distributive shock, 125
Diverticulosis, 241-242, 242f
DNA, 96
DNA viruses, 83
Dowager's hump, 419
Down's syndrome, 97-98, 97f, 98f, 135
Drowning, 183-184
Drugs
    as carcinogens, 79
    liver diseases induced by, 276, 276t
    skin eruptions caused by, 404
Dry gangrene, 18, 18f, 141-142
Dual-energy x-ray absorptiometry, 419
Duchenne's muscular dystrophy, 106-107,
        184, 441-442, 441t, 442f

Ductal carcinoma in situ, 372
Dwarfism, 94
Dysgerminomas, 355, 358t
Dyspepsia, 231, 237-238
Dysphagia, 231, 235
Dysplasia, 349
Dysplastic nevi, 406
Dyspnea, 33, 117, 163, 170, 183, 184t
Dysraphic anomaly, 108
Dysraphic disorders, 455, 456f
Dystrophia myotonica protein kinase, 443
Dystrophic calcification, 18, 18f
Dystrophin, 436, 441
Dysuria, 305

E

Ear(s)
  anatomy of, 485, 485f
  noise exposure effects on, 488
  physiology of, 485
Ear diseases
  deafness, 488-489, 489f
  Ménière's disease, 488
  otitis externa, 486, 487f
  overview of, 485-489
Ear-nose-throat surgeon, 485
Eburnation, 426-427
Eccrine sweat glands, 396
Eclampsia, 362
Ectopic pregnancy, 360, 360f
Eczema, 403-404
Edema, 115-117
  forms of, 115-117, 115t
  of heart failure, 116, 116f
  hydrostatic, 115-116, 115t
  hypervolemic, 116
  inflammatory, 115, 115t
  lymphedema, 116
  oncotic, 116
  pathogenesis of, 115f
  pulmonary, 126-127
Ehler-Danlos syndrome, 423
Ejaculation, 322-323
Electrical injury, 399
Electrocardiogram, 146
Electroencephalography, 469
Elephantiasis, 116
Elliptocytosis, 202-203
Embolism, 122-124
  arterial, 122, 124
  clinicopathologic correlations of, 122-124
  definition of, 122
  description of, 120
  forms of, 122
  pulmonary, 120-121, 123-124
  saddle, 123-124, 124f
  venous, 122-124, 123f
Embryonal carcinoma, 328-329, 330, 358t
Embryonic development
  malformations of, 94-112
    causes of, 94f
    genetic factors, 94
    normal, 92-94, 93f
Emphysema, 174-175, 175f
Empyema, 32, 170
Encephalitis, 461-462, 462f
Encephalomalacia, 459

Endarterectomy, 141
Endocardial cushions, 135
Endocardial mural thrombus, 143-144
Endocarditis, 150, 152-153, 152f, 153f
Endochondral ossification, 412
Endocrine diseases, 380-393. *See also*
    specific disease
Endocrine glands
  hormonal control of, 380
  hyperfunctioning, 380, 380f
  hypofunctioning, 380, 380f
  illustration of, 378f
  parathyroid. *See* Parathyroid glands
  pituitary. *See* Pituitary gland
  thyroid. *See* Thyroid gland
  trophic hormones, 380
Endocrine stimulation, 7
Endocrine system
  anatomy of, 378-380, 379f
  definition of, 378
  function of, 378
  parathyroid glands. *See* Parathyroid
    glands
  physiology of, 378-380, 379f
  pituitary gland. *See* Pituitary gland
  thyroid gland. *See* Thyroid gland
Endocrinologists, 378
Endometrial biopsy, 353
Endometrial carcinoma, 351-353
  definition of, 351
  description of, 340-341
  etiology of, 351-352
  pathogenesis of, 351-352
  pathology of, 352, 352f
  staging of, 352, 353f
Endometrioid adenocarcinomas, 352
Endometrioid carcinomas, 357
Endometriosis, 354-355, 354f
Endometritis, 343
Endometrium
  anatomy of, 340
  hyperplasia of, 14, 340, 346-347, 347f
Endomysium, 434
Endophthalmitis, 478f, 478-479
Endoplasmic reticulum, 4
  rough, 4, 44, 45f, 75
  smooth, 4
Endothelial cells, 119-120, 139f
End-stage glomerulopathy, 312-313, 312f
Entamoeba histolytica, 248, 280
Enteric saprophytes, 168
Enterohepatic circulation, 262
Enzymatic fat necrosis, 18, 18f
Eosinophilia, 47-48
Eosinophils
  functions of, 199-200
  in inflammation, 29, 29f
Ependymal cells, 452-453
Ependymomas, 471-472
Ephelis, 406
Epicanthus, 97, 477
Epidemiology/epidemiologic studies, 78,
    88-90
Epidermal growth factor receptor, 376
Epidermis, 395f
Epidermolysis bullosa, 398
Epididymitis, 326
Epidural hematomas, 455-456, 457f

Epiglottitis, 167, 167f
Epilepsy, 469, 469t
Epimysium, 434
Epinephrine, 380
Epithelial tumors, 73t, 404-406, 405t
Epithelioid cells, 33, 52
Epitope, 46-47, 50
Epstein-Barr virus, 83, 212-213
Erosive gastritis, 238
Erythroblastosis fetalis, 57
Erythrocytes. *See also* Red blood cells
  description of, 195
  function of, 198
  life cycle of, 199, 200f
  measurements of, 199
  microcytic, 202
  normocytic, normochromic, 202
  schematic diagram of, 199f
Erythroplakia, 234
Erythroplasia, 347
Erythropoietin, 197-198, 304
Esophageal atresia, 230
Esophageal diseases, 235-237
  carcinoma, 236-237, 237f
  circulatory disturbances, 236
  developmental, 235
  hiatal hernia, 235
  motility, 235-236
Esophageal varices, 236, 275
Esophagitis, 235-236
Esophagotracheal fistula, 235, 236f
Estradiol, 80f
Estrogens, 79
Ethylenediaminetetraacetic acid, 198
Eustachian tube, 486
Ewing's sarcoma, 75, 423-424, 426f
Excoriation, 397
Exocrine pancreatic insufficiency, 294
Exotoxins, 11
Experimental allergic encephalomyelitis,
    463-464
Experimental oncologists, 68
Experimental studies, 78
External auditory canal, 486
External ear
  anatomy of, 485-486, 485f
  diseases of, 486
  otitis externa, 486, 487f
Extracellular matrix, 36, 414
Extramedullary hematopoiesis, 195
Extrauterine pregnancies, 340
Exudate, 115
Eye(s)
  anatomy of, 475-476, 475f
  functions of, 476t
  myasthenia gravis of, 440
  physiology of, 475-476
  traumatic injuries of, 478
Eye diseases
  cataracts, 476, 481-482
  circulatory disorders, 479-480, 480f, 481f
  conjunctivitis. *See* Conjunctivitis
  developmental, 477-478
  glaucoma, 480-481, 481f
  immunologic, 479
  infections, 476, 478-479, 478f
  malignant melanoma, 482
  neoplasms, 482

513

Eye diseases (Continued)
  overview of, 476-483
  pathology of, 476-477
  retinoblastoma, 482, 482f
Eye tumors, 477, 482
Eyeglasses, 476

F

Facial nerve palsy, 111
Factor VIII deficiency, 106, 224
Factor IX deficiency, 106, 224
Factor Xa, 221
Fallopian tubes, 346
Familial adenomatous polyposis coli, 85,
    85f, 253
Familial hypercholesterolemia, 101-102,
    101f, 102f
Fanconi's syndrome, 85
Farsightedness, 476
Fascicular atrophy, 438, 438f
Fatty liver, 276
Female reproductive system
  anatomy of, 339-340, 339f. See also specific
      anatomy
  functions of, 340, 341f
  hypothalamic-pituitary-ovarian axis
      control of, 341f
  physiology of, 339-340, 339f
Female reproductive system diseases and
    disorders
  developmental, 343
  hormonally induced lesions, 346-347, 347f
  infections, 345-346
  inflammatory, 343-346, 344f
  overview of, 340-359
  sexually transmitted diseases. See Sexually
      transmitted diseases
Femoral hernia, 249
Ferritin, 203-204
Ferruginous bodies, 182-183
Fertilization
  disorders of, 359-360
  in vitro, 92
Fetal alcohol syndrome, 95, 95f, 135
Fetal hemoglobin, 206-207
Fever
  definition of, 34
  pathogenesis of, 34f
  prostaglandin mediation of, 34
Fibrillin, 101
Fibrin, 31, 119
Fibrinoid necrosis, 51-52
Fibrinous inflammation, 31, 31f
Fibroadenomas, 366, 369, 370f
Fibroblasts
  description of, 6
  extracellular matrix production by, 36
  wound healing role of, 36
Fibrocystic change in breast, 368-369, 369f
Fibroids, 353
Fibroma, 72
Fibronectin, 36
Fibrosarcoma, 72
Fibrosis, 33
Fibrothorax, 191-192
First-degree burns, 398
First-intention wound healing, 36, 36f

Fissure, 397
Fistula
  cholecystoenteric, 281
  definition of, 31-32, 32f
Floppy child syndrome, 443, 444f
Floppy mitral valve, 416
Flow cytometry, 217
Fluid(s)
  compartments for, 114f
  description of, 114
  edema. See Edema
Foam cells, 137
Focal epilepsy, 469
Focal segmental glomerulosclerosis, 311
Folic acid deficiency, 201, 205
Follicle-stimulating hormone, 340
Follicular adenomas, 385
Follicular carcinoma, 385-386, 386f
Follicular cells, 379
Follicular lymphoma, 217f, 218
Folliculitis, 401, 401f
Foregut, 228
Foreign bodies
  granuloma, 30
  suffocation caused by, 183
Formaldehyde, 181t
Fractures, 111, 419, 421-423, 422f, 423f
Fragile X syndrome, 107
Free ribosomes, 4
French-American-British classification
    system, 214
Frontal lobe, 450
Frostbite, 399, 399f
Full-thickness burns, 398
Fulminant hepatitis, 269
Fungal infections
  respiratory, 173
  skin, 401-402
Furuncle, 401
Fusiform aneurysm, 140, 141f

G

G cells, 7
Gallbladder
  carcinoma of, 282t, 283-285, 284f
  hydrops of, 281
Gallstone(s), 280-282, 290
  acute pancreatitis caused by, 290
  complications of, 282f
  definition of, 280
  description of, 265
  pathogenesis of, 280-281
  pathology of, 281, 281f
Gallstone ileus, 281
Gangliosides, 12
Gangrene, 18, 18f, 141-142
Gardner's syndrome, 253
Gastric carcinoma, 232
Gastric neoplasms, 240-241
Gastrin, 7, 229-230, 238
Gastrinomas, 296-297
Gastritis, 238
Gastroenteritis, viral, 247-248
Gastroenterologists, 228
Gastrointestinal carcinoids, 257, 258f
Gastrointestinal diseases, 230-259. See also
    specific disease

Gastrointestinal infections
  acute appendicitis, 248, 249f
  diarrhea, 247, 247f
  peritonitis, 248-249
  protozoal enteritis, 248
  pseudomembranous colitis, 241-257
  viral gastroenteritis, 247-248
Gastrointestinal lymphoma, 241
Gastrointestinal neuroendocrine system,
    229-230
Gastrointestinal tract
  adenomas of, 72
  anatomy of, 228-230, 229f
  blood supply to, 228
  cancer of, 88
  carcinogen exposure in, 232
  digestive functions of, 229
  functions of, 228-230
  layers of, 228
  lymphatic system of, 228
  mucosa of, 230-231
  physiology of, 228-230
  secretions of, 230t
Gaucher's disease, 104
Gene amplification, 83
Generalized epilepsy, 469
Genetic bone diseases, 415-416, 415f
Genetic counseling, 109
Genetic disorders
  chromosomal abnormalities.
      See Chromosomal abnormalities
  multifactorial inheritance, 107-109, 107t
  prenatal diagnosis of, 109, 109f, 110f
  single-gene. See Single-gene disorders
Genetic hypothesis, of aging, 16
Genital herpes, 326-327, 345
Genital infections, 345-346, 345t
Germ cell tumors
  description of, 73-75, 73t
  ovarian, 355, 357, 358t, 359
  testicular, 329b, 330-332
Gestational trophoblastic disease, 361
Ghon's complex, 172, 172f
Giant cell arteritis, 156
Giant cell tumor of bone, 423, 424t
Giardia lamblia, 248
Gigantism, 382, 415
Gilbert's disease, 266, 266t, 277
Glaucoma, 476, 480-481, 481f
Glial acidic fibrillary protein, 5
Glial cells, 452-453
Glioblastoma, 471
Gliomas, 72, 454, 471-472, 471f
Gliosis, 454
Glisson's capsule, 262-263
Global aphasia, 459
Global ischemia, 458-459
Glomerular diseases, 307-313
  classification of, 307-308
  end-stage glomerulopathy, 312-313, 312f
  focal segmental glomerulosclerosis, 311
  lipoid nephrosis, 310-311, 312f
  membranous nephropathy, 310, 311f
  metabolic disorders, 307-308
  multiple mechanisms of, 308
Glomerulonephritis, 305
  acute, 308-309, 309f
  chronic proliferative, 311-312

Glomerulonephritis *(Continued)*
  crescentic, 309-310, 310f
  poststreptococcal, 308
  rapidly progressive, 308, 310
Glomerulosclerosis, 305
Glomerulus, 309f
Glucagon, 289
Glucosuria, 306
Glucuronide, 265-266
Glue ear, 487-488
Gluten-sensitive enteropathy. *See* Celiac sprue
Glycogenesis, 298
Glycolysis, 298
Goiter, 385, 385f
Golgi apparatus, 2f, 4
Gonadotropin-releasing hormone, 340
Gonococcal conjunctivitis, 346
Gonorrhea, 327, 345t, 346
Goodpasture's syndrome, 50, 50f, 310
Gout, 430-432, 431b, 431f
Graafian follicle, 355
Grading of tumors, 75
Granulation tissue, 36, 37f
Granulocytosis, 212
Granuloma
  composition of, 53f
  definition of, 33
  noncaseating, 33, 178
  periapical, 233, 233f
Granulomatous inflammation, 33, 34f
Granulosa cell tumors, 359
Granulosa cells, 340
Graves' disease, 51, 383-384
Greenstick fracture, 422
Growth hormone hypersecretion, 381f, 382
Guillain-Barré syndrome, 437
Gumma, 328
Gynecologists, 340
Gynecomastia, 99, 367-368

H

H1N1, 165
Hageman factor, 24-25, 25f, 221-222
Hair diseases, 409-410
Hair follicles, 396
Hamartoma, 254
Haptens, 46
Hashimoto's thyroiditis, 384
Hay fever, 48-49
Hearing loss, 488-489
Heart
  anatomy of, 130-133, 131f
  atria of, 130, 131f
  blood supply to, 130
  chambers of, 130, 131f
  conduction of, 130
  dystrophic calcification of, 18f
  embryologic development of, 135
  fetal, 135
  hypertrophy of, 14, 14f
  iatrogenic lesions of, 155-156
  metabolic diseases that affect, 134
  physiology of, 130-133
  tumors of, 155-156
  valves of, 18, 18f
  ventricles of
    anatomy of, 130, 131f
    aneurysm of, 143, 144f

Heart diseases
  congenital. *See* Congenital heart disease
  congestive heart failure. *See* Congestive
    heart failure
  coronary. *See* Coronary heart disease
  endocarditis, 150, 152-153, 152f,
    153f
  infectious, 151-153, 154
  myocarditis, 33, 134, 151, 154
  pericarditis, 154, 154f
  rheumatic, 150-151, 150f, 151f
Heart murmurs, 131
Heart transplantation, 155-156
Heavy chains, 45
Heavy metals, 10-11, 79t
Heberden's nodules, 428
HeLa, 78
Helicobacter pylori, 238, 240
Helper T lymphocytes, 44, 52, 62
Hemangioblastomas, 470-471
Hemangiosarcomas, 134
Hemarthrosis, 106
Hematemesis, 118, 231
Hematochezia, 118, 231
Hematocrit, 197
Hematologic diseases
  anemia. *See* Anemia
  overview of, 198-226
Hematologists, 195
Hematology, 195
Hematomas
  definition of, 118
  epidural, 455-456, 457f
  subdural, 456-457, 457f
Hematopoiesis, 195, 196f, 201
Hematopoietic growth factors, 198
Hematopoietic stem cells, 195-197
Hematopoietic system, 195-198
Hematuria, 118, 306, 308
Heme, 198
Hemiparesis, 459-460
Hemiplegia, 438, 459-460
Hemochromatosis, 277
Hemodynamic disorders
  hemorrhage. *See* Hemorrhage
  hyperemia, 117, 117f
  thrombosis. *See* Thrombosis
Hemoglobin
  definition of, 198
  fetal, 206-207
  schematic diagram of, 199f
Hemoglobin S, 198, 206
Hemolysis, 47
Hemolytic anemia, 50, 206-210
  definition of, 206
  description of, 201
  hereditary spherocytosis, 206, 209-210,
    209f
  immune, 210-211, 210f, 211f
  sickle cell anemia, 198, 202-203,
    206-208, 207f, 208f
  thalassemia, 202, 208-209, 208f
Hemolytic crisis, 206-207
Hemolytic disease of the newborn,
  57-58
Hemopericardium, 143, 144f
Hemoperitoneum, 118
Hemophilia, 106, 107f, 223-224

Hemoptysis, 118
Hemorrhage, 117-119, 118f
  aortic, 117
  arterial, 118
  capillary, 118
  cardiac, 117
  definition of, 117
  intracerebral, 457, 459-460
  periventricular, 111, 111f
  retroretinal, 478
  subarachnoid, 457
  subdural, 111
  venous, 118-119
Hemorrhoids, 242-243
Hemosiderin, 15, 203
Hemosiderosis, 15, 15f
Hemostasis
  definition of, 221
  normal, 221-222, 221f
Hepatic encephalopathy, 265, 275, 454
Hepatitis, 267-271
  alcoholic, 276
  autoimmune, 278, 278t
  chronic, 269, 270-271, 271f
  definition of, 267
  etiology of, 267
  fulminant, 269
  jaundice caused by, 269
  pathogenesis of, 267
Hepatitis A, 267-268, 268t
Hepatitis B, 83, 268-269, 268t, 269f,
  270f
Hepatitis B core antigen, 268
Hepatitis B *e* antigen, 268
Hepatitis C, 268t, 269-270, 270f
Hepatitis D, 268t, 269
Hepatitis E, 268t, 270-271
Hepatization, 169
Hepatobiliary neoplasms, 282-285, 282t,
  284f, 285f
Hepatoblastoma, 73
Hepatocellular adenomas, 282-283
Hepatocellular carcinoma, 265, 269, 282t,
  283
Hepatocytes, 262, 262f, 270
Hepatorenal syndrome, 275-276
Hereditary hemochromatosis, 15, 15f
Hereditary liver diseases, 277-278
Hereditary nonpolyposis colorectal cancer,
  253
Hereditary spherocytosis, 206, 209-210,
  209f
Hermaphroditism, 343
Hernia, 249-250, 250f
  diaphragmatic, 250
  femoral, 249
  hiatal, 235, 250
  inguinal, 249
  periumbilical, 250
Herniation of brain, 454, 455f
Herpesvirus, 326, 345, 461
Heterophagosomes, 4-5
Heterozygotes, 99-100
Hexosaminidase A, 464
HFE, 277
Hiatal hernia, 235, 250
Hilar tumors, 188-189
Hindgut, 228

Hirschsprung's disease, 230, 241, 242f
Hirsutism, 409
Histaminase, 24
Histamine, 24, 48f
Histoplasmosis, 173
Hodgkin's lymphoma, 75, 216, 218-219,
        218f, 219f
Homeostasis, 7
Homografts, 54
Hordeolum, 479
Human chorionic gonadotropin, 329-330,
        340
Human immunodeficiency virus, 61, 62f.
        See also Acquired immunodeficiency
        syndrome
Human leukocyte antigens
        description of, 46, 54
        HLA-B27, 414
Human papillomaviruses, 83, 341, 345,
        345f, 345t, 402
Human T-cell lymphoma/leukemia virus 1,
        83, 213
Hunchback deformity, 416
Hunter's syndrome, 104
Huntington's disease, 465, 468
Hurler's syndrome, 104
Hyaline membranes, 110, 111f
Hyaloplasm, 3-4, 5
Hydatidiform mole, 361-362, 361f,
        362f
Hydrocephalus, 454
Hydrocephalus ex vacuo, 13
Hydrochloric acid, 7
Hydroperitoneum, 115, 274-275
Hydropic change, 8
Hydrops fetalis, 56, 57f
Hydrostatic edema, 115-116, 115t
Hydrothorax, 115, 187f, 191
Hyperacute reaction, 54
Hyperaldosteronism, 388, 389-390
Hyperbilirubinemia, 207, 265-266
Hypercalcemia, 306, 387
Hypercoagulability, 88, 120
Hypercortisolism, 388-389, 389f
Hyperemia, 23, 117, 117f
Hyperextension injury, 460-461
Hyperflexion injury, 460-461
Hyperglycemia, 298, 298f
Hyperkalemia, 306
Hyperlipidemia, 140
Hyperopia, 476
Hyperparathyroidism, 386-387, 388f
Hyperplasia
        cell, 13-14, 13f
        chronic irritation as cause of, 14
        hypertrophy with, 14
        prostate, 14f
Hyperplastic polyps, 254
Hyperprolactinemia, 381-382
Hypersensitivity pneumonitis, 179, 179t,
        180f
Hypersensitivity reactions, 47-53
        definition of, 47
        type I, 46, 47-50, 477, 479
        type II, 50-51, 50f
        type III, 51-52, 51f, 52f, 479
        type IV, 52-53, 53f, 479
Hypersplenism, 201, 275

Hypertension, 147-150, 316
        arterial, 459
        atherosclerosis and, 134, 139
        benign, 149
        cardiomegaly secondary to, 149
        etiology of, 147-149, 147t
        malignant, 149
        pathogenesis of, 147-149, 147t
        pathology of, 149-150, 149f
        portal, 242, 263, 274-275
        pulmonary, 135-136
        secondary, 147
        vascular effects of, 149
Hypertensive encephalopathy, 149-150
Hypertensive hemorrhage, 460f
Hypertensive retinopathy, 150, 479, 480f
Hypertensive stroke, 149-150
Hyperthyroidism, 383-384, 383f
Hypertrophic cardiomyopathy, 155, 155f
Hypertrophy
        cell, 13-14, 13f
        heart, 14, 14f
        with hyperplasia, 14
        skeletal muscles, 14
Hyperuricemia, 430-431, 431b
Hypervolemic edema, 116
Hypoalbuminemia, 116
Hypochromic, microcytic anemia, 204
Hypodermis, 395f, 396
Hypofibrinogenemia, 224
Hypogonadism, 380
Hypokalemic periodic paralysis, 436
Hypoparathyroidism, 388
Hypophosphatemia, 420
Hypopigmentation, 396
Hypospadias, 325
Hypothalamic-pituitary-ovarian axis, 341f
Hypothalamus, 450, 451f
Hypothyroidism, 383f, 384-385
Hypotonic shock, 125-127
Hypovitaminosis C, 222
Hypovolemia, 118
Hypovolemic shock, 125
Hypoxia
        anemia and, 200
        causes of, 10, 11f
        cell injury caused by, 8, 10, 10t
Hysterectomy, 351t, 353
Hysteroscope, 360

I

Iatrogenic heart lesions, 155-156
Ichthyosis, 397-398
Idiopathic thrombocytopenic purpura, 223
IgA deficiency, 60-61
IgA nephropathy, 307, 311-312
Immersion foot, 399
Immune hemolytic anemia, 210-211, 210f,
        211f
Immune response, 86, 86f
Immune system cells, 43-44
        lymphocytes, 43-44
        plasma cells, 44, 45f
Immunity
        acquired, 42
        definition of, 41
        innate, 41-42, 42f

Immunocompetence, 42
Immunodeficiency diseases, 59-64
        acquired. See Acquired immunodeficiency
                syndrome
        characteristics of, 59-60
        DiGeorge syndrome, 61
        IgA deficiency, 60-61
        primary, 60-61
        severe combined, 60
Immunoglobulins
        features of, 45-46, 134
        IgA, 46, 231
        IgE, 46, 47-48
        IgG, 46, 50, 463-464
        IgM, 46, 429
        schematic diagram of, 45f
Immunohistochemistry, 217
Immunosuppressive drugs, 53-54, 55
Impetigo, 401, 401f
Inborn errors of metabolism, 272, 443,
        464
Incomplete abortion, 361
Increased intracranial pressure, 454
Industrial carcinogens, 78-79
Infarction, 124-125
        definition of, 124
        myocardial. See Myocardial infarction
        outcome of, 125
        pale infarcts, 124
        red infarcts, 124-125, 125f
        white infarcts, 124, 124f
Infections. See also specific infection
        central nervous system, 461-463
        chlamydial, 327, 345-346, 345t
        eyes, 476, 478-479, 478f
        female reproductive system, 345-346
        gastrointestinal. See Gastrointestinal
                infections
        genital, 345-346, 345t
        male reproductive system, 324, 325-328,
                326f
        skin. See Skin infections
Infectious arthritis, 430
Infectious esophagitis, 235
Infectious mononucleosis, 212
Infectious myositis, 445, 445f
Infectious vaginitis, 344f, 345t, 346
Infertility, 324, 340, 343, 354
Inflammation
        acute, 22, 30, 34
        arachidonic acid derivatives in, 26-27, 26f
        bradykinin's role in, 24-25, 25f
        breast, 366-367, 367f
        cells involved in, 28-30, 29f
                basophils, 29, 29f
                eosinophils, 29, 29f
                leukocytes, 23-24, 24f, 27, 27f
                macrophages, 29
                platelets, 29
                polymorphonuclear neutrophils, 27-28,
                        29f
        cellular events in, 24f, 27-30
        characteristics of, 22
        chronic, 22, 30, 33
        circulatory changes associated with,
                23-27, 23f
        classification of, 30
        complement system's role in, 25-26, 25f

Inflammation *(Continued)*
  constitutional symptoms of, 34
  definition of, 22
  duration of, 30
  etiology of, 30
  fibrinous, 31, 31f
  granulomatous, 33, 34f
  histamine's role in, 24
  localized, 34
  location of, 30
  mediators of, 22, 24-27, 30, 34, 119
  pathogenesis of, 23-27
  pathology of, 30-32, 33
  phagocytosis in, 27-28, 28f
  pseudomembranous, 32, 33f
  purulent, 31-32, 32f
  resolution of, 34
  serous, 30-31, 31f
  signs and symptoms of, 22-27, 22f, 34
  ulcerative, 32, 33f
  vessel wall changes associated with, 24, 24f
  as vital reaction, 22-23
Inflammatory bowel disease, 243-246
  Crohn's disease, 244-246, 244f, 246t
  etiology of, 244
  pathogenesis of, 244
  ulcerative colitis, 245-246, 245f, 246t
Inflammatory edema, 115, 115t
Inflammatory polyps, 254
Inguinal hernia, 249
Innate immunity, 41-42, 42f
Inner ear
  anatomy of, 485, 485f
  diseases of, 488
  Ménière's disease, 488
Insect infestations and bites, 402
Insulin, 289-290
  functions of, 298
  secretion of, 7
Insulinomas, 296
Interleukins
  description of, 23-24
  IL-1, 181
Intermediate filaments, 5-6, 5t
Intermittent claudication, 141
Interstitial fluid, 114f
Interstitial pneumonia, 167, 168f, 169-170
Intestinal neoplasms, 253-257
  classification of, 253b
  dietary factors, 253-254
  etiology of, 253-254
  genetic factors, 253
  pathogenesis of, 253-254
Intestinal obstruction, 249-250, 250b, 250f
Intestinal strictures, 244-245
Intracellular fluid, 114f
Intracerebral hemorrhage, 457, 459-460
Intracranial hemorrhages, 455-457
  during childbirth, 111
  epidural hematomas, 455-456, 457f
  intracerebral hemorrhage, 457
  subarachnoid hemorrhages, 457
  subdural hematomas, 456-457, 457f
Intramembranous ossification, 412
Intramural thrombi, 120
Intratubular germ cell neoplasia, 328-329
Intravascular fluid, 114f
Intrinsic pathway, 221

Intussusception, 250, 250f
Involution, 12
Iodine deficiency, 384
Ionizing radiation, 400
Iridocyclitis, 478f, 479
Iris, 476t
Iron
  accumulation of, 15
  food sources of, 203
  metabolism of, 204f
Iron deficiency anemia, 198, 203-204, 204f
Irreversible cell injury, 9-10, 9f, 10t
Irreversible shock, 127
Ischemic bowel disease, 243
Ischemic colitis, 243
Islet cell tumors, 72-73, 289, 296
Islets of Langerhans, 288-289, 294, 297
Isograft, 54

J

Japanese B encephalitis, 461
Jaundice, 57, 206, 261f, 265-267, 266b, 266t, 267b, 269
"Jelly-belly," 359
Joint
  definition of, 413
  dislocation of, 422-423
  immobilization effects on, 414
  synovial, 413-414, 414f
  types of, 413
Joint diseases, 425-432
  degenerative, 425-426
  gout, 430-432, 431b, 431f
  infectious arthritis, 430
  osteoarthritis, 415, 426-428, 427f, 427t
  overview of, 414-432
  rheumatoid arthritis, 415, 428-429, 429f, 430b, 430f
Junctional nevus, 406
Juvenile rheumatoid arthritis, 429

K

Kaposi's sarcoma, 62, 63-64, 75, 408, 408f
Karyolysis, 9
Karyorrhexis, 9
Kayser-Fleischer rings, 277
Keloids, 37, 38f
Keratinocytes, 395
Keratins, 5-6, 395
Keratitis, 478f, 479
Kernicterus, 57, 453
Ketoacidosis, 298
Ketogenesis, 298
Kidneys
  agenesis of, 306
  circulatory disturbances, 315-316
  coagulative necrosis of, 17f
  diabetes mellitus effects on, 299-300, 313
  function of, 304-305
  infarcts of, 124f
  nephron of, 303, 304f
  transplantation of, 55
Klinefelter's syndrome, 98-99, 98f, 99f, 324, 367-368
Köhler's disease, 417

Koilocytes, 349
Koilonychia, 409
Korsakoff's syndrome, 464-465
Krukenberg tumors, 241, 359
Kupffer cells, 262, 265-266
Kyphoscoliosis, 101, 184

L

Labyrinthitis, 488
Laceration, 398
Lactate dehydrogenase, 10
Lactation, 365
Lactic acid, 75
Laetrile, 11
Langerhans' giant cells, 52
Large intestine diseases
  diarrhea, 246t
  diverticula of, 243
  hemorrhoids, 242-243
  intestinal, 242-246
  ischemic bowel disease, 243
  neoplasms. *See* Intestinal neoplasms
  obstruction, 249-250, 250b, 250f
  volvulus, 250, 250f
Larynx
  anatomy of, 161-162
  carcinoma of, 187-188, 187f
  croup, 166-167, 167f
Left-sided congestive heart failure, 145f
Legg-Calvé-Perthes disease, 417
Legionella pneumophila, 168-169
Legionnaire's disease, 168-169
Leiomyoma, 72, 353-354, 353f, 354f
Leiomyosarcoma, 72, 240, 447, 447t
Lens, 476t
Lentigo, 406
Lentigo maligna, 407
Leukemia, 213-221
  acute, 212-213
  acute lymphoblastic, 213-214, 215f
  acute myelogenous, 213-214
  age distribution of, 214f
  chronic, 212-213
  chronic lymphocytic, 213, 215f, 216
  chronic myelogenous, 213, 214-216, 215f
  classification of, 212
  clinical features of, 213
  complications of, 213
  etiology of, 213
Leukocytes, 195
  emigration of, 27, 27f
  in inflammation, 23-24, 24f, 27, 27f
  pavementing of, 23-24, 24f
Leukocytosis, 34, 212
Leukopenia, 212
Leukoplakia, 234, 347
Leukotrienes, 26, 177
Lewy's bodies, 468
Leydig cells
  description of, 322-323
  tumors involving, 332
Lichenoid eruptions, 404
Limb-girdle muscular dystrophy, 441t, 443
Lines of Zahn, 120
Lip cancer, 234, 234f
Lipase, 250-252, 288

Lipids
  cellular accumulation of, 15
  liver accumulation of, 15
Lipofuscin, 4-5
Lipogenesis, 298
Lipoid nephrosis, 310-311, 312f
Lipoma, 72, 73f
Liposarcoma, 72, 447, 447t
Lipoxins, 26
Lipoxygenase, 26
Liquefactive necrosis, 17, 17f
Lithotripsy, 314
Liver
  alcoholic fatty, 15, 16f
  anastomoses, 263, 264f, 275
  anatomy of, 261-263, 261f, 262f
  apoptosis in, 19f
  blood supply to, 261-262, 263
  functions of, 262-263
  lipid accumulation in, 15
  metastases to, 285
  necrosis in, 19f
  physiology of, 261-263
  plasma proteins, 265
Liver cells, 265
Liver diseases
  alcoholic, 276-277, 277f
  bacterial infections, 280
  chronic, 265
  cirrhosis. See Cirrhosis
  drug-induced, 276, 276t
  Gilbert's disease, 266, 266t, 277
  hemochromatosis, 277
  hepatitis. See Hepatitis
  hereditary, 277-278
  immune, 278-279
  jaundice, 261f, 265-267, 266b, 266t,
    267b, 269
  overview of, 263-285
  parasitic infections, 280
  primary biliary cirrhosis, 278-279, 279f
  primary sclerosing cholangitis, 277-278,
    279
  protozoal infections, 280
  toxin-induced, 276
  Wilson's disease, 272, 277
Liver transplantation, 285
Lobar pneumonia, 167, 168f, 169
Long bones, 412, 413f
Loop electrosurgery excision procedure, 350
Lou Gehrig's disease. See Amyotrophic
    lateral sclerosis
Low-density lipoprotein, 101-102
Lower esophageal sphincter, 235
Lower motor neurons, 437f, 451
Ludwig's angina, 445
Lumpectomy, 375
Lung(s)
  acid–base balance function of, 164
  blood supply to, 163, 165
  function of, 163, 164f
  gas exchange in, 163, 164f
  pleura of, 161
  prematurity effects on, 110
Lung abscess, 173
Lung cancer, 188-191
  asbestos exposure as cause of, 183
  carcinogens that cause, 165

Lung cancer (Continued)
  clinical features of, 190-191, 190f
  deaths from, 188
  etiology of, 188
  metastasis of, 189, 190f, 191, 191f
  non–small-cell, 189-190
  pathogenesis of, 188, 189f
  pathology of, 188-190
  prevention of, 88
  smoking as cause of, 188
  symptoms of, 190
  treatment of, 191
Lung silicosis, 30
Lupus. See Systemic lupus erythematosus
Luteinizing hormone, 340
Luxations, 425-426
Lyme disease, 430
Lymph, 133
Lymphadenopathy, 212
Lymphangitis, 158
Lymphatic system
  of breast, 365
  of cardiovascular system, 133
  of gastrointestinal tract, 228
Lymphedema, 116
Lymphocytes, 43-44
  B. See B lymphocytes
  definition of, 43-44
  description of, 200
  T. See T lymphocytes
Lymphogranuloma venereum, 326
Lymphoid cells, 43
Lymphoid organs, 43-44
Lymphoma, 216-219
  acquired immunodeficiency syndrome-
    related, 63
  Burkitt's, 83-84, 218
  definition of, 72
  description of, 200
  diffuse large B-cell, 218
  etiology of, 213
  extranodal, 216
  follicular, 217f, 218
  forms of, 213
  gastrointestinal, 241
  Hodgkin's, 75, 216, 218-219, 218f,
    219f
  non-Hodgkin's, 216-218, 217f
Lymphopenia, 59-60, 212
Lysosomal storage diseases, 104, 104f
Lysosomes, 4-5, 5f
Lysozyme, 41-42

M

Macroadenomas, 382
Macroglossia, 97
Macrophages
  alveolar, 163
  in fibrinous exudate, 31
  in inflammation, 29
  wound healing role of, 35
Macula lutea, 475, 476t
Macule, 397, 397f
Maculopapular rash, 402
Main pancreatic duct, 290
Major histocompatibility complex, 46
Malabsorption, 231

Malabsorption syndromes, 250-253
  causes of, 252b
  celiac sprue, 252
  clinical features of, 253
  pathophysiology of, 251f
  tropical sprue, 252
  Whipple's disease, 252-253
Malaria, 201
Male breast
  gynecomastia, 367-368
  lesions of, 376
Male reproductive system
  anatomy of, 322-323, 322f
  diseases of
    cryptorchidism, 324-325, 325f, 328
    infections, 324, 325-328, 326f
    infertility, 324
    overview of, 324-337
    sexually transmitted diseases.
      See Sexually transmitted diseases
    tumors, 324-325
Malignant hypertension, 149, 316
Malignant melanoma, 407-408, 407f, 482
Malignant peripheral nerve sheath tumor, 447
Malignant tumors, 69-71, 69f, 71t, 87-88, 87f
Mallory's hyaline, 276, 277f
Mallory-Weiss syndrome, 236
Mammography, 368, 373-374, 375f
Marfan's syndrome, 100-101, 101f
Mast cells, 29, 47-48
Mastectomy, 375
Mastication, 229
Mastitis, 366-367, 367f
Mastoiditis, 487f
Maternofetal Rh incompatibility, 56
McBurney's point, 248
Mean corpuscular hemoglobin, 199
Mean corpuscular hemoglobin
  concentration, 199
Mean corpuscular volume, 199
Mechanical trauma to skin, 398
Meckel's diverticulum, 241
Meconium peritonitis, 103
Medulla oblongata, 450-451, 451f
Medullary carcinoma, 386, 386f
Medulloblastoma, 470, 472
Megacolon, 231, 241
Megaesophagus, 231
Megaloblastic anemia, 201, 204-206, 205f
Megaloblasts, 204-205
Melancholy, 263
Melanocytes, 395
Melena, 118, 237
Membrane attack complex, 25-26, 25f
Membranous nephropathy, 310, 311f
MEN1, 381
Mendelian genetics, 100
Ménière's disease, 488
Meninges, 451
Meningiomas, 470-471, 472, 472f
Meningitis, 453-454, 462, 462f
Meningocele, 108, 455, 456f
Meningomyelocele, 108
Meniscus, 413-414
Menopause, 346-347, 418
Menorrhagia, 340, 352
Menstrual cycle, 342f
Mesenchymal cells, 72

Mesenchymal tumors, 72, 73t
Mesenteric thrombosis, 243, 243f
Mesothelioma, 192, 192f
Mesothelium, 163
Messenger RNA, 3, 3f
Metabolic bone diseases, 417-420, 421
Metabolic glomerulopathy, 307-308
Metaphysis, 412
Metaplasia, 14
Metastases
   brain tumors, 469-470, 473
   breast cancer, 372
   description of, 71-72, 71f, 72f
   hepatocellular carcinoma, 283
   liver, 285
   lung cancer, 189, 190f, 191, 191f
   ovarian tumors, 359
   pancreatic cancer, 295-296
   prostate cancer, 335, 336f
Metastatic calcification, 18
Metastatic cascade, 71, 71f
Methicillin-resistant *Staphylococcus aureus*, 401
3-Methylcholanthrene, 80f
Metrorrhagia, 118
Microadenomas, 381-382
Microangiopathy, 299-300
Microbial pathogens, 10t, 11
Microbial teratogens, 95-96, 96f
Microcephaly, 96
Microfilaments, 5, 5t
Microglia, 452-453
Microphthalmia, 477
Microtubules, 5-6, 5t
Microvascular thrombi, 120
Micturition, 304
Midbrain, 450-451, 451f
Middle ear
   anatomy of, 485, 485f
   diseases of, 486-488
   otitis media, 486-488, 487f
   otosclerosis, 488
Middle respiratory syndromes, 166-167
Midgut, 228
Miliary tuberculosis, 172
Minerals, 7
Minimal change disease, 310-311
Missed abortion, 361
Mitochondria, 2f, 4
Mitochondrial myopathies, 443
Mitosis, 2
Mitotic cells, 35, 35f
Mitral stenosis, 150-151
Mixed germ cell tumors, 356
Monocytes, 200
Monosomy, 96-97
Mons pubis, 339-340, 339f
Morula, 92
Mucopolysaccharidoses, 104
Mucosa-associated lymphoid tissue, 43-44, 163, 230, 241
Mucosal ulcers, 35
Multifactorial inheritance disorders, 107-109, 107t
Multinucleated giant cells, 33, 34f
Multiple endocrine adenomatosis type II, 470-471
Multiple endocrine neoplasia, 381

Multiple myeloma, 219-221, 220f
Multiple sclerosis, 453-454, 463-464, 464f
Mumps, 234
Murmurs, heart, 131
Muscle
   anatomy of, 434-436
   mechanical injury of, 444-445
   physiology of, 434-436
   skeletal. *See* Skeletal muscle
Muscle cells, 435-436, 437
Muscle diseases
   characteristics of, 436
   dystrophies. *See* Muscular dystrophies
   myasthenia gravis, 439-441, 440f
   myopathies. *See* Myopathies
   myositis, 445-446, 445b, 445f
   neurogenic atrophy, 437-439, 437f, 438b, 438f
   overview of, 436-448, 436b
   soft tissue tumors, 446-447, 447f
Muscle fibers, 434f, 439, 439f
Muscular dystrophies, 106-107, 441-443
   Becker's, 106-107, 441, 441t, 442-443
   characteristics of, 441t
   definition of, 106, 441
   Duchenne's, 106-107, 441-442, 441t, 442f
   inheritance patterns of, 441
   limb-girdle, 441t, 443
   myotonic, 441t, 443, 444f
Muscular dystrophy, 184
Myalgia, 445
Myasthenia gravis, 51, 184
Mycobacterium spp.
   description of, 52-53
   M. avium intracellulare, 63
   M. tuberculosis, 168-169, 171-172
Mycoplasma trachomatis, 477
Mycosis fungoides, 408
Mydriasis, 475
Myelitis, 462
Myeloid stem cells, 195-197
Myeloid:erythroid ratio, 200
Myelomeningocele, 455, 456f
Myelophthisic anemia, 201
Myeloproliferative disorders, 211
Myenteric plexus, 228
Myocardial infarction, 146-147
   complications of, 143-144, 144f
   coronary heart disease as cause of, 142
   definition of, 146
   description of, 134
   diagnosis of, 146-147, 147f
   distribution of, 143f
   heart failure secondary to, 146
   outcome of, 146f
   secondary liquefaction of infarcts, 17
   treatment of, 147
Myocardial ischemia, 142, 142f
Myocarditis, 33, 134, 151, 154
Myofibroblasts, 36
Myoglobin, 146-147
Myometrium, 340
Myopathia rheumatica, 444
Myopathies
   acquired, 444
   congenital, 443-444, 443b, 443f

Myopia, 476
Myosis, 475
Myositis, 445-446, 445b, 445f
Myotonic dystrophy, 441t, 443, 444f
Myxedema, 384

N

Na+/K+-adenosine triphosphatase pump, 8
Nail diseases, 409, 409f
Naphthylamine, 78-79, 80f
Natural biologic carcinogens, 81
Natural killer cells, 44
Near-drowning, 183-184
Nearsightedness, 476
Necrosis, 17-20
   apoptosis vs., 19f, 20t
   caseous, 17, 33
   coagulative, 17, 17f
   enzymatic fat, 18, 18f
   liquefactive, 17, 17f
   in liver, 19f
   word origin of, 17
Needle biopsy, 374-375, 375f
Negri bodies, 461-462
Neisseria spp.
   N. gonorrhoeae, 327
   N. meningitidis, 461
Nemaline bodies, 436
Neolipogenesis, 15
Neonatal respiratory distress syndrome, 110-111, 111f
Neoplasia. *See also* Adenocarcinoma; Cancer; Carcinoma; Tumor(s)
   clinical manifestations of, 86-88
   definition of, 68
   epidemiology of, 88-90
   prevention of, 87b
   symptoms of, 87-88, 87f
   terminology associated with, 68
Neoplasms. *See also* Adenocarcinoma; Cancer; Carcinoma; Tumor(s)
   gastric, 240-241
   hepatobiliary, 282-285, 282t, 284f, 285f
   ovarian. *See* Ovarian tumors
   skin. *See* Skin neoplasms
   thyroid, 385-386, 386f
   tumors vs., 68
Neoplastic cells, 68
Neoplastic polyps, 254-255, 255f
Neoplastic stem cells, 213
Nephritic syndrome, 308
Nephroangiosclerosis, 12, 316
Nephroblastoma, 73
Nephrologists, 303
Nephron, 303, 304f
Nephrotic syndrome, 308, 313
Nerve sheath tumors, 470-471
Nervous system
   anatomy of, 450-453, 451f
   cells of, 452f
   central. *See* Central nervous system
   infections of, 461-463
   peripheral, 451
   physiology of, 450-453
   traumatic injuries to, 460-461, 460f

Nervous system diseases
alcoholism, 465, 465f
autoimmune, 463-464
cerebrovascular diseases. *See* Cerebrovascular diseases
developmental disorders, 455
epilepsy, 469, 469t
inborn errors of metabolism, 272, 443, 464
intracranial hemorrhages. *See* Intracranial hemorrhages
multiple sclerosis, 463-464, 464f
neoplasms. *See* Brain tumors; Central nervous system tumors
neurodegenerative diseases. *See* Neurodegenerative diseases
nutritional diseases, 464-465
overview of, 453-473
Neural hearing loss, 489, 489f
Neural stimulation, 7
Neuroblastoma, 83, 86, 391-392, 392f
Neurodegenerative diseases, 465-468
Alzheimer's disease, 466-467
amyotrophic lateral sclerosis, 468
definition of, 465
Huntington's disease, 468
Parkinson's disease, 467-468, 467f
Neurofibrillary tangles, 466
Neurofibroma, 100, 408, 472
Neurofibromatosis, 85
Neurogenic atrophy, 437-439, 437f, 438b, 438f
Neuromas, 472
Neuromuscular junction, 435
Neurosyphilis, 461, 463
Neutropenia, 212
Neutrophils. *See also* Polymorphonuclear neutrophils
bone marrow production of, 200
function of, 199-200
Nevus, 397-398, 406, 477
Nevus flammeus, 397-398
NF1, 84t, 85
Nicotinic acid deficiency, 465
Niemann-Pick disease, 464
Nitrosamines, 79t, 240
Nodular goiter, 384-385, 385f
Nodular melanoma, 407
Nodule, 397, 397f
Noise exposure, 488
Noncaseating granulomas, 33, 178
Non-Hodgkin's lymphoma, 216-218, 217f
Nonseminomatous germ cell tumors, 330-332, 331f
Non–small-cell lung carcinoma, 189-190
Norepinephrine, 380
Norovirus, 248
Nuclear dust, 9
Nuclear-to-cytoplasmic ratio, 70
Nucleocytoplasmic ratio, 3
Nucleolus, 2
Nucleus
cells, 2-3, 2f
DNA of, 2-3
Nutcracker esophagus, 235
Nutrient arteries, 416-417
Nutritional diseases, 464-465

O

Oat-cell carcinomas, 188
Occipital lobe, 450
Occult blood, 257
Oligoastrocytomas, 471-472
Oligodendroglia, 452-453
Oligodendrogliomas, 471-472
Oligominerals, 7
Oligospermia, 359
Oliguria, 127, 305-306
Onchocerca volvulus, 477
Oncogenes, 83-84
activation of, 83f
definition of, 77
intestinal tumors, 254
leukemias caused by, 213
lymphomas caused by, 213
proto-oncogene transformation into, 83-84
viral, 83
Oncogenic viruses, 82
Oncology, 68
Oncotic edema, 116
Oncotic pressure, 115-116
Onychomyces, 409
Oocytes, 340
Oophoritis, 343
Open-angle glaucoma, 480-481, 481f
Ophthalmologists, 476
Opisthorchis sinensis, 81
Opsonins, 25-26, 27
Oral cancer, 88, 234, 234f
Oral cavity diseases and disorders, 232-234
cleft lip, 230, 232, 232f
dental caries, 232-233, 233f
developmental, 232
periodontal disease, 232, 233-234, 233f
stomatitis, 232, 234
Orchitis, 325-326
Organogenesis, 92-94, 93f
Organs, 6. *See also specific organ*
Osteitis cystica, 420
Osteitis deformans. *See* Paget's disease
Osteoarthritis, 415, 426-428, 427f, 427t
Osteoblasts, 413
Osteoclasts, 413
Osteogenesis imperfecta, 100, 414, 415-416, 415f
Osteoid, 414
Osteoma, 423
Osteomalacia, 414, 419-420
Osteomyelitis, 416-417, 416f
Osteons, 412
Osteopenia, 414
Osteopetrosis, 414
Osteophytes, 426-427
Osteoporosis, 417-419, 418f
Osteosarcoma, 84, 421, 423-424, 424t, 425f
Osteosclerosis, 420
Otitis externa, 486, 487f
Otitis interna, 487f
Otitis media, 30, 486-488, 487f
Otorhinolaryngologists, 161, 485
Otosclerosis, 486, 488
Ovarian cancer, 355
Ovarian cysts, 347, 355

Ovarian neoplasms, 355-356, 356f
Ovarian tumors, 355-356
classification of, 357t
etiology of, 355-356
germ cell, 355, 357, 358t, 359
metastases, 359
pathogenesis of, 355-356
sex cord stromal tumors, 356, 357-359
surface epithelial tumors, 356-357
teratocarcinomas, 356
Ovaries
anatomy of, 340
tumors of. *See* Ovarian tumors
Ovulation, 340
Oxidative phosphorylation, 4
Oxygen radicals, 10, 11f
Oxygen toxicity, 10
Oxytocin, 379

P

Paget's disease, 421, 421f
Pale infarcts, 124
Panacinar emphysema, 174, 175f
Pancreas
anatomy of, 288-289, 288f
physiology of, 288-289
Pancreatic cancer, 295-296
clinical features of, 295-296, 296f
deaths caused by, 289
diagnosis of, 296
incidence of, 295
pathology of, 295, 295f
Pancreatic diseases
cancer. *See* Pancreatic cancer
overview of, 289-301
pancreatitis. *See* Pancreatitis
Pancreatic pseudocysts, 289, 292, 293f
Pancreatic tumors
classification of, 295
endocrine, 296-297
risk factors for, 295
Pancreatitis
acute. *See* Acute pancreatitis
acute edematous, 290
chronic, 292, 293-294, 294f
Panhypopituitarism, 382
Pannus, 428
Panophthalmitis, 479
Papanicolaou test, 341-343, 343f, 351t
Papilla of Vater, 288, 290
Papillary carcinoma, 385, 386f
Papillary urothelial carcinomas, 318-319
Papilledema, 479
Papillomas, 72
Papillomatosis, 368
Papule, 397, 397f
Paracrine effect, 378
Paracrine stimulation, 7
Paradoxical embolism, 122
Paralysis, 438
Paraneoplastic syndromes, 88, 191, 283, 444
Paraplegia, 438
Parathyroid adenoma, 380-381, 387
Parathyroid glands
anatomy of, 379
diseases of, 386-388

Parathyroid glands (Continued)
  hyperparathyroidism, 386-387, 388f
  hyperplasia of, 387, 387f
  hypoparathyroidism, 388
Parathyroid hormone, 379, 386-387, 413
Parathyroid hormone-related polypeptide, 88, 381
Parietal lobe, 450
Parkin, 468
Parkinsonism, 467
Parkinson's disease, 465, 467-468, 467f
Paronychia, 409, 409f
Passive hyperemia, 117, 117f
Patch, 397, 397f
Pathologic apoptosis, 20
Pathologic atrophy, 12
Pathologic fracture, 422
Pavementing, 23-24, 24f
Pelvic exenteration, 351t
Pelvic inflammatory disease, 33, 340, 344f, 346
Penile carcinoma, 337, 337f
Peptic esophagitis, 235-236
Peptic ulcer, 33f, 238-240, 239f
Peptidases, 288
Periapical abscess, 233
Periapical granuloma, 233, 233f
Pericarditis, 151, 154, 154f
  bacterial, 31, 31f
  constrictive, 33
Perifascicular atrophy, 446
Perikaryon, 452
Perimysium, 434
Periodontal disease, 232, 233-234, 233f
Periodontitis, 233
Periosteum, 412
Peripheral blood, 197-198, 197b
Peripheral nervous system, 451
Peripheral neuropathy, 300
Peripheral resistance, 148-149
Peripheral vascular disease, 137, 137f, 141-142
Peristalsis, 229
Peritonitis, 248-249
Periumbilical hernia, 250
Periventricular hemorrhage, 111, 111f
Pernicious anemia, 205
Peutz-Jeghers polyps, 254
Phagocytosis, 27-28, 28f, 199-200
Pharynx, 161-162
Phenylalanine hydroxylase, 104
Phenylketonuria, 104-105, 105f
Pheochromocytoma, 392-393, 393f
Philadelphia chromosome, 72, 213
Phocomelia, 95
Phospholipase, 27
Phyllodes tumor, 369-370
Physical carcinogens, 80-81
Physiologic apoptosis, 20
Physiologic atrophy, 12
Pickwickian syndrome, 184
Pigmented nevus, 477
Pigmented villonodular synovitis, 425-426
"Pink puffers," 175, 176f, 176t
"Pinkeye." See Conjunctivitis
Pituitary adenomas, 381, 382f

Pituitary gland
  anatomy of, 378
  anterior, 379
  diseases of, 381-383, 381f, 382f
  hormones produced by, 379, 379f
  hyperfunction of, 381-382
  hypofunction of, 382
  posterior, 379
  tumors of, 382-383
Placenta accreta, 361
Placenta previa, 361
Placental anomalies, 360-362
Plaque, 405
Plasma, 119, 195
Plasma cells, 44, 45f
Plasma membrane
  anatomy of, 6, 6f
  semipermeability of, 8f
Plasma proteins, 265
Plasmacytoma, 212
Plasmapheresis, 441
Plasmin, 119-120
Plasminogen, 24-25, 25f
Plasmodium spp., 201
Platelet(s)
  description of, 195
  functions of, 119-120, 200
  in inflammation, 29
  normal levels of, 223
Platelet disorders, 223
Platelet-derived growth factor, 29
Pleomorphic adenoma, 235
Pleomorphism, 69-70
Pleura, 161
Pleural cavity, 191
Pleural diseases, 187f, 191-192, 192f
Pleural effusion, 144-146, 190, 191-192
Pleural tumors, 192, 192f
Pleuritis, 170, 173, 187
Pneumoconioses, 180-183
  asbestosis, 182-183
  coal-workers' lung disease, 164-165, 181, 182f
  definition of, 180
  silicosis, 181-182
Pneumocystis jiroveci, 171
Pneumocytes, 162-163
Pneumonia, 167-171
  alveolar, 167, 168f, 169
  atypical, 171
  clinical features of, 170-171
  community-acquired, 170
  complications of, 170, 170f
  definition of, 167
  description of, 164
  etiology of, 168-169, 169t
  forms of, 171
  interstitial, 167, 168f, 169-170
  lobar, 167, 168f, 169
  pathogenesis of, 169
  pathology of, 169-170
  physical examination findings, 171
  signs and symptoms of, 170-171
  sputum analysis, 171
Pneumothorax, 187f, 191, 192f
Poikilocytosis, 202
Point mutation, 83
Poison ivy reaction, 53

Poliomyelitis, 184, 437
Polyarteritis nodosa, 51-52, 156, 157f
Polychlorinated biphenyls, 181t
Polycyclic aromatic hydrocarbons, 79, 79t, 80f, 188
Polycystic kidney disease, 306-307, 306f
Polycystic ovary syndrome, 355
Polycythemia, 211-212, 211f
Polydipsia, 300
Polymastia, 366
Polymorphonuclear leukocytes, 27. See also Leukocytes
Polymorphonuclear neutrophils, 27-28, 29f, 142, 166, 416-417. See also Neutrophils
Polymorphous sarcoma, 447, 447f, 447t
Polymyositis, 444-445, 446
Polyphagia, 300
Polyps
  definition of, 254
  hyperplastic, 254
  inflammatory, 254
  juvenile, 254
  neoplastic, 254-255, 255f
  non-neoplastic, 254
  Peutz-Jeghers, 254
Polysomes, 4
Polythelia, 366
Polyuria, 300, 305-306
Pons, 450-451, 451f
Pontine myelinolysis, 465
Portal cirrhosis, 271-272
Portal hypertension, 242, 263, 274-275
Posterior pituitary gland, 379
Postperfusion myocardial injury, 10, 11f
Poststreptococcal glomerulonephritis, 52, 308
Potassium cyanide, 10, 11b
Pott, Percival, 78
Pott's disease, 416
Precocious puberty, 324
Preeclampsia, 362
Pregnancy
  acquired immunodeficiency syndrome during, 109
  birth injuries, 111-112
  ectopic, 360, 360f
  normal duration of, 109
  pathology of, 359-362
  premature labor, 109-111
  toxemia of, 362
Prematurity, 109-111
Premenstrual syndrome, 366
Prenatal development, 93f
Prenatal diagnosis of genetic disorders, 109, 109f, 110f
Presbycusis, 488
Presbyopia, 476
Primary biliary cirrhosis, 278-279, 279f
Primary sclerosing cholangitis, 277-278, 279
Primitive neuroectodermal tumors, 424
Prions, 461-462
Procarcinogens, 79-80, 188
Proenzymes, 289
Programmed cell death, 18
Prolactin, 365
Prolactinomas, 381-382
Proliferative breast disease, 369

Properdin, 41-42
Prostacyclin, 26
Prostaglandins
    description of, 26
    fever mediation by, 34
Prostate cancer, 335-337
    clinical features of, 336-337
    etiology of, 335
    incidence of, 335
    metastases, 335, 336f
    pathogenesis of, 335
    pathology of, 335-336, 335f
    prevention of, 88
    sex hormones in, 325
Prostate gland
    benign hyperplasia of, 332-335, 333f, 334f
    hyperplasia of, 14f
    tumors of, 324
Prostatectomy, 337
Prostate-specific antigen, 336
Prostatic acid phosphatase, 336
Prostatitis, 326
Proteasomes, 13
Protein synthesis, 3
Proteinuria, 306
Prothrombin time, 221-222
Proto-oncogenes
    definition of, 83
    functions of, 84
    oncogene transformation of, 83-84
Protozoal enteritis, 248
Protozoal infections
    of central nervous system, 462
    of gastrointestinal tract, 248
    of heart, 134
    of liver, 280
    of vagina, 345
Pseudocysts, 233, 289, 291-292, 293f
Pseudohermaphroditism, 343
Pseudomembranous colitis, 241-257
Pseudomembranous inflammation, 32, 33f
Pseudomonas aeruginosa, 168, 171
Pseudopolyps, 245, 245f, 254
Psoriasis, 404, 404f
PTEN, 352
Puberty
    breast changes in, 367
    delayed, 324
    precocious, 324
Pulmonary edema, 126-127
Pulmonary embolism, 120-121, 123-124
Pulmonary hypertension, 135-136
Pulmonary stenosis, 135
Pulmonary tuberculosis, 171-173, 172f
Pulmonologists, 161
Pulpitis, 233f
Punch biopsy, 351t
Purulent inflammation, 31-32, 32f
Pus, 28, 31, 32f
Pustule, 397, 397f
Pyelonephritis, 305, 314-315, 315f
Pyknosis, 9
Pylephlebitic abscess, 280
Pyloric stenosis, 237
Pyorrhea, 233
Pyothorax, 170
Pyrogens, 34
Pyuria, 306

R

Rabies, 461-462
Radiation injury, 399-400
Radicular cyst, 233
Radioactive materials, 81
Rapidly progressive glomerulonephritis, 308, 310
Raynaud's disease, 156-157
RB1, 84, 84t
Red blood cells. *See also* Erythrocytes
    anemia caused by loss and destruction of, 201
    antibodies to, 47, 47f
    bilirubin excretion by, 264
Red infarcts, 124-125, 125f
Reed-Sternberg cells, 218, 218f
Reiter's syndrome, 326
Renal cell carcinoma, 317, 317f
Renal failure, 305
    acute, 308
Renal osteodystrophy, 420
Renin, 149, 304
Renin-angiotensin system, 149, 380
Respiratory diseases
    allergic rhinitis, 175
    asthma, 176-178, 176b, 177f, 178f
    bronchiolitis, 167
    croup, 166-167, 167f
    epiglottitis, 167, 167f
    fungal, 173
    hypersensitivity pneumonitis, 179, 179t, 180f
    immune, 175-179
    lung abscess, 173
    middle respiratory syndromes, 166-167
    overview of, 164-192
    pneumonia. *See* Pneumonia
    pulmonary tuberculosis, 171-173, 172f
    sarcoidosis, 178-179, 179f
    upper, 165-166, 166b, 166f
Respiratory syncytial virus, 167
Respiratory system. *See also* Upper respiratory tract
    anatomy of, 161-164, 162f
    functions of, 161
Respiratory tract neoplasms, 187-191, 187f.
    See also Upper respiratory tract
Restrictive cardiomyopathy, 155, 155f
Retinitis pigmentosa, 478
Retinoblastoma, 73, 84, 482, 482f
Retinoblastoma suppressor gene, 84, 84t, 85f, 96, 381, 482
Retroretinal hemorrhages, 478
Reverse transcriptase, 81-82
Reversible cell injury, 8-9, 8f, 9f
Rh factor incompatibility, 56-58, 57f
Rhabdomyolysis, 444
Rhabdomyoma, 72
Rhabdomyosarcoma, 72, 446-447, 447t
Rheumatic fever, 150f
Rheumatic heart disease, 150-151, 150f, 151f
Rheumatoid arthritis, 415, 428-429, 429f, 430b, 430f
Rheumatoid nodules, 429
Rhinorrhea, 166
Rhinovirus, 165
RhoGAM, 57

Ribosomal RNA, 3, 3f
Ribosomes, 4
Rickets, 414, 420
Right ventricular failure, 144-146
RNA tumor viruses, 81-82, 82f
Rods, 476t
Rotavirus, 248
Rough endoplasmic reticulum, 4, 44, 45f, 75
Rouleaux, 23-24
Rous sarcoma, 81-82, 82f
Rubella, 96f, 135
"Rule of nines," 399f

S

Saccular aneurysm, 140, 141f
Saddle embolism, 123-124, 124f
Salivary glands
    diseases of, 234-235
    neoplasms of, 234-235
    secretions of, 230t
    sialadenitis, 234
    tumors of, 234-235
Salpingitis, 343, 344f
Sarcoidosis, 33, 178-179, 179f, 445
Sarcoma
    angiosarcoma, 447, 447t
    chondrosarcoma, 423-424, 424t, 425f
    Ewing's, 75, 424, 424t, 426f
    hemangiosarcomas, 134
    histopathology of, 74f
    Kaposi's, 62, 63-64, 75, 408, 408f
    leiomyosarcoma, 447, 447t
    liposarcoma, 447, 447t
    osteosarcoma, 423-424, 424t, 425f
    polymorphous cell, 447, 447f, 447t
    rhabdomyosarcoma, 446-447, 447t
    synovial, 447, 447t, 448f
    types of, 72
    vimentin expression by, 5
Sarcoptes scabiei, 402
Scabies, 402
Scales, 397, 397f
Scar
    deficient formation of, 37
    definition of, 36
    excessive formation of, 37
Schistosoma haematobium, 81, 314
Schwann cells, 438-439
Schwannomas, 472
Scirrhous carcinomas, 372
Sclera, 475, 475f, 476t
Scleritis, 429
Scleroderma, 396
Sclerosing adenosis, 368
Scurvy, 118, 222
Seborrheic dermatitis, 404
Seborrheic keratosis, 404
Secondary-intention wound healing, 37, 38f
Second-degree burns, 398
Secretin, 290
Sella turcica, 378
Semicircular canals, 485
Semilunar valves, 130
Seminoma, 72, 328-329, 330, 331f
Senile cataracts, 481
Sensory hearing loss, 488, 489f
Septic emboli, 121-122, 134

Septicemia, 134
Serous inflammation, 30-31, 31f
Sertoli cells
    description of, 322-323, 324-325
    tumors involving, 332
Sertoli-Leydig cell tumors, 359
Serum amyloid A protein, 65, 65f
Serum sickness, 51, 51f
Severe combined immunodeficiency, 60
Sex chromosome abnormalities, 98-99, 98f,
    99f
Sex cord stromal tumors, 356, 357-359
Sex hormones
    in prostate cancer, 325
    sebaceous gland stimulation by, 402-403
    tumors induced by, 79
Sexually transmitted diseases, 326-328
    acquired immunodeficiency syndrome.
        See Acquired immunodeficiency
        syndrome
    bacterial infections as causes of, 345
    chlamydia, 327, 345-346
    genital herpes, 326-327, 345
    gonorrhea, 327, 345t, 346
    human immunodeficiency virus.
        See Human immunodeficiency virus
    syphilis, 327-328, 327f, 345t, 346
    in women, 340
Sheehan's syndrome, 382
Shock, 125-127
    cardiogenic, 125, 146
    compensated, 127
    decompensated, 127
    definition of, 125
    distributive, 125
    hypotonic, 125-127
    hypovolemic, 125
    irreversible, 127
    pathogenesis of, 126f
Sialadenitis, 234
Sialolithiasis, 234
Sialorrhea, 234
Sickle cell anemia, 198, 202-203, 206-208,
    207f, 208f
SIDS. See Sudden infant death syndrome
Sigmoid colon
    carcinoma of, 256f
    diverticula of, 241, 242f
Silicosis, 30, 181-182
Simian immunodeficiency viruses, 61
Simple fracture, 422, 422f
Single-gene disorders, 99-107
    autosomal dominant, 100-102, 100f, 100t,
        101f
    autosomal recessive, 101f, 102-105,
        102b, 102f
    cystic fibrosis, 102-104, 103f
    familial hypercholesterolemia, 101-102,
        101f, 102f
    fragile X syndrome, 107
    hemophilia, 106, 107f
    lysosomal storage diseases, 104, 104f
    Marfan's syndrome, 100-101, 101f
    phenylketonuria, 104-105, 105f
    Tay-Sachs disease, 104, 105f
    X-linked recessive, 105-107, 106b
Sinus, 31-32, 32f
Sjögren's syndrome, 234

Skeletal muscle
    anatomy of, 434
    histology of, 435f
    hypertrophy of, 14
Skeleton. See also Bone(s)
    anatomy of, 412-414, 413f
    physiology of, 412-414
Skin
    anatomy of, 395-396, 395f
    bacteria on, 396
    dermis of, 395f
    epidermis of, 395f
    function of, 396
    hypodermis of, 395f, 396
    immune functions of, 396
    physiology of, 395-396
    sunbathing effects on, 399-400, 400f
    sunlight exposure, 396
Skin appendages, 396. See also Hair
        diseases; Nail diseases
Skin cancer
    prevalence of, 89-90
    prevention of, 88
Skin diseases
    congenital, 397-398
    eczema, 403-404
    idiopathic, 403-404
    immune, 403-404
    overview of, 396-410
    psoriasis, 404, 404f
    seborrheic dermatitis, 404
Skin grafts, 398
Skin infections, 400-403
    acne, 402-403, 403f
    bacterial, 401f
    fungal, 401-402
    insect infestations and bites, 402
    viral, 402
Skin lesions, 397, 397f
Skin neoplasms, 404-409
    basal cell carcinoma, 404-405, 405f
    dermal connective tissue tumors, 408, 408f
    epithelial tumors, 404-406, 405t
    malignant melanoma, 407-408, 407f
    pigmented lesions, 406-409
    seborrheic keratosis, 404
    squamous cell carcinoma, 405-406, 406f
Skin trauma
    cold, 399, 399f
    description of, 396
    electrical, 399
    ionizing radiation, 400
    mechanical, 398
    radiation, 399-400
    sunlight, 399-400
    thermal, 398-399, 399f
Skull
    anatomy of, 453
    birth-related fracture of, 111
Slow-reacting substances of anaphylaxis, 48
Small intestine
    diseases of, 241-257
        developmental, 241
        diarrhea, 246t
        diverticulosis, 241-242, 242f
        inflammatory bowel disease. See
            Inflammatory bowel disease
        intestinal, 242-246

Small intestine (Continued)
        ischemic bowel disease, 243
        neoplasms. See Intestinal neoplasms
        obstruction, 249-250, 250b, 250f
        volvulus, 250, 250f
    secretions of, 230t
Smegma, 337
Smoking
    atherosclerosis and, 140
    bladder cancer caused by, 318
    lung cancer caused by, 188
Smooth endoplasmic reticulum, 4
Somatotropic adenomas, 382
Spherocytes, 209-210
Spherocytosis, 202-203, 206, 209-210, 209f
Sphingomyelinase, 464
Spina bifida, 108, 455, 456f
Spinal cord
    anatomy of, 451
    injuries to, 460-461
Spinal nerve tumors, 472-473
Splenomegaly, 201, 275
Spondylosis, 428
Spongiform encephalopathies, 461
Spontaneous abortion, 361
Squames, 397
Squamous cell carcinoma
    of bladder, 319
    definition of, 72
    histopathology of, 74f
    of skin, 405-406, 406f
Staghorn calculi, 313-314
Staphylococcal osteomyelitis, 416
Stasis dermatitis, 158
Statins, 102
Status asthmaticus, 177
Steady state, 7-8, 7f
Steatohepatitis, 276
Steatorrhea, 102-103, 253
Steatosis, 15
Stem cells
    bone marrow, 43
    definition of, 35
    hematopoietic, 195-197
    myeloid, 195-197
Stethoscope, 171
Stomach
    diseases and disorders of, 237-241
        carcinoma, 240-241, 240f
        developmental, 237
        gastric neoplasms, 240-241
        gastritis, 238
        peptic ulcer, 238-240, 239f
    secretions of, 230t
Stomatitis, 232, 234
Streptococcus pneumoniae, 171, 461
Stridor, 49-50
Stroke, 149-150, 458
Struvite stones, 313, 314f
Stye, 479
Subarachnoid hemorrhages, 457
Subdural hematomas, 456-457, 457f
Subdural hemorrhage, 111
Substantia nigra, 467
Sudden cardiac death, 156
Sudden infant death syndrome, 112
Suffocation, 183
Suicide genes, 18

Sulci, 450
Sulfur dioxide, 181t
Sunbathing, 399-400, 400f
Sundowning, 467
Sunlight injury, 399-400
Superficial spreading melanoma, 407
Superinfection, 269
Supernumerary breasts, 366
Superoxide dismutase, 10, 468
Suppurative osteomyelitis, 417
Surface adhesion molecules, 23-24
Swallowing, 229
Sweat glands, 396
Synarthroses, 413
Syndactyly, 19f, 20
Synovial joint, 413-414, 414f
Synovial sarcoma, 447, 447t, 448f
Syphilis, 327-328, 327f, 345t, 346
Systemic lupus erythematosus, 58-59
    antibodies associated with, 58
    butterfly rash associated with, 59, 59f
    chronic proliferative glomerulonephritis
        associated with, 312
    clinical features of, 59, 59b, 60f
    description of, 52
    joint involvement, 415
    myositis of, 445
    pathogenesis of, 58-59
    pathology of, 59
    prevalence of, 58
Systole, 130

T

T cell receptor, 44
T helper cells, 44, 52, 62
T lymphocytes, 44
    B lymphocytes vs., 44
    cytokine secretions by, 6
    origins of, 43-44
    subsets of, 44
T suppressor cells, 44
Tabes dorsalis, 328
Tachycardia, 127
Tachypnea, 127, 170
Tay-Sachs disease, 12, 104, 105f, 464
Temporal lobe, 450
Teratocarcinomas, 329-330, 356, 358t
Teratogens
    chemical, 95, 95f
    definition of, 94
    exogenous, 95-96
    microbial, 95-96, 96f
    physical, 95
Teratomas, 73-75, 75f, 324-325, 329-330,
    355-356, 357, 358t
Terminal duct lobular units, 365
Testes
    anatomy of, 322
    histologic features of, 323f
Testicular cancer, 328f
Testicular tumors
    description of, 324
    etiology of, 328-330
    germ cell, 329b, 330-332
    pathogenesis of, 328-330
    self-examination of, 334
    types of, 329b

Testosterone, 323
Tetanus, 437, 445
Tetany, 436
Tetralogy of Fallot, 136-137, 136f
Thalamus, 450, 451f
Thalassemia, 202, 208-209, 208f
Thalidomide, 95
Theca cells, 340
Thermal injuries, 398-399, 399f
Thiamine deficiency, 464-465
Third-degree burns, 398
Threatened abortion, 361
Thrombasthenia, 223
Thrombin, 221
Thrombocytes, 200
Thrombocytopenia, 223
Thromboembolism, 122-123
Thrombophlebitis, 88, 134, 158
Thrombosis, 119-122
    arterial, 120
    clinicopathologic correlations of, 120-122
    intramural, 120
    microvascular, 120
    outcome of, 120, 122f
    pathogenesis of, 119-120
    pathology of, 120, 121f, 122f
    sites of, 121f
    valvular, 120
    venous, 120
Thrombus, 118
Thrush, 402
Thymomas, 440
Thymus, 43-44, 195
Thyroid adenomas, 384
Thyroid carcinoma, 385, 386f
Thyroid diseases, 383-386
    hyperthyroidism, 383-384, 383f
    hypothyroidism, 383f, 384-385
    neoplasms, 385-386, 386f
    nodular goiter, 385, 385f
Thyroid gland
    anatomy of, 379
    diseases of. See Thyroid diseases
Thyroidectomy, 384
Thyroiditis, 384
Thyroid-stimulating hormone, 51
Thyrotoxicosis, 383
Thyroxine, 379, 383
Tinea, 401-402, 402f
Tissue
    cellular organization of, 6
    reoxygenation of, 10
TNM staging system, 75, 319-320
Tophi, 431
TORCH syndrome, 95-96, 477
Toxemia of pregnancy, 362
Toxins
    bacterial production of, 11
    cell injury caused by, 10-11, 10t
    liver diseases induced by, 276
Toxoplasma gondii, 462
Toxoplasmosis, 462
TP53, 84
Trachea, 161
Tracheobronchitis, purulent, 32f
Trachoma, 479
Transduction, 82
Transfection, 77

Transfer RNA, 3, 3f
Transferrin, 203, 277
Transitional cell carcinomas, 72
Transplantation, 53-55
    allografts, 54
    autograft, 54
    bone marrow, 55
    clinical use of, 55
    donor–recipient match, 55
    heart, 155-156
    homografts, 54
    immunosuppressive drugs for, 53-54, 55
    isograft, 54
    kidney, 55
    liver, 285
    rejection after, 54-55, 54f
    types of, 54
    xenografts, 54
Transudate, 115
Transudation, 27, 191
Traumatic injuries
    to bone, 421-423, 423f
    to brain, 460, 460f
    to eyes, 478
    to muscle, 444-445
    to neck, 460-461
    to nervous system, 460-461, 460f
    to skin. See Skin trauma
    to spinal cord, 460-461
Traveler's diarrhea, 247
Trench foot. See Immersion foot
Treponema pallidum, 325-326, 327, 461
Trichinella spiralis, 437, 445
Trichinosis, 445f, 446
Trichomonas vaginalis, 345
Trichotillomania, 409
Triiodothyronine, 379, 383
Trilineage-myeloid stem cells, 195-197
Trisomy 21, 97-98, 97f, 98f, 135
Trophic hormones, 380
Trophic ulcer, 158
Trophoblast, 92
Tropical sprue, 252
Troponin I, 146-147
Troponin T, 146-147
Trousseau, Armand, 296
Trousseau's syndrome, 88
Trypanosoma cruzi, 134, 154
Trypsin, 294
Trypsinogen, 289
Tuberculin, 53, 173
Tuberculosis
    granulomas of, 33
    pulmonary, 171-173, 172f
Tuberculous pneumonia, 173
Tubo-ovarian abscess, 346
Tubular adenomas, 72, 254-255
Tubulovillous adenomas, 255
Tumor(s)
    adrenocortical, 388-389, 390f
    angiogenesis induced by, 72, 72f
    benign
        breast, 369-370
        description of, 69-71, 69f, 71t
    biliary tract, 263
    biologic features of, 70-71, 71t
    bladder, 316, 318
    blood cells, 73t

Tumor(s) *(Continued)*
  bone. *See* Bone tumors
  brain. *See* Brain tumors
  cardiac, 155
  cellular features of, 69-70, 70f, 75-77, 76f
  chromosomal studies of, 70, 71f
  classification of, 69-75
  clinical classification of, 69
  definition of, 68, 397
  epithelial, 73t
  eye, 477, 482
  germ cell, 73-75, 73t
  glial cells, 73t
  grading of, 75
  histologic classification of, 69, 72-75, 73t, 74f, 75f
  immune response to, 86, 86f
  immunotherapy of, 86
  laryngeal, 187, 187f
  liver, 263
  macroscopic features of, 69, 69f
  male reproductive system, 324-325
  malignant, 69-71, 69f, 71t, 87-88, 87f
  mesenchymal, 72, 73t
  metastasis, 71-72, 71f, 72f
  microscopic features of, 69
  muscle, 446-447, 447f
  neoplasms vs., 68
  neural cell precursors, 73t
  ovarian. *See* Ovarian tumors
  pancreatic. *See* Pancreatic tumors
  phyllodes, 369-370
  pituitary, 382-383
  pleural, 192, 192f
  salivary glands, 234-235
  staging of, 75
  testicular. *See* Testicular tumors
  thyroid, 385-386, 386f
Tumor antigens, 86
Tumor necrosis factor, 23-24, 181
Tumor protein p53, 84, 84t
Tumor suppressor genes, 84, 84t, 85f, 254
Turner's syndrome, 98-99, 98f, 99f, 343, 355
Tympanic membrane
  description of, 485
  functions of, 486
  perforation of, 486
Tympanocentesis, 487
Type I hypersensitivity, 46, 47-50, 477, 479
Type II hypersensitivity, 50-51, 50f
Type III hypersensitivity, 51-52, 51f, 52f, 479
Type IV hypersensitivity, 52-53, 53f, 479
Typhoid fever, 247
Tyrosine kinase inhibitors, 215

U

Ubiquitin, 13
Ulcer
  aphthous, 244-245
  Curling's, 238
  Cushing's, 238
  definition of, 32, 397, 397f
  mucosal, 35
  peptic, 33f, 238-240, 239f
  trophic, 158

Ulcerative colitis, 245-246, 245f, 246t
Ulcerative inflammation, 32, 33f
Ultrasound, 109, 109f
Unconjugated hyperbilirubinemia, 266
Undifferentiated large-cell carcinoma, 188
Upper motor neurons, 437f, 451
Upper respiratory tract
  anatomy of, 161, 162f
  infections of, 165-166
    characteristics of, 165
    clinical features of, 166
    description of, 164
    etiology of, 165-166
    pathogenesis of, 165-166
    pathology of, 166
    sites of, 166f
Ureaplasma urealyticum, 326
Uremia, 306
Urethra, 322
Urethritis, 326
  chlamydial, 327
  gonococcal, 327
Uric acid, 431
Uric acid stones, 313
Urinary stones, 313-314, 314f
Urinary tract
  anatomy of, 303-304
  diseases and disorders of, 304-320
    circulatory disturbances, 315-316
    developmental, 306-307
    glomerular diseases. *See* Glomerular diseases
    polycystic kidney disease, 306-307, 306f
    symptoms of, 305-306
  neoplasms of, 316-320, 316f
    renal cell carcinoma, 317, 317f
    urothelial carcinoma, 318
  tumors of, 305
Urinary tract infection, 305, 314-315, 314f, 315f
Urine
  chemical composition of, 306
  formation of, 303
Urobilinogen, 262
Urolithiasis, 313
Urothelial carcinoma, 318
Urticaria pigmentosa, 408-409
Uterine tumors, 351-355
  endometrial carcinoma. *See* Endometrial carcinoma
  endometriosis, 354-355, 354f
  leiomyoma, 353-354, 353f, 354f
Uterus
  agenesis of, 343
  anatomy of, 339-340, 339f
UV light, 80, 81f
Uveitis, 479

V

Vagina
  agenesis of, 343
  anatomy of, 339-340, 339f
  carcinoma of, 348
  protozoal infections of, 345
Vaginitis, 344f, 345t, 346
Valvular thrombi, 120
Vanillylmandelic acid, 392-393

Varicose veins, 157, 158f
Vascular endothelial growth factor, 362
Vasculitis, 134
Vasodilation, 23
Veins
  anatomy of, 132, 132f
  characteristics of, 157
  diseases of, 157-158, 158f
  varicose, 157, 158f
Venereal Disease Research Laboratory, 328
Venous embolism, 122-124, 123f
Venous hemorrhage, 118-119
Venous thrombi, 120
Ventilation
  disturbances of, 183-184
  physiology of, 183
Ventilatory failure, 184
Ventricular aneurysm, 143, 144f
Ventricular septal defect, 135-136, 136f
Venules, 132-133
Verruca vulgaris, 402
Verrucous endocarditis, 152, 152f
Vertebral fractures, 419
Vertigo, 486, 488
Vesicle, 397, 397f
Vibrio cholerae, 230, 247
Villous adenomas, 72, 255
Vimentin, 5
Viral carcinogens, 81-83
Viral gastroenteritis, 247-248
Viral genome, 84
Viral hepatitis, 267-271. *See also* Hepatitis
Viral meningitis, 462
Viral myocarditis, 134
Viral oncogenes, 83
Virchow, Rudolf, 22-23, 214
Virchow-Robin spaces, 462, 462f
Virchow's nodes, 241
Virilization, 359
Viruses. *See also specific virus*
  cell injury caused by, 11, 12f
  cytopathic, 11
  DNA, 83
  upper respiratory infections caused by, 165-166
Visual system, 475-476, 475f. *See also* Eye(s)
Vitamin B$_{12}$
  absorption of, 205
  deficiency of, 201, 465
Vitamin C, 36, 118
Vitamin D
  active form of, 420
  deficiency of, 253, 415, 419-420
  dietary intake of, 418
  metabolism of, 419f
Vitamin K, 224
Vitiligo, 396
Vitreous cavity, 475
Volvulus, 124-125, 250, 250f
Vomiting, 237
von Hippel–Lindau syndrome, 317, 470-471
von Willebrand factor, 120, 224
Vulva
  anatomy of, 339-340
  carcinoma of, 341, 347-348, 348f, 348t
Vulvectomy, 348
Vulvitis, 344f
Vulvovaginitis, 345

INDEX

W

WAGR syndrome, 96
Wallerian degeneration, 438-439, 439f
Waterhouse-Friderichsen syndrome, 391
Watershed infarcts, 459
Wear-and-tear hypothesis, 16, 426
Wegener's granulomatosis, 307, 310
Wernicke-Korsakoff syndrome, 464-465
Wernicke's encephalopathy, 464-465
West Nile virus, 461
Wet gangrene, 18
Whipple's disease, 252-253
White blood cell diseases, 212-221
    classification of, 212-213
    leukemia. *See* Leukemia
    lymphoma. *See* Lymphoma
    multiple myeloma, 219, 220f
White blood cells, 199-200
White infarcts, 124, 124f
White matter, 450

Wilms' tumor, 85, 305, 318
Wilson's disease, 272, 277
Wound dehiscence, 37
Wound healing, 34-37
    cells involved in, 35-36
    clinical, 36-37, 36f, 37f, 38f
    complications of, 37
    delayed, 37
    factors that affect, 37
    by first intention, 36, 36f
    granulation tissue in, 36, 37f
    by secondary intention, 37, 38f
WT1, 84t

X

Xanthomas, 101-102, 279
Xenografts, 54
Xeroderma pigmentosum, 80, 85
Xerophthalmia, 234

Xerostomia, 231-232, 234
X-linked recessive disorders, 105-107, 106b
    hemophilia, 106, 107f
    inheritance pattern of, 105f
X-rays, 80-81, 95

Y

Yolk sac carcinomas, 356, 358t
Yolk sac tumors, 330, 332

Z

Z deformity, 429
Zollinger-Ellison syndrome, 296-297
Zona fasciculata, 380
Zona glomerulosa, 379
Zona reticularis, 380
Zygote, 340